# Evaluating Research
# in Communicative Disorders

**FIFTH EDITION**

# Evaluating Research in Communicative Disorders

**Nicholas Schiavetti**

*State University of New York at Geneseo*

**Dale Evan Metz**

*State University of New York at Geneseo*

PEARSON

Boston ■ New York ■ San Francisco
Mexico City ■ Montreal ■ Toronto ■ London ■ Madrid ■ Munich ■ Paris
Hong Kong ■ Singapore ■ Tokyo ■ Cape Town ■ Sydney

*Executive Editor and Publisher:* Stephen D. Dragin
*Editorial Assistant:* Meaghan Minnick
*Marketing Manager:* Kris Ellis-Levy
*Editorial-Production Service:* Omegatype Typography, Inc.
*Manufacturing Buyer:* Andrew Turso
*Composition and Prepress Buyer:* Linda Cox
*Cover Administrator:* Linda Knowles
*Electronic Composition:* Omegatype Typography, Inc.

For related titles and support materials, visit our online catalog at www.ablongman.com.

Between the time Website information is gathered and then published, it is not unusual for some sites to have closed. Also, the transcription of URLs can result in typographical errors. The publisher would appreciate notification where these occur so that they may be corrected in subsequent editions.

**Library of Congress Cataloging-in-Publication Data**

Schiavetti, Nicholas
    Evaluating research in communicative disorders / Nicholas Schiavetti, Dale Evan Metz.
        p.   cm.
    Includes bibliographical references and index.
    ISBN 0-205-44961-1
        1. Speech disorders—Research—Evaluation.   2. Audiology—Research—Evaluation.
    I. Metz, Dale Evan.   II. Title.

    RC423.V45   2006
    616.85'5'0072—dc22

                                                                    2005042918

Printed in the United States of America
10   9   8   7   6   5   4   3   2   1       10   09   08   07   06   05

Dedicated to the Memory of

**Ira M. Ventry**
*1932–1983*

"Technical progress evolves through applied scientific research and propagation of the knowledge acquired. It is not enough to pursue the knowledge of wine in the laboratory alone, it must be spread through the wineries in order for this knowledge to become part of daily practice. Moreover, the faster scientific progress advances, the greater risk there is of widening the gap between what we know and what we do. It is necessary to narrow this gap and speed up evolution."

—Emile Peynaud, *Knowing and Making Wine,*
New York: John Wiley & Sons, 1984, p. vii

# Contents

# Preface

The fifth edition of *Evaluating Research in Communicative Disorders* remains faithful to the basic purpose of the earlier editions, with changes primarily evident in the updating of material and examples, as well as the addition of new content.

The main audience for the previous editions proved to be master's degree students in communicative disorders. The original intent was to help them prepare for a clinical career that would be guided by developments in the field reported in the research literature published in the professional journals. We also hoped to introduce those master's degree students who planned to pursue doctoral study to some of the basic concepts and terminology that they would encounter in the more rigorous research training that doctoral programs provide for potential producers of research.

The vast majority of professionals in communicative disorders are not producers of research but most of them are consumers of research in their professional activities. Therefore, this is not a book that describes how to do research. It is a book about how to read, understand, and evaluate research that someone else has done. It should be apparent, however, that the ability to read, understand, and evaluate the research done by others is a basic prerequisite to doing good research.

Most of the revisions that have been incorporated into the fifth edition have resulted from our experiences in teaching and conducting research in recent years. The text has also been revised in places where reviewers, colleagues, and students have suggested improvements. Many of the examples have been changed, particularly excerpts in Part II of the book. Some of the older examples were replaced by newer ones that either illustrated points more clearly or related to current research topics that were not prevalent at the time of the previous editions. Some new examples were added to illustrate concepts that were not discussed in the first four editions. A new example is not always better than an old one, however, so classic examples that have illustrated important points well over the years have been retained.

The fifth edition, like "all of Gaul," is divided into three parts. Part I includes basic information on research strategies and design in communicative disorders, measurement issues, evaluation criteria, treatment efficacy research, and organization and analysis of data. Part II reflects the four typical parts of a research article: introduction, method, results, and conclusions. The excerpted examples in Part II are intended to illustrate the points made in

Part I. Part III contains two complete research articles reprinted with evaluation checklists to guide students in evaluating the important features of research discussed in Parts I and II.

We gratefully acknowledge permission granted by the American Speech-Language-Hearing Association and by the authors to reprint selections from the journal articles. We are especially indebted to Peter Fitzgibbons, Sandra Gordon-Salant, Shari Brand Robertson, and Susan Ellis Weismer for allowing us to reprint their articles *in toto*. We also wish to thank the many colleagues, students, and reviewers who have offered constructive criticisms and suggestions for the five editions of this book.

The senior author of the first edition of this book was Ira Ventry, who died in 1983. Although there have been many revisions made in the subsequent editions, his influence remains obvious to those who knew him or his work. We thank Nona Ventry for graciously affording us access to Ira's notes and files from the first edition.

Five people who have been instrumental in helping us to complete this book deserve special thanks. Our department chair, Linda House, has provided a working environment that fosters creativity, independence, and accomplishment: we couldn't ask for a better boss. Steve Dragin has proved to be an intelligent, perceptive, and proactive editor: we couldn't ask anyone to be more supportive of our work. Ray O'Connell has been the guardian angel of this book for more than two decades: no one understands better than he does why it is still being read. Finally, we thank our wives, Carolyn Schiavetti and Wendy Metz, for offering the love, encouragement, forbearance, and support that we needed to complete this task in time again for the favorite holiday. The mountain echoes our thanks to all of you.

Nicholas Schiavetti
Dale Evan Metz
Geneseo, New York

# Evaluating Research
# in Communicative Disorders

# Basic Considerations in Evaluating Research

## Overview

The six chapters of Part I introduce basic principles for evaluating communicative disorders research. Part I lays the foundation for evaluation of the excerpts from research articles that are presented in Part II and the complete articles found in Part III.

Chapter 1 discusses principles of scientific method, empirical and rational knowledge, theory construction, the relationship between clinical and research enterprises, and the improvement of clinical practice through the application of research findings.

As Kent (1983, p. 76) has said:

A profession that provides its own research base is much more in charge of its own destiny than a profession that doesn't. . . . As clinical practice changes, it will change in large part in response to new knowledge gained through research.

Common ground in clinical and research activities and in basic and applied research is considered in Chapter 1 and emphasis is placed on the critical evaluation of research as an important activity for all professionals in the field: clinicians and researchers, consumers and producers of research. As Kent (1983, p. 76) further stated:

It is tempting to cast a discussion of research into a simple framework in which master's graduates are viewed as users of research and Ph.D. graduates are seen as the producers of research. However, this simplistic framework has important exceptions, and failure to recognize these exceptions may lead us into a faulty first step.

The tension between basic research and practical application is not unique to our field. Gershenfeld (1995, p. 50) clearly expressed it in his essay "Why I Am/Am Not a Physicist":

There is a vigorous battle being fought between the defenders of curiosity-driven basic research and the proponents of applied development to solve practical problems. I would like to suggest that this polarization risks satisfying neither camp, because it misses the deeper and much more interesting interrelationship between research and application. *Neither curiosity nor practice arises in a vacuum* [emphasis ours].

1

Such polarization does not need to exist. An excellent example of the blending of curiosity and practice in our field can be seen in the series of articles on physical examination of speech breathing structures that was published in the *American Journal of Speech-Language Pathology* by Hixon and Hoit. Donald A. Robin, editor of the journal, made the following remarks in his "From the Editor" overview of the August 2000 issue that included the third Hixon and Hoit article (Robin, 2000, p. 178):

> I would like to point the readership to a series of papers on clinical examination of the diaphragm, abdominal wall, and rib cage by Hixon and Hoit. In this issue is the third and last paper (examination of the rib cage wall) in a series that presents up-to-date clinical examination of the breathing-for-speech mechanism. The previous two papers can be found in *AJSLP,* 7 (4), 37–45, and *AJSLP,* 8, 335–346. This series of papers represents what I think are among the best examples of the integration between science and clinic. The research foundations of the clinical methods described is well known and has been the focus of Tom Hixon's since the late 1960's; since the 1980's, Jennifer Hoit has been part of this impressive systematic research program. The three papers in this *Journal* guide the clinician in the clinical examination of the speech breathing system and provide a strong basis for the assessment procedures described. The protocols arise from the combined science and clinical efforts of Hixon and Hoit. I will leave to you to read these excellent papers but want to point out to the readership what I think are superlative efforts in merging clinic and science with the highest degree of scholarship.

Robin's comments exemplify the basic theme of this book that is presented in Chapter 1: *Scientific research is the foundation upon which sound clinical practice should rest.*

The primary focus of Chapter 2 is research strategies in communicative disorders. Commonalities and differences among various experimental and descriptive research strategies are discussed and examples are presented of various approaches. Relationships among independent and dependent variables are discussed and different strategies for examining different kinds of variables are explored. Chapter 3 discusses research design in communicative disorders and examines some basic principles of many group and single-subject designs commonly encountered in the research literature. Measurement issues in communicative disorders are the topic of Chapter 4. Measurement is defined, different levels of measurement are specified, and some general and specific factors that affect the quality of measurements, especially reliability and validity, are discussed.

Chapter 5 considers the important topic of evaluating treatment efficacy research, which, perhaps more than any other area, exemplifies the linkage of research and clinical enterprise. Using the framework of Campbell and Stanley (1966) for the evaluation of research designs in educational psychology, this chapter discusses the important criteria of internal and external validity and factors that may jeopardize them. Some specific treatment efficacy research designs are reviewed relative to these factors and some matters concerning meta-analysis and research ethics are also considered.

Chapter 6 concludes Part I with an overview of important principles in the organization and analysis of data for consumers of research. The purpose of this chapter is to familiarize readers with some terminology, concepts, and statistical methods, without a lengthy discussion of calculation procedures. The material in this chapter, along with the examples in Part II, is intended to assist students in the reading of the results section of a research article. It is beyond the scope of this book to teach statistics *per se* and it is assumed that graduate students in communicative disorders will have at least a one-semester introductory course in statistics. Chapters 6 and 9 review the major terms and concepts of a semester's survey of statistics and provide relevant examples from the communicative disorders literature.

Part II will follow with excerpts from the communicative disorders research literature that provide specific examples of the concepts discussed in Part I. Part III will then follow with two complete articles reprinted, one in speech-language pathology and one in audiology, for students to evaluate on the basis of the concepts presented in Part I and exemplified in Part II.

Throughout their reading of this book, students should be mindful of the statement made by Kent (2001, p. 457):

> Research is intrinsically futuristic, always directed to the next experiment, the next theoretical advance, the next challenge to the standard view. Research is a frontier phenomenon, and its practitioners work on the horizon of possibilities.

We hope that you will open your eyes wide to these possibilities.

# REFERENCES

Campbell, D. T., & Stanley, J. C. (1966). *Experimental and quasi-experimental designs for research.* Chicago, IL: Rand McNally.

Gershenfeld, N. (1995). Why I am/am not a physicist. *Physics Today, 48*(7), 50–51.

Kent, R. D. (1983). How can we improve the role of research and educate speech-language pathologists and audiologists to be competent users of research? In N. S. Rees & T. L. Snope (Eds.), *Proceedings of the 1983 National Conference on Undergraduate, Graduate, and Continuing Education* (pp. 76–86). St. Paul, MN: American Speech-Language-Hearing Association.

Kent, R. D. (2001). The future of science. In R. Lubinski & C. Frattali (Eds.), *Professional issues in speech-language pathology and audiology* (2nd ed., pp. 457–469).

Robin, D. A. (2000). From the editor. *American Journal of Speech-Language Pathology, 9,* 178.

# The Consumer of Research in Communicative Disorders

*Beliefs are tentative, not dogmatic; they are based on evidence, not on authority.*
—Bertrand Russell (1945)
*History of Western Philosophy*

The purpose of this book is to help practitioners and students in communicative disorders become critical readers of the quantitative research literature in the field.[1] A *critic* is "one who forms and expresses judgments of the merits, faults, value, or truth of a matter" and the word *critical* is used, here and throughout, to mean "characterized by careful, exact evaluation and judgment" (*The American Heritage College Dictionary,* 1997). Practitioners should be able to evaluate published research critically. The book, then, facilitates the practitioner's use of the research literature to improve, modify, and update clinical practice through reasoned assessment and evaluation of the literature relevant to clinical practice. Our goal stems from the basic premise that sound clinical practice should be based, in large part, on the relevant basic and applied research rather than on pronouncements by authorities, intuition, or dogma. As Siegel (1993, p. 36) stated:

> Clinicians need to have enough familiarity with research to judge whether the claims are reasonable and to determine just how closely the proposed clinical procedures adhere to the research methods and the underlying theory. Informed clinicians need not be sophisticated researchers, but they should have had first-hand experience with research during their graduate education to help them understand the limitations and the possibilities of research and the decisions that face researchers at so many turns in the conduct of a study.

---

[1]Qualitative research will not be discussed in this text and the rationale for limiting our discussion to quantitative research is summarized cogently by Cizek (1995). Readers interested in a popular treatment of qualitative research are referred to Dilollo and Wolter (2004). Readers interested in a more detailed treatment of qualitative research are referred to Babbie (2004) and the Special Forum on Qualitative Research that was published in the May 2003 issue of the *American Journal of Speech-Language Pathology: A Journal of Clinical Practice.*

Let's first consider a basic question asked by Reynolds (1975): "What is research?" Reynolds goes on to answer his question as follows (p. 13):

> Research is the cornerstone of an experimental science. Both the certainty of the conclusions and the rapidity of the progress of an experimental science depend intimately and ultimately on its research. As its root meaning ("to search again") implies, most research either results in a rediscovery, and hence a confirmation, of already known facts and principles or represents another painstaking attempt to answer a formerly unanswered question in an objective and repeatable fashion. But research also means the search for and the discovery of formerly misunderstood or unconceived principles and facts. Research is, in practice, a two-pronged fork with one tine in the past and the other in the future. An experiment attempts to confirm or deny what is already believed to be true and at the same time to go beyond existing knowledge toward either a more comprehensive body of facts or, if possible, toward a general principle around which all the known and verifiable facts about a subject may cluster in a logical, predictable, and sensible whole.

The whole point of the text is to assist the clinician and student to arrive at reasoned decisions about the adequacy of the research reported in our journals and to make independent judgments about the relevance of the research to their clinical activities. In the process, we hope to dispel some of the more common myths about the research article, myths such as "You must be a statistician to read the literature" or "If it is in print, it must be good" or "The more difficult to read, the more scholarly an article must be."

In addition to our goal of helping clinicians develop the critical skills required in reading research, we have two additional goals: we hope the book serves as a bridge between clinician and researcher; and we view the text as a foundation, as a *first* course for the student who plans a career in research or for practitioners interested in conducting research within a clinic or school setting. It must be emphasized, however, that this is not a book on how to do research; it is a book on how to *read* research. It will become apparent, however, that intelligent evaluation of research has much in common with the intelligent conduct of research.

## Research-Practice Relationships in Communicative Disorders

It is generally accepted that advances in diagnostic and treatment protocols for a particular disorder are derived from scholarly research. A simplified example from the field of medicine illustrates this point. Scholarly research to map the human genome has shed light on previously unexplained causes of certain disorders. Many forms of cancer, manic-depressive illness, obesity, and other abnormal conditions are now known to be, at least partially, genetically based (Shprintzen, 1997). Such research leads to potential advances in diagnostic procedures like the identification of individuals with a predisposition to a particular disorder and advances in treatment procedures like gene replacement therapy.

In the above scenario, the research-practice relationship appears straightforward and cooperative; research leads to advances in practice. The research-practice relationship in communicative disorders, however, may not be quite so straightforward or cooperative. Dr.

Jeri Logemann, President of the American Speech-Language-Hearing Association in the year 2000, discussed the research-practice relationship in communicative disorders in *The ASHA Leader.* She stated:

> There are comments that I find disturbing, but luckily, hear only occasionally. The clinician, for instance, who says, "I don't read journals because they're all research and that's over my head." Or the researcher who says, "It's unimportant whether a clinician reads my research or not, because it's really for other researchers." (Logemann, 2000, p. 2)

This apparent disconnection between research and clinical practice is not unique to the discipline of communicative disorders and it is not a new problem. Debate on this topic has appeared frequently in the communicative disorders literature since the early 1960s and "is as keen now as ever" (Robin, 1999, p. 194). The essence of this disconnection appears to be due to a conventional notion that research does little to inform clinical practice and an idealized model that segregates producers of research from consumers of research in communicative disorders.

The currency and relevance of the research-practice relationship in communicative disorders was underscored poignantly in a special February 1998 issue of the journal *Topics in Language Disorders.* This special issue, subtitled *New Directions: Science and Service for the 90's and Beyond,* featured seven articles devoted to discovering methods to bridge the gap between research and clinical practice. The underlying theme of and motivation for each article was expressed succinctly in the journal's lead article in which Ingram (1998, p. 1) stated:

> Effective communication between research and practice is as fundamental in the field of speech-language pathology as in any field that provides services to the community.

He went on to say:

> ...there needs to be an effective means for reliable results from research to be communicated to... clinicians. Further, clinicians must have confidence in the researchers in their field and in ways to communicate their needs to them.

Ingram (1998) proposed that three distinct relationships, or lines of communication, exist between research and practice and that effective use of these lines of communication would mutually benefit research efforts and clinical practice. The three lines of communication proposed by Ingram are (a) *shared-interest communication,* (b) *research-driven communication,* and (c) *practice-driven communication.*

Shared-interest communication is based on the reasonable assumption that a continuum of interests exists between researchers and practitioners and that the most effective communication will occur where interests overlap the most. Ingram suggested that shared-interest communication could be enhanced by initiating a regular survey of research and researchers that addresses the types and nature of research being conducted in the field. Such surveys could inform both researchers and clinicians about research directions and, perhaps, encourage collaborative efforts. Ingram pointed out that a number of professional organizations, such as ASHA, attempt to provide a broad range of clinical research presentations at their annual conventions in an effort to foster research-practice relationships. Also, ASHA's Special Interest Groups serve as a vehicle that encourages researcher/clinician interactions.

Research-driven communication regards the manner "in which research findings are reported and converted into practice" (Ingram, 1998, p. 2). Ingram suggested that adequate outlets for the distribution of research findings currently exist in the form of books, professional conventions, printed and online journals, and the Internet. He added the caveat, however, that there is so much research information available that clinicians may feel overwhelmed and not know how to use it effectively in their practice. Ingram (1998, p. 9) offered some suggestions that could assist clinicians in the application of current research findings to their practices, and, consistent with the philosophy of this book, stressed that.

> Graduate programs need to continue to focus on training students to access and reach judgments on their own about applied research.

Practice-driven communication concerns the manner in which clinicians express their interests to researchers regarding their information needs and the input they provide to the initiation of research (Ingram, 1998). To facilitate practice-driven communication, Ingram suggested a survey of clinicians that would examine the extent of satisfaction, or lack thereof, with research in the field. He also proposed the establishment of Internet bulletin boards that would enable clinicians to express their needs directly to researchers. Such an effort might also facilitate clinician-initiated research proposals. ASHA's American Speech-Language-Hearing Foundation has taken an active role in fostering practice-driven communication by awarding grants to individuals conducting germane clinical research.

Additionally, ASHA has taken a proactive stance regarding the integration of research and clinical practice. Three articles published recently in *The ASHA Leader* stress the need and potential for such integration (Katz, 2003; Ramig, 2002; Wambaugh & Bain, 2002). A related and important ASHA initiative regards the call to instantiate mandates in the Code of Ethics that require clinicians to "provide services that are based on careful, professional reasoning" (Apel & Self, 2003, p. 6). Apel and Self (2003, p. 6) state that, "By engaging in evidence-based practices, clinicians abide by these ethical codes while best serving their clients."

## Evidence-Based Practice (EBP)

Evidence-based practice (EBP) requires clinicians to integrate high-quality scientific clinical research evidence with individual clinical expertise to ensure ethical and optimal client management (Dollaghan, 2004; Sackett, Straus, Richardson, Rosenberg, & Haynes, 2000). Dollaghan (2004, p. 12) asserts that "EBP offers us a framework and a set of tools by which we can systematically improve in our efforts to be better clinicians, colleagues, advocates, and investigators." ASHA has recently established the National Center for Treatment Effectiveness in Communicative Disorders and is currently coordinating a National Institutes of Health–funded effort to promote clinical research that will support EBP.

Evidence-based practice is hardly unique to communicative disorders. Consider the following quotation by Poggi (2003, p. 4):

Every day we expect people to base their practices on evidence that demonstrates proven results—doctors diagnosing patients, lawyers advising clients, and educators teaching our children. In fact, the U.S. Congress that passed the No Child Left Behind Act of 2001 believes so strongly in the use of scientifically based research that it is referenced over 100 times within the pages of the legislation—in every section and on every topic.

Despite the widespread acclaim for EBP, at least two fundamental issues confront clinicians who wish to establish an EBP. The first issue confronting the individual who wants to establish an EBP is locating relevant, germane sources of clinical evidence in a timely fashion. Dollaghan (2004, p. 4) suggests that "no practitioner has the time" to scour hundreds of journals and textbooks for clinical evidence. Dollaghan and other EBP proponents like Schlosser (2004) suggest using "high-yield sources" that are easily accessible via the Internet. For example, the Agency for Healthcare Research and Quality supports a website (www.guideline.gov) that is a compilation of clinical evidence reviews from a large number of disciplines on a wide variety of topics. Seven additional high-yield source websites are cited in Dollaghan's (2004) article. Additional EBP-related websites are provided by Goldstein (2004).

The second issue regards the clinician's understanding of the "levels of evidence" used in treatment efficacy research and EBP. The term *levels of evidence* refers to a classification system that establishes a hierarchy of evidence based on scientific quality and rigor (Robey, 2004). Consistent with the purpose of this book, levels of evidence are discussed in detail in Chapter 5.

## Knowledge Acquisition

How does one acquire knowledge? On what basis does one accept new information as accurate or truthful? Such questions are the broad concern of *epistemology,* the study of the nature and grounds of knowledge. Knowledge can be acquired in various ways, and Kerlinger and Lee (2000, pp. 6–8) discussed Charles Sanders Pierce's notion of "four general ways of knowing" as an approach to understanding the ways in which knowledge has been acquired historically.

The first way of knowing is called the *method of tenacity.* In this method of knowing, people hold firmly to certain beliefs because they have always known them to be true and frequent repetition of the belief enhances its ostensible validity. Perpetuating the notion that the world is flat, even in the face of overwhelming contradictory evidence, is an example of the method of tenacity.

The second way of knowing is called the *method of authority.* Within the method of authority, people accept knowledge from an individual or group of individuals who have been, in some way, designated as authoritative producers of knowledge. An example of the method of authority is believing that the sun revolves around the earth because a historical institution such as a government or religion insists that it is true. The method of authority is not necessarily unsound, depending on how the authority acquired its knowledge. In the United States, for example, citizens generally accept the authority of the U.S. Food and Drug Administration regarding prescription medicines and food safety—but much of its authority is based on sound scientific evidence. The method of authority may be unsound, however, if everyone merely accepts the word of authority without examining or questioning the qualifications of the *source* of its knowledge (Kerlinger & Lee, 2000).

The third way of knowing is called the *a priori method.* It is also called the *method of pure rationalism* or the *method of intuition.* This method of knowing relies on the use of pure reason based on prior assumptions that are considered to be self-evident with little or no consideration given to the role of experience in the acquisition of knowledge. A serious limitation of intuition is that experience may show that a self-evident truth is not a valid assumption in a logical system and if an a priori assumption is incorrect, the conclusion will be incorrect. For example, a conclusion drawn from basing a purely logical argument on the a priori assumption that the earth, not the sun, is the center of our galaxy, will be incorrect. With the exception of mathematics, pure rationalism is not used exclusively to develop scientific principles. Despite the limitations of pure rationalism, elements of rationalistic thinking are important to scientific inquiry in communicative disorders and other disciplines. We will discuss the relationship of rationalism and experience and their roles in scientific inquiry further in the following section.

The fourth method of knowing is the *method of science.* The word *science* is derived from the Latin word *scire,* which means "to know" and the method of science is widely heralded as the most powerful and objective means available to gain new knowledge. Scientific knowledge is gained from scientific research, which is defined by Kerlinger and Lee (2000, p. 14) in the following manner:

> Scientific research is systematic, controlled, empirical, amoral, public, and critical investigation of natural phenomena. It is guided by theory and hypotheses about the presumed relations among such phenomena.

The words used in the above definition have conceptual importance and they refer to many of the themes and concepts that will be introduced in this text. As such, it is worthwhile to examine briefly Kerlinger and Lee's (2000, p. 14) explanations of their intended meanings. The words *systematic* and *controlled* imply that scientific investigation is tightly disciplined and conducted in a manner that methodically rules out alternative explanations of a particular finding. Systematic control over events during the execution of a scientific investigation engenders confidence in the research findings. The word *empirical* implies that the beliefs must be subjected to outside independent tests; subjective beliefs must "be checked against objective reality." The word *amoral* implies that knowledge obtained from scientific research does not have moral value. Research findings are not "good" or "bad." Rather, research findings are considered in terms of their reliability and validity. Finally, the word *public* implies that scientific research is evaluated by other independent individuals of equal knowledge and training prior to being published in a professional journal. This process is called "peer review" and we will have more to say about the peer review process later in this chapter.

Scientific research depends on a complex interplay of two distinct lines of inquiry, namely, empiricism and rationalism. Empiricism is a philosophy that assumes that knowledge must be gained through experience. Empiricists generally rely on inductive reasoning; that is, they use evidence from particular cases to make inferences about general principles. To be accepted into the realm of knowledge, explanations of phenomena must be based on evidence gained from observations of phenomena, and critical evaluation of the accuracy of observations is necessary before the observations can be accepted as evidence. This critical, self-correcting activity of empiricism is the core of scientific endeavor and is a necessary requisite of sound research.

Rationalism is a philosophy that assumes that knowledge must be gained through the exercise of logical thought. Rationalists generally rely on deductive reasoning, that is, the use of general principles to make inferences about specific cases. Rationalism is often referred to as a *schematic, formal,* or *analytic* endeavor because it deals with abstract models, and the logical criticism of propositions is necessary for the acceptance of explanations into the realm of knowledge.

Various schools of thought differ in the extent to which they rely on empirical and rational endeavors. In linguistics, for instance, Chomsky (1968) insisted that rational consideration rather than empirical inquiry is necessary for the development of a theory of language. In psychology, Skinner (1953) relied on empirical evidence for a functional analysis of behavior and eschewed the exclusively rational approach. Although these two examples illustrate the extreme ends of the continuum of rational and empirical thought, many positions regarding the integration of empirical evidence and rational inquiry exist along this continuum. Stevens (1968, p. 850) suggested the term *schemapiric* for the "proper and judicious joining of the schematic with the empirical," and concluded (p. 856):

> Science presents itself as a two-faced, bipartite endeavor looking at once toward the formal, analytic, schematic features of model-building, and toward the concrete, empirical, experiential observations by which we test the usefulness of a particular representation. Schematics and empirics are both essential to science, and full understanding demands that we know which is which.

## Scientific Method

Siegel and Ingham (1987, p. 100) argued that the discipline of communicative disorders, as a science, "shares models, methods, and concepts with a larger community." They went on to say that most people "in the field of communicative disorders belong to the community of behavioral science."

Although not all research findings may impact directly and immediately on the clinical enterprise, there are many research topics and paradigms that show great promise for both the researcher and the clinician. For example, Siegel (1993, p. 37) argued that treatment efficacy research "makes a natural bridge between the requirements of careful research and the needs of clinical practice." Similarly, Olswang (1993) suggested that clinical efficacy research can address both applied clinical questions and questions of a more theoretical nature. Specifically, Olswang (1993, p. 126) stated:

> For those of us driven by both clinical practice and theory, we have found our playground. Efficacy research allows us to function within our split interests—addressing practice and the needs of the individual while investigating theory and the underlying mechanisms of communication. What we need is further research with this two-pronged approach, advancing our clinical and theoretical knowledge. Our profession and discipline indeed depend on both.

There are potentially hundreds of legitimate research questions that fall under the general rubric of treatment efficacy research. Carefully controlled group studies could investigate the relative efficacy of two or more intervention paradigms designed to improve dysarthric speech, time-series designs could be employed to investigate the immediate and long-term effectiveness of fluency-enhancing protocols, and single-subject designs could be used to investigate clinical strategies for increasing language output in children who are language delayed. It goes beyond the scope of this text to discuss all the potential treatment efficacy investigations, but the area is rich with research potential. Wertz (1993, p. 38) asked if the question "Does therapy work?" serves as a legitimate research question and proceeded to answer the question by responding:

> It seems to me that the question is not only appropriate for research; it is essential for clinical practice. The rationale for not asking appears weak.

In summary, we see the communicative disorders profession as primarily a clinical enterprise. It is an enterprise that is changing, growing, and developing. To ensure that the growth of the knowledge base is truly substantive, it must rest, we believe, on a scientific and research basis, a basis that must be understood and incorporated into clinical practice.

Behavioral science, which has been differentiated from physical and natural sciences in the past, is that branch of science that deals with the development of knowledge concerning human or animal behavior. In recent years, physical and natural sciences (e.g., physics and biology) have been combined with the traditional behavioral sciences (e.g., psychology and sociology) for interdisciplinary research on many aspects of behavior. Areas of study such as sociobiology, neuropsychology, psychoacoustics, and vocal physiology illustrate considerable overlap among the behavioral, physical, and natural sciences in the study of human or animal behavior. Similarly, many disciplines contribute to the scientific underpinnings of communicative disorders. Physics, biology, physiology, computer science, speech science, hearing science, psychology, and psycholinguistics contribute directly or indirectly to the discipline of communicative disorders. These disciplines provide the knowledge and tools required to attack and solve clinical problems in communicative disorders.

To understand the research enterprise (i.e., common knowledge gathering) in communicative disorders, it is necessary to understand the general framework of behavioral science within which these research activities operate. Science is a search for knowledge concerning general truths or the operation of general laws, and it depends on the use of a systematic method for the development of such knowledge. This systematic method is commonly called the *scientific method.* The scientific method includes the recognition of a problem that can be studied objectively, the collection of data through observation or experiment, and the drawing of conclusions based on an analysis of the data that have been gathered.

Scientific research may be directed toward the development of knowledge *per se,* in which case it is called *basic research,* or it may be undertaken to solve some problem of immediate social or economic consequence, in which case it is called *applied research.* In recent years, professionals in many disciplines have realized that basic and applied research are not entirely separate or opposed activities. A piece of research that was done for the sake of basic knowledge may turn out to have an important application; a piece of research done to solve an immediate problem may provide basic information concerning the nature of some phenomenon. In the past, there have been instances of acrimonious opposition between people identified with the so-called basic and applied schools, and such opposition has resulted in communication failures that have retarded rather than advanced the development of knowledge. Today, many people recognize the importance of both basic and applied research, as well as the need for clear communication between researchers with more basic orientations and professionals with more applied orientations.

Within the framework of behavioral science, two major types of research may be identified: *descriptive* and *experimental*. Descriptive research examines group differences, developmental trends, or relationships among variables through the use of laboratory measurements, various kinds of tests, and naturalistic observations. Experimental research examines causation through observation of the effects of the manipulation of certain variables on other variables under controlled conditions. These two types of research are different empirical approaches to the development of knowledge.

## Theory Construction in Behavioral Science

Empirical and rational inquiry leads to the development of theories that are statements formulated to explain phenomena. Kerlinger and Lee (2000, p. 11) stated that theory is the "ultimate aim of science" and defined a theory as

> a set of interrelated constructs (concepts), definitions, and propositions that presents a systematic view of phenomena by specifying relations among variables, with the purpose of explaining and predicting the phenomena.

Rummel (1967) discussed the relationship of rational and empirical inquiry in theory construction and stated that empirical facts alone are meaningless unless they are linked through propositions that confer meaning on the facts. According to Rummel (1967, p. 454):

> A scientific theory consists of two components: *analytic* and *empirical*. The analytic component is the linking of symbolic statements through chains of reasoning that obey logical or mathematical rules but that have little or no operational-empirical content.... This analytic component of theories can be the creation of the scientist's imagination, the distillation of a scholar's experience with the subject matter, or a tediously built structure slowly erected on a foundation of numerous experiments, investigations, and findings. The empirical component of theories is operational. It fastens the abstract analytic part of a theory to the facts.

Theories generally fall into one of two broad categories (Sidman, 1960). First, they may be generalizations, developed after the facts are in, that try to synthesize the available empirical evidence into a coherent explanation of a phenomenon. Skinner (1972, p. 100) has called such a theory "a formal representation of the data reduced to a minimal number of terms." Second, theories may be tentative generalizations or conjectures that can be subjected to future empirical confirmation—as such, they are often called *hypotheses*. The first kind of theory looks back at available data and employs a formal logic to synthesize this empirical evidence; the second kind looks ahead to future empirical and rational inquiry for verification of the theory. Empirical and rational inquiry is necessary for verification of a theory or for its modification if observed facts do not fit the theory. A knowledgeable consumer of research should recognize the theoretical organization of empirical evidence and the empirical confirmation of theories as two activities that coalesce to form the "schema-piric view" in the behavioral sciences.

Bordens and Abbott (2002, p. 44) suggested that some theories have "stood the test of time, whereas others have fallen by the wayside." Many factors contribute to the longevity, or lack thereof, of any particular theory, and Bordens and Abbott (2002, pp. 44–46) have listed five essential factors that can figure centrally in the life of theory. The first is the theory's ability to "account for most of the existing data within its domain." They explained that the amount of data accounted for is *most* not *all* because some of the data germane to the theory may be unreliable. Second, theories must have *explanatory relevance.* Explanatory relevance means that the "explanation for a phenomenon provided by a theory must offer good grounds for believing that the phenomenon would occur under the specified conditions" of the theory. The third condition is that of *testability.* Bordens and Abbott (2002, p. 44) stated:

> A theory is testable if it is capable of failing some empirical test. That is, the theory specifies outcomes under particular conditions, and if these outcomes do not occur, then the theory is rejected.

The theory's ability to predict novel events or new phenomena is the fourth characteristic of a sound theory. A theory should predict phenomena "beyond those for which the theory was originally designed." Such new phenomena were not taken into account when the theory was originally formulated. Finally, the theory should be *parsimonious* (i.e., it should adopt the fewest and/or simplest set of assumptions in the interpretation of data).

## Common Steps in Behavioral Science Research

Examination of articles in the behavioral science literature reveals some common steps taken in empirical research. These steps exemplify the nature of the scientific approach discussed more thoroughly in texts such as Kerlinger and Lee (2000) and Bordens and Abbott (2002). Consideration of this simplified outline may enable consumers to understand the general framework underlying empirical research and to realize that the different types of research to be discussed here are variations on a common theme of empirical inquiry.

The common steps in empirical research are

Statement of a *problem* to be investigated
Delineation of a *method* for investigation of the problem
Presentation of the *results* of this investigation
Drawing *conclusions* from the results about the problem

### Statement of the Problem

The researcher usually begins with the formulation of a general problem, a statement of purpose, a research question, or a hypothesis. In some cases, there may be a general statement followed by its breakdown into a number of specific subproblems or subpurposes. Whether researchers choose to present their topics with a statement of the problem, a purpose, a research question, or a hypothesis seems to be a matter of personal preference and, in fact, there is disagreement among researchers as to which of these linguistic vehicles is best for conveying the nature of the topic under investigation. We are not interested here in the polemics surrounding the choice of wording in presenting the topic to be investigated. We are more concerned that researchers provide a *clear and concise statement of what it is they are investigating.*

The problem statement should also contain some material on the meaningfulness or relevance of the topic under investigation by placing it in context. This is generally accomplished by establishing a *rationale* for the study through a review of the literature that has already been published on the particular topic to be investigated. This review may provide a historical background of the research to date and perhaps provide a summary or organization of the existing data so that the reader has an overview of what is known, what is not known, and what is equivocal concerning this general topic. Eventually, the review should culminate in a statement of the need for the particular study and a statement of the significance of the particular study.

## Method of Investigation

After stating the research problem and providing its rationale by placing it in perspective relative to the existing literature, the researcher outlines a *strategy* for investigating the problem. This is accomplished through the description of the method of investigation. It is common to find the Method section of an article divided into three subsections: (1) participants, (2) materials, and (3) procedures. Although there are variations on these subsections, the important questions we are concerned with are *How was the study carried out? Did the method provide valid and reliable results?*

*Participants.* In this section of the research article, the researcher describes the people (or animals) that were studied. A careful description is generally provided of the relevant characteristics of the participants (e.g., number of participants, age, gender, intelligence, type of speech or hearing disorder, etc.). The important point is how well the general population under consideration is defined and how well the sample of participants represents the population the researcher wishes to study.

*Materials.* In this section, the researcher describes the various tests, instruments, apparatus, or training materials used and may also describe the situation or environment in which the study took place. Information about the calibration, reliability, and validity of tests or instruments used is also presented here.

*Procedure.* In this section, the researcher describes how the *materials* were used to study the *participants.*

## Results of Investigation

Here, the researcher presents the results of the collection of data by means of the method of investigation just described. Tables and figures are often used to summarize and organize the data. Tables and figures are usually easier to understand than a simple listing of all the individual or raw data. It is important for a researcher to present a specific breakdown of the results as they relate to the specific subcomponents of the problem presented at the beginning of the article.

## Conclusions

After presenting the results, the researcher draws conclusions from them that reflect on the original statement of the problem. The conclusions are often cast in the form of a discussion of the results in relation to previous research, theoretical implications, practical implications, and suggestions for further research.

This simplified discussion of the manner in which the common steps in empirical research are reported in a journal article may give beginning readers the impression that research is a drab activity that follows a single pattern. It is difficult to understand the excitement and creativity inherent in the design and execution of an empirical study unless the student experiences it directly. In fact, all researchers may not necessarily follow the orderly steps just outlined in doing their research; adjustments may be made to meet the needs of a researcher in a particular situation. Skinner (1959, p. 363) has captured some of the flavor of scientific creativity and excitement in his famous statement:

> Here was a first principle not formally recognized by scientific methodologists: when you run onto something interesting, drop everything else and study it.

The common steps just outlined, then, are meant to illustrate the major components of the scientific method as reflected in the structure of most journal articles that report empirical research and should not be construed as an inviolate set of rules for defining *the* scientific method.

We also want to point out that readers are likely to encounter some articles that do not report original empirical research data, but, instead, review the existing literature on a particular topic in communicative disorders. These reviews are usually much more comprehensive and detailed than the literature review found in the introduction to a typical research article. They provide a historical perspective of trends in the development of thought about a particular topic and demonstrate how these trends may have shaped research approaches to these topics. Discussion of method and theory in historical research is beyond the scope of this book and readers are referred to Barzun and Graff (1970) for a general overview of historical research. A few brief points should be made about literature reviews as they relate to the commonalities of empirical research.

First, such reviews are important in synthesizing research developments to date, organizing our thinking regarding how past research has contributed to our present knowledge, and suggesting new avenues for exploration. Second, such devices are valuable in theory construction and in placing data into theoretical perspective. Third, such reviews are important sources of *critical* evaluation of the research literature.

For example, Cacace and McFarland (1998) wrote a critical review regarding the lack of empirical evidence supporting central auditory processing disorders (CAPD) as a specific auditory dysfunction. They contended that the evaluation of CAPD in school-aged children is based on an assumption that an auditory-specific deficit underlies many learning problems and language disabilities. From their extensive review of the extant research literature on the topic, Cacace and McFarland (1998, p. 355) concluded that there is insufficient evidence to support the unimodal auditory-specific deficit assumption and suggested that multimodal perceptual testing be used to help clarify the true underlying nature of CAPD.

Finally, comprehensive reviews of the research literature also help to illuminate what Boring (1950) has referred to as the *zeitgeist* (German: "time spirit"), or the prevailing outlook that is characteristic of a particular period or generation. The zeitgeist influences research trends along particular lines and may proscribe other directions, but it may also shift to generate new research trends.

An example of a potential zeitgeist change is an article published by Hixon and Weismer (1995) in which they reexamined published data from a complex study of speech breathing (Draper, Ladefoged, & Whitteridge, 1959) that has become known as the Edinburgh study. Hixon and Weismer (1995, p. 42) asserted that

> The Edinburgh study has had a forceful, pervasive, and lasting impact on the speech sciences and is considered by many to be the definitive account of speech breathing function. Indeed, it is widely afforded the status of a classic.

In a detailed critique, Hixon and Weismer (1995) pointed out several measurement and interpretive flaws in the Edinburgh study that serve to invalidate the study. In a sense, Hixon and Weismer's critique serves as a strong impetus to conduct new research in speech breathing processes. Hixon and Weismer (1995, p. 58), in fact, stated:

> There is still much to be learned about speech breathing and its role in human communication. Our hope for this article is that it will stimulate thinking and serve a useful tutorial purpose for those who will follow.

The best way for students of communicative disorders to appreciate the common steps in empirical research that we have discussed thus far is to read journal articles that report empirical research. Sustained experience in the reading of empirical research will enable the student to eventually assimilate the concept or process of moving from the formulation of a problem that can be attacked empirically to the drawing of conclusions based on empirical evidence. Many students report that the reading of literature reviews is as important as the reading of original empirical articles in developing an appreciation of the common steps in empirical research.

## The Nature of Research in Communicative Disorders

It is extremely difficult to paint a complete picture of the research enterprise in communicative disorders. No one has done it and we will not do it here. The data that would form the basis of such a picture are simply not available. A few generalizations should help, however, in understanding the broad scope of research activities that impinge, either directly or indirectly, on communicative disorders.

Although relatively few communicative disorders specialists are involved in full-time research (American Speech-Language-Hearing Association, 1999), the research enterprise in communicative disorders is much broader than would appear from surveys of the ASHA membership. One obvious reason is that not all people who are involved in communicative disorders research are members of ASHA. More important, though, is that many people are involved in research activities on less than a full-time basis. Perhaps the best example of such a person is the academician whose primary job responsibility is teaching. Such an individual is often involved in his or her own research or supervises doctoral dissertations or master's theses. The same person publishes the results of his or her research not only to advance knowledge but also to advance his or her own standing in the academic community because "publish-or-perish" is still commonplace in university life. Other part-time researchers include doctoral students and clinicians working in a variety of clinical settings. Finally, much of the research appearing in the periodical literature is done by people working outside of communicative disorders. These include individuals such as otolaryngologists, experimental psychologists, psycholinguists, and neurophysiologists. The numbers of published articles that relate directly or tangentially to the interests of professionals in communicative disorders attest to the numbers and different interests and backgrounds of individuals involved in the communicative disorders research enterprise.

The areas investigated are equally diverse, ranging, for example, from the study of the effects of noise on the hearing sensitivity of chinchillas to the study of hearing-aid evaluation procedures, from a study of infant respiration to a study of the most efficient way to teach esophageal speech, from the study of how children acquire language to the study of how people with aphasia relearn speech and language. The areas studied are almost as numerous as the people involved in their study.

The settings in which research is conducted are equally varied. Language acquisition of a typically developing child is studied in the naturalistic environment of the child's home; the efficiency of an auditory site-of-lesion test is evaluated in the audiology clinic. The chinchilla's hearing sensitivity is investigated within the confines of a laboratory; the effects of noise on human hearing sensitivity may be studied in a factory setting. Stuttering behavior may be investigated in a laboratory, clinic, or school. In broad terms, normal processes are usually but not always studied in a laboratory setting; the study of disordered communication is frequently but not always carried out in a clinical setting.

Finally, as we will see in Chapter 2, the research strategies in communicative disorders are also diverse, ranging from survey studies performed in the field to experimental research performed in the laboratory.

## Research Ethics

In addition to having a responsibility to communicate relevant findings, the researcher has other important ethical responsibilities—responsibilities that are inherent in the research process. Several professional associations have codes of ethics that specify the ethical constraints placed on investigators who do research with human participants. For example, participants must have the freedom to decline to participate in a research project or to withdraw from the project at any time. The welfare and dignity of participants must be protected at all times. The investigator must protect the confidentiality of information obtained during the course of the study. The investigator must protect participants from physical and mental discomfort, harm, and danger. Investigators must honor all agreements and commitments made to participants. More complete descriptions of these ethical obligations can be found in such sources as *Ethical Principles of Psychologists and Code of Conduct* (American Psychological Association [APA], 2002) and in Part III of the November 23, 1982, *Federal Register.*

The ethical responsibilities placed on the researcher are as stringent as those required of clinicians, especially when the researcher is using human participants. In fact, researchers have both ethical *and* legal responsibilities to protect the rights of both human and nonhuman living participants. Many institutions are required to have an Institutional Review Board that studies research proposals to ensure that the welfare of participants is scrupulously maintained, especially if the institution is interested in obtaining governmental funds for the conduct of the research. Suffice it to say that researchers have important obligations to a varied constituency—to their audience, their participants, their institutions, their profession, and themselves.

## The Editorial Process in the Publication of a Research Article

One common myth that needs to be dispelled early is that if an article appears in print, it must be worthwhile, valuable, and a significant contribution to the literature and to our knowledge. This is simply not the case. Inadequate research is reported, trivial problems are investigated, and articles vary tremendously in quality and value. Perhaps a brief description of the publication process will help the reader understand how an article gets published and how the quality of research can vary from one article to the next.

Although the editorial process differs from journal to journal, there are commonalities in the review process that cut across most journals. (For a description of the editorial process for articles published by the American Psychological Association, the reader should consult the Association's *Publication Manual* [American Psychological Association, 2001]). Let us use, as an example, a clinical research article submitted for publication to the *American Journal of Speech-Language Pathology: A Journal of Clinical Practice (AJSLP),* one of the journals published by ASHA. At the time of writing, the journal was directed to professionals who provide services to persons with communicative disorders. Manuscripts that deal with the nature, assessment, prevention, and treatment of communicative disorders were invited. Note that the *Journal of Speech, Language, and Hearing Research (JSLHR),* also published by ASHA, "invites papers concerned with theoretical issues and research in the communication sciences." Manuscripts submitted to *AJSLP* are considered on the basis of clinical significance, conformity to standards of evidence, and clarity of writing. The journal welcomes philosophical, conceptual, or synthesizing essays, as well as reports of clinical research. The details are contained in the Information for Authors section of each issue, a section that defines, in a general way, the scope and emphasis of the journal, thus helping potential contributors to decide whether *AJSLP* is the appropriate journal for their manuscript.

The editorial staff of *AJSLP* consists of an editor and several associate editors in areas such as fluency and fluency disorders, neurogenic communication disorders, dysphagia, voice disorders, and communication disorders in early childhood. In addition, there are more than one hundred editorial consultants, all of whom are knowledgeable in one or more areas of communicative disorders. Overall editorial policy is established by the editor and must be consistent with the general guidelines set by the Publication Board of ASHA.

On receipt of a manuscript, a decision is made into whose purview the manuscript falls. An associate editor is then assigned to oversee the review process and to serve as a reviewer. Next, the manuscript is forwarded by the associate editor to two editorial consultants who, after careful evaluation of the manuscript, recommend one of four alternatives: (1) accept for publication as is, (2) accept contingent on the author agreeing to make certain revisions recommended by the reviewers, (3) defer decision pending major revisions and another review by two different editorial consultants, and (4) reject outright. No matter which alternative is recommended, the final decision to accept or reject lies with the editor. If a decision to reject is reached, the evaluations by the reviewers are forwarded to the author, sometimes with a marked copy of the manuscript. The editorial consultants are not identified to the author and the editorial consultants do not know the name of the author or the author's institutional affiliation. That is, manuscripts are subjected to a "blind" review in which reviewers are ostensibly unaware of the identity of the author.

Although every effort is made to arrive at a publication decision quickly, the review process can be time consuming, especially if extensive revision is requested. The revisions may require considerable work on the part of the author, data may have to be reanalyzed or displayed differently, tables and figures may have to be added or deleted, and portions of the manuscript may have to be rewritten. Obviously, the more revisions required, the less likely is a manuscript to be accepted, particularly if a journal has a backlog of manuscripts already accepted for publication. All of this necessitates considerable correspondence between the author and the editor and, perhaps, even another review by two more editorial consultants. It is for these reasons that considerable time may elapse between the date the manuscript is received and the date it is finally accepted.

How do inadequate or marginal manuscripts end up being published? Despite the care that is taken to select knowledgeable and informed editorial consultants, not all editorial consultants have the same level of expertise, have comparable research or evaluative skills, are equally familiar with a given area, use the same standards in evaluating a manuscript, and give the same amount of time and energy to the evaluation process. One journal in the field of communicative disorders, the *Journal of Fluency Disorders,* periodically surveys the consulting editors regarding their interests and expertise in an attempt to provide competent and balanced manuscript reviews.

Finally, the research sophistication found among members of a profession or discipline can have a pronounced effect on the character and excellence of its journals. Equally important, however, is the great care of the journal staff to ensure a high degree of excellence in the review process. Despite everyone's devotion to quality, journal articles indeed differ in excellence, and educated consumers of research have the responsibility of being able to identify those differences.

## Some Myths and a Caveat

One of our goals is to explode some of the myths surrounding research and the evaluation of research. We have noted already that the appearance of an article in a journal is no guarantee of the article's quality. There is good research and there is poor research, both of which may be published. The objective of the critical evaluation is to discern which is which. A stance of healthy skepticism is good both for the reader and, in the long run, for the researcher and the profession.

A major obstacle standing in the path of the consumer of research is the attitude that one must have a solid background in statistics before one can intelligently read the research literature. A similar attitude is that research and statistics are synonymous. Nothing could be further from the truth. For example, Plutchik (1983) stated that statistical analysis is not an end in itself and cannot ensure meaningful conclusions simply by its application to experimental data. This view continues to be held by current authors of research design textbooks such as DePoy and Gitlin (1994, p. 237), who pointed out that "conducting statistical analysis is just one action process in research." No matter how excellent and sophisticated the statistical treatment, a major weakness in any other part of the research study or article vitiates the value of the statistical analysis. A trivial problem is still trivial no matter how sophisticated the statistical analysis. A poorly conceived research design remains poorly conceived, despite a complex statistical approach. The inferences and generalizations drawn from the data may be appropriate and fair but the statistical analysis does not ensure this.

Statistical analysis is an essential tool for the researcher, but research and statistical treatment are not the same. A serious weakness in *any* part of a research article—introduction (rationale), method, data analysis, or discussion—weakens the whole.

Another myth, perhaps less widely held, is that the researcher is characteristically a recluse in a white coat isolated in the ivy-covered laboratory working on problems that have little relevance to human life, no less to the practicing clinician. Again, this is not true. Most researchers are concerned about people with communicative disorders, and it is this concern that continues to motivate their research. In fact, many of today's researchers have strong clinical backgrounds and extensive clinical experience. Many researchers, while perhaps not involved in research that has immediate application, are doing research that tomorrow may have considerable relevance to clinical practice. Researchers usually do not go out of their way to be obtuse or uncommunicative; some may not write well, but the poor writing is unintentional. A number of leading researchers have played important roles in the nonresearch professional aspects of communicative disorders. Some researchers are haughty and aloof; so, too, are some clinicians.

Now for the caveat. Although we are attempting to lead the interested clinician through the process of research evaluation, a fundamental prerequisite to intelligent consumership is the fund of substantive information possessed by the reader. To illustrate, let us take a research article on stuttering and, further, let us consider the introductory section devoted to developing the need for the study and the purpose of the study. How can one evaluate the author's rationale without some knowledge of the literature on stuttering? Have important citations been omitted because they are inconsistent with the author's purpose? Can the reader understand the theoretical framework within which the author is operating? Has the author misinterpreted or misunderstood previous research? The only way the reader can answer these questions is to have a strong background in the subject of stuttering. The identical problem exists for the editorial consultant; that is why journals have large rosters of reviewers. The information explosion in communicative disorders has made it almost impossible for one person to be truly knowledgeable in all substantive areas.

This is not a book on stuttering, aphasia, cleft palate, or audiometry; therefore, we have made the assumption that practitioners and students will approach a journal article with some background on the topic dealt with in the article. Although we have provided a framework for evaluation, the framework must rest on a substantive foundation that the reader must have.

## Study Questions

1. Read the following article:

   Phillips, S. L., Gordon-Salant, S., Fitzgibbons, P. J., & Yeni-Komshian, G. (2000). Frequency and temporal resolution in elderly listeners with good and poor word recognition. *Journal of Speech, Language, and Hearing Research, 43,* 217–228.

   Examine the relationship between the physical and behavioral measurements used in this study.

2. Read the following article:

   Cacace, A. T., & McFarland, D. J. (1998). Central auditory processing disorder in school-aged children: A critical review. *Journal of Speech, Language, and Hearing Research, 41,* 355–373.

   What are the major issues raised by Cacace and McFarland regarding the empirical evidence that suggests central auditory processing disorders are related deficits in the auditory system exclusively?

3. Read the following article:

   Stevens, S. S. (1968). Measurement, statistics, and the schemapiric view. *Science, 161,* 849–856.

   Summarize Stevens's viewpoint on the relationship between the schematic and empirical aspects of science. What is the meaning of Stevens's reference to the two faces of Janus?

4. Read the following articles:

   Hixon, T. J., & Weismer, G. (1995). Perspectives on the Edinburgh study of speech breathing. *Journal of Speech and Hearing Research, 38,* 42–60.

   Folkins, J. W., & Bleile, K. M. (1990). Taxonomies in biology, phonetics, phonology, and speech motor control. *Journal of Speech and Hearing Disorders, 55,* 596–611.

   Discuss the manner in which the authors deal with the relationship of empirical evidence to theory. Are theories cited that represent a synthesis of previous evidence? Are new theories advanced that need to be confirmed by future empirical evidence?

5. Read the following article:

   Perkins, W. H. (1990). What is stuttering? *Journal of Speech and Hearing Disorders, 55,* 370–382.

   What does Perkins say about the relationships among research, theory, and therapy?

**6.** Read the following article:

Schlosser R. W. (2004). Evidence-based practice in AAC: 10 points to consider. *The ASHA Leader, 9(12),* 6–7, 10.

Contrast the "myths and realities" of EBP discussed by Schlosser.

**7.** Read the following article:

Justice, L. M., & Fey, M. E. (2004). Evidence-based practice in schools: Integrating craft and theory with science and data. *The ASHA Leader, 9(17),* 4–5, 30–31.

From the example provided in the text, explain why a clinician's decision *not* to use a new treatment program is evidence-based practice.

**8.** Read the following article:

Caswell, E. (2004). The latest and best research at your fingertips—literally. *The ASHA Leader, 9(16),* 4–5, 21.

Discuss why it is important to have a solid research base in communicative disorders. What is the future for online publishing of ASHA journals?

# REFERENCES

*The American heritage college dictionary.* (1997). Boston: Houghton Mifflin.

American Psychological Association. (2001). *Publication manual of the American Psychological Association* (5th ed.). Washington, DC: American Psychological Association.

American Psychological Association. (2002). *Ethical principles of psychologists and code of conduct.* Washington, DC: American Psychological Association. Retrieved June 17, 2004, from www.apa.org/ethics/code2002.html.

American Speech-Language-Hearing Association. (1999). *ASHA database.* Unpublished document.

Apel, K., & Self, T. (2003). Evidence-based practice: The marriage of research and clinical service. *The ASHA Leader, 8(16),* 6–7.

Babbie, E. (2004). *The practice of social research* (10th ed). Belmont, CA: Wadsworth.

Barzun, J., & Graff, H. F. (1970). *The modern researcher.* New York: Harcourt Brace.

Bordens, K. S., & Abbott, B. B. (2002). *Research design and methods: A process approach* (5th ed.). New York: McGraw-Hill.

Boring, E. G. (1950). *A history of experimental psychology.* New York: Appleton-Century-Crofts.

Cacace, A. T., & McFarland, D. J. (1998). Central auditory processing disorder in school-aged children: A critical review. *Journal of Speech, Language, and Hearing Research, 41,* 355–373.

Chomsky, N. (1968). *Language and mind.* New York: Harcourt, Brace, & World.

Cizek, G. J. (1995). Crunchy granola and the hegemony of the narrative. *Educational Researcher, 24(3),* 26–28.

DePoy, E., & Gitlin, L. N. (1994). *Introduction to research: Multiple strategies for health and human services.* St. Louis: Mosby.

Dilollo, A., & Wolter, J. (2004). Qualitative research in communicative disorders. *The ASHA Leader, 9(11),* 4–5, 16–17.

Dollaghan, C. (2004). Evidence-based practice: Myths and realities. *The ASHA Leader, 9(7),* 4–5, 12.

Draper, M., Ladefoged, P., & Whitteridge, D. (1959). Respiratory muscles in speech. *Journal of Speech and Hearing Research, 2,* 16–27.

Goldstein, B. A. (2004). From the editor. *Language, Speech, and Hearing Services in Schools, 35(3),* 199.

Hixon, T. J., & Weismer, G. (1995). Perspectives on the Edinburgh study of speech breathing. *Journal of Speech and Hearing Research, 38,* 42–60.

Ingram, D. (1998). Research-practice relationships in speech-language pathology. *Topics in Language Disorders, 18(2),* 1–9.

Katz, W. F. (2003). From basic research in speech science to answers in speech-language pathology. *The ASHA Leader, 8(1),* 6–7, 20.

Kerlinger, F. N., & Lee, H. B. (2000). *Foundations of behavioral research* (4th ed.). New York: Harcourt Brace.

Logemann, J. A. (2000). Are clinicians and researchers different? *The ASHA Leader, 5(8),* 2.

Olswang, L. B. (1993). Treatment efficacy research: A paradigm for investigating clinical practice and theory. *Journal of Fluency Disorders, 18,* 125–134.

Plutchik, R. (1983). *Foundations of experimental research* (3rd ed.). New York: Harper & Row.

Poggi, S. (2003, Spring). Facing the challenge to use scientifically based research in schools. *NCREL's Learning Point,* 4–7.

Ramig, L. (2002). The joy of research. *The ASHA Leader, 7(8),* 6–7, 19.

Reynolds, G. S., (1975). *A primer of operant conditioning.* Glenview, IL: Scott Foresman.

Robey, R. R. (2004). Levels of evidence. *The ASHA Leader, 9(7),* 5.

Robin, D. A. (1999). From the editor. *American Journal of Speech-Language Pathology, 8,* 194.

Rummel, R. J. (1967). Understanding factor analysis. *Journal of Conflict Resolution, 11,* 444–480.

Russell, B. (1945). *History of western philosophy.* New York: Simon & Schuster.

Sackett D. L., Straus, S. E., Richardson, W. S., Rosenberg, W., & Haynes, R. B. (2000). *Evidence-based medicine: How to practice and teach EBM* (2nd ed.). Edinburgh: Churchill Livingstone.

Schlosser, R. W. (2004). Evidence-based practice in AAC: 10 points to consider. *The ASHA Leader, 9(12),* 6–7, 10.

Shprintzen, R. (1997). *Genetics, syndromes, and communication disorders.* San Diego, CA: Singular.

Sidman, M. (1960). *Tactics of scientific research.* New York: Basic Books

Siegel, G. M. (1993). Research: A natural bridge. *Asha, 35,* 36–37.

Siegel, G. M., & Ingham, R. J. (1987). Theory and science in communication disorders. *Journal of Speech and Hearing Disorders, 52,* 99–104.

Skinner, B. F. (1953). *Science and human behavior.* New York: Macmillan.

Skinner, B. F. (1959). A case history in the scientific method. In S. Koch (Ed.), *Psychology: A study of a science* (Vol. 2, pp. 359–379). New York: McGraw-Hill.

Skinner, B. F. (1972). *Cumulative record* (3rd ed.). New York: Appleton-Century-Crofts.

Stevens, S. S. (1968). Measurement, statistics, and the schemapiric view. *Science, 161,* 849–856.

Wambaugh, J., & Bain, B. (2002). Make research methods an integral part of your clinical practice. *The ASHA Leader, 7(21),* 1, 10–13.

Wertz, R. T. (1993). Adult-onset disorders. *Asha, 35,* 38–39.

# Research Strategies
# in Communicative Disorders

This chapter reviews research strategies that are prevalent in the communicative disorders literature. Classification of research studies into mutually exclusive categories is difficult because of the variety of research strategies employed and the overlap among them. In addition, it is common for a single journal article to report the results of a large study that uses different research strategies simultaneously to study different aspects of the same research problem. Therefore, our categorization will be arbitrary as are those of other research textbooks. It is intended to illustrate common principles of empirical research in communicative disorders, some of the differences among various research strategies, and the appropriateness of certain strategies for the study of different problems.

Bordens and Abbott (2002) make a clear distinction between research strategy and research design. In their scheme, a research strategy is the general plan of attack, whereas the specific tactics used to carry out the strategy constitute the research design. Before choosing a specific research design, an investigator must first select an overall research strategy. This chapter will outline some of the more common research strategies used in communicative disorders research, and the next chapter will describe some specific research designs employed to carry out these major research strategies.

## Variables in Empirical Research

Empirical research is concerned with the relationships among *variables.* Variables are measurable quantities that vary or change under different circumstances rather than remain constant. In geometry, for example, the radius and circumference of a circle are two variables: draw a large and a small circle and you can measure the different values of the radius and circumference of each circle. However, the formula that relates the radius and the circumference of a circle ($c = 2\pi r$) contains the term $\pi$ (pi), which has a constant value of approximately 3.14159. Thus, $\pi$ is a constant; it never varies regardless of the size of the circle. However, the radius and the circumference are variables, or measurable quantities that may differ from one circle to the next. In behavioral science, the variables studied are often common measurable quantities such as stimulus characteristics (tone intensity or frequency), environmental conditions (background noise level), speech behavior (rate of speech or number of nonfluencies), language performance (mean length of utterance or number of embedded clauses found in a language sample), or hearing ability (speech reception threshold). Kerlinger and Lee (2000) have outlined three classifications of variables that are important for understanding the ways in which behavioral research attempts to understand the relationships among important variables.

## Independent and Dependent Variables

Kerlinger and Lee's most important notion is the distinction between *independent* and *dependent* variables. Indeed, this concept forms the core of the material in this chapter and underlies everything discussed in the rest of the book. According to Kerlinger and Lee (2000, p. 46):

> The most useful way to categorize variables is either as independent or dependent. This categorization is highly useful because of its general applicability, simplicity, and special importance, both in conceptualizing and designing research and in communicating the results of research. An *independent variable* is the *presumed* cause of the *dependent variable,* the *presumed* effect. The independent variable is the antecedent; the dependent is the consequent.

Independent variables, then, can often be conceptualized as conditions that cause changes in behavior; dependent variables can be seen as the behavior that is changed. For example, delayed auditory feedback (independent variable) may cause a change in speech rate (dependent variable). Masking noise (independent variable) may cause a change in auditory threshold (dependent variable). Kerlinger and Lee caution us, however, on the use of "the touchy word *cause* and related words" in discussing independent and dependent variables. One problem is the level of causation that we talk about: the variable that we manipulate may cause a change in a variable that is unknown to us, and the change of the unknown variable is what causes the change we observe in our dependent variable.

Another problem facing researchers in discussing cause-and-effect relations among variables will be seen in our discussion in this chapter of the distinctions between experimental and descriptive research. Cause–effect relations are more logically inferred from the results of experiments than from the results of descriptive research because of the nature of the independent variables in these two kinds of research. In experimental research, the experimenter manipulates an independent variable (while holding other potential independent variables constant) to examine what effect the manipulation of the independent variable has on the dependent variable. In descriptive research, however, it is not possible for the researcher to manipulate the independent variable to see what effect that manipulation will have on the dependent variable. Independent variables in descriptive research usually include factors such as participant classification (e.g., normal vs. language-delayed children) that the researcher cannot manipulate. The descriptive researcher may be able to compare a group of normal children with a group of language-delayed children on some dependent variable, but the participant classification of the children cannot be directly manipulated to observe the effect of manipulation on their behavior. (Some authors call such descriptive research "experiments of nature" because nature has manipulated the independent variable in determining the children's classification.) Thus, direct cause–effect relations are difficult to infer from the results of descriptive research.

Kerlinger and Lee (2000) have also pointed out that the distinction between independent and dependent variables is really a distinction that is based on our *use* of variables rather than on some inherent property of a variable. We conceive of a certain variable as the antecedent that causes a change in another variable and, therefore, use that first variable as the independent variable and the second variable as the dependent variable. It is sometimes possible for researchers to conceive of a particular variable as being an independent variable in one situation and a dependent variable in another situation. For example, mean length of utterance is sometimes used (instead of chronological age) to classify children into groups that vary in degree of language development; mean length of utterance, thereby, becomes the measure of the values of the independent variable. In another study, however, a researcher may study the effect of manipulation of an independent variable on children's mean length of utterance; mean length of utterance thereby becomes the dependent variable. We must always look carefully at how a researcher employs the variables studied to determine the independent and dependent variables.

Kerlinger and Lee (2000) advocate thinking of independent and dependent variables in mathematical terms where $X$ is an independent variable and $Y$ is a dependent variable, and we may specify the relationship between $X$ and $Y$ as a mathematical *function.* Jaeger and Bacon (1962, p. 6) state that

> If two variables are related in such a way that the value of one is determined whenever the other is specified, the one is said to be a *function* of the other.

Thus, if we know the functional relationship of $X$ and $Y$, we know how $Y$ varies whenever $X$ is varied. When we know the value of $X$, we can determine the value of $Y$ from the functional relation of the two variables. In other words, if we know how the independent variable and the dependent variable are related and we know the value of the independent variable, we can determine the value of the dependent variable.

Functions can be demonstrated graphically by plotting the values of $X$ and $Y$ on the coordinate axes of a graph. Functions can also be demonstrated by writing an equation that shows how to calculate the value of $Y$ for any value of $X$. The equation can be used to generate a line that connects all the plotted values of $X$ and $Y$ on the graph. The equation and the graph are just two different ways of displaying the same function—the equation with mathematical symbols and the graph with a line that connects the coordinate values of $X$ and $Y$.

It is useful to exemplify this concept by examining the manner in which research results may often be presented in a graph. For example, the results of a research study examining the relationship of two variables might look like the hypothetical data shown in Figure 2.1. The values of the independent variable are indicated on the *abscissa* (horizontal or $X$-axis), and the values of the dependent variable are indicated on the *ordinate* (vertical or $Y$-axis). The values of the independent variable increase from left to right on the abscissa and the values of the dependent variable increase from bottom to top on the ordinate. The dots indicate coordinate points of average values of the dependent variable ($Y$) that were found for each value of the independent variable ($X$), and the line drawn to connect these dots graphically shows the function relating the changes in the dependent variable to changes in the independent variable.

Figure 2.1 shows how the dependent variable varies as a function of changes in the independent variable in a graphic fashion. The function could also be shown with an equation

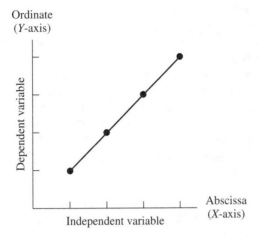

Ordinate
(*Y*-axis)

Dependent variable

Independent variable

Abscissa
(*X*-axis)

**FIGURE 2.1   Hypothetical Data Illustrating a Dependent Variable That Increases as a Function of Increases in the Independent Variable.**

relating the values of *Y* to the values of *X*. Because the function shown in Figure 2.1 is a straight line, a simple linear equation can be used to show the function

$$Y = a + bX$$

This equation states that values of the dependent variable (*Y*) can be calculated by taking the value of the independent variable (*X*) and multiplying it by a value (*b*) and adding to it another value (*a*). The *b* term is the slope of the line that indicates how fast *Y* increases as *X* is increased. The *a* term is the value of *Y* at the point where the line intercepts the *Y* axis when the value of *X* is zero and is called the *Y*-intercept. The formula can be used to calculate the value of *Y* for any value of *X* and can also be used to generate the line drawn through the data points. The values of *a* and *b* are calculated from the actual *X* and *Y* data. The particular function shown in Figure 2.1 is a positive linear function: *Y* increases linearly as a function of increases in *X*. There are many other possible functions that can be seen in actual research data. For example, *Y* in a negative function, decreases as a function of increases in *X,* in which case, the line would slope downward to the right rather than upward as in Figure 2.1. Or the data points may not fall along a straight line; they may show a curvilinear relationship between *X* and *Y.* In any case, the function is a mathematical or graphic way of depicting the relationship between the independent variable and the dependent variable by demonstrating how the dependent variable changes as a function of changes in the independent variable. Readers should note that the function may also be flat; that is, there may be no functional relationship between *X* and *Y.* If there is no effect of the independent variable on the dependent variable, then as *X* increases there is no change in *Y.*

An option that is sometimes included with such a graph is to indicate the variability of the *Y* values in addition to the average *Y* value at each value of *X*. This is accomplished by drawing a vertical bar at each coordinate *XY* point, the height of which indicates the variability of the *Y* values around the average. Homogeneous *Y* values at each *X* will show a small variability bar indicating a tight clustering of the dependent variable values at each value of the independent variable. Heterogeneous *Y* values at each *X* will show a large variability bar indicating more spread of the dependent variable values at each value of the independent variable. Some of the examples that are used in this book include this variability option with line graphs (see, for example, Figure 2.6) and some do not. A discussion of some specific indices of variability and their use is found in Chapters 6 and 9.

Tabachnick and Fidell (2001, p. 2) have nicely summarized the issues covered in this discussion of the relationship between independent and dependent variables as follows:

> Variables are roughly dichotomized into two major types—independent and dependent. Independent variables (IVs) are the differing conditions (treatment vs. placebo) to which you expose your subjects, or characteristics (tall or short) the subjects themselves bring into the research situation. IVs are usually considered either predictor or causal variables because they predict or cause the DVs—the response or outcome variables. Note that IV and DV are defined within a research context; a DV in one research setting may be an IV in another.

## Active and Attribute Variables

A second notion about classifying variables that Kerlinger and Lee (2000) discuss is the distinction between *active* and *attribute* variables. A variable that can be *manipulated* is an active variable. Thus, the independent variable in an experiment is an active variable because the experimenter can manipulate it or change its value. For example, an experimenter can change the intensity of a tone presented to a listener by manipulating the hearing-level dial on an audiometer.

There are many independent variables, however, that cannot be manipulated by an experimenter. Variables such as participant characteristics cannot be manipulated. An experimenter cannot change things such as a participant's age, gender, intelligence, type of speech disorder, degree of hearing loss, or history. Such variables have already existed for each participant—or have been "manipulated by nature." These variables are attributes of the participants.

Some variables may be either active or attribute variables, depending on the circumstances of the research or how the researcher uses the variable. Kerlinger and Lee (2000, pp. 51–52) use the example of anxiety as a variable that may be either active or attribute. Anxiety may be thought of as an attribute of participants—yet, anxiety could also be manipulated by inducing different degrees of anxiety in different participants to see what effect the manipulation of anxiety has on some dependent variable. For example, anxiety could be raised in some participants by telling them that the task they are about to undertake is a difficult one that will require great concentration, while telling other participants not to worry about the task that they are about to complete because it is very easy.[1]

---

[1]Kerlinger and Lee (2000, p. 52) however, state that "Actually, we cannot assume that the measured (attribute) and the manipulated (active) 'anxieties' are the same. We may assume that both are 'anxiety' in a broad sense, but they are certainly not the same." Nevertheless, the example points out the principle that what may be an attribute variable in one situation may be an active variable in another.

The important point is that the independent variable in an experiment is active—it can be manipulated in some way by an experimenter to see what effect it has on a dependent variable. However, the independent variable in descriptive research is an attribute—it cannot be manipulated by the researcher to see what effect it has on the dependent variable. In descriptive studies, the researcher must rely on comparisons of values of the dependent variable that correspond to some existing value of an attribute independent variable.

## Continuous and Categorical Variables

A third notion about classifying variables discussed by Kerlinger and Lee (2000) is the distinction between *continuous* and *categorical* variables. A continuous variable is one that may be measured along some continuum or dimension that reflects at least the rank ordering of values of the variable and possibly reflects even more refined measurement of the actual numerical values of the variable. The intensity of a tone, for example, is measured along a numerical continuum from low to high values of sound pressure level. Stuttering frequency can vary from zero nonfluencies to a high number of nonfluencies.

Categorical variables, however, cannot be measured along a continuum. Instead, different values of the variable can only be categorized or named. For example, tones can be presented to a listener binaurally or monaurally. Participants can be classified as "stutterers" or "nonstutterers" (although the degree of stuttering *severity* of the stutterers can be measured along some continuum from mild to severe). The ways in which we measure continuous and categorical variables differ—more will be said about this in Chapters 4 and 6 when we discuss measurement and data organization and analysis.

One immediate concern in this chapter is the way that continuous and categorical variables are displayed graphically. This is especially important in distinguishing between continuous and categorical independent variables. When graphing the change in a dependent variable as a function of changes in a continuous independent variable, it is common to use a line graph like the one in Figure 2.1. The line drawn through the data points in Figure 2.1 is an interpolation and intended to demonstrate what the values of the dependent variable ought to be for intermediate values of the independent variable that are not actually used. However, when graphing the changes in a dependent variable as a function of changes in a categorical independent variable, it is customary to use a bar graph in which the height of the bar that is aligned at each categorical value of the independent variable on the X-axis is meant to indicate the value of the dependent variable on the Y-axis for that categorical value of the independent variable. Several examples of both types of graphs are seen in this and later chapters, but it may be useful to illustrate briefly the way in which a categorical independent variable is presented in a bar graph.

Figure 2.2 shows the same hypothetical data that are illustrated in Figure 2.1, except that the four values of the independent variable are shown as four categories of a categorical variable rather than as four ordered values on a continuous variable. The data in Figure 2.1 show a dependent variable that increases as the values of the independent variable increase along a continuum. The data in Figure 2.2 show the differences in the values of the dependent variable for four different categories of an independent variable. In general, throughout the rest of the book, we follow the convention of presenting data for a continuous independent variable with a line graph and data for a categorical independent variable with a bar graph. The option to include the variability of the Y values in addition to the average Y value at each

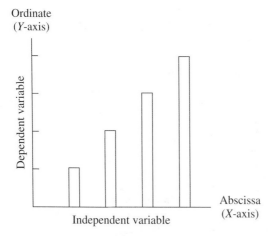

**FIGURE 2.2  Hypothetical Data Illustrating Differences in the Values of the Dependent Variable for Four Different Categories of an Independent Variable.**

value of *X* can also be used with this type of bar graph by drawing a thinner vertical bar on top of each bar in the graph to show the spread of the dependent variable values at each value of the independent variable. Some of the examples that will be used in this book include this variability option with bar graphs (see, for example, Figure 2.5) and some do not.

Tabachnick and Fidell (2001, pp. 6–8) have nicely summarized the issues covered in this discussion of the relationship between continuous and categorial ("discrete") variables as follows:

> Continuous variables are measured on a scale that changes values smoothly rather than in steps. Continuous variables take on any value within the range of the scale, and the size of the number reflects the amount of the variable. Precision is limited by the measuring instrument, not by the nature of the scale itself. Some examples of continuous variables are time as measured on an old-fashioned analog clock face, annual income, age, temperature, distance, and grade point average (GPA).... Discrete variables take on a finite and usually small number of values and there is no smooth transition from one value or category to the next. Examples include time as displayed by a digital clock, continents, categories of religious affiliation, and type of community (rural or urban).... The distinction between continuous and discrete variables is not always clear. If you add enough digits to the digital clock, for instance, it becomes for all practical purposes a continuous measuring device, while time as measured by the analog device can also be read in discrete categories such as hours or half hours. In fact, any continuous measurement may be rendered discrete (or dichotomous) by specifying cutoffs on the continuous scale.

Now that we have discussed the concept of variables in empirical research, we will examine some different research strategies in communicative disorders and consider their similarities and differences. We will outline various research strategies by presenting a description of the general purpose of each strategy, giving an example of its application to problems in the field of communicative disorders, and discussing some advantages and disadvantages of each one.

# Experimental Research

Experimental research is the appropriate method for investigating cause-and-effect relations among variables. With regard to the investigation of cause and effect, Underwood and Shaughnessy (1975, p. 15) state:

> The critical strength of the experiment lies in the fact that when it is properly executed we learn about cause–effect relationships existing in nature. It is as near a foolproof technique for making these discoveries as has yet been devised. Those who have sought other approaches for determining cause–effect relationships in behavior have usually become discouraged.

The ability to make conclusions about cause–effect relationships among variables, then, is a hallmark of experimental research. Shaughnessy, Zechmeister, and Zechmeister (2000, p. 210) define *experiment* as follows:

> A true experiment involves the *manipulation* of one or more factors and *measurement* (observation) of the effects of this manipulation on behavior. The factors the researcher controls or manipulates are called the *independent variables*. The measures that are used to observe the effect (if any) of the independent variables are called *dependent variables*.

There are numerous kinds of research problems in communicative disorders that have been studied through the use of experimental research. Experiments have been carried out to examine the effects of treatment on the behavior of persons with speech or hearing disorders. The experimental question in such cases would be "Does treatment cause a change in behavior?" In addition to such rather long-term treatment experiments, many experiments have examined more short-term cause–effect relationships in laboratories or clinics. For example, the research question "What effect does delayed auditory feedback have on speech behavior?" has been submitted to considerable experimental scrutiny over the years. Psychophysical experiments have been used to examine stimulus–response relationships to determine what effects certain changes in stimulus characteristics may have on people's responses. Psychophysical experiments of this nature have been especially common in audiology and underlie the development of most of the clinical tests used in audiometry. Questions such as "What effect does change in pure-tone frequency have on auditory threshold?" or "What effect does presentation level of phonemically balanced (PB) words have on speech intelligibility?" have been answered by psychophysical experiments.

In reality, there are so many potential uses of the experimental approach that it is difficult to classify all of its possible applications. As Kling and Riggs (1971, p. 3) comment in attempting to define the experimental method in psychology:

> . . . contemporary methodology has become so highly specific that it is difficult to lay down general rules applicable to all experiments. However, a few characteristics of the experimental method may be mentioned.

The four characteristics of experimental research that Kling and Riggs list (1971, p. 3) are (1) experimenters start with some purpose, question, or hypothesis that allows them to know when to observe certain specific aspects of behavior; (2) experimenters can control the occurrence of events and, thus, observe changes in behavior when they are best prepared to make the observations; (3) because of this, experimenters (or others) can repeat these observations under the same conditions; and (4) because experimenters can control the conditions of observation, they can systematically manipulate certain conditions to measure the effects of these manipulations on behavior.

The experimenter, then, can manipulate an independent variable to study its effect on the dependent variable. However, a change in an independent variable may be considered to cause a change in a dependent variable only if other potential independent variables have been controlled or held constant so that they will not be able to have a simultaneous effect on the dependent variable. Other potential independent variables are often called "extraneous" or "nuisance" variables because they may confuse the picture of a cause–effect relationship if left uncontrolled. Therefore, a major purpose of experimentation is to control potential extraneous variables while manipulating the independent variable of interest to the experimenter. We discuss several potential nuisance variables and how they may be controlled in Chapter 5. In this chapter, though, we are concerned mainly with the way in which the independent variable is manipulated as the basis for identifying different types of experiments.

Plutchik (1983) outlines a classification of types of experiments that is based on the structure of the independent variables used. Plutchik's classification is useful as a first step toward understanding experimental research and appreciating the strategies that an experimenter might use to study the effects of manipulating an independent variable on some dependent variable. Not every experiment found in the literature falls into an exact niche in Plutchik's classification, but an understanding of the classification enables consumers of research to grasp the overall concept of how independent variables affect dependent variables and how experimenters go about studying these effects. Plutchik's classification is based on the number of independent variables studied and the number of manipulated values of the independent variable. Although it may seem trivial at first merely to count variables and their values, it eventually becomes apparent that the number of independent variables and the number of values of an independent variable can be critical in enabling an experimenter to determine the nature of the functional relationship of an independent and a dependent variable.

## Bivalent Experiments

The first type of experiment that Plutchik (1983) identifies is the bivalent experiment in which the experimenter studies the effects of two values of one independent variable on the dependent variable. This type of experiment is called bivalent ("two values") because the independent variable is manipulated by the experimenter in a manner that allows for only two values of the independent variable to be presented to the participants. In the case of a continuous independent variable, this means that the experimenter has selected only two of the many values that fall along the continuum of the independent variable to be the manipulated values of the independent variable. For example, an experimenter may wish to manipulate the intensity of tones presented to listeners and selects only two intensities to present to them: a "low" and a "high" intensity. In the case of a categorical independent variable, the experimenter may select two of the many categories of the independent variable that are available. In some cases, the independent variable may be dichotomous and, therefore, classifiable into only two categories. For example, the experimenter may wish to study the effects of binaural versus monaural listening. In any case, regardless of the potential number of values of the independent variable at the experimenter's disposal, only two are employed in the bivalent experiment.

The study by Marvin and Privratsky (1999) of the effects of materials sent home from preschool on children's conversational behavior is an example of a bivalent experiment. In this experiment, preschool children were recorded under two conditions: (A) while traveling home with child-focused material and (B) while traveling home with material that was not child-focused. One result of this bivalent experiment is illustrated in Figure 2.3, which shows the average percent of school-related talk in each of the two conditions. A bar graph is used to display these results because the two conditions (child-focused versus non-child-focused material) represent categorical manipulations of the independent variable rather than manipulations that fall along a continuum of values of the independent variable.

In another example of a bivalent experiment, Tye-Murray, Spencer, Bedia, and Woodworth (1996) examine differences in children's sound production when speaking with cochlear implants turned on versus turned off. Speech samples were elicited from twenty children in two conditions: (A) after several hours with their cochlear implants turned off and (B) after one to four hours with their cochlear implants turned on. The results of the experiment show essentially no differences in speech production between the two conditions. Figure 2.4 illustrates one result of this bivalent experiment for total percent correct vowels in the two conditions. Inspection of Figure 2.4 reveals that the children pro-

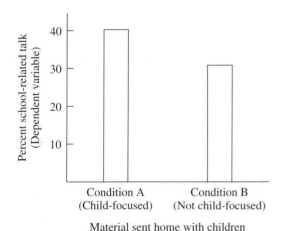

**FIGURE 2.3   Results of a Bivalent Experiment Showing the Effect of Child-Focused Material on School-Related Talk of Preschool Children.**

Drawn from the data of Marvin and Privratsky, 1999.

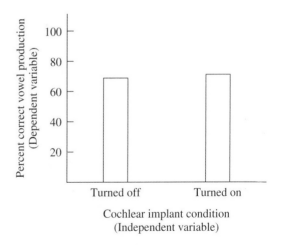

**FIGURE 2.4   Results of a Bivalent Experiment Showing No Effect of Cochlear Implant Condition on Vowel Production.**

Drawn from the data of Tye-Murray, Spencer, Bedia, and Woodworth, 1996.

duced about the same percentage of correct vowel production in both conditions; 71 percent with the cochlear implants turned on versus 70 percent with the cochlear implants turned off. Again, the result of this bivalent experiment is illustrated with a bar graph because the independent variable was manipulated categorically (cochlear implant on versus off) rather than along a continuum of values.

Many experiments examine the effect of the independent variable on more than one dependent variable. In the Marvin and Privratsky (1999) experiment, several dependent variables were compared in the two conditions, including past, present, and future time referents, initiations, references to school and to the materials, as well as school talk. In the Tye-Murray et al. (1996) experiment, several dependent variables were compared in the two conditions, including phonemic features such as place of articulation, vowel height, or consonant voicing. It is actually fairly common to examine the effects of an independent variable on several related dependent variables. The graphs in Figure 2.5 illustrate some results from an experiment by Sapienza and Stathopoulos (1994) on the effect of changing vocal intensity from a comfortable to a loud level on various respiratory and laryngeal variables. The figure demonstrates the effect of increasing intensity from comfortable to loud speech (bivalent independent variable) on six respiratory and laryngeal functions (dependent variables). Each of the six panels in the figure shows a different dependent variable plotted as a function of changing vocal intensity from the comfortable to the loud level. Many of the studies used throughout the rest of this chapter to illustrate various experimental and descriptive research strategies also use more than one dependent variable, but we will generally discuss only the single dependent variable that illustrates the point under consideration in each example.

Other examples of bivalent experiments might include studies of the effect of treatment versus no treatment on the articulation performance of articulation-impaired children, studies of the effect of binaural versus monaural stimulation on speech perception, studies of the effect of fluency reinforcement versus no reinforcement on stuttering, or studies of the effect of delayed versus normal feedback on speech rate. All of these examples represent problems for which bivalent experiments could be valuable in examining the effects of dichotomous independent variables on these dependent variables because the independent variables can be dichotomized to form two values for manipulation.

Some categorical independent variables comprise more than two categories. In that case, an experimenter may select two of them to form a dichotomous independent variable, either because two of the categories are of more interest or because two of the categories seem to be opposed in a dichotomous fashion. For example, we could conceive of binaural versus monaural stimulation as a dichotomous independent variable because stimuli can be presented to either one ear or both. However, we could also conceive of a more general categorical independent variable, mode of auditory stimulation, that includes values such as monaural left, monaural right, true binaural (dichotic), pseudobinaural (diotic), and so on. We could then select various apparent dichotomies from the available categories such as left-ear versus right-ear monaural stimulation, monaural versus binaural, dichotic versus diotic, and so on to form the two values of a bivalent experiment. On the other hand, an experimenter may decide to select more than two categories for manipulation and not do a simple bivalent experiment.

An experimenter may also take a continuous independent variable and use it to form a more or less artificial dichotomy in order to conduct a bivalent experiment. For example, the

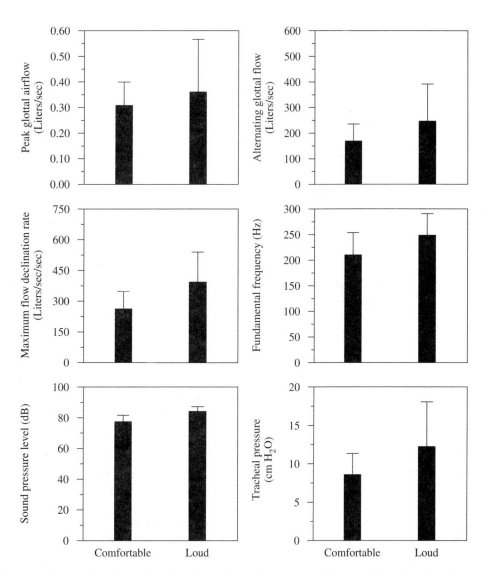

**FIGURE 2.5    Results of a Bivalent Experiment Showing the Effect of Changing Vocal Intensity from a Comfortable to a Loud Level on Six Dependent Variables.**

From "Respiratory and Laryngeal Measures of Children and Women with Bilateral Vocal Fold Nodules," by C. M. Sapienza and E. Stathopoulos, 1994, *Journal of Speech and Hearing Research, 37,* p. 1236. Copyright 1994 by the American Speech-Language-Hearing Association. Reprinted with permission.

experimenter might study the effect of the presence versus the absence of reinforcement on nonfluencies. Amount of reinforcement could be conceptualized as a continuous independent variable that could be artificially dichotomized into values of zero versus a large amount, or "present" versus "absent."

Although bivalent experiments are valuable in examining the effects of categorical independent variables (especially those that reflect true dichotomies), Plutchik (1983) indicates that they are limited in scope and may even lead to erroneous conclusions when the independent variable is continuous. Bivalent experiments are limited in scope because they do not always encompass as much of the potential range of values of the continuous independent variable as may be possible. In other words, presenting only two values of a continuous independent variable may not give as clear a picture of the function relating it to a dependent variable as presenting a larger number of values of the independent variable might. Bivalent experiments can lead to erroneous conclusions when the function being studied is not linear. Discussion of the next type of experiment in Plutchik's classification will help to clarify these two problems.

## Multivalent Experiments

The second type of experiment that Plutchik (1983) identifies is the multivalent experiment in which the experimenter studies the effects of several values of the independent variable on the dependent variable. This type of experiment is called multivalent ("many values") because the independent variable is manipulated in a manner that allows for at least three (and usually more) values of the independent variable to be presented to the participants. When the independent variable is continuous, a multivalent experiment is more appropriate than a bivalent experiment for two reasons.

First, the multivalent experiment gives a broader picture of the relationship between the independent and dependent variables than the bivalent experiment does, because the experimenter samples the range of possible values of the independent variable more completely. If the dependent variable changes linearly as a function of changes in the independent variable (i.e., the graph slopes upward or downward in a straight-line fashion), then the bivalent experiment would show a pattern of results similar to the multivalent experiment. The results of the bivalent experiment, however, would be limited in scope, and the multivalent experiment would broaden the picture of the functional relationship between the independent and dependent variables.

A second and more serious problem occurs when the function takes the form of a curve rather than a straight line on the graph relating changes in the dependent variable to manipulations of the independent variable. At least three values of the independent variable must be used to identify a curvilinear function, because at least three coordinate points on a graph must be used to plot a curve. Because a bivalent experiment examines only two values of the independent variable, its resultant graph cannot reveal the shape of a curvilinear function. A multivalent experiment must be performed to reveal a curvilinear function. We now examine some examples from the research literature to demonstrate the appropriateness of multivalent experiments for studying the effects of a continuous independent variable on a dependent variable.

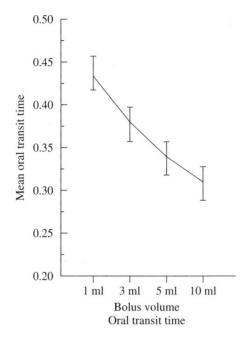

**FIGURE 2.6   Results of a Multivalent Experiment Showing the Effect of Bolus Volume on Oral Transit Time.**

From "Age and Volume Effects on Liquid Swallowing Function in Normal Women," by A. W. Rademaker, B. R. Pauloski, L. A. Colangelo, and J. A. Logemann, 1998, *Journal of Speech, Language, and Hearing Research, 41,* p. 281. Copyright 1998 by the American Speech-Language-Hearing Association. Reprinted with permission.

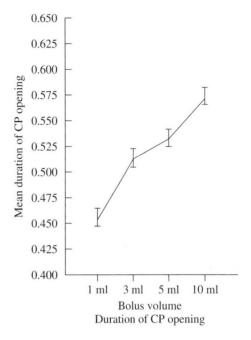

**FIGURE 2.7   Results of a Multivalent Experiment Showing the Effect of Bolus Volume on Duration of Cricopharyngeal Opening.**

From "Age and Volume Effects on Liquid Swallowing Function in Normal Women," by A. W. Rademaker, B. R. Pauloski, L. A. Colangelo, and J. A. Logemann, 1998, *Journal of Speech, Language, and Hearing Research, 41,* p. 282. Copyright 1998 by the American Speech-Language-Hearing Association. Reprinted with permission.

The swallowing research conducted by Rademaker, Pauloski, Colangelo, and Logemann (1998) includes a multivalent experiment concerning the effects of liquid bolus volume on a number of dependent variables. Figure 2.6 shows their results for the effect of bolus volume on oral transit time and Figure 2.7 shows their results for the effect of bolus volume on duration of cricopharyngeal opening. As bolus volume is manipulated across values from 1 to 10 ml, oral transit time is reduced but duration of cricopharyngeal opening increased. Thus, Figure 2.6 shows a negative effect of bolus volume on oral transit time, whereas Figure 2.7 shows a positive effect of bolus volume on duration of cricopharyngeal opening.

Although both of these functions are roughly linear, it is not uncommon to encounter functions in multivalent experiments that are non-linear, as is the case with two of the other dependent variables that Rademaker et al. studied. Figures 2.8 and 2.9 show their results for the effects of bolus volume on duration of velopharyngeal closure and pharyngeal tran-

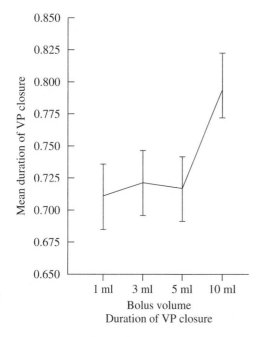

**FIGURE 2.8    Results of a Multivalent Experiment Showing the Effect of Bolus Volume on Duration of Velopharyngeal Closure.**

From "Age and Volume Effects on Liquid Swallowing Function in Normal Women," by A. W. Rademaker, B. R. Pauloski, L. A. Colangelo, and J. A. Logemann, 1998, *Journal of Speech, Language, and Hearing Research, 41,* p. 282. Copyright 1998 by the American Speech-Language-Hearing Association. Reprinted with permission.

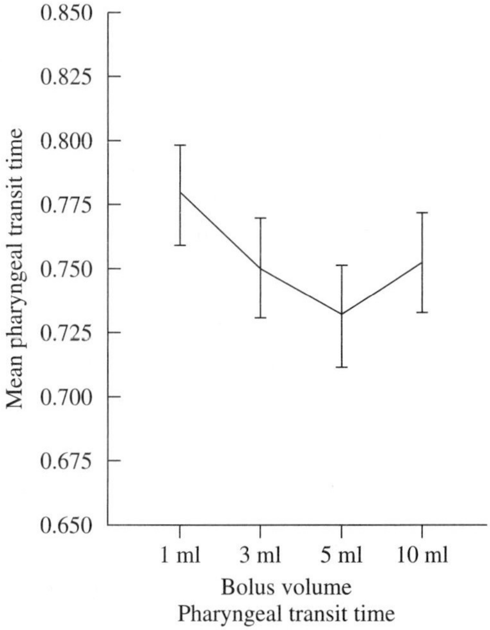

**FIGURE 2.9    Results of a Multivalent Experiment Showing the Effect of Bolus Volume on Pharyngeal Transit Time.**

From "Age and Volume Effects on Liquid Swallowing Function in Normal Women," by A. W. Rademaker, B. R. Pauloski, L. A. Colangelo, and J. A. Logemann, 1998, *Journal of Speech, Language, and Hearing Research, 41,* p. 281. Copyright 1998 by the American Speech-Language-Hearing Association. Reprinted with permission.

sit time. Note that the effect of bolus volume on duration of velopharyngeal closure is a positive non-linear function and the effect of bolus volume on pharyngeal transit time is a negative non-linear function.

The example shown in Figure 2.8 clearly indicates that a multivalent experiment is necessary to discover the shape of this function. If a bivalent experiment is performed using the values of 1 ml and 5 ml for the independent variable, the conclusion will be that there is no effect of bolus volume on duration of velopharyngeal closure. If a bivalent experiment is performed using the values of 1 ml and 10 ml for the independent variable, the function will seem to rise sharply but there will be no indication of the curvilinearity of the effect of bolus volume on duration of velopharyngeal closure. Thus, a bivalent experiment will not be appropriate for examining the effect of bolus volume on duration of velopharyngeal closure, because the dependent variable changes as a non-linear function of the independent variable. The same comments will be true for the effects of bolus volume on pharyngeal transit time, even though this is a negative rather than a positive non-linear function.

In summary, a multivalent experiment is more appropriate than a bivalent experiment in the case of a continuously manipulable independent variable. Consumers of research should be cautious in drawing conclusions from bivalent experiments unless the independent variable can be dichotomized. When the independent variable can be manipulated along some continuum of values for presentation to the participants, bivalent experiments suffer from two disadvantages. First, the picture of the functional relation of the dependent to the independent variable is limited in scope. Plutchik (1983) cautions that this limitation may force readers to overgeneralize the effects of other possible values of the independent variable. Second, when the function is curvilinear, a bivalent experiment could lead to incorrect conclusions because at least three values of the independent variable (and preferably more) are necessary to determine the shape of the curve. These disadvantages can be overcome by conducting a multivalent experiment in which several values of the independent variable are manipulated or presented to the participants. The multivalent experiment, then, is a much more comprehensive type of experiment for studying the functional dependence of one variable on another variable, especially when examining non-linear functions.

## Parametric Experiments

The third type of experiment Plutchik (1983) describes is the *parametric* experiment in which the experimenter studies the simultaneous effects of more than one independent variable on the dependent variable. It is called a parametric experiment because the second independent variable is referred to as the parameter.[2] The main effect of one independent variable on the dependent variable can be examined at the same time that the main effect of another independent variable on the dependent variable is studied. In addition, the *interaction* of the two independent variables in causing changes in the dependent variable can also be determined.

Why are parametric experiments important and what are their advantages over bivalent and multivalent experiments? First, parametric experiments can be more economical and efficient than bivalent or multivalent experiments because they examine effects of more independent variables in a single experiment. However, there is a rationale for parametric experiments that is even more compelling than conservation of time, effort, and money. The communication behaviors that we study in this complex world are multivariate in nature, and it is rare to encounter a single independent variable that can account for the entire causation of change in any dependent variable. In trying to explain the communication between a talker and a hearing-impaired listener, for example, it would be important to consider several variables that would affect the intelligibility of the speaker's message to the listener: acoustical characteristics of the talker's speech, the noise level in the background, distance between talker and listener, reverberation in the room, type and severity of the listener's hearing loss, amplification properties of the listener's hearing aid (e.g., gain, distortion), familiarity of the listener with the speaker and the topic, and so forth.

---

[2]This is a special use of the term *parameter,* a word that has several uses. In mathematics, parameter means a variable quantity that may be arbitrarily held constant or changed to generate a family of curves. In statistics, parameter means a variable population characteristic; this statistical use of the word will be explained in more detail in Chapter 6.

Therefore, it is important in research concerning the nature and treatment of communicative disorders to design experiments that examine the simultaneous effects of many relevant independent variables that may cause changes in the dependent variables of interest.

An example of a parametric experiment is the study by Erber (1971) of the simultaneous effects of distance (independent variable) and syllabic pattern of words (parameter) on visual recognition of speech through lipreading by deaf children (dependent variable). The results of this experiment are illustrated in Figure 2.10. Inspection of the figure reveals that recognition of words by lipreading decreased as the talker moved farther away from the receiver and that this function held true for three types of words differing in syllabic pattern. Also demonstrated was the fact that at any given distance, spondees were easiest to recognize by lipreading, trochees were somewhat more difficult, and monosyllables were most difficult. Therefore, there were two main effects operating on lipreading recognition: distance of talker from receiver and syllabic pattern of words spoken.

In a parametric experiment that was part of a research program for the development of a reliable computer assisted speech recognition assessment (CASRA), Gelfand (1998) examines the simultaneous effects of signal-to-noise ratio and scoring method on speech recognition performance. Figure 2.11 shows his results for normal listeners with signal-to-noise ratio indicated on the abscissa (independent variable) and scoring method (parameter) indicated by different symbols (circles versus triangles) in the field of the graph.

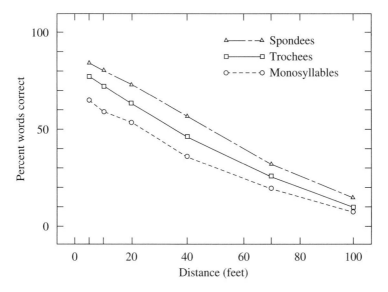

**FIGURE 2.10   Results of a Parametric Experiment Showing the Main Effects of Distance of Talker from Receiver and Syllabic Pattern of Words on Recognition of Words by Lipreading.**

From "Effects of Distance on the Visual Perception of Speech," by N. P. Erber, 1971, *Journal of Speech and Hearing Research, 14,* p. 852. Copyright 1971 by the American Speech-Language-Hearing Association. Reprinted with permission.

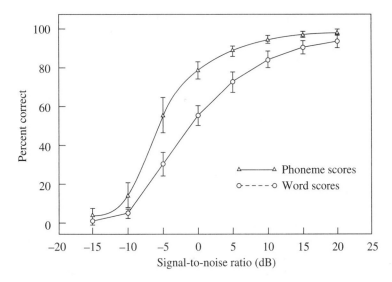

**FIGURE 2.11   Results of a Parametric Experiment Showing the Effect of Signal-to-Noise Ratio and Scoring Method on Speech Recognition Performance.**

From "Optimizing the Reliability of Speech Recognition Scores," by S. A. Gelfand, 1998, *Journal of Speech, Language, and Hearing Research, 41,* p. 1092. Copyright 1998 by the American Speech-Language-Hearing Association. Reprinted with permission.

Inspection of Figure 2.11 reveals the effect of signal-to-noise ratio on speech recognition (both phoneme and word-recognition performance improve as the signal intensity increases relative to the noise) and the effect of the parameter (phoneme recognition performance is better than word-recognition performance across the range of signal-to-noise ratios). It should be noted that, whereas the three functions shown in Figure 2.10 in Erber's parametric experiment are essentially linear, the two functions shown in Figure 2.11 are both curvilinear. In addition, note that the difference between word scoring and phoneme scoring shown in Figure 2.11 is not uniform across all levels of signal-to-noise ratio. This leads us to a discussion of the most important issue in parametric experiments: the main and interaction effects of the independent variables on the dependent variable.

The individual effect of each independent variable and each parameter on the dependent variable is called the *main effect* of that independent variable or that parameter. The simultaneous effect of the independent variable and parameter is called the *interaction* effect. An interaction effect occurs when the independent variable affects the dependent variable in a different manner for different levels of the parameter. In the Erber (1971) experiment, there is no interaction between distance and syllabic pattern. Lipreading is always better at shorter than longer distances, regardless of syllabic pattern. Participants lipread spondees better than trochees and trochees better than monosyllables regardless of distance. The three lines in Figure 2.10 are roughly parallel and, with the exception of a slight difference at 100 feet for trochees and monosyllables, the difference between the three syllabic patterns is uniform across distances. In the Gelfand (1998) experiment, however, there is an interaction between signal-to-noise ratio and scoring method because the difference between phoneme and word scores is not uniform across the levels of signal-to-noise ratio.

An interaction effect can be observed only when two (or more) independent variables are studied *simultaneously* in a parametric experiment. An interaction effect cannot be observed when two separate experiments are conducted, one to study the effect of each independent variable, even if the two independent variables would have interacted in a parametric experiment. The independent variables must be *crossed* with each other in that each level of the independent variable and each level of the parameter occur together in the experiment. Gelfand could have studied the effect of signal-to-noise ratio on speech recognition and then conducted a second experiment on the effect of scoring method, seeing each main effect, but not observing the interaction between the independent variable and the parameter. Similarly, Erber could have studied the effect of distance on lipreading and then conducted a second experiment on the effect of syllabic pattern, observing each main effect but not observing the lack of an interaction between the independent variable and the parameter. There are many different kinds of interaction effects observed in parametric experiments and we will discuss a few common examples here.

An interaction effect occurs when the function, relating changes in the dependent variable to changes in the independent variable, is not the same form for all values of the parameter. For example, the dependent variable may *increase* as a function of increases in the independent variable for one value of the parameter, but the dependent variable might show *no change* as a function of increases in the independent variable for another value of the parameter. In fact, the dependent variable may increase with increases in the independent variable for one value of the parameter and *decrease* with increases in the independent variable for another value of the parameter. Whenever the form of the function relating changes in the dependent variable to changes in the independent variable is different for different values of the parameter, an interaction between the independent variable and the parameter occurs.

An example of a parametric experiment that illustrates an interaction between two independent variables in their effect on the dependent variable is seen in the study by De Filippo, Sims, and Gottermeier (1995) on the effects of linking visual and kinesthetic imagery in lipreading instruction. Figure 2.12 shows their pretraining versus posttraining results for deaf adults who received two different kinds of lipreading training: viewing their own speech versus viewing the trainer's speech. In this graph, the time of testing (pre versus post) is plotted as the independent variable, and type of training is plotted as the parameter. The figure reveals that participants who viewed their own speech made greater pre–post gains than participants who viewed the trainer's speech. The interaction can be visualized best by considering the crossing of the graphic lines. This crossing indicates that the self-viewing participants scored slightly below the trainer-viewing participants before training, but the self-viewing participants scored above the trainer-viewing participants after training. This reversing of the order of groups from before to after training is sometimes referred to as a *reversal-shift* interaction because of the shifting order of the group scores from one condition to another.

Another example of a parametric experiment with an interaction between two independent variables is seen in the study of Camarata, Nelson, and Camarata (1994) on imitative

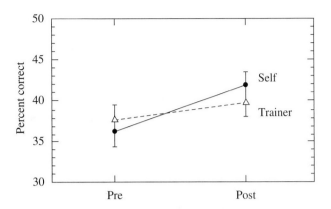

**FIGURE 2.12    Results of a Parametric Experiment Showing the Main and Interaction Effects of Time of Test and Type of Training on Lipreading Performance.**

From "Linking Visual and Kinesthetic Imagery in Lipreading Instruction," by C. L. De Filippo, D. G. Sims, and L. Gottermeier, 1995, *Journal of Speech and Hearing Research, 38,* p. 250. Copyright 1995 by the American Speech-Language-Hearing Association. Reprinted with permission.

versus conversational–interactive language interventions. They found that although imitation treatment was more effective than conversational–interactive treatment in producing elicited productions, the conversational–interactive treatment was more effective in producing spontaneous productions. This interaction of treatment type and production condition is illustrated in Figure 2.13, which shows fewer clinician presentations needed to generate elicited production for the imitation treatment but fewer clinician presentations needed to generate spontaneous production for the conversational treatment.

In the previous two examples of interaction effects in parametric experiments, both independent variables are bivalent; that is, both the independent variable and the parameter have only two levels. Parametric experiments often include a multivalent independent variable and a bivalent parameter. Figure 2.14 shows the results of an experiment by Schiavetti, Whitehead, Whitehead, and Metz (1998) that illustrate this pattern with a study of the effect of fingerspelling task length and communication mode on perceived speech naturalness (dependent variable measured on a 9-point scale, with 1 equal to most natural and 9 equal to most unnatural). Fingerspelling task length (four levels from shortest to longest number of letters to be fingerspelled in the words) is the multivalent independent variable and communication mode (speech-only versus simultaneous communication) is the bivalent parameter. There is a main effect of communication mode: speakers are always perceived as more unnatural sounding when they use simultaneous communication than when they use speech-only. There is a main effect of fingerspelling task length: as length increases, perceived unnaturalness increases. However, this increased unnaturalness holds for only the simultaneous communication condition. There is essentially no increase in the perceived unnaturalness for the speech-only condition (even though the higher level words are longer)

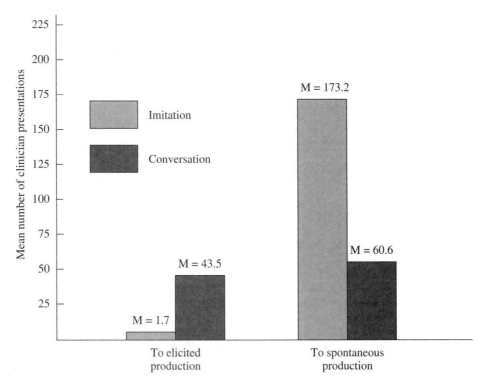

**FIGURE 2.13   Results of a Parametric Experiment Showing the Main and Interaction Effects of Type of Treatment and Mode of Generalization on Number of Clinician Presentations Needed for Client to Produce a Target Utterance.**

From "Comparison of Conversational-Recasting and Imitative Procedures for Training Grammatical Structures in Children with Specific Language Impairment," by S. M. Camarata, K. E. Nelson, and M. N. Camarata, 1994, *Journal of Speech and Hearing Research, 37,* p. 1419. Copyright 1994 by the American Speech-Language-Hearing Association. Reprinted with permission.

but there is a marked increase in perceived unnaturalness for the simultaneous communication mode. The function for the speech-only level of the parameter is essentially flat, but for simultaneous communication perceived speech, unnaturalness increases as a positive function of fingerspelling task length. The interaction effect is illustrated by the two different forms of the functions for the two levels of the parameter.

Interaction effects are also encountered in parametric experiments in which both the independent variable and the parameter are multivalent. Figure 2.15 shows the results of an experiment by Loven and Collins (1988) on the effects of signal-to-noise ratio (shown on the abscissa as the independent variable with six levels) and reverberation time (plotted as the parameter with three levels) on speech recognition. An interaction effect between the two variables is reported by the authors because speech recognition is not greatly affected by reverberation time at signal-to-noise ratios below 0 dB, but above 0 dB, speech recognition at

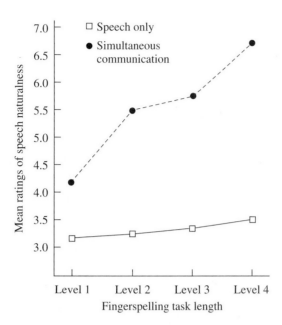

**FIGURE 2.14    Results of a Parametric Experiment Showing the Effect of Fingerspelling Task Length and Communication Mode on Perceived Speech Naturalness.**

From "Effect of Fingerspelling Task on Temporal Characteristics and Perceived Naturalness of Speech in Simultaneous Communication," by N. Schiavetti, R. L. Whitehead, B. H. Whitehead, and D. E. Metz, 1998, *Journal of Speech, Language, and Hearing Research, 41,* p. 13. Copyright 1998 by the American Speech-Language-Hearing Association. Reprinted with permission.

the 1.2 second reverberation time is deteriorated relative to the other two reverberation times. This interaction effect can be seen clearly in the figure: below 0 dB the three lines are close and overlapping; above 0 dB the three lines separate and the line showing the function for 1.2 seconds drops well below the other two lines.

An interaction occurs, then, when the function, relating performance on the dependent variable to manipulation of the independent variable, is not the same for all of the levels of the parameter. As a general rule of thumb, when the lines on a line graph are roughly parallel, there is no interaction between the independent variables, but when lines deviate grossly from parallelism, there is an interaction effect. Parallel lines on the graph indicate that the functions relating the changes in the dependent variable to manipulation of the independent variable are the same for each level of the parameter. Lines that are not parallel indicate that the functions relating the changes in the dependent variable to the manipulations of the independent variable are not the same for each level of the parameter.

Parametric experiments may employ more than one parameter, so it is not uncommon to encounter experiments that examine the simultaneous effects of three, four, or five inde-

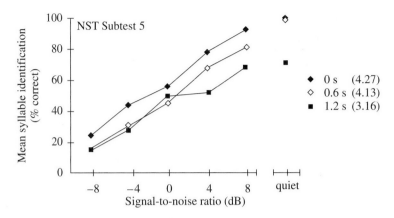

**FIGURE 2.15   Results of a Parametric Experiment Showing the Main and Interaction Effects of Signal-to-Noise Ratio and Reverberation Time on Syllable Identification.**

From "Reverberation, Masking, Filtering, and Level Effects on Speech Recognition Performance," by F. C. Loven and M. J. Collins, 1988, *Journal of Speech and Hearing Research, 31,* p. 689. Copyright 1988 by the American Speech-Language-Hearing Association. Reprinted with permission.

pendent variables. It is much less common to find experiments that examine six or more independent variables, because they may become cumbersome and difficult to analyze and interpret, especially when considering the complexity of the potential interactions among so many independent variables. Figure 2.16 shows the results of a parametric experiment using three independent variables (i.e., one independent variable and two parameters). In this study Helfer (1994) examines the effects of (1) presentation mode (monaural, diotic, binaural), (2) listening condition (noise, reverberation, both), and (3) consonant position (initial, final) on the accuracy of consonant identification. Figure 2.16 shows that the combination of reverberation and noise reduces consonant identification more than either condition alone; that final consonants are affected more than initial consonants by reverberation and the combined condition, although not by noise; and that monaural, diotic, and binaural presentation modes do not differ markedly in this task.

To summarize Plutchik's (1983) classification, experiments may be categorized as bivalent, multivalent, or parametric. Bivalent experiments examine the effects of two values of one independent variable on a dependent variable and are appropriate when the independent variable can be dichotomized. These experiments are inappropriate for studying independent variables that can be continuously manipulated, especially when examining non-linear functions. Multivalent experiments examine the effects of several values of one independent variable on the dependent variable. They are more comprehensive and accurate than bivalent experiments in determining functional relationships when the independent variable is continuous. When there is the possibility of more than one independent variable having an effect on the dependent variable, the parametric experiment is appropriate for simultaneously manipulating an independent variable and a parameter to study their

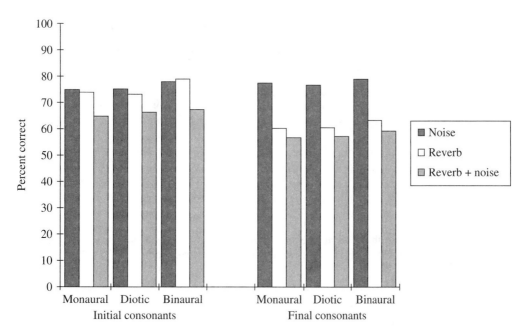

**FIGURE 2.16    Results of a Parametric Experiment Showing the Main Effects of Presentation Mode, Listening Condition, and Consonant Position on Consonant Identification.**

From "Binaural Cues and Consonant Perception in Reverberation and Noise," by K. S. Helfer, 1994, *Journal of Speech and Hearing Research, 37,* p. 433. Copyright 1994 by the American Speech-Language-Hearing Association. Reprinted with permission.

combined effects on the dependent variable. Any of these types of experiments could employ more than one dependent variable.

## Descriptive Research

Descriptive research is used to observe group differences, developmental trends, or relationships among variables that can be measured by the researcher. Research of this type provides an empirical picture of what was observed at one time or of observed changes over a period of time, without manipulation of independent variables by the researcher. Shaughnessy, Zechmeister, and Zechmeister (2000, p. 85) contrast the processes of scientific and nonscientific observation:

> What distinguishes scientific observation from nonscientific observation is the manner in which observations are made. Nonscientists are likely to observe casually and are often unaware of personal and situational biases that may influence their observations.... Scientific observation, on the other hand, is made under precisely defined conditions, in a systematic and objective manner, and with careful record keeping. When observations are made in this manner, valuable information about behavior and its antecedents can be obtained.

In descriptive research, researchers are essentially passive observers who try to be as unobtrusive as possible so that their presence (or the presence of their measuring instruments or techniques) causes minimal alteration of the naturalness of the phenomena under investigation. As Shaughnessy et al. (2000, p. 87) state:

> Observation of behavior in a more or less natural setting, without any attempt by the observer to intervene, is frequently called *naturalistic observation.* An observer using this method of observation acts as a passive recorder of what occurs. The events witnessed are those occurring naturally and have not been manipulated or in any way controlled by the observer.... The major goals of observation in natural settings are to describe behavior as it ordinarily occurs and to investigate the relationship among variables that are present.

As pointed out earlier in this chapter, experimental research involves manipulation of an active independent variable to determine its effect on a dependent variable, whereas descriptive research involves the observation of relations between attribute independent variables and dependent variables. But, according to Shaughnessy et al. (2000, p. 209):

> The distinction between experimental methods and descriptive methods should not be drawn too sharply.

McGuigan (1968, p. 149) also illuminated this point of view concerning the similarity of experimental and observational research when he wrote:

> There are essentially two ways in which an investigator may exercise independent variable control: (1) purposive manipulation of the variable; and (2) selection of the desired values of the variable from a number of values that already exist. When purposive manipulation is used, we say that an experiment is being conducted; but when selection is used, we say that the method of systematic observation is being used.

Descriptive research is an important endeavor in behavioral science and constitutes a large portion of the research found in the communicative disorders literature. There are, however, some common misunderstandings of descriptive research that should be discussed.

First, descriptive research results should not lead to the formulation of cause-and-effect statements. The description of differences between groups or of relationships among variables does not provide sufficient grounds for establishing *causal* relations. The discovery of cause and effect falls within the purview of experimental research, and the experimenter's ability to make things happen under controlled conditions is simply not possible in descriptive research. It is difficult, therefore, to draw conclusions from descriptive research about cause–effect relations because many factors beyond the control of the researcher may confound the results.

Second, statements, such as the foregoing, have led some people to disparage descriptive research as an inferior method. It is not an inferior method. There are situations in which descriptive research is more appropriate and situations in which experimental research is more appropriate. Descriptive research is more appropriate in a situation in which the researcher is interested in behaviors as they occur naturally without the interference of an experimenter. In other situations, when the researcher wishes to manipulate conditions to study cause–effect relations, experimental research is more appropriate.

There are, however, situations in which experimental research is desired, but ethical concerns such as the regard for protection of human participants preclude the use of certain experimental techniques. For example, it would be unethical to conduct an experiment that would produce a conductive hearing loss in humans in order to study the effects of middle ear pathology on auditory perception or academic achievement. Therefore, researchers must rely on descriptive studies of children with and without middle ear pathology. Such descriptive research is not equal to experiments in determining cause–effect relationships, but it must be relied on as the best available compromise because of the ethical concern that forbids experimental studies of the effects of pathology on humans. The problems inherent in such a situation have led to much controversy concerning descriptive research such as investigations of the relations between middle ear pathology and auditory perception (Ventry, 1980). An exchange of letters in the *Journal of Speech and Hearing Disorders* between Ayukawa and Rudmin (1983) and Karsh and Brandes (1983) illustrates the dilemma facing researchers who must substitute a descriptive study for an experiment that is impossible to conduct. A review of problems inherent in the design of descriptive studies of variables such as otitis media and speech disorder is provided by Shriberg, Flipsen, Thielke, Kwiatkowski, Kertoy, Katcher, Nellis, and Block (2000). Casby (2001) applied meta-analysis, a technique described in Chapter 5 for reviewing the results of studies of treatment efficacy, to provide an objective and quantitative evaluation of the research literature on the relationship of otitis media and language development, and he offered an important critique of the descriptive methods used in this body of descriptive research.

Another example concerns research on the etiology of stuttering. It has been hypothesized that various conditions in the child's speaking environment may be responsible for the onset of stuttering. However, it would be unethical to manipulate systematically environmental conditions in an attempt to cause stuttering in children. Therefore, much research concerned with environmental factors related to the onset of stuttering has focused on descriptions of stuttering and nonstuttering children around the time of typical onset.

In summary, when observation of natural phenomena is necessary to solve a particular problem, descriptive research is appropriate. When the researcher wishes to examine cause-and-effect relations by manipulating variables, experimental research is appropriate. There may be situations in which experimental research is desirable but impossible. When descriptive research is substituted for experimental research in such a situation, the ensuing investigation is unable to determine the kind of direct cause-and-effect links that the experiment might have found.

Before discussing the different strategies used in descriptive research, it is worth commenting on the various terms that are used to describe independent and dependent variables in descriptive research. As stated previously, experimental independent variables are active and can be manipulated by the experimenter to examine their effects on dependent variables. The independent variables of descriptive research, however, are attribute variables that cannot be manipulated.

In certain kinds of descriptive research, participants can be *classified* according to certain variables and comparisons can be made between the classifications with regard to some *criterion* variable. The terms *classification variable* and *criterion variable* are analogous, respectively, to the terms *independent variable* and *dependent variable*. For example, persons with aphasia might be compared to persons without aphasia on some measure of linguistic performance. In such a case, the classification variable would be language status (aphasic versus nonaphasic) and linguistic performance would be the criterion variable.

In certain other kinds of descriptive research, participants of one classification are measured on a number of criterion variables to determine the relationships among these variables and the ability to predict one variable from another. In such a case, one of the variables can be designated the *predictor variable* and the other can be designated the *predicted variable.* Again, the terms *predictor variable* and *predicted variable* are analogous to the terms *independent variable* and *dependent variable.* The real difference between the two sets of terms lies in the ability of the researcher to manipulate the independent variable.

It might help consumers of research to differentiate experimental and descriptive research if they would examine the manipulability of the variables used in a research study. If the independent variable can be manipulated to determine its effect on the dependent variable, then the study is experimental. If the participants are classified according to some nonmanipulable dimension and compared on some criterion, or if relationships are examined between nonmanipulable predict*or* and predict*ed* variables, then the research is descriptive. It should be pointed out to consumers that many authors use the terms independent and dependent variables for *both* experimental and descriptive research, so an analysis of the manipulability of variables is often necessary to determine whether a given research study is experimental or descriptive. As will be seen later, much research in communicative disorders is a *combination* of experimental and descriptive research.

Tabachnick and Fidell (2001, pp. 2–3) have nicely summarized the issues covered in this discussion of the relationship between experimental and descriptive research as follows:

> A critical distinction between experimental and nonexperimental research is whether the researcher manipulates the levels of the IVs. In an experiment, the researcher has control over the levels (or conditions) of at least one IV to which a subject is exposed. Further, the experimenter randomly assigns subjects to levels of the IV, and controls all other influential factors by holding them constant, counterbalancing, or randomizing their influence.... In nonexperimental (correlational or survey) research, the levels of the IV(s) are not manipulated by the researcher. The researcher can define the IV, but has no control over the assignment of subjects to levels of it. In this type of research the distinction between IVs and DVs is usually arbitrary and many researchers prefer to call IVs predictors and DVs criterion variables.

Many different strategies for descriptive research can be found in the literature and those outlined as follows illustrate some of the common approaches found in communicative disorders. Five different strategies of descriptive research will be considered: (1) *comparative,* (2) *developmental,* (3) *correlational,* (4) *survey,* and (5) *retrospective* research.

## Comparative Research

Comparative research is a strategy used to measure the behavior of two or more types of participants at one point in time in order to draw conclusions about the similarities or differences between them. For example, Rescorla and Ratner (1996) studied vocalization patterns, phonetic profiles, and syllable formation patterns of thirty toddlers with specific

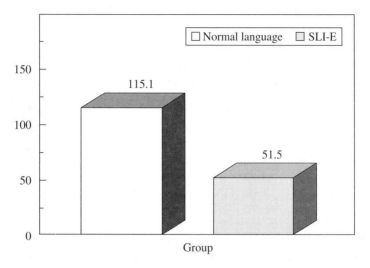

**FIGURE 2.17    Results of a Bivalent Comparison of the Number of Vocalizations of Children with Normal Language and Children with Specific Expressive Language Impairment (SLI-E).**

From "Phonetic Profiles of Toddlers with Specific Language Impairment (SLI-E)," by L. Rescorla and N. B. Ratner, 1996, *Journal of Speech and Hearing Research, 39,* p. 157. Copyright 1996 by the American Speech-Language-Hearing Association. Reprinted with permission.

expressive language impairment (SLI-E) versus thirty typically developing toddlers. The average number of vocalizations in each ten-minute mother–child interaction for the two groups of participants is illustrated in Figure 2.17. Inspection of Figure 2.17 shows that the SLI-E toddlers vocalized at less than half the rate of the typically developing toddlers. The figure also reveals that comparative research that examines dichotomous groups is analogous to a bivalent experiment, but involves the selection of participants from dichotomous classifications rather than manipulation of a dichotomous independent variable. In other words, the independent variable is an attribute rather than an active variable.

As pointed out earlier in the section on experimental research, many experiments have more than one dependent variable. The same is true for many descriptive studies. Figure 2.18 shows more results from the same example used to illustrate this point earlier. In this study by Sapienza and Stathopoulos (1994), a comparison was made of the performance of children versus adults on a number of respiratory and laryngeal functions; these bivalent descriptive comparisons are illustrated in the bar graphs of Figure 2.18. It is interesting to note the similarity of this figure to the example in Figure 2.5. Both figures show multiple dependent variables influenced by a single bivalent independent variable. In the experimental case the independent variable is an active variable manipulated by the experimenter by instructing speakers to talk at different loudness levels. In the descriptive case the independent variable is an attribute variable that cannot be manipulated by the experimenter: the speakers' ages. This example is an excellent illustration from the same study of two different types of independent variables that may influence the same dependent variables. The active variable may

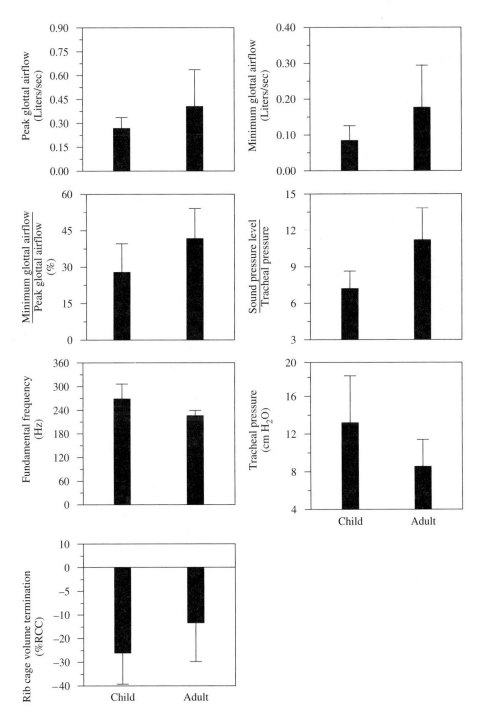

**FIGURE 2.18    Results of a Bivalent Comparison of Children versus Adults on Seven Respiratory and Laryngeal Variables.**

From "Respiratory and Laryngeal Measures of Children and Women with Bilateral Vocal Fold Nodules," by C. M. Sapienza and E. Stathopoulos, 1994, *Journal of Speech and Hearing Research, 37,* p. 1235. Copyright 1994 by the American Speech-Language-Hearing Association. Reprinted with permission.

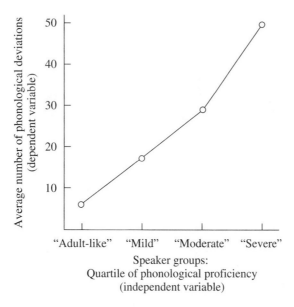

**FIGURE 2.19    Results of a Multivalent Comparison
of Number of Phonological Deviations Produced
by Children at Four Different Levels of Phonological
Proficiency.**

Drawn from the data of Gordon-Brannan and Hodson, 2000.

be studied experimentally, but the attribute variable may be observed only in a descriptive study.

Comparative research studies may also be found that are analogous to multivalent and parametric experiments. A comparative research study analogous to a multivalent experiment would involve comparison of three or more groups of participants who could be classified along some continuum. For example, Gordon-Brannan and Hodson (2000) compared several intelligibility/severity measurements for forty-eight prekindergarten children who were ranked into four groups of varying levels of phonological proficiency based on the intelligibility of their continuous speech. The children were divided into four quartile groups of twelve children each that included I. children with "adult-like" speech (91–100 percent intelligible), II. children with mild involvement (83–90 percent intelligible), III. children with moderate involvement (68–81 percent), and IV. children with severe involvement (16–63 percent intelligible).

To illustrate the analogy between this comparative study and a multivalent experiment, their data on the average number of phonological deviations of the four groups are shown in Figure 2.19. The similarity between Figure 2.19 and Figure 2.7 illustrates the analogy between a multivalent comparison and a multivalent experiment. The graph relating the criterion variable to the classification variable can be evaluated in much the same manner as the graph relating the dependent variable to the independent variable in experimental research.

The major difference between the multivalent comparison and the multivalent experiment concerns the ability to manipulate the independent variable in the experiment versus the need to select already existing members of the classifications in the descriptive comparison.

A comparative study that is analogous to a parametric experiment involves comparisons of groups that differ simultaneously with respect to two or more classification variables. The study by Caselli, Vicari, Longobardi, Lami, Pizzoli, and Stella (1998) of gesture and word development in children with Down syndrome provides an excellent illustration. Children with Down syndrome and normally developing children are classified into five levels of word comprehension ability based on the Italian MacArthur parental questionnaire. Figure 2.20 shows their results for gesture production of children at the five different levels of word comprehension (independent variable) with group classification (normally developing children, ND, versus children with Down syndrome, DS) indicated as the parameter in the field of the graph. Inspection of Figure 2.20 reveals that gesture production increased as a function of word comprehension level, that normally developing and Down syndrome children in the two lowest word comprehension groups used about the same number of gestures, and that children with Down syndrome used more gestures than normally developing children as word comprehension increased beyond the second level. In other words, there is an interaction between word comprehension level and group classification in the gesture use of these children. It is interesting to compare these results to the results of the parametric experiments illustrated in Figures 2.14 and 2.15 to see the analogy between parametric experiments and parametric comparative research. The same concepts of main and interaction effects apply to both research strategies. The difference between them is that the independent variable and parameter in the parametric experiment are manipulable active variables, whereas the independent variable and parameter are nonmanipulable attribute variables in the descriptive research.

Another good example of a parametric comparative study can be seen in the article by Geers and Moog (1992), which uses degree of hearing impairment as the independent variable and incorporates type of communication mode used in their educational program (oral versus total communication [TC]) as the parameter. Table 2.1 illustrates the composition of the groups of children arranged by pure tone average as an index of hearing-impairment severity and by communication mode indexed as oral, TC with hearing parents, or TC with deaf parents. Figure 2.21 shows the results for lipreading performance and indicates a main effect of hearing impairment, communication mode, and an interaction of the two variables. The main effects demonstrate that children with less severe hearing impairment have better lipreading scores than children with more severe hearing impairment, and children with oral communication mode have better lipreading than children with TC. The interaction effect is seen clearly as a wider gap between oral and TC students at the higher levels of hearing-impairment severity. In fact, the oral students showed no diminution in lipreading performance as a function of level of hearing impairment, so the interaction between educational program and hearing impairment severity indicates that the decrease in lipreading performance was evident for only the two groups of TC children.

Another good example of a parametric comparative study can be seen in the results from Riddel, McCauley, Mulligan, and Tandan (1995) shown in Figure 2.22 on the intelligibility of speakers with amyotrophic lateral sclerosis (ALS). The two attribute independent variables are dysarthria and gender, and the figure shows no difference in phonetic

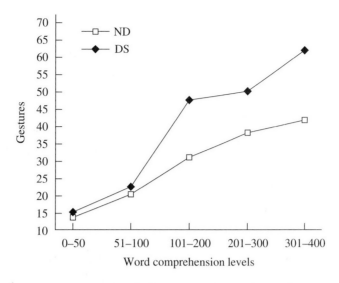

**FIGURE 2.20    Results of a Parametric Comparison of Gesture Production by Children with Normal Development (ND) and Down Syndrome (DS) at Five Levels of Word Comprehension.**

From "Gesture and Words in Early Development of Children with Down Syndrome," by M. C. Caselli, S. Vicari, E. Longobardi, L. Lami, C. Pizzoli, & G. Stella, 1998, *Journal of Speech, Language, and Hearing Research, 41,* p. 1131. Copyright 1998 by the American Speech-Language-Hearing Association. Reprinted with permission.

**TABLE 2.1    Number and Percentage of Subjects in Each Communication Mode and Hearing-Impairment Group**

| | Hearing-Impairment Group[a] | | | | | | | |
| | *80–90 dB* | | *91–100 dB* | | *101–110 dB* | | *>110 dB* | |
| **Communication Mode Group** | *n* | *%* | *n* | *%* | *n* | *%* | *n* | *%* |
|---|---|---|---|---|---|---|---|---|
| ORAL (*n* = 100) | 10 | 10 | 43 | 43 | 37 | 37 | 10 | 10 |
| TC-HP (*n* = 63) | 8 | 13 | 14 | 22 | 25 | 40 | 16 | 25 |
| TC-DP (*n* = 64) | 13 | 20 | 13 | 20 | 25 | 40 | 13 | 20 |

From "Speech Perception and Production Skills of Students with Impaired Hearing from Oral and Total Communication Education Settings," by A. E. Geers and J. S. Moog, 1992, *Journal of Speech and Hearing Research, 35,* p. 1388. Copyright 1992 by the American Speech-Language-Hearing Association. Reprinted with permission.

*Note:* ORAL = oral education program; TC-HP = total communication program—hearing parents; TC-DP = Total communication program—deaf parents.

[a]In dB HL (ANSI, 1969).

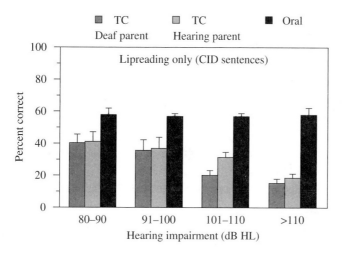

**FIGURE 2.21  Results of a Parametric Comparison Showing Differences in Lipreading Scores for Children Classified According to Severity of Hearing Impairment and Communication Mode.**

From "Speech Perception and Production Skills of Students with Impaired Hearing from Oral and Total Communication Education Settings," by A. E. Geers and J. S. Moog, 1992, *Journal of Speech and Hearing Research, 35,* p. 1390. Copyright 1992 by the American Speech-Language-Hearing Association. Reprinted with permission.

contrast errors between male and female speakers without dysarthria but a large difference between males and females with dysarthria. This example illustrates another interaction effect, where gender and clinical classification have interacted: the pattern of errors for males versus females is different in the two different clinical classification groups.

Comparative research, then, involves the examination of differences and similarities among existing variables or participant classifications that are of interest to the researcher. This descriptive research strategy has the advantage of allowing researchers to study variables that cannot be manipulated experimentally. Sometimes these experiments are called "experiments of nature" because participants belong to the classifications as a result of the vagaries of nature. These experiments may also be referred to as "natural-group" research studies for the same reason.

There are two disadvantages of comparative research that should be mentioned. First, it is difficult to draw conclusions about the causes of criterion-variable differences that may be found. This difficulty in attributing causation is due to the possibility that other variables may concurrently operate with the classification variable to influence the criterion variable. The lack of experimental control in the descriptive approach makes it difficult to preclude such a possibility.

Second, Young (1976, 1993, 1994) criticizes the use of group-difference data for generating knowledge about the performance of different groups of subjects on various criterion measures. He suggests correlational strategies and analysis of variation accounted

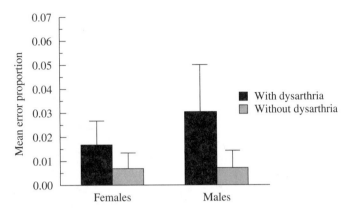

**FIGURE 2.22    Results of a Parametric Comparison Showing Differences in Phonetic Contrast Error Proportions for Participants Classified According to Gender and Dysarthria.**

From "Intelligibility and Phonetic Contrast Errors in Highly Intelligible Speakers with Amyotrophic Lateral Sclerosis," by J. Riddel, R. J. McCauley, M. Mulligan, and R. Tandan, 1995, *Journal of Speech and Hearing Research, 38,* p. 310. Copyright 1995 by the American Speech-Language-Hearing Association. Reprinted with permission.

for in dependent variables and group compositions as better strategies for assessing performance of participants who differ in classification variables and has emphasized the difficulties of using descriptive comparisons for the development of conclusions about cause-and-effect relationships.[3]

## Developmental Research

Developmental research strategies measure changes in behavior or characteristics of people over time to examine the influence of aging. Developmental research tends to concentrate on very young and very old populations because it is concerned with the emergence of behavior as children grow and the changes in performance that accompany the normal aging processes in the geriatric population. The independent variable in developmental research is maturation (e.g., physical, cognitive, and emotional growth and experience) and is usually indicated by general measurements of chronological or mental age or by some index of specific maturation, such as mean length of utterance as an index of language age. Developmental research has focused on such topics as physiological development of speech motor control in young children (Green, Moore, Higashikawa, & Steeve, 2000), changes in hearing as adults progress through old age (Wiley, Cruikshanks, Nondahl, Tweed, Klein, & Klein, 1998), and development of abstract entities in the language of

[3]Young uses the term *retrospective* to describe what we call comparative research, and our use of the term *retrospective* later in this chapter has a more restricted meaning than the one Young implied.

pre-adolescents, adolescents, and young adults (Nippold, Hegel, Sohlberg, & Schwarz, 1999). Three different developmental plans of observation may be encountered in the literature: *cross-sectional, longitudinal, and semilongitudinal.*

A cross-sectional plan of observation involves selection of participants from various age groups and comparison of differences among the average behaviors or characteristics of the different groups. The study of swallowing function in normal women by Rademaker et al. (1998) referred to earlier in this chapter as a multivalent experiment also has a cross-sectional developmental component to it. In addition to studying the effect of bolus size on dependent variables such as oral transit time (multivalent experiment), these researchers are also interested in the influence of the aging process on these same dependent variables (developmental research). They use a cross-sectional plan of observation to examine the influence of aging by selecting women participants for the study from four different age ranges: 20–39, 40–59, 60–79, and 80–89 years of age. Figure 2.23 shows a graph from their study illustrating changes in oropharyngeal swallow efficiency as a function of age.

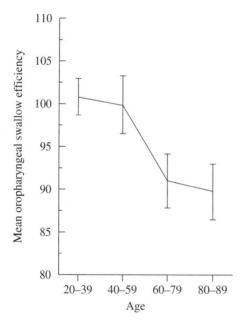

**FIGURE 2.23  Results of a Cross-Sectional Developmental Study of Oropharyngeal Swallow Efficiency.**

From "Age and Volume Effects on Liquid Swallowing Function in Normal Women," by A. W. Rademaker, B. R. Pauloski, L. A. Colangelo, and J. A. Logemann, 1998, *Journal of Speech, Language, and Hearing Research, 41*, p. 278. Copyright 1998 by the American Speech-Language-Hearing Association. Reprinted with permission.

Average oropharyngeal swallow efficiency decreased across the four age groups and these differences between age groups may be interpreted as evidence of the influence of the aging process on swallowing. Note that the function shown in Figure 2.23 is similar to the functions shown in Figures 2.6 and 2.7 illustrating the experimental data from the same study. The difference is that the independent variable shown in Figures 2.6 and 2.7 is a manipulable, active variable (bolus volume), whereas the independent variable shown in Figure 2.23 is age used as an index of maturation.

The cross-sectional developmental study by Rademaker et al. (1998) could be considered multivalent, because the independent variable (maturation, as indexed by chronological age) varies across four levels. Figures 2.24 and 2.25 show two graphs from studies by Wohlert and Smith (1998) and Smith and Goffman (1998) that illustrate bivalent and multivalent cross-sectional developmental studies. Figure 2.24 shows results from a bivalent study of strength of perioral musculature in young adults (20–35 years) versus older (76–83 years) adults. The three bars for each group reflect pressure of bilabial compression, and inward pressure on the right and left sides of the mouth. The graph indicates that younger participants demonstrate greater perioral musculature strength than older participants do. Age, as an index of the independent variable of maturation, then, is dichotomized into "young" and "old" in this bivalent study.

Figure 2.25 shows the results of a study of the development of stability and patterning of speech movement sequences in four- and seven-year-old children and young adults. Absolute values of peak velocities for opening and closing lip movements for syllables initiated and closed with voiced and voiceless plosives are plotted for four- and seven-year-old children and young adults. Adults showed higher peak velocity for all four movements than did the two groups of younger children, but all three groups showed the same pattern of higher velocities for voiced than voiceless consonants and for closing than opening movements. Age as an index of the independent variable of maturation, then, was sampled across three increasing levels in this multivalent study.

A weakness of cross-sectional research is that observations are made of differences *between* participants of different ages in order to generalize about developmental changes that would occur *within* participants as they mature. Direct observation of how participants actually develop as they age and mature are made with a *longitudinal* plan of observation that involves following participants as they mature or age and observing changes in their behavior. Longitudinal studies have the advantage of directly showing how participants mature in their behavior while they are aging.

A good example of longitudinal research can be found in the study by Shriberg, Gruber, and Kwiatkowski (1994) that followed ten children with developmental phonological disorders for seven years. Figure 2.26 shows the averaged performance of the children at twelve age points (spaced about a half-year apart when the children were younger and about one year apart when the children were older) on five dependent variables that are observed over the seven-year span of the study. The figure depicts the developmental progress of the children's performance on these variables as they actually age.

Despite their advantage of direct observation of actual development, longitudinal studies have the disadvantages of being expensive, time-consuming, and more subject to attrition than cross-sectional studies. Longitudinal studies may take years for data collection, resulting in high costs of data collection and loss of participants or researchers from

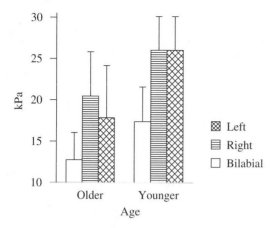

**FIGURE 2.24   Results of a Bivalent Cross-Sectional Developmental Study of Perioral Musculature Strength.**

From "Spatiotemporal Stability of Lip Movements in Older Adult Speakers," by A. B. Wohlert and A. Smith, 1998, *Journal of Speech, Language, and Hearing Research, 41,* p. 47. Copyright 1998 by the American Speech-Language-Hearing Association. Reprinted with permission.

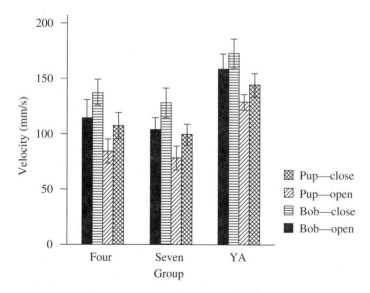

**FIGURE 2.25   Results of a Multivalent Cross-Sectional Developmental Study of Peak Velocity of Lip Movements.**

From "Stability and Patterning of Speech Movement Sequences in Children and Adults," by A. Smith and L. Goffman, 1998, *Journal of Speech, Language, and Hearing Research, 41,* p. 24. Copyright 1998 by the American Speech-Language-Hearing Association. Reprinted with permission.

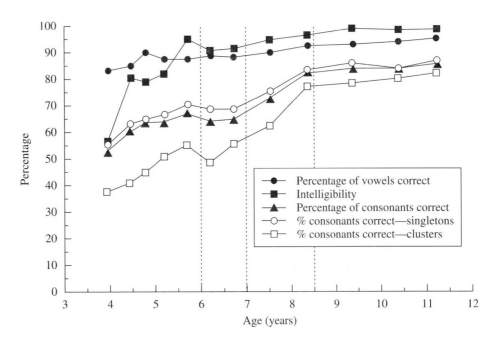

**FIGURE 2.26   Results of a Longitudinal Developmental Study Showing Five Dependent Variables Plotted as a Function of Age.**

From "Developmental Phonological Disorders III: Long-Term Speech-Sound Normalization," by L. D. Shriberg, F. A. Gruber, and J. Kwiatkowski, 1994, *Journal of Speech and Hearing Research, 37,* p. 1164. Copyright 1994 by the American Speech-Language-Hearing Association. Reprinted with permission.

the study. As a result of their expense, attrition, and time consumption, longitudinal studies often include only small numbers of participants, somewhat limiting generalization relative to cross-sectional studies. Although longitudinal studies are more desirable because they directly observe development, cross-sectional studies are often substituted for longitudinal plans because they are more cost-effective and practical.

A logical compromise to minimize the weaknesses and maximize the strengths of cross-sectional and longitudinal studies is a *semilongitudinal* plan of observation, also called *cohort-sequential* research (Bordens & Abbott, 2002, p. 308). This plan involves dividing the total age span to be studied into several overlapping age spans, selecting participants whose ages are at the lower edge of each new age span and following them until they reach the upper age of the span. Wilder and Baken (1974), for example, were interested in observing respiratory parameters underlying infant crying behavior with a technique called impedance pneumography to record thoracic and abdominal movements. Ten infants entered the study at ages ranging from 2 to 161 days, and each was observed over a period of four months. Rather than making one observation of infants of different ages or waiting for infants to be born and then following them for a year, a semilongitudinal approach was adopted that allowed Wilder and Baken to make observations between *and* within participants over a period of time in a more efficient manner. Figure 2.27 shows the time schedule for observation of the ten infants used by Wilder and Baken in their semilongitudinal developmental study and demonstrates that each infant was observed four times over the total time span from 2 to 255 days of age at time intervals that averaged 28 days. Bordens and Abbott (2002, pp. 303–309) provide a detailed comparison of the relative advantages and disadvantages of cross-sectional, longitudinal, and cohort-sequential approaches to developmental research.

In addition, it is not uncommon to see longitudinal and cross-sectional data put together for comparison to capitalize on the practical advantages of the cross-sectional plan and the scientific advantages of the longitudinal plan. Figure 2.28 shows such a comparison from the Shriberg et al. (1994) article of their longitudinal data for speech-delayed children with cross-sectional data for speech-normal developing age-mates on early-8, middle-8, and late-8 sounds. The six trends plotted in the graph illustrate the developmental progress on the three classes of sounds for the two groups of participants.

As indicated in the previous comparison of longitudinal and cross-sectional data, developmental studies may be concerned with the comparison of developmental trends of normally developing and late developing populations on dependent variables that may be late in developing as a result of various disorders and conditions. Therefore, it is common for a developmental strategy to be combined with a comparative strategy in examining the developmental delay of one group of participants compared to normative data for their peers. The longitudinal study of Ellis Weismer, Murray-Branch, and Miller (1994) illustrates this combined strategy in the study of language development in late talkers versus typically developing talkers. Children were observed at three-month intervals for a year

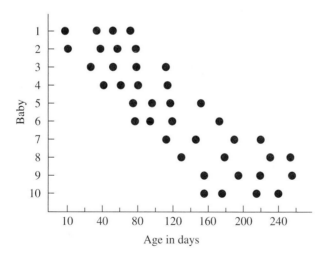

**FIGURE 2.27 Time Scheduling of Four Recordings of Cry Samples for Each of Ten Infants in a Semilongitudinal Developmental Study.**

From "Respiratory Patterns in Infant Cry," by C. N. Wilder and R. J. Baken, 1974, *Human Communication, 3,* p. 31.

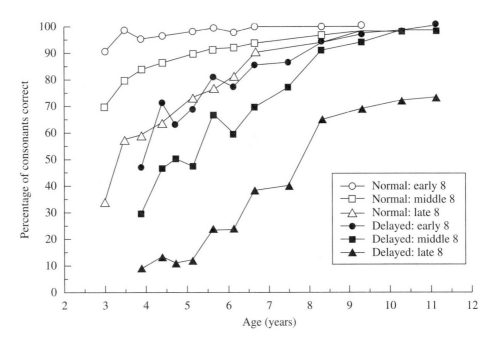

**FIGURE 2.28    Longitudinal Data on Delayed Development (Filled Symbols) Compared with Cross-Sectional Data on Normal Development (Open Symbols) for Early, Middle, and Late Groups of Speech Sounds.**

From "Developmental Phonological Disorders III: Long-Term Speech-Sound Normalization," by L. D. Shriberg, F. A. Gruber, and J. Kwiatkowski, 1994, *Journal of Speech and Hearing Research, 37,* p. 1167. Copyright 1994 by the American Speech-Language-Hearing Association. Reprinted with permission.

starting at about thirteen to fourteen months of age. Figure 2.29 shows the data on the number of different words produced at each observational visit over the course of the study for the late and typically developing talkers. This figure provides a ready picture of the developmental trends of the two subject groups. In this sense, including the clinical classification variable into the study adds this attribute to the independent variable as a parameter, making the research a combined developmental-comparative study with two nonmanipulable independent variables.

## Correlational Research

A correlational research strategy is used to study the relationships among two or more variables by examining the degree to which changes in one variable correspond with or can be predicted from variations in another. Details of the statistical procedure called *correlation and regression analysis* will be discussed in Chapter 6, but the logical framework of correlational research should be considered as a descriptive research strategy. Correlational research may range from a simple problem in which only two variables are studied to complex research in which the interrelation of a large number of variables is considered.

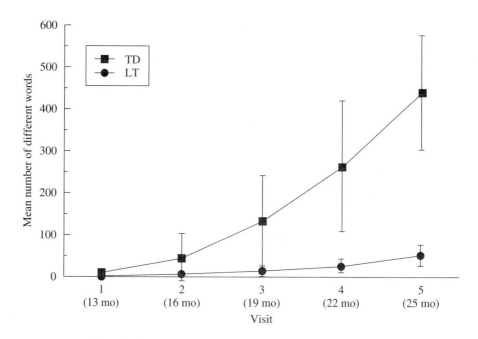

**FIGURE 2.29  Results of a Longitudinal Developmental Study Comparing Vocabulary Size of a Group of Typically Developing (TD) Children to a Group of Late Talkers (LT) at Various Ages.**

From "A Prospective Longitudinal Study of Language Development in Late Talkers," by S. Ellis Weismer, J. Murray-Branch, and J. F. Miller, 1994, *Journal of Speech and Hearing Research, 37,* p. 858. Copyright 1994 by the American Speech-Language-Hearing Association. Reprinted with permission.

There are two basic questions asked in correlational research. First, how closely related are the variables? This question is answered by examining the performance of a group of participants on the variables. The appropriate correlation coefficient is computed to indicate the strength of the relationship with regard to how much variation the two share. The correlation also indicates the direction of the relationship. A positive correlation indicates that increases in one variable are associated with increases in the other, whereas a negative correlation indicates that increases in one variable are associated with decreases in the other. A zero correlation indicates that the two variables are unrelated.

The concept of the correlation between variables can also be depicted visually on a graph called the *scatterplot* or *scattergram,* which will be discussed in more detail in Chapters 6 and 9. The scattergram will be mentioned here only to illustrate correlational research. Briefly, the scattergram shows the pairs of scores on the two variables that are attained by each participant. The graph is a plot of the functional relationship between the two variables and is similar to the functions plotted for the data of experimental, comparative, and developmental research.

The second question that can be asked in correlational research is how well performance on one variable can be predicted from knowledge of performance on the other for a typical participant. This question is answered by completing a regression analysis that develops an equation for predicting the expected score (with a margin of error for the prediction) on one variable from knowledge of a participant's score on the other variable.

In the regression problem, one variable (or set of variables) is designated as the predictor and another variable (or set of variables) is designated as the predicted variable. As mentioned previously, some researchers designate the predictor and predicted variables as independent and dependent variables, respectively. The terms *predictor* and *predicted variables* may provide a more accurate description of the nature of the variables studied in correlational research than do the terms *independent* and *dependent variables*. In correlational research, an independent variable is not manipulated to examine its effect on a dependent variable. Rather, two variables are measured and then one is used to try to predict the other one. Consumers should be aware, however, that they may encounter the terms *independent* and *dependent variables* used interchangeably with the terms *predictor* and *predicted variables* in correlational studies.

An example of such a prediction problem is found in the task of the college admissions office in predicting how well an applicant should do in college, given the applicant's high school background and performance on standardized tests. Variables such as high school grade-point average, college board aptitude and achievement test scores, and interview ratings are designated as predictor variables, and college grade-point average is designated as the predicted variable. The admissions office has correlated the predictor and predicted variables of college students from previous years and developed a regression equation for predicting college grade-point average from high school grade-point average, college board scores, and interview rating. This equation can then be applied to a new applicant's record to predict the expected college grade-point average to help in deciding whether to admit the applicant.

An example of an investigation of the correlation between two variables can be seen in part of the study by Turner and Weismer (1993) concerning speaking rate in the dysarthria associated with amyotrophic lateral sclerosis (ALS). This study includes four research questions, one of which deals with the relationship between physical and perceptual measures of speech rate in persons with ALS and with normal speech. The authors were concerned with this relationship because of previous suggestions that physical measures of speech rate might not predict perceptual measures of speech rate in some instances of dysarthria. Figure 2.30 shows the scatterplots, correlation coefficients, and regression equations for the two variables of speaking rate (in words per minute) and magnitude estimation of perceived speaking rate for twenty-seven normal speakers and twenty-seven speakers with dysarthria. Correlations for both speaker groups were strong and positive, and the slightly different regression equations show that perceived speaking rate increased slightly faster with increases in physical speaking rate for the dysarthrics than for the normal speakers.

Carhart and Porter (1971) provide an example of multiple-regression analysis in their study of the predictive relation between pure-tone thresholds and speech reception threshold (SRT) with six groups of patients classified according to audiometric configuration. A separate regression analysis was performed for each group: patients with flat, gradual, marked high-tone, rising, trough-shaped, and atypical pure-tone configurations. Predictor variables were pure-tone thresholds at 250, 500, 1,000, 2,000, and 4,000 Hz; the predicted variable was SRT measured with spondees. Pure-tone threshold at 1,000 Hz emerged as the most

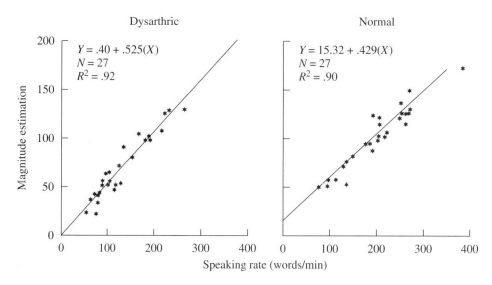

**FIGURE 2.30** **Results of a Correlational Study of Speaking Rate in Words per Minute and Magnitude Estimation of Perceived Speaking Rate of Normal and Dysarthric Speakers.**

From "Characteristics of Speaking Rate in the Dysarthria Associated with Amyotrophic Lateral Sclerosis," by G. S. Turner and G. Weismer, 1993, *Journal of Speech and Hearing Research, 36,* p. 1141. Copyright 1994 by the American Speech-Language-Hearing Association. Reprinted with permission.

important predictor variable for all groups except those patients with marked high-tone loss; for them, 500 Hz was the best single predictor of SRT. Combinations of frequencies in the multiple prediction equations were also studied, and a noticeable, although not dramatic, improvement in prediction of SRT was achieved by adding a second frequency to the equation; adding a third frequency did not significantly improve the prediction. Also, the second frequency that most improved the prediction differed for various categories of audiometric configuration. The authors summarized the best combinations of predictor variables for each audiometric configuration and suggest an optimal combination for use if separation of patients by audiometric configurations could not be accomplished.

Monsen (1978) provides another excellent example of a multiple correlation study with his research on the relationship between physical characteristics of deaf children's speech (predictor variables) and their speech intelligibility (predicted variable). His multiple-regression analysis reveals that the voice onset time differences between /t/ and /d/, the second format difference between /i/ and /ɔ/, and a liquid/nasal contrast measure are the three best predictors of the intelligibility of the deaf children's speech. A number of complex extensions of correlational research strategies are discussed in more detail in Monge and Cappella (1980) and Pedhazur (1999).

One advantage of correlational research has already been pointed out in referring to Young's (1976, 1993, 1994) criticism of comparative research. Correlational research can be used to estimate the amount of variation in a criterion measure that can be accounted for on the basis of knowledge of group classification rather than simply looking at average differences in a criterion measure between two groups of participants. Correlational research can be a powerful tool for learning what aspects of human behavior share common properties. If a strong relationship exists between two variables, then a researcher can predict one variable from knowledge of the value of the other. But there are also disadvantages. Correlation does not imply causation, and many people have seemed to miss this fact in applying cause-and-effect statements to correlational data. In addition, correlational studies suffer from problems in the interpretation of the meaning of correlation coefficients. Two variables may be significantly correlated, but this may occur because both variables are correlated with a third variable that may be unknown to the researcher. Knowledge of the third variable may be crucial to understanding the true nature of the correlation between the original two variables. For these and other more technical reasons, it may be difficult to assess the theoretical or practical implications of a correlation. Sometimes correlational studies use a "shotgun" approach in an attempt to intercorrelate many variables, and a large number of significant but fairly small correlation coefficients are found that make it difficult to assess the meaning of the complex interrelation of the variables.

## Survey Research

A survey research strategy is used to provide a detailed inspection of the prevalence of conditions, practices, or attitudes in a given environment by asking people about them rather than observing them directly. The instruments used in survey research include questionnaires, interviews, and, sometimes, a combination of the two. From a practical point of view, questionnaires are generally more appropriate for collecting relatively restricted information from a wide range of persons, whereas interviews are generally more appropriate for gathering more detailed information from a more restricted sample. When a balance of depth of information and breadth of respondents is desired, a combination of the two methods may be appropriate. For example, a relatively restricted or superficial questionnaire may be administered to a large number of people and a follow-up interview of a sample of these persons may be conducted.

Surveys do not usually encompass the entire population of interest for a number of practical reasons. For example, the population may be enormous and widely distributed geographically so that the time and expense necessary to study the entire population would be prohibitive. Therefore, a sample is usually drawn from the population for study, and inferences are made concerning the entire population by studying the sample. Such surveys are often called sample surveys, and problems may arise in determining how well the data of the sample survey can be applied to make a generalization about the entire population. A particular problem with the use of questionnaires should be mentioned. Regardless of whether a questionnaire is sent to the whole population or to a sample of the population, not all the questionnaires are returned, so the ones that are returned may not be an unbiased representation of the population. Interviews and questionnaires may both suffer from problems in determining the accuracy and the veracity of respondents' answers to various questions. Surveys have been used frequently in the communicative disorders research literature to study professional issues such as salaries, caseloads, or working conditions.

Surveys have been used frequently in communicative disorders research to study professional issues such as caseloads or working conditions. For example, Blood, Ridenaur, Thomas, Qualls, and Hammer (2002) presented questionnaire results regarding job satisfaction among professionals in the field. In addition to surveys of professional issues, the survey research strategy is often applied to clinical issues, such as prevalence of disorders, client self-reports of conditions, parental reports of children's conditions, or long-term follow-up of the consequences of disorders. Examples of survey studies of these clinical issues include the prevalence survey of voice disorders among schoolteachers by Roy, Merrill, Thibeault, Parsa, Gray, and Smith (2004); the life span epidemiology survey of stuttering by Craig, Hancock, Tran, Craig, and Peters (2002); the Gomez, Hwang, Sobotova, Stark, and May (2001) survey concerning self-reported hearing loss and audiometry among farmers; the Anderson, Pellowski, Conture, and Kelly (2003) survey of parental reports of temperament of children who stutter; the Watson and Gabel (2002) national survey of clinical practices in assessment of phonemic awareness; and the Felsenfeld, Broen, and McGue (1994) interview survey of educational and occupational accomplishments of adults who had been identified as either phonologically normal or phonologically disordered as children twenty-eight years before in the 1960s. Blood (1993) used both interview and questionnaire instruments together in survey research for the development of a scale for assessing the communication needs of persons who have had laryngectomies.

## Retrospective Research

Retrospective research is designed to examine data already on file before the formulation of the research problem. A clinic may keep routine records of patients with a particular disorder and a researcher may review these records to study important independent and dependent variables. Or a researcher may look back at data collected in a previous research study to reexamine old data or to examine some aspect of the data that had not been previously examined.

Some authors (e.g., Plutchik, 1983; Young, 1976) use the term *retrospective* to describe what we have called comparative research in this chapter, but we believe that a distinction should be made between the two strategies. In comparative research, the investigator has control over the selection of participants and the administration of criterion-variable measures. In retrospective research, however, the investigator depends on participant classifications and criterion-variable measurements that are performed at a different time and possibly by a different person. Thus, there arises the danger in retrospective research that the investigator may not know the reliability and validity of these file data. For example, audiograms in patients' files may have been obtained by a new and unpracticed graduate student who committed procedural errors; the equipment may have been out of calibration on the day of testing; or shortcuts in measurement method may have been taken to save time on a busy day.

Such shortcomings may be overcome to ensure reliable and valid measures in the files if the researcher is responsible for all of the measurements in the first place or is absolutely certain of the conditions under which the data were collected. This could be documented by keeping careful records of calibration and measurement methods. Otherwise, the records used in retrospective research may provide the researcher with incorrect or inaccurate information that, in turn, will be passed on to the profession. Retrospective research, then, should be conducted when the researcher has had administrative control over the collection of the data and when it would be very difficult to collect new data because of financial or other administrative considerations.

Yaruss, LaSalle, and Conture (1998) performed a retrospective analysis of diagnostic data collected from clinical files between 1978 and 1990. They reviewed clinical records of 100 two- to six-year-old children seen for fluency evaluations and found that those referred for treatment differed from the other children on a number of variables, but that there was also significant overlap among the groups. Their method section specified that details of the diagnostic procedures had been described in previous publications by the third author and that all data were collected "by teams of six master's level student-clinicians under the supervision of the third author and at least one Ph.D.-level, licensed, ASHA-certified supervisor." Nevertheless, Cordes (2000) raised several questions about this retrospective study, especially concerning the arrangements to control for examiner training over the years, and Yaruss et al. (2000) responded to that critique with a defense of their clinical procedures and data. This exchange illustrates the controversial nature of retrospective research and the need to carefully document the conditions under which clinical data have been collected in the past. The detailed discussion of research design issues in the retrospective study by Shriberg, Flipsen, Thielke, Kwiatkowski, Kertoy, Katcher, Nellis, and Block (2000) of otitis media and risk for speech disorder in two different populations illustrates many of these difficulties of conducting retrospective research based on data collected in different environments over many years and the care that must be taken to describe retrospective data collection procedures.

An alternate source of data for retrospective analysis can be the data of previous research studies. Using old research data may, in fact, be a better approach than using clinical file data because it is probable that old research data would have been collected under more rigorous and standardized conditions than old clinical file data. An example of the use of previously collected research data in retrospective research can be seen in the study of Colburn and Mysak (1982) of developmental disfluency and emerging grammar in young children. Audiotapes of their subjects were available from a previous study of normal language development (Bloom, 1970), and Colburn and Mysak did a retrospective analysis of the development of disfluencies in these longitudinal data. An extra advantage of the retrospective approach in this study is that the participants proved to have followed a normal course in development of language and fluency over the subsequent ten years between the original data collection and the retrospective analysis, thus allowing the researchers to specify long-term participant characteristics.

The study of speaking fundamental frequency of women's voices by Russell, Penny, and Pemberton (1995) illustrates the combining of retrospective research with currently collected data for a longitudinal study of voice change with aging. Archival recordings made of the women's voices in 1945 and 1981 were available for comparison with recordings made in 1993. Russell et al. presented a method for verification of the accuracy of the recordings in their method section as a rationale for use of the older recordings for comparison of speaking fundamental frequencies at different ages. However, they described why certain measures such as shimmer and jitter could not be used because of lack of information about mouth-to-microphone distance, microphone quality, and microphone angle in the 1945 and 1981 recordings, because these factors had been previously shown to affect perturbation measures. This article is an example of the judicious use and rejection of different retrospective data based on the analysis of the quality and appropriateness of the data for fulfilling specific research purposes.

## Combined Experimental and Descriptive Research

As mentioned in the beginning of this chapter, it is difficult to classify research articles into mutually exclusive categories of research strategies. In reality, many articles that are published in the communicative disorders journals report research that is based on some combination of experimental and descriptive strategy. Because of the prevalence and importance of such investigations in the literature, several examples will be discussed in the following paragraphs.

These articles generally summarize the investigation of the effects of manipulation of one or more independent variables on the performance of participants who have been selected from groups that differ on the basis of classification variables such as age, gender, or pathology. The effect of the experimental manipulation on the dependent variable for one group is compared with the effect of the experimental manipulation for the other group. The research is partly descriptive because the experimenter cannot directly manipulate the classification of participants—that is, the experimenter cannot cause a disorder or accelerate maturation or change the gender of a participant. Therefore, the experimenter has to select participants who fall into preexisting classifications of age, gender, or pathology.

Examination of some illustrative data from combined experimental–descriptive studies may aid consumers in understanding the importance of combining active and attribute independent variables in this common research strategy. A good example of the combination of attribute and active independent variables in combined experimental–descriptive research is seen in the study by Tomblin, Abbas, Records, and Brenneman (1995) of evoked responses to frequency-modulated (FM) tones in children with specific language impairment versus children with no language impairment. Averaged cortically evoked potentials were elicited under two conditions: presentation of an unmodulated steady tone of 1,000 Hz and presentation of a modulated tone that varied in frequency between 900 and 1,100 Hz. Frequency modulation was an active independent variable that was manipulated in a bivalent experiment with two levels: modulated versus unmodulated. Children who were normal language learners were compared to children with specific language impairment in the comparative part of the study. The results showed greater amplitude of auditory evoked response to the modulated than to the unmodulated stimuli for both groups of participants with no apparent differences found between the two groups. Figure 2.31 shows their results plotting evoked response amplitude in microvolts for the control (normal language learners) and SLI (specific language impairment) participants for the modulated and unmodulated conditions.

Rochon, Waters, and Caplan (2000) studied the relation between working memory and sentence comprehension in patients with Alzheimer's disease. As part of this study they compared older volunteers without Alzheimer's disease and patients with Alzheimer's disease in their reaction times to auditory tones under two experimental conditions: (A) while listening to tones alone and (B) while simultaneously tracking a visual stimulus on a computer screen and listening to the tones. Figure 2.32 shows the effect of the tone alone versus tone plus tracking task on reaction time for the two groups (volunteer control participants without Alzheimer's disease versus patients with Alzheimer's disease). Inspection of Figure 2.32 reveals two main effects and an interaction effect. There is a main effect of the experimental condition—reaction time is slower in the tones plus tracking condition than in the tone alone condition. There is also a main effect of groups—patients

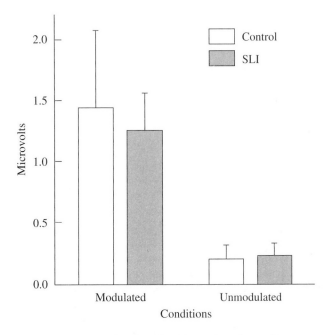

**FIGURE 2.31   Results of a Combined Experimental–
Descriptive Study of the Effects of Frequency Modulation
on Evoked Responses of Children with Specific Language
Impairment versus Children with Normal Language.**

From "Auditory Evoked Responses to Frequency-Modulated Tones in
Children with Specific Language Impairment," by B. Tomblin, P. Abbas,
N. L. Records, and L. M. Brenneman, 1995, *Journal of Speech and Hear-
ing Research, 38,* p. 391. Copyright 1995 by the American Speech-
Language-Hearing Association. Reprinted with permission.

with Alzheimer's disease perform more slowly than control participants. There is also an
interaction effect between experimental condition and group because there is very little
difference between the performance of the control participants on the two tasks but the
patients with Alzheimer's disease perform much slower on the tones plus tracking task
than on the tones alone task.

     In another example, Montgomery (1995) reports two experiments with children exhib-
iting normal language (NL) versus children with specific language impairment (SLI). In the
first experiment, he studied the effect of syllable length (multivalent continuous independent
variable) on the children's ability to repeat nonsense words; in the second, he studied the
effect of redundancy (bivalent categorical independent variable) on a sentence comprehension task. Figure 2.33 shows his results for the first experiment. The figure reveals that the
NL children outperformed the SLI participants, longer stimuli were more difficult, and there
was an interaction between stimulus length and participants classification in which the SLI
children fell further behind the NL children as stimulus length increased. That is, the graph

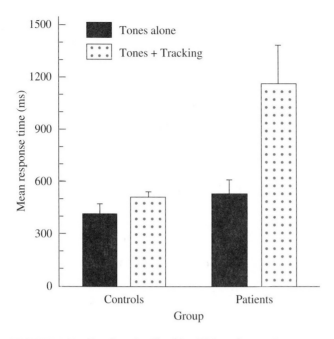

**FIGURE 2.32    Results of a Combined Experimental–Descriptive Study of the Effect of Tracking on Reaction Time to Tones for Control Participants versus Patients with Alzheimer's Disease.**

From "The Relationship between Measures of Working Memory and Sentence Comprehension in Patients with Alzheimer's Disease," by E. Rochon, G. S. Waters, and D. Caplan, 2000, *Journal of Speech, Language, and Hearing Research, 43,* p. 407. Copyright 2000 by the American Speech-Language-Hearing Association. Reprinted with permission.

showing performance on the task as a function of stimulus length fell more sharply for the SLI children than for the NL children. Figure 2.34 shows Montgomery's results for his second experiment with these children. The figure shows (a) NL children outperformed SLI children; (b) NL children performed about the same for both redundant and nonredundant material; (c) SLI children had more difficulty with the redundant than the nonredundant material. Thus, another interaction effect occurred in which the active redundancy variable differentially affected the participants who differed on the attribute language classification variable.

In another example of a combined experimental–descriptive study, Boike and Souza (2000) examine the effect of varying compression ratio on speech recognition for two groups of participants with normal hearing and hearing impairment. Participants in both groups listened to speech in noise under a no compression (1:1 ratio) condition and under three different compression ratios ranging from 2:1 to 10:1. Figure 2.35 shows speech recognition (RAU transformed scores on the ordinate) plotted as a function of compression

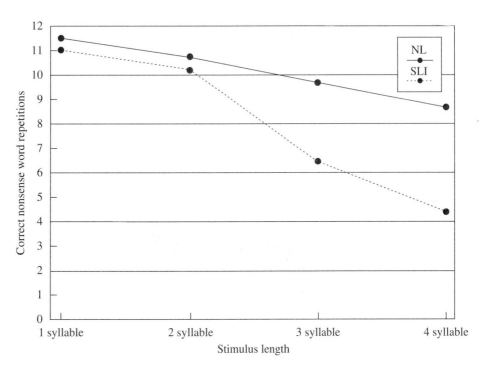

**FIGURE 2.33    Results of a Combined Experimental–Descriptive Study of the Effect of Stimulus Length on Word Repetition of Children with Normal Language (NL) versus Children with Specific Language Impairment (SLI).**

From "Sentence Comprehension in Children with Specific Language Impairment: The Role of Phonological Working Memory," by J. W. Montgomery, 1995, *Journal of Speech and Hearing Research, 38,* p. 191. Copyright 1995 by the American Speech-Language-Hearing Association. Reprinted with permission.

ratio for the hearing-impaired and normal hearing participants. The graph shows an obvious main effect of group—the normal hearing listeners outperformed the hearing-impaired listeners at each compression ratio; a main effect of compression—speech recognition decreased as compression increased; and most important, an interaction effect in which this decrease in speech recognition as a function of compression is evident for the hearing-impaired listeners but not for the normal hearing listeners. In other words, there are two different functions showing the effect of compression on speech recognition in noise for the two different groups of listeners.

The final example in this section shows the application of a parametric experiment with the manipulation of two active independent variables to four groups of participants varying in age as part of a series of experiments examining developmental changes in audition in old age. The results of the experiment by Takahashi and Bacon (1992) are shown in Figure 2.36. Four age groups of listeners (young persons in their twenties, and persons in their fifties, sixties, and seventies) listened to speech in modulated and in unmodulated broadband noise at four different signal-to-noise ratios (SNR). The active,

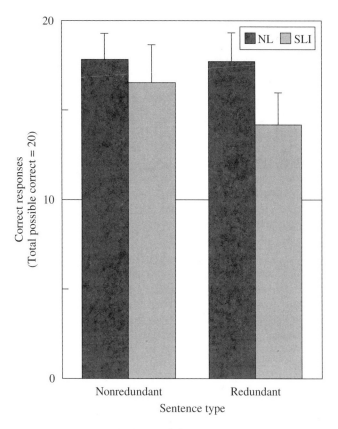

**FIGURE 2.34 Results of a Combined Experimental–Descriptive Study of the Effect of Redundancy on Sentence Comprehension of Children with Normal Language (NL) versus Children with Specific Language Impairment (SLI).**

From "Sentence Comprehension in Children with Specific Language Impairment: The Role of Phonological Working Memory," by J. W. Montgomery, 1995, *Journal of Speech and Hearing Research, 38,* p. 192. Copyright 1995 by the American Speech-Language-Hearing Association. Reprinted with permission.

manipulated independent variables, then, were noise modulation and SNR, and the attribute variable was age of the participants. The dependent variable was the percentage of correct speech understanding. The left panel of the figure shows the results of the four groups of participants at each SNR for the modulated noise condition, and the right panel shows the results for the unmodulated condition. Inspection of the figure reveals main effects of SNR, noise modulation, and age and interactions between SNR and modulation, as well as between modulation and age. As SNR increased, so did speech understanding, as indicated by the slope of the lines upward to the right. Speech understanding was generally better with modulated than with unmodulated noise as indicated by the

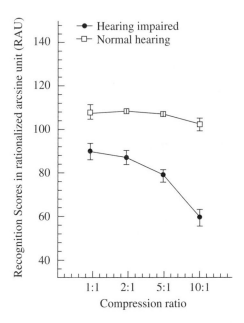

**FIGURE 2.35    Results of a Combined Experimental–Descriptive Study of the Effect of Compression Ratio on Speech Recognition of Participants with Normal Hearing versus Those with Hearing Impairment.**

From "Effect of Compression Ratio on Speech Recognition and Speech-Quality Ratings with Wide Dynamic Range Compression Amplification," by K. T. Boike and P. E. Souza, 2000, *Journal of Speech, Language, and Hearing Research, 43,* p. 464. Copyright 2000 by the American Speech-Language-Hearing Association. Reprinted with permission.

higher scores in the left panel. The interaction of SNR and modulation is seen in the steeper slope of the functions in the right panel than in the left panel, indicating that the modulated and unmodulated functions converged as SNR increased. Finally, the interaction of modulation and age group is seen in the separation of the young listeners from the older listeners in the modulated condition but not in the unmodulated condition—that is, modulated noise facilitated young listeners' performance relative to older listeners more than did unmodulated noise. Such combined experimental–descriptive studies can become quite complex and revealing as more independent variables are introduced and their importance in communicative disorders cannot be stressed enough. Because combined experimental–descriptive research is both a common and an important strategy in communicative disorders research, considerable attention will be devoted to it in subsequent chapters of this book.

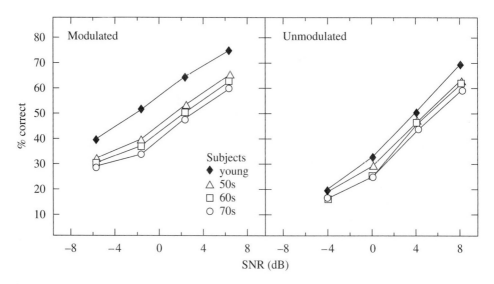

**FIGURE 2.36  Results of a Combined Experimental–Descriptive Study of the Effects of Signal-to-Noise Ratio (SNR) and Noise Modulation on Speech Understanding of Participants in Four Different Age Groups.**

From "Modulation Detection, Modulation Masking, and Speech Understanding in Noise in the Elderly," by G. A. Takahashi and S. P. Bacon, 1992, *Journal of Speech and Hearing Research, 35,* p. 1418. Copyright 1992 by the American Speech-Language-Hearing Association. Reprinted with permission.

## Study Questions

**1.** Read the following articles:

Ertmer, D. J. (2004). How well can children recognize speech features in spectrograms? Comparisons by age and hearing status. *Journal of Speech, Language, and Hearing Research, 47,* 484–495.

Johnson, C. E. (2000). Children's phoneme identification in reverberation and noise. *Journal of Speech, Language, and Hearing Research, 43,* 144–157.

Solomon, N. P., Robin, D. A., & Luschei, E. S. (2000). Strength, endurance, and stability of the tongue and hand in Parkinson's disease. *Journal of Speech, Language, and Hearing Research, 43,* 256–267.

Write a brief abstract of each article that outlines the four common steps in empirical research as described in Chapter 1 and identifies the research strategies as described in Chapter 2.

2. Read the following article:

   Solomon, N. P., & Munson, B. (2004). The effect of jaw position on measures of tongue strength and endurance. *Journal of Speech, Language, and Hearing Research, 47,* 584–594.

   **a.** What research strategy did the authors employ?
   **b.** Identify the dependent variables that were measured in the different bite block conditions.
   **c.** What differences were observed as a function of manipulation of the independent variable?

3. Read the following article:

   Redmond, S. M. (2003). Children's productions of the affix *-ed* in past tense and past participle contexts. *Journal of Speech, Language, and Hearing Research, 46,* 1095–1109.

   **a.** What three groups of subjects were compared (i.e., what was the classification variable)?
   **b.** Identify the dependent variables that were used to compare them.
   **c.** What differences were found among the three groups?

4. Read the following article:

   Roy, N., Merrill, R. M., Thibeault, S., Parsa, R. A., Gray, S. D., & Smith, E. M. (2004). Prevalence of voice disorders in teachers and the general population. *Journal of Speech, Language, and Hearing Research, 47,* 281–293.

   **a.** What research strategies were combined in this article?
   **b.** Identify the dependent variables that were measured.
   **c.** What differences were observed among the two groups of participants?

5. Read the following article:

   Hillenbrand, J., Cleveland, R. A., & Erickson, R. L. (1994). Acoustic correlates of breathy voice quality. *Journal of Speech and Hearing Research, 37,* 769–778.

   **a.** What research strategy did the authors employ?
   **b.** Identify the variables that were most highly correlated with breathy voice quality.

6. Read the following article:

   McCathren, R. B. (1999). The relationship between prelinguistic vocalization and later expressive vocabulary in young children with developmental delay. *Journal of Speech, Language, and Hearing Research, 42,* 915–924.

   **a.** What were the predictor and predicted variables in this correlational study?
   **b.** Which variables were identified as the best predictors of each predicted variable?

**7.** Read the following article:

Anderson, J. D., & Conture, E. G. (2004). Sentence-structure priming in young children who do and do not stutter. *Journal of Speech, Language, and Hearing Research, 47,* 552–571.

   **a.** What research strategies were combined in this study?

   **b.** Identify the active and attribute independent variables that were used.

   **c.** What effect did the independent variable have on the dependent variables for the different groups of participants?

**8.** Read the following article:

Turner, C., Chi, S., & Flock, S. (1999). Temporal factors and speech recognition performance in young and elderly listeners. *Journal of Speech, Language, and Hearing Research, 42,* 773–784.

   **a.** What research strategies were combined in this study?

   **b.** Identify the active and attribute independent variables that were used.

   **c.** Examine the functions in Figure 4 and identify the manipulated independent variable, the parameter, and the dependent variables.

**9.** Read the following article:

Nippold, M. A., & Rudzinski, M. (1993). Familiarity and transparency in idiom explanation: A developmental study of children and adolescents. *Journal of Speech and Hearing Research, 36,* 728–737.

   **a.** What research strategies were combined in this study?

   **b.** Identify the dependent variables that were used.

   **c.** Explain the effects of idiom familiarity and maturation that are shown in Figure 1.

# REFERENCES

Anderson, J. D., Pellowski, M. W., Conture, E. G., & Kelly, E. M. (2003). Temperamental characteristics of young children who stutter. *Journal of Speech, Language, and Hearing Research, 46,* 1221–1233.

Ayukawa, H., & Rudmin, F. (1983). Does early middle ear pathology affect auditory perception skills and learning? Comment on Brandes and Ehinger (1981). *Journal of Speech and Hearing Disorders, 48,* 222–223.

Blood, G. (1993). Development and assessment of a scale addressing communicative needs of patients with laryngectomies. *American Journal of Speech-Language Pathology, 2(3),* 82–90.

Blood, G. W., Ridenour, J. S., Thomas, E. A., Qualls, C. D., & Hammer, C. S. (2002). Predicting job satisfaction among speech-language pathologists working in public schools. *Language, Speech, and Hearing Services in Schools, 33,* 282–290.

Bloom, L. (1970). *Language development: Form and function in emerging grammars.* Cambridge, MA: MIT Press.

Boike, K. T., & Souza, P. E. (2000). Effect of compression ratio on speech recognition and speech-quality ratings with wide dynamic range compression amplification. *Journal of Speech, Language, and Hearing Research, 43,* 456–468.

Bordens, K. S., & Abbott, B. B. (2002). *Research design and methods: A process approach* (5th ed.). New York: McGraw-Hill.

Camarata, S. M., Nelson, K. E., & Camarata, M. N. (1994). Comparison of conversational-recasting and imitative procedures for training grammatical structures in children with specific language impairment. *Journal of Speech and Hearing Research, 37,* 1414–1423.

Carhart, R., & Porter, L. S. (1971). Audiometric configuration and prediction of threshold for spondees. *Journal of Speech and Hearing Research, 14,* 486–495.

Casby, M. W. (2001). Otitis media and language development: A meta analysis. *American Journal of Speech-Language Pathology, 10(1),* 65–80.

Caselli, M. C., Vicari, S., Longobardi, E., Lami, L., Pizzoli, C., & Stella, G. (1998). Gesture and words in early development of children with Down syndrome. *Journal of Speech, Language, and Hearing Research, 41,* 1125–1135.

Colburn, N., & Mysak, E. D. (1982). Developmental disfluency and emerging grammar: I. Disfluency characteristics in early syntactic utterances. *Journal of Speech and Hearing Research, 25,* 414–420.

Cordes, A. K. (2000). Comments on Yaruss, LaSalle, and Conture (1998). *American Journal of Speech-Language Pathology, 9(2),* 162–165.

Craig, A., Hancock, K., Tran, Y., Craig, M., & Peters, K. (2002). Epidemiology of stuttering in the community across the life span. *Journal of Speech, Language, and Hearing Research, 45,* 1097–1105.

De Filippo, C. L., Sims, D. G., & Gottermeier, L. (1995). Linking visual and kinesthetic imagery in lipreading instruction. *Journal of Speech and Hearing Research, 38,* 244–256.

Ellis Weismer, S., Murray-Branch, J., & Miller, J. F. (1994). A prospective longitudinal study of language development in late talkers. *Journal of Speech and Hearing Research, 37,* 852–867.

Erber, N. P. (1971). Effects of distance on the visual perception of speech. *Journal of Speech and Hearing Research, 14,* 848–857.

Felsenfeld, S., Broen, P. A., & McGue, M. (1994). A 28-year follow-up of adults with a history of moderate phonological disorder: Educational and occupational results. *Journal of Speech and Hearing Research, 37,* 1341–1353.

Geers, A. E., & Moog, J. S. (1992). Speech perception and production skills of hearing-impaired children from oral and total communication education settings. *Journal of Speech and Hearing Research, 35,* 1384–1393.

Gelfand, S. A. (1998). Optimizing the reliability of speech recognition scores. *Journal of Speech, Language, and Hearing Research, 41,* 1088–1102.

Gomez, M. I., Hwang, S., Sobotova, L., Stark, A. D., & May, J. J. (2001). A comparison of self-reported hearing loss and audiometry in a cohort of New York farmers. *Journal of Speech, Language, and Hearing Research, 44,* 1201–1208.

Gordon-Brannan, M., & Hodson, B. W. (2000). Intelligibility/severity measurements of prekindergarten children's speech. *American Journal of Speech-Language Pathology, 9(2),* 141–150.

Green, J. R., Moore, C. A., Higashikawa, M., & Steeve, R. W. (2000). The physiological development of speech motor control: Lip and jaw coordination. *Journal of Speech, Language, and Hearing Research, 43,* 239–255.

Helfer, K. S. (1994). Binaural cues and consonant perception in reverberation and noise. *Journal of Speech and Hearing Research, 37,* 429–438.

Jaeger, C. G., & Bacon, H. M. (1962). *Introductory college mathematics.* New York: Harper & Row.

Karsh, D. E., & Brandes, P. (1983). Response to Ayukawa and Rudmin. *Journal of Speech and Hearing Disorders, 48,* 223–224.

Kerlinger, F., & Lee, H. B. (2000). *Foundations of behavioral research* (4th ed.). New York: Harcourt Brace.

Kling, J. W., & Riggs, L. A. (Eds.). (1971). *Woodworth and Schlossberg's experimental psychology.* New York: Holt, Rinehart and Winston.

Loven, F. C., & Collins, M. J. (1988). Reverberation, masking, filtering, and level effects on speech recognition performance. *Journal of Speech and Hearing Research, 31,* 681–695.

Marvin, C. A., & Privratsky, A. J. (1999). After school talk: The effects of materials sent home from preschool. *American Journal of Speech-Language Pathology, 8(3),* 231–240.

McGuigan, F. J. (1968). *Experimental psychology: A methodological approach* (2nd ed.). Englewood Cliffs, NJ: Prentice Hall.

Monge, P. R., & Cappella, J. N. (1980). *Multivariate techniques in human communication research.* New York: Academic Press.

Monsen, R. (1978). Toward measuring how well hearing-impaired children speak. *Journal of Speech and Hearing Research, 21,* 197–219.

Montgomery, J. W. (1995). Sentence comprehension in children with specific language impairment: The role of phonological working memory. *Journal of Speech and Hearing Research, 38,* 187–199.

Nippold, M. A., Hegel, S. L., Sohlberg, M. M., & Schwarz, I. E. (1999). Defining abstract entities: Development in pre-adolescents, adolescents, and young adults. *Journal of Speech, Language, and Hearing Research, 42,* 473–481.

Pedhazur, E. J. (1999). *Multiple regression in behavioral research* (3rd ed.). New York: Harcourt Brace.

Plutchik, R. (1983). *Foundations of experimental research* (3rd ed.). New York: Harper & Row.

Rademaker, A. W., Pauloski, B. R., Colangelo, L. A., & Logemann, J. A. (1998). Age and volume effects on liquid swallowing function in normal women. *Journal of Speech, Language, and Hearing Research, 41,* 275–284.

Rescorla, L., & Ratner, N. B. (1996). Phonetic profiles of toddlers with specific expressive language impairment

(SLI-E). *Journal of Speech and Hearing Research, 39,* 153–165.

Riddel, J., McCauley, R. J., Mulligan, M., & Tandan, R. (1995). Intelligibility and phonetic contrast errors in highly intelligible speakers with amyotrophic lateral sclerosis. *Journal of Speech and Hearing Research, 38,* 304–314.

Rochon, E., Waters, G. S., & Caplan, D. (2000). The relationship between measures of working memory and sentence comprehension in patients with Alzheimer's disease. *Journal of Speech, Language, and Hearing Research, 43,* 395–413.

Roy, N., Merrill, R. M., Thibeault, S., Parsa, R. A., Gray, S. D., & Smith, E. M. (2004). Prevalence of voice disorders in teachers and the general population. *Journal of Speech, Language, and Hearing Research, 47,* 281–293.

Russell, A., Penny, L., & Pemberton, C. (1995). Speaking fundamental frequency changes over time in women: A longitudinal study. *Journal of Speech and Hearing Research, 38,* 101–109.

Sapienza, C. M., & Stathopoulos, E. (1994). Respiratory and laryngeal measures of children and women with bilateral vocal fold nodules. *Journal of Speech and Hearing Research, 37,* 1229–1243.

Schiavetti, N., Whitehead, R. L., Whitehead, B. H., & Metz, D. E. (1998). Effect of fingerspelling task on temporal characteristics and perceived naturalness of speech in simultaneous communication. *Journal of Speech, Language, and Hearing Research, 41,* 5–17.

Shaughnessy, J. J., Zechmeister, E. B., & Zechmeister, J. S. (2000). *Research methods in psychology* (5th ed.). New York: McGraw-Hill.

Shriberg, L. D., Flipsen, P., Thielke, H., Kwiatkowski, J., Kertoy, M. K., Katcher, M. L., Nellis, R. A., & Block, M. G. (2000). Risk for speech disorders associated with early recurrent otitis media with effusion: Two retrospective studies. *Journal of Speech, Language, and Hearing Research, 43,* 79–99.

Shriberg, L. D., Gruber, F. A., & Kwiatkowski, J. (1994). Developmental phonological disorders III: Long-term speech sound normalization. *Journal of Speech and Hearing Research, 37,* 1151–1177.

Smith, A., & Goffman, L. (1998). Stability and patterning of speech movement sequences in children and adults. *Journal of Speech, Language, and Hearing Research, 41,* 18–30.

Tabachnick, B. G., & Fidell, L. S. (2001). *Using multivariate statistics* (4th ed.). Boston: Allyn & Bacon.

Takahashi, G. A., & Bacon, S. P. (1992). Modulation detection, modulation masking, and speech understanding in the elderly. *Journal of Speech and Hearing Research, 35,* 1410–1421.

Tomblin, B., Abbas, P., Records, N. L., & Brenneman, L. M. (1995). Auditory evoked responses to frequency-modulated tones in children with specific language impairment. *Journal of Speech and Hearing Research, 38,* 387–392.

Turner, G. S., & Weismer, G. (1993). Characteristics of speaking rate in the dysarthria associated with amyotrophic lateral sclerosis. *Journal of Speech and Hearing Research, 36,* 1134–1144.

Tye-Murray, N., Spencer, L., Bedia, E. G., & Woodworth, G. (1996). Differences in children's sound production when speaking with a cochlear implant turned on and turned off. *Journal of Speech and Hearing Research, 39,* 604–610.

Underwood, B. J., & Shaughnessy, J. J. (1975). *Experimentation in psychology.* New York: John Wiley & Sons.

Ventry, I. M. (1980). Effects of conductive hearing loss: Fact or fiction. *Journal of Speech and Hearing Disorders, 45,* 143–156.

Watson, M., & Gabel, R. (2002). Speech-language pathologists' attitudes and practices regarding the assessment of children's phonemic awareness skills: Results of a national survey. *Contemporary Issues in Communication Science and Disorders, 29,* 173–184.

Wilder, C. N., & Baken, R. J. (1974). Respiratory patterns in infant cry. *Human Communication, 3,* 18–34.

Wiley, T. L., Cruickshanks, K. J., Nondahl, D. M., Tweed, T. S., & Klein, R., & Klein, B. E. K. (1998). Aging and high-frequency hearing sensitivity. *Journal of Speech, Language, and Hearing Research, 41,* 1061–1072.

Wohlert, A. B., & Smith, A. (1998). Spatiotemporal stability of lip movements in older adult speakers. *Journal of Speech, Language, and Hearing Research, 41,* 41–50.

Yaruss, J. S., LaSalle, L. R., & Conture, E. G. (1998). Evaluating stuttering in young children: Diagnostic data. *American Journal of Speech-Language Pathology, 7 (4),* 62–76.

Yaruss, J. S., LaSalle, L. R., & Conture, E. G. (2000). Understanding stuttering in young children: A response to Cordes. *American Journal of Speech-Language Pathology, 9(2),* 165–171.

Young, M. A. (1976). Application of regression analysis concepts to retrospective research in speech pathology. *Journal of Speech and Hearing Research, 19,* 5–18.

Young, M. A. (1993). Supplementing tests of statistical significance: Variation accounted for. *Journal of Speech and Hearing Research, 36,* 644–656.

Young, M. A. (1994). Evaluating differences between stuttering and nonstuttering speakers: The group difference design. *Journal of Speech and Hearing Research, 37,* 522–534.

# CHAPTER 3

# Research Design in Communicative Disorders

This chapter considers research designs that are commonly used in communicative disorders. The topics to be discussed are (1) the meaning of research design, (2) the purposes of research design, (3) general research design principles in experimental and descriptive research, (4) some specific principles of group research design, (5) some specific principles of single-subject research design, and (6) some issues regarding generalization.

## Meaning of Research Design

As mentioned in Chapter 2, Bordens and Abbott (2002) distinguished between research design and research strategy by stating that strategy is the general plan of attack and design is the specific set of tactics used to carry out the strategy. Kerlinger (1979, p. 83) has more specifically defined research design as follows:

> The plan and structure of research are often called the design of research. The word "design," as used here, focuses on the manner in which a research problem is conceptualized and put into a structure that is a guide for experimentation and for data collection and analysis. We define *research design,* then, as the plan and structure of investigation conceived so as to obtain answers to research questions. Modern conceptions of the design of research are founded in experimental research.

Research design, then, is the development of a plan for selecting and measuring the independent and dependent variables in order to answer research questions about their relationships. As Kerlinger stated previously, modern research designs are rooted in the concept of the experiment in which an independent variable is manipulated to determine its effect on a dependent variable. As pointed out in Chapter 2, the *structure* of nonmanipulable independent variables in descriptive research is similar to the *structure* of manipulable independent variables in experiments. Thus, the structure of descriptive research design will be similar in many ways to the structure of experimental design, with the main difference being the manipulability of the independent variables.

# Purposes of Research Design

Kerlinger and Lee (2000, p. 450) state that

> Research design has two basic purposes: (1) to provide answers to research questions and (2) to control variance. Design helps the investigator obtain answers to the questions of research and also helps him to control the experimental, extraneous, and error variances of the particular research problem under study.

In order to accomplish the first purpose, the investigator must develop an experimental or descriptive research design for obtaining empirical data about the relationship of the independent and dependent variables of interest. In order to accomplish the second purpose, the investigator must structure the research plan in such a way that contamination of the answer to the research question by extraneous variables and measurement error is minimized. Because the relationship between the independent and dependent variable is quantified by describing the degree to which variation or change in one variable is linked to variation or change in the other variable, control of variance is necessary to produce answers to research questions that are as free as possible of contamination by extraneous variables and measurement error. Kerlinger and Lee (2000, pp. 455–463) describe in detail the concept of research design as variance control by outlining the manner in which efficient research design is used (a) to maximize the systematic variance associated with the independent and dependent variables of interest to the investigator, (b) to minimize error or random variance (including errors of measurement), and (c) to control variance attributable to the influence of extraneous variables on the dependent variable.

The two basic purposes of research design are common to both experimental and descriptive research, but some specific objectives are different for these two types of research. In experimental research, the first design objective is to manipulate the independent variable in order to answer the question "What effect does this have on the dependent variable?" The second design objective is to arrange the experiment so that extraneous variables are controlled and, therefore, cannot have a confounding effect on the dependent variable. In descriptive research, the first objective is to select the variables for observation in order to answer questions such as "What are the dimensions or differences or relationships found in the natural phenomena?" The second objective is to make these observations in a systematic and unobtrusive fashion so that the dimensions, differences, or relationships of the criterion variables are not confounded by extraneous variables.

We have merely rephrased the general purposes of research design into specific objectives to fit the descriptive and experimental models. The main point is that both types of research should be designed to (1) answer the research question empirically and (2) reduce or eliminate contamination of the answer by extraneous variables.

Kerlinger and Lee (2000, p. 450) have indicated that it may be tempting to omit the first purpose (because it is so obvious) and concentrate on the second. They point out, however, that this is a dangerous delimitation because research design can then degenerate into a "sterile technical exercise" in which one may lose sight of the importance of uniting the research questions, the empirical evidence, and the conclusions of the study. The research question should be a common unifying element in the design of research.

# General Research Design Principles

As Kerlinger and Lee (2000) point out, theoretically at least, there are as many research designs as there are hypotheses to be tested. Therefore, rather than attempt to present an exhaustive taxonomy of descriptive and experimental research designs, we have limited our discussion to some basic principles of research design that have broad applicability in communicative disorders research. Two major classes of research designs are considered here: group designs and single-subject designs.[1] In group designs, one or more groups of participants are exposed to one or more levels of the independent variable, and the average performance of the group of participants on the dependent variable is examined to determine the relationship between the independent and dependent variable. Single-subject designs focus on the individual behavior of participants rather than considering the average performance of a group of participants. Single-subject designs may, in fact, examine the behavior of more than one person, but the data of each person will be evaluated individually rather than as part of a group average.

In evaluating any research design, there are two important criteria suggested by Campbell and Stanley (1966): *internal validity* and *external validity.* The internal validity of any research design concerns the degree to which the design meets Kerlinger and Lee's two purposes within the confines of the study. That is, did the study answer the research question and control variance appropriately to provide an uncontaminated picture of the relationship between independent and dependent variables? The external validity of any research design concerns the degree to which generalizations can be made outside of the confines of the study. Some general comments on the internal and external validity of research designs will be made in this chapter, and a more detailed analysis of the application of these two criteria in treatment efficacy research will be included in Chapter 5.

# Group Research Designs

This section will consider group designs for both experimental and descriptive research and briefly address the primary issues affecting internal validity of the major group designs.

## Between-Subjects Designs

In between-subjects research designs, the performances of separate groups of participants are measured and comparisons are made between the groups. In experimental between-subjects designs, different groups of participants are exposed to different treatments or levels of the independent variable. In descriptive between-subjects designs, different groups of participants are compared with each other with regard to their performance on some criterion

---

[1]Although the current terminology identifies persons who participate in research as "participants" rather than as "subjects," we will continue to use the traditional terms for "group design" and "single-subject design" in order to be consistent with the terminology found in the extant body of research literature.

variable. We will first discuss some issues in between-subjects experimental designs and then consider points concerning between-subjects descriptive research designs.

In between-subjects experimental designs, the independent variable or experimental treatment is applied to one group of participants (experimental group) but not applied to another group of participants (control group). The difference between the performance of the two groups is taken as an index of the effect of the independent variable on the dependent variable. This would be the case, for example, in a treatment experiment in which the experimental group is given treatment and the control group is not given treatment. The two groups are then compared on some dependent variable that is usually some measure of performance improvement.

Ferguson and Takane (1989, p. 238) summarize the process of designing a between-subjects experiment:

> In developing the design for an experiment, the investigator (1) selects the values of the independent variable, or variables, to be compared; (2) selects the subjects for the experiments; (3) applies rules or procedures whereby subjects are assigned to the particular values of the independent variable; (4) specifies the observations or measurements to be made on each subject.

Between-subjects experimental designs may be bivalent, in which case one experimental group is compared to one control group to study the effect of the presence versus the absence of the experimental treatment (independent variable). These designs may also be multivalent, in which case each of several experimental groups is exposed to a different value of the independent variable and the control group receives no treatment. Finally, between-subjects designs may be parametric, in which case several groups can receive different values of the different independent variables in different combinations and can also be compared with a control group that receives no treatment.

Experimental design is concerned with the manipulation of an active independent variable and the measurement of the effect of this manipulation on the dependent variable. Descriptive research design is concerned with the selection of levels of an attribute independent variable (such as group classifications in comparative studies or maturation levels in developmental studies), and the measurement of the dependent variable to assess group differences or developmental trends in the dependent variables, or to study the relationships among these variables. Both experimental and descriptive research designs are usually classified as *between-subjects, within-subjects,* or *mixed* (both between-subjects and within-subjects) designs.[2]

In between-subjects designs, different groups of participants are compared to each other. Within-subjects designs involve the comparison of the same group of participants in different situations. Mixed designs include both types of comparison in the same study. Some problems are well suited to between-subjects designs, whereas other problems are more logically attacked through within-subjects designs. In some cases, a combination of the two in a mixed design is necessary in order to study the problem appropriately. The selection of an appropriate design is dependent, to a large extent, on a clear understanding of the research problem and a logical analysis of the alternate means for studying the problem.

---

[2]Although the current terminology identifies persons who participate in research as "participants" rather than as "subjects," we will continue to use the traditional terms for "between-subjects" and "within-subjects" designs in order to be consistent with the terminology found in the extant body of research literature.

In between-subjects designs, the levels of the independent variable are varied across different groups of participants, and averages on the dependent variable of each of the groups are compared to each other. In within-subjects designs the levels of the independent variable are varied across different conditions and the group averages on the dependent variable in each of the conditions are compared to each other. Mixed designs include both types of comparison in the same study because they include two independent variables: a between-subjects design is used to analyze one independent variable, and a within-subjects design is used to analyze the other.

A major consideration in the evaluation of the design of between-subjects experiments is the equivalence of the experimental and control groups. If the two groups of participants that are exposed to two levels of the independent variable are different from each other in characteristics such as age, intelligence, gender, and prior experience, they may perform differently on the dependent variable because of these participant characteristic differences rather than because they have been exposed to two different levels of the independent variable. The participant characteristic difference, then, is an extraneous, or nuisance, variable that can compete with the independent variable as an explanation for any difference in the dependent variable between the two groups of participants. In other words, differences in the relative performances of experimental and control groups might be attributable to differences in participant characteristics of the two groups in addition to, or instead of, the effects of the independent variable.

Experimenters, then, must attempt to ensure that participants in the experimental and control groups are equivalent in all respects except for the varied distribution of the independent variable to these groups. There are basically two techniques for attempting to equate experimental and control groups for between-subjects experimental designs: *randomization* and *matching.*

Randomization is usually considered the better of these two techniques and will be discussed first. Christensen (2004, p. 234), in commenting on the importance of randomization as a technique for equating groups, states:

> Randomization, the most important and basic of all the control methods, is a statistical control technique designed to assure that extraneous variables, known or unknown, will not systematically bias the study results. It is the only technique for controlling unknown sources of variation.

Randomization is the assignment of participants to experimental and control groups on a random basis. Random, in this sense, does not mean that participants are assigned in a haphazard fashion. Rather, randomization is a technique for group assignment that ensures each subject has an equal probability of being assigned either to the experimental group or to the control group. Christensen (2004, p. 237) summarizes the objective of randomization in dealing with extraneous variables in experimental and control groups:

> Random assignment produces control by virtue of the fact that the variables to be controlled are distributed in approximately the same manner in all groups (ideally the distribution would be exactly the same). When the distribution is approximately equal, the influence of the extraneous variables is held constant, because they cannot exert any differential influence on the dependent variable.

With a random assignment of participants to experimental and control groups, extraneous variables (e.g., age, gender, intelligence, or socioeconomic status), which could affect the participants' performance on the dependent variable, should be balanced among the groups so that there will be no systematic bias favoring one group over another. In such a case, then, the two groups may be considered equivalent at the start of the experiment.

Christensen (2004) points out, however, that randomization may not always result in the selection of experimental and control groups that are equivalent in all respects, especially when a small number of participants is used. Because random chance determines the assignment of participants to experimental and control groups (and, therefore, the distribution of extraneous variables to experimental and control groups), it is possible occasionally for the two groups to differ on some variables. Experimenters often check this possibility by examining the groups after randomization to ascertain the equivalence of the groups on known extraneous variables. Christensen (2004) indicates, however, that the probability of experimental and control groups being equivalent on extraneous variables is greater with randomization than with other methods of group selection and, therefore, randomization is a powerful technique for reducing systematic bias in assignment to experimental and control groups. In addition, randomization is an important prerequisite to unbiased data analysis, and many of the statistical techniques to be described in Chapter 6 are based on the assumption of random assignment to experimental and control groups.

A second technique for attempting to equate experimental and control groups in between-subjects experimental designs is matching. The experimenter could attempt to match the members of the two groups on all extraneous variables that are considered relevant to the experiment. Two groups could be assembled that would be equivalent at the start of the experiment on extraneous variables known to be correlated with the dependent variable. Because the rationale for matching groups is to reduce the possibility of group differences mimicking the effect of the independent variable on the dependent variable, it makes sense to match the groups on extraneous variables that could influence performance on the dependent variable. Thus, differences between the experimental and control groups on the dependent variable at the end of the experiment would not be attributable to differences between the groups on these extraneous variables.

A number of techniques are available for matching experimental and control groups on extraneous variables. Two common techniques that are used are *matching the overall distribution* of the extraneous variables in the groups and *matching pairs of participants* for assignment to experimental and control groups. Christensen (2004) calls the first matching technique the "frequency distribution control technique" because the two groups are matched in their overall frequency distribution (i.e., the frequency of cases occurring at each value of the extraneous variable) rather than comparing participants on a case-by-case basis on a number of characteristics. Christensen (2004) calls the second matching technique the "precision control technique" because matching participants on a case-by-case basis not only reduces participant differences as an extraneous variable but also increases the sensitivity of the experiment to small effects of the independent variable on the dependent variable when participants are equated on extraneous variables that are highly correlated with the dependent variable.

Overall matching is accomplished by assembling experimental and control groups that have similar distributions of the extraneous variables—that is both groups have about the same average and spread of each of the extraneous variables. For example, factors, such as age, intelligence, level of education, and gender, would be distributed about equally in the experimental and control groups. Each group could be assembled so that it would contain equal numbers of males and females; the age range and average age would be the same in each group; the average IQ and the range from the lowest to the highest IQ in each group would be about the same, and so on.

Although overall matching on the surface may appear to be an adequate technique for ensuring group equivalence, consumers of research should be aware that there are disadvantages to this technique. For example, one distinct disadvantage is that the combinations of extraneous variables in individual participants may not be well matched for two groups. Although age and IQ may be the same on the average in the two groups, the older participants may be more intelligent than the younger participants in one group, whereas the younger participants may be more intelligent than the older participants in the other group. Although individual nuisance variables may seem to be equivalent in the two groups, the interaction of the nuisance variables in each participant in the two groups may not necessarily be the same.

Matching pairs of participants for subsequent assignment to experimental and control groups is a more effective technique than overall matching. Matching pairs is accomplished by first selecting a participant for assignment to one group and then searching for another participant whose constellation of extraneous variables is essentially the same as for the first participant. Because no two people are exactly alike in all respects, matching is usually accomplished within certain limits on the extraneous variables. For example, the first participant may be a twenty-one-year-old female college senior with an IQ of 115. To find her matched pair member for assignment to the other group, the experimenter would then look for a female college senior with an IQ between 112 and 118 in the age range from twenty to twenty-two years. The rest of the participants would be paired in a similar fashion, with each pair having a unique pattern of the extraneous variables.

Once matched pairs are assembled, the next step is to assign the pair members to the experimental and control groups. Although pair matching will equate experimental and control groups on the known extraneous variables selected for matching, it will not equate them with respect to any other extraneous variables overlooked by the experimenter. Therefore, assigning pair members to experimental and control groups only on the basis of some convenience may result in nonequivalent groups with respect to unknown extraneous variables. Suppose, for example, that the pairs were assembled by selecting participants from two different clinical settings and matching one member from each setting to one member of the other setting. Then, for the sake of convenience, all pair members from one setting are assigned to the experimental treatment, and all pair members from the other setting are assigned to the control group. The problem is that if there are any differences between the groups of participants in the two settings on unknown extraneous variables, then these differences will result in a threat to internal validity, despite the matching of the groups on the known extraneous variables.

Campbell and Stanley (1966) and Van Dalen (1966) suggest, however, that matching pairs can be a powerful technique for ensuring group equivalence if that technique is *combined with randomization*. Members of matched pairs can be subsequently assigned *at random,* one pair member being assigned randomly to the experimental group and the other pair member to the control group. This combination of matching pairs and randomization will be used (1) to match pairs on extraneous variables that are known to be correlated with the dependent variable, and (2) to reduce the probability of group differences on unknown extraneous variables through the random assignment of pair members to the two groups.

Consumers of research should be aware of some of the advantages and disadvantages both of randomization and of matching. Randomization is often preferred, for example, if a large number of participants is available because it is difficult to match numerous pairs, especially if they must be matched on several extraneous variables. Therefore, it would be more efficient to randomize group assignment at the outset, because randomization alone decreases the probability of group differences with respect to both known and unknown extraneous variables.

Randomization is also generally preferred when more than one experimental group is to be compared with the control group. If, for example, three experimental groups are to be compared with one control group, then matched quadruplets rather than matched pairs will be needed. Matching quadruplets of participants will present considerable difficulty to any experimenter, especially if the quadruplets are to be matched on several extraneous variables. It will be much more efficient to assign participants randomly to each of the four groups at the outset than to try to match groups of four participants for subsequent randomization.

The combination of matching pairs with subsequent randomization of pair members to experimental and control groups may be preferred by some experimenters when only a small number of participants is available for inclusion in the experiment. As indicated by Christensen (2004), the risk for failure to equate groups as a result of randomization is greater with a small number of participants than it is with a larger number of participants. Therefore, experimenters may often feel more confident about group equivalence on known extraneous variables if pair matching is combined with subsequent randomization. Despite the disadvantages of overall matching and pair matching, many experimenters apparently believe that matching alone is better than nothing at all, as evidenced by the prevalence of articles in the research literature that use matching alone for assembling experimental and control groups.

Between-subjects designs have been discussed so far only with regard to experimental research. Between-subjects designs are also common in descriptive research, and some of the foregoing considerations are applicable to descriptive research designs. In addition, there are other specific considerations unique to descriptive research that need to be addressed.

Between-subjects designs are found in comparative research, cross-sectional developmental research, and surveys that compare the responses of different groups. Comparative research involves the description of dependent variable differences between groups of participants who differ with respect to some classification variable (e.g., children with palatal clefts versus children without palatal clefts). Cross-sectional developmental research uses a between-subjects design because separate groups of participants who differ with respect to age are compared. Some surveys are conducted for the purpose of comparing the interview or questionnaire responses of participants who fall into different classifications (e.g., hearing-aid users versus nonusers).

Between-subjects descriptive research designs may be bivalent, in which case the classification variable is broken into two mutually exclusive categories (e.g., speakers who have had laryngectomies versus speakers with normal larynges). Between-subjects descriptive designs may also be multivalent, in which case the classification variable is divided into categories that are ordered along some continuum (e.g., mild versus moderate versus severe hearing loss). Finally, between-subjects descriptive designs may include comparisons of participants who are simultaneously categorized with respect to more than one classification variable (e.g., male versus female; mild versus moderate versus severe mental retardation).

As is the case with between-subjects experimental designs, participant selection is the major consideration in between-subjects descriptive research designs. Consumers should recognize, however, that researchers cannot randomly assign participants to different classifications in a descriptive study. Instead, the researcher has to select participants who already fall within the various classifications (e.g., normal hearing versus hearing impaired). The main strategy in between-subjects descriptive research design, then, is selection of participants who fall into distinctly different categories of the classification variable but who are otherwise equivalent with regard to known extraneous variables. This is, indeed, a formidable task. A comparison of some problems encountered and some strategies used in designing between-subjects research studies with manipulable independent variables versus classification variables may be found in Ferguson and Takane (1989, pp. 237–247).

The first step in this design is the definition of criteria for selecting participants from each category of the classification variable. Consumers of research should pay careful attention to the manner in which selection criteria are defined. Classifications must be constructed that are mutually exclusive, that is, participants should fall into only one category with regard to each classification variable. For example, in a comparison of patients with cochlear hearing loss and patients with conductive hearing loss, all participants must fit the definition of only one of the two groups. Patients who are found to have both a cochlear and a conductive component to their losses would have to form a third comparison group, that is, patients with mixed hearing losses. Consumers are likely to notice that researchers vary in the strictness with which they define selection criteria. Compromises are often necessary in trying to establish well-defined groups and remain reasonably consistent with the actual characteristics of the participants that are available for study.

Although some classification variables are relatively easy to categorize, others may require more elaborate criteria for defining mutually exclusive groups of participants. Sometimes it may be necessary to use several measures in a battery of selection tests in order to classify participants. In many cases, a range of scores on a particular measure may be used to define arbitrary boundaries for classification. Consumers should examine the reliability and validity of tests used for classification in order to evaluate the effectiveness with which the researcher has assembled the groups of participants.

The second design step in between-subjects descriptive research is the attempt to equate participants on extraneous variables. Because participants cannot be assigned randomly to the various classifications, consumers of research should realize that equivalence of groups on all extraneous variables is quite difficult to achieve. The inability to eliminate this threat to internal validity is one of the reasons that many researchers are reluctant to infer cause–effect relationships from descriptive studies.

Because random assignment to classifications is impossible, the best alternative is to try to minimize group differences on extraneous variables known to correlate with the dependent variable. A common method for reducing extraneous variable differences is to match the various groups on the extraneous variables known to be most highly correlated with the dependent variable. Both overall matching and pair matching have been used for this purpose in between-subjects descriptive research. The advantages and disadvantages of these two techniques were discussed earlier. Neither technique fully eliminates characteristic differences between comparison groups, but many researchers consider using these techniques to be better than ignoring the problem of extraneous variables. The greatest problem, of course, is in overlooking relevant extraneous variables that can influence performance on the dependent variable.

In summary, between-subjects designs compare the performance of different groups of participants in experimental or descriptive research. In experimental work, the comparison is made between groups of participants who are exposed to different treatments or levels of the independent variable. In descriptive research, the performances of participants in different classifications are compared. Effective between-subjects designs include efforts to select groups that are equivalent regarding extraneous variables.

## Within-Subjects Designs

In within-subjects designs, the performance of the *same* participants is compared in different conditions. In experimental research, the participants are exposed to all levels of the independent variable. Longitudinal developmental studies are within-subjects descriptive designs because the same participants are studied as they mature. Correlational studies also include within-subjects designs because each participant is measured on all of the variables that are correlated. Experimental within-subjects design will be considered first, and additional comments will be made about within-subjects descriptive research designs.

In the preceding discussion of between-subjects experimental design, emphasis was placed on evaluation of attempts to equate groups of participants on extraneous variables. There is no problem with extraneous variables affecting the performance of one group of participants and not the other in a within-subjects design because only one group of participants participates. In other words, assignment of participants to experimental and control groups is not a problem. The basic concern in evaluation of a within-subjects design is that all conditions should be equivalent except for the application of the various levels of the independent variable. Action should be taken to ensure that observed changes in the dependent variable can be attributed to the effect of the independent variable rather than to the effect of nuisance or extraneous variables that can emulate the effect of the independent variable.

Many of these threats to internal validity may be related to the temporal arrangements or sequence of the conditions of a within-subjects experiment. Therefore, a necessary tactic in within-subjects experimental design is the attempt to control what is sometimes termed *sequencing effect* or *order effect.* Sequencing effect and order effect are not used consistently in the various textbooks on research design, but two distinct effects are usually identified regarding the temporal arrangement of experimental conditions. We will use the terminology employed by Christensen (2004, pp. 248–250) in describing these effects.

Christensen uses *sequencing effect* to describe the overall problem that occurs when participants participate in a number of treatment conditions and their participation in an earlier condition may affect their performance in a subsequent condition. He differentiates between two types of sequencing effects. The first effect is called an *order effect,* that is, a general performance improvement or decrement that may occur between the beginning and end of an experiment. For example, performance might improve toward the end of an experiment because of the practice in the task that they receive or because of familiarity with the experimental environment. On the other hand, participants may show a decrease in performance in the latter part of an experiment because of fatigue.

Christensen (2004) calls the second sequencing effect a *carry-over effect.* A carry-over effect is not a general performance change from the beginning to the end of an experiment but rather the result of the influence of a specific treatment condition on performance in the next condition. In other words, the results of one treatment condition may be carried over into the next condition. For example, in studies of temporary threshold shift (TTS) induced by presentation of intense noise, it is important that participants be given sufficient time to recover from TTS before experiencing a subsequent noise exposure. Otherwise, performance in the subsequent condition would be affected by the carryover of TTS remaining from the first exposure. This carry-over effect may occur whenever exposure to one treatment condition either permanently or temporarily affects performance in subsequent conditions. Temporary carryover can often be minimized with a rest period between experimental conditions, but permanent carryover is a more serious problem that will be discussed later in this section.

There are two major techniques for reducing sequencing effects: *randomizing* and *counterbalancing* the sequence of experimental treatments. Randomization is the presentation of the experimental treatment conditions to the participants in a random sequence. Random distribution of the treatments in the time course of the experiment will essentially wash out most sequencing effects in a within-subjects design. Sometimes, however, the experimenter may wish to examine the nature of a sequencing effect, and this cannot be done with randomization. Counterbalancing is a technique that enables the experimenter to control and measure sequencing effects by arranging all possible sequences of treatments and, then, randomly assigning subjects to each sequence. Any differences in performance attributable to the sequencing of treatment conditions can then be measured by examining the performances of participants who participate in the different sequences. In a sense, the sequence of treatment conditions will become another independent variable that is manipulated by the experimenter.

In some cases, sequencing effects may involve such severe or permanent carryover that within-subjects designs are not appropriate. For example, Underwood and Shaughnessy (1975) list experiments on the effects of instructions as being generally inappropriate for within-subjects designs. Suppose an experimenter wishes to study the differential effect of two types of instructions on participants' performance of a certain task. One set of instructions contains information that may influence performance, but this information is withheld from the other set of instructions. If participants always receive the informative instructions last, a possible order effect might be introduced (i.e., participants might warm up or become fatigued from the first to the second condition). If the sequence of instructions is randomized or counterbalanced, however, those participants who received the informative instructions first will not be likely to forget those instructions when tested later with the noninformative instructions. In other words, there will be a permanent carry-over effect from the informative to the noninformative instructions.

Whenever carryover is likely to be permanent, a between-subjects design is more appropriate than a within-subjects design. In the example of the effects of instructions on performance, participants can be randomly assigned to one of two groups: one group will receive the informative instructions, and the other group will receive the noninformative instructions. Whenever a sequencing effect cannot be controlled by randomization or counterbalancing, between-subjects designs are usually considered more appropriate. Whenever sequencing can be well controlled, within-subjects designs are often considered to be more powerful than between-subjects designs because the participants act as their own control group by participating in all experimental conditions.

Longitudinal developmental research is an example of the application of a within-subjects design to descriptive research. The longitudinal design differs from the between-subjects cross-sectional design because the researcher follows the same participants as they age or mature rather than measuring the performance of different groups of participants selected from each age range. This within-subjects developmental design allows the researcher to study the rate of development directly for each participant as time passes and the participants age or mature.

Correlational studies are also examples of within-subjects designs in descriptive research because they involve the application of a number of different measures to a group of participants. Sequencing effects can usually be controlled through randomization or counterbalancing the sequence of the tests administered.

## Mixed Designs

In many research studies, more than one independent variable is considered. The effects of two or more independent variables on a dependent variable may be examined in an experimental study. More than one classification variable may be investigated in a descriptive study. In many of these cases, one independent variable is studied with a between-subjects comparison, and the other independent variable is studied with a within-subjects comparison. Hence, a mixed design that incorporates each of the two tactics is used.

In an experiment in which two independent variables are manipulated, it may sometimes be better to measure the effects of one independent variable with a between-subjects design and measure the effects of the other independent variable with a within-subjects design. A descriptive study may incorporate a comparison of the correlation between two variables in one type of participant with the correlation between these two variables in another type of participant. A descriptive study may also incorporate a comparison of the longitudinal development of two different types of participants. Combined descriptive–experimental studies often involve a within-subjects experimental study of the effect of an independent variable on a dependent variable with two different types of participants. The experimental effect for one group would be compared to the experimental effect for the other group. All of these research studies would involve mixed designs because they incorporate both within-subjects and between-subjects comparisons.

Because mixed designs incorporate the tactics of both between-subjects and within-subjects designs, the foregoing discussion of both types of designs applies to the mixed designs. The cautions required to ensure group equivalence for between-subjects designs apply to groups compared in mixed designs. Similarly, the comments on randomizing or counterbalancing techniques apply to the within-subjects component of a mixed design.

It is important for consumers of research to be aware of the nature of mixed designs because of their prevalence in the communicative disorders literature. Consumers should be able to identify which part of a mixed design is a within-subjects comparison and which part is a between-subjects comparison, in order to evaluate the attempts made by the researcher to minimize the influence of extraneous variables.

## Single-Subject Research Designs

In addition to the group research designs discussed previously, there are many single-subject research designs that are prevalent in the research literature in communicative disorders. Single-subject designs may be applied to only one participant or to a small number of participants who are evaluated as separate individuals rather than as members of a larger group to be averaged together.

Although these designs are often referred to as single-subject designs, they do not necessarily employ just one participant. A study may employ more than one participant; however, if the analysis of the effect of the independent variable manipulation on the dependent variable focuses on one participant at a time, the study is usually considered to be a single-subject design. As Ingham and Riley (1998, p. 758) state:

> The term *single-subject* is actually a misnomer for such designs when they are used to test treatment outcome because the generality of findings based on only one subject is, of course, unknown. The number of subjects required is fewer than for group studies, but the exact number cannot be determined a priori. It is up to researchers to examine their results with individual subjects and judge how many replicated findings are needed to demonstrate to themselves, and to potential users, whether the generality of the treatment effect is adequately substantiated (Sidman, 1960). Single-subject designs earn their name because findings across multiple subjects are individually reported, and each subject is studied in depth over time (hence the term "time series").

Group research designs are based on comparison of the average behavior of one group of participants to the average of another group in between-subjects designs or are based on the comparison of the average behavior of one group of participants in two different conditions in a within-subjects design. Usually there is only one measurement of the dependent variable made per participant in each group or condition. Statistical comparisons of the averages of these measurements in different groups or different conditions form the basis for conclusions about the relationships of the independent and dependent variables. In single-subject designs, however, the focus is on a detailed analysis of the behavior of each individual participant under highly controlled and specified conditions. Rather than measuring each participant's behavior just once in each condition, multiple measurements of the dependent variable are made under different experimental conditions. Single-subject designs are often called *time-series* designs because a series of measurements of the dependent variable are made over a period of time.

Single-subject designs are similar in some respects to within-subjects designs in the sense that each participant participates in all conditions of the experiment that represent all levels of the independent variable. However, single-subject designs differ from within-subjects designs in that the focus is on the analysis of the performance of the individual participant in each condition rather than on how the group performs on the average in each condition. Single-subject designs include at least two time segments: a *baseline* segment of behavioral observation and a *treatment* segment in which the independent variable is manipulated. A simple time-series design with one baseline and one treatment segment is often referred to as an *AB* design, with the letter *A* referring to the first, or baseline, segment and the letter *B* referring to the second, or treatment, segment. Figure 3.1 diagrams a hypothetical AB single-subject design and illustrates the kind of small fluctuation in the dependent variable often seen in baseline and a dramatic increase in the dependent variable during the treatment segment. Single-subject designs often include other segments that incorporate design elements to improve control over extraneous variables; some of these design elements will be discussed later in this section and in Chapter 5.

In a baseline segment, the participant's behavior is measured over time with no intervention, changing of conditions, or manipulation of the independent variable. Some variability over time is expected in behavior, but the baseline segment is continued until reasonable stability is observed in the participant's behavior. Setting criteria for baseline stability is a controversial issue, but several characteristics of behavior in the baseline segment have been considered including *level, trend, slope,* and *variability* (Christensen, 2004; Kratochwill & Levin, 1992; McReynolds & Kearns, 1983; Barlow & Hersen, 1984). Level refers to the overall value of the dependent variable. Trend refers to whether the graph of the behavior in the baseline segment is flat, increasing, or decreasing over time. Slope is the rate of change over time, if any trend is evident. Variability is the range over which behavior fluctuates during the baseline segment. In general, a stable baseline implies no extensive changes in level and a reasonably small range of variability. Sidman (1960) has suggested a range of 5 percent as acceptable baseline variability, but this criterion may be too stringent for research in clinical, as opposed to laboratory, settings (Christensen, 2004). Baseline stability also implies either no systematic trend upward or

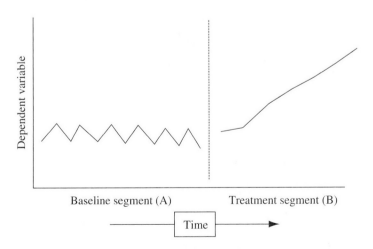

**FIGURE 3.1   Results of a Hypothetical Single-Subject Experiment.**

downward in the behavior or, if a trend is evident, a constant slope against which changes in behavioral trend during a treatment segment can be compared. Figure 3.2 illustrates hypothetical baseline data showing upward trends with different slopes (lines 1 and 2), a change in level (line 3), and large variability (line 4) and small variability (line 5) without a systematic level change or directional trend. More detailed analyses of possible outcomes of baseline measurements and their effects on the validity of single-subject designs can be found in Campbell and Stanley (1966; see especially Figure 3 on page 38), Barlow and Hersen (1984; see especially pages 71–79), and Kratochwill and Levin (1992; see especially Chapters 2 and 3).

Once the baseline segment has been completed, the treatment segment is introduced and the participant is exposed to the independent variable. Measurement of the dependent variable at specific intervals is continued during treatment in the same manner as during the baseline segment. Changes in the participant's behavior over time during the treatment are compared to the measurements taken during the baseline segment as an indication of the effect of the independent variable on the dependent variable. In group within-subjects designs, each participant's behavior is measured once under each level of the independent variable, and the average behavior of the group of participants is compared among conditions to see the effect of the independent variable on the dependent variable. In the single-subject design, the participant's behavior is measured several times under each level of the independent variable but no averaging takes place: the pattern of behavior over time is compared between the baseline and treatment conditions.

As stated previously, the simple time-series design with one baseline and one treatment segment is often referred to as an *AB* design. A common extension of this simple

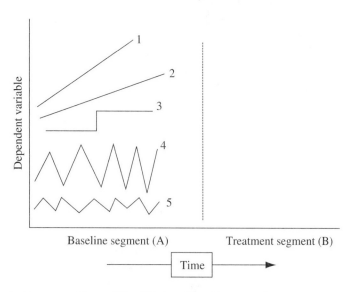

**FIGURE 3.2    Several Possible Baseline Outcomes in a Hypothetical Single-Subject Experiment.**

design is the *ABA* (or *reversal*) design in which a reversal to a second baseline condition is made after behavior change has been observed in the treatment condition. The ABA design is commonly used to determine whether behavior that has been temporarily changed will revert to baseline level if the treatment is removed. Another common extension is the *ABAB* design in which the reversal includes a second treatment segment following the second baseline segment. In an ABAB design, behavior changed during the first treatment segment should revert to baseline level in the second *A* segment and should show change again in the second *B* segment if the independent variable introduced during the treatment segment affected the dependent variable. Figure 3.3 diagrams a hypothetical ABAB single-subject design and illustrates a first baseline with moderate variability and no systematic level changes or trends, increase in the dependent variable during the first treatment segment, return to the original baseline level during the second baseline segment, and another increase in the dependent variable during the second treatment segment.

In addition to these reversal designs, a number of other design elements are available for incorporation into single-subject designs to examine changes in one dependent variable as a result of application of different independent variables or to examine changes across different dependent variables, people, or settings caused by introduction of an independent variable. A variety of alternating treatment designs, changing-criterion designs, and multiple baseline designs for accomplishing these objectives are discussed in more detail in a number of texts on single-subject design (e.g., Christensen, 2004; Kratochwill & Levin, 1992; McReynolds & Kearns, 1983; Barlow & Hersen, 1984). Christensen (2004) outlines methodological considerations in the design of single-subject experiments and compares them to considerations in the group designs. Whereas the group designs achieve control over extraneous variables by random assignment of groups or randomization and counter-balancing of conditions, single-subject designs use multiple time-series measures in both baseline and treatment segments to compare treatment effects to temporal fluctuations in

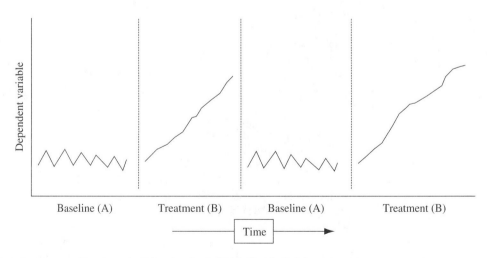

**FIGURE 3.3    Results of a Hypothetical ABAB Single-Subject Experiment.**

behavior without treatment. In addition, reversal designs are implemented to compare withdrawal of the independent variable to its application.

Christensen (2004) outlines the specifics of several other variations commonly employed in single-subject designs. Briefly, alternating treatment designs examine the effects of more than one independent variable (and their interactions) by applying different treatments to a single participant in alternating sequences that are counterbalanced after baseline measurement. Multiple baseline designs involve collection of baseline data on different behaviors of the same participant or on the same behavior of different participants. After baseline measurement, treatment is introduced at staggered times to different participants or different behaviors. The effects of treatments on different behaviors or participants are then examined in the various treatment segments. In changing criterion designs, treatment is introduced in successive segments with a higher criterion for improvement of behavior introduced in each segment as treatment continues. The effectiveness of the independent variable is demonstrated by successive replications of changes in the dependent variable as the standard for acceptance of a change in behavior increases (i.e., more is expected of the participant as a result of treatment in each successive segment).

Some recent articles in the literature comparing group and single-subject research designs illustrate some of the relative advantages and disadvantages of these two approaches in communicative disorders research. Prins (1993) discusses models for treatment efficacy in stuttering research with adults and considers a number of important research design issues. He states that (1993, p. 342)

> Depending on the questions asked, single-subject or group designs are appropriate.... A distinctive advantage of single-subject approaches, whenever appropriate, is that each subject serves as his own control, allowing the experimenter to escape subject matching problems and uncontrollable intersubject effects.

With regard to the subject matching that is necessary in group designs, Prins admonishes (1993, p. 342):

> When group designs are used, subjects who undergo different treatment conditions should be matched on measures of various behavioral and constitutional dimensions that could affect outcome ... for example: disorder, treatment, and family history; sex and age; speech variability under different conditions; personal-social attributes; speech motor functions, and the like.

However, Prins also points out the necessity to specify subject characteristics of participants in single-subject designs, especially with regard to external validity (1993, p. 342):

> Similarly, the description of subject characteristics could be extraordinarily important for the interpretation of outcomes in single-subject experiments. In fact, the erratic results of some studies in the response-contingent literature may have been a function of such factors....

Ingham and Riley (1998) outline four guidelines for treatment efficacy research with young children who stutter. In their guideline for verification of the relationship between treatment and outcome, they discuss several issues with regard to group and single-subject designs for evaluating treatment efficacy. They stress the ability of the single-subject design to study individual participants in depth through protracted pretreatment measures, to examine behavior changes over time, and to evaluate the effect of withdrawal of treatment on behavior. They also state that group designs are useful for following up single-subject studies that have demonstrated a treatment effect in order to compare different treatments and study factors, such as average time course of treatment or cost-benefit analysis. Robey (1999) and Wambaugh (1999) in an ASHA "Speaking Out Column" exchange views comparing the relative merits of group and single-subject designs from two different perspectives. Robey (1999) noted the importance of group data in nomothetic inquiry with its emphasis on generalization from a representative sample, as well as the usefulness of having an independent reference with a randomly assigned no-treatment group for comparison to a treatment group. Wambaugh identifies several values of single-subject designs, including the flexibility to modify the design in progress and the use of continuous measurement to highlight and control individual participant variability. Wambaugh concludes by saying (1999, p. 15):

> Despite their divergent approaches to examining relationships among variables, single-case and randomized group design are not incompatible in the study of communication disorders. The designs can be used in a complementary fashion or in a combination. Both offer important contributions to the establishment of empirically supported treatments in communication disorders.

Obviously these comments indicate that there is a place in communicative disorders research for both group and single-subject designs and that consumers of research need to be aware of the relative merits of both approaches. All of these articles (Prins, 1993; Ingham & Riley, 1998; Robey, 1999; Wambaugh, 1999) note both pros and cons of the two approaches and Table 3.1 summarizes several of the main issues discussed in these articles concerning the positive and negative aspects of group and single-subject designs.

Single-subject designs have become more prevalent in communicative disorders literature in both basic and applied research, and the popularity of this approach is likely to continue. Several research method books (e.g., Christensen, 2004; Kratochwill & Levin, 1992; McReynolds & Kearns, 1983; Barlow & Hersen, 1984) are available that cover single-subject design in more detail than can be presented here. Interested readers are referred to these sources for further detail concerning the single-subject approach to research design.

## External Validity Issues in Research Design

The preceding discussion has focused on issues of internal validity in research design. Some comments are now in order regarding external validity or generalizability of results. Campbell and Stanley (1966, p. 5) state that

> ...*external validity* asks the question of generalizability: To what populations, settings, treatment variables, and measurement variables can this effect be generalized?

**TABLE 3.1    Relative Merits of Group versus Single-Subject Research Designs[1]**

| Design | Advantages | Disadvantages |
| --- | --- | --- |
| Group | Nontreatment group provides independent reference | Not as flexible as single-subject design |
| | Participants can be randomly assigned to treatment groups | Intraparticipant variation not measured or controlled |
| | Can generalize from representative sample by inductive inference | Random sampling or close matching of participants needed for inference |
| | Can calculate effect size with meta-analysis | Does not reveal extended temporal measures of dependent variable |
| | Attrition has less effect on overall results | Needs larger number of participants |
| Single Subject | Smaller number of participants who act as their own controls | Less generalizable than group designs |
| | Avoids participant matching problems | Greater need for direct or systematic replications |
| | Examines behavior at level of individual participant over time | Interparticipant variability not well accounted for |
| | Flexible design can be modified during experiment | Needs more time and effort per participant to collect measurements |
| | Intraparticipant variation can be measured and controlled | Attrition has more effect on overall results |

[1]Table entries based on factors discussed in Prins (1993), Ingham and Riley (1998), Robey (1999), and Wambaugh (1999).

Much of the effort to strengthen the internal validity of a research design is aimed at specifying the independent and dependent variables, reducing the influence of extraneous variables, controlling random variability and measurement error, narrowing participant characteristics, limiting the setting involved, and following a strict measurement protocol. These efforts constrain the ability to generalize results to other people, settings, measurements, or treatment variables. Efforts to extend the generalizability of results can weaken the internal validity of a single study through relaxation of control over relevant extraneous variables. Yet both types of validity are important in any area of research, particularly in communicative disorders and other fields in which generalization to a variety of populations in different settings is critical. As Campbell and Stanley (1966, p. 5) state:

> While *internal validity* is the *sine qua non*, and while the question of *external validity*, like the question of inductive inference, is never completely answerable, the selection of designs strong in both types of validity is obviously our ideal. This is particularly the case for research on teaching, in which generalization to applied settings of known character is the desideratum.

Internal validity, as the *sine qua non,* must be dealt with in any study before external validity can be considered. Trying to generalize results that are not internally valid would waste both time and effort. As Pedhazur and Schmelkin (1991, p. 229) have said:

> Clearly, when internal validity of a study is in doubt, it makes little sense to inquire *to* what or *across* what, are its findings generalizable.

External validity is more difficult to deal with than internal validity in a single research study and often better addressed in a series of studies as part of a systematic research program. As Reynolds has stated (1975, pp. 13–14):

> The ultimate goal of research is always a general principle. Rarely, however, does a single experiment directly establish a general principle. A single experiment is concerned with the relation between a specific *independent variable,* which is manipulated by the experimenter, and a specific *dependent variable,* which changes as a result of changes in the independent variable. Each of such relations, established repeatedly in laboratories around the world, contributes to the formulation of the general principle.

Although researchers try to limit their generalizations, their results *may be* generalizable. However, external validity cannot be assumed until some evidence for generalization is presented. In the interim, consumers of research need to *limit* the degree to which they try to generalize the results of an individual research article.

The main concern for consumers of research is the manner in which researchers try to find solutions to the problem of generalizing results beyond the confines of an individual study. There are basically two ways of conceptualizing generalization. Pedhazur and Schmelkin (1991, p. 229) characterize them as follows:

> External validity refers to generalizability of findings *to* or *across* target populations, settings, times, and the like.

Pedhazur and Schmelkin (1991, p. 229) further specify the process of "generalizing to":

> The term *generalizing to* concerns validity of generalizations from samples to populations of which the samples are presumably "representative." Consequently, whatever the target population (e.g., people, times, settings), the validity of this type of generalization is predicated on the sample-selection procedures.

There are basically two procedures for improving the external validity of results for generalizing to other populations such as people, settings, and times. The first is selecting random samples of people, settings, and times to be included in the study. Random sampling helps to improve generalization to the specific target because all of the participants (or stimuli) in the population have an equal probability of being selected for inclusion in the study. A random sample comprises a group of participants that is likely to be more representative of the characteristics of the target population than a nonrandom sample. Random sampling is often discussed only with respect to participants in a study but can also be considered for settings, values of the independent variable, times of measurement, stimulus materials, measurement procedures, and so on.

Unfortunately, most investigators are unable to select random samples from the population of interest because of practical constraints. Pedhazur and Schmelkin (1991, p. 329) summarize this problem as follows:

> In spite of its appeal and seeming simplicity, simple random sampling is not used often in research. From a practical point of view, the task of selecting a random sample from a list can be extremely tedious and time consuming. More often than not, lists (let alone numbered lists) of elements of relatively large populations are difficult, if not impossible, to come by. Additional constraints arise when the population of interest resides in geographically wide areas. For example, a simple random sample of the population of the United States would probably yield a sample so dispersed as to make it an economic and physical nightmare.

Despite the practical constraints that limit the ability of most researchers to select simple random samples, there are alternate tactics for improving generalizability. First, there are several techniques for targeting a specific subpopulation by examining clusters or stratified groups of people and then taking random samples within local subgroups (see, for example, Kerlinger and Lee, 2000, pp. 163–187 or Pedhazur and Schmelkin, 1991, pp. 318–341 for discussion of these methods). Second, generalization can also be improved by increasing sample size; in general, a larger sample more closely approximates the characteristics of a population. The specific concern of how large a sample should be may be approached with a technique called *power analysis* that can determine a sample size based on the notion of what the probability is of detecting a hypothesized degree of effect of an independent variable on a dependent variable, or *effect size*. In general, increasing to a larger sample size leads to a higher probability of detecting an effect of a given size in the population. Power analysis is discussed in more detail in Pedhazur and Schmelkin (1991) and Cohen (1988).

Third, generalization can be improved with replication. A finding that can be replicated in a subsequent study is stronger in external validity than a finding that has not yet been replicated. Sidman (1960) discusses two major types of replication and calls the replication that would extend generalization to the same population, setting, or variables a *direct replication*. In a direct replication, the investigator repeats the research with the same participants or a new group of participants to confirm the reliability of the original results and test their generality within the limits of type of participants, settings, and measurements. Direct replication is an important and practical technique for improving generalization when it is impractical for an investigator to select a large or random sample.

In summary, generalization *to* the population, setting, or other variables is a difficult task, but this type of external validity can be improved with larger and more representative samples of the population of interest. Now we turn to the problem of generalization *across* populations, settings, or other variables of interest.

Pedhazur and Schmelkin (1991, p. 229) further specify the process of "generalizing across":

> *Generalizing across* concerns the validity of generalizations *across* populations. For example, results obtained with a sample from a given population (e.g., males, blacks, blue-collar workers), are generalized to other populations (e.g., females, whites, white-collar workers), or results obtained in one setting (e.g., classroom, laboratory) are generalized to another setting (e.g., playground).

Generalizing across populations, settings, or other variables should be limited until evidence is presented that indicates the validity of a result beyond the confines of an individual study. Evidence for generalization across these variables of interest may be derived from *systematic replication* studies (Sidman, 1960).

In systematic replication, the research may be repeated under different conditions or with different types of participants in order to extend generalization to other participants, settings, measurements, or treatments. Some aspect of the participants, setting, measurement, or treatment would be varied to include some new population, setting, measurement, or treatment to which the investigator would like to generalize results. Systematic replication is, therefore, a powerful tool for extending external validity beyond the limits of a single research study. Consumers of research should consider the generalizability of research results as limited to the particular kinds of participants, settings, measurements, and treatments used until such time as systematic replications demonstrate that the results are, in fact, more general. In some cases, of course, the limited generality of results may not pose a problem to consumers of research. The results of a study that use a particular measurement with a particular type of participant in a specific setting may be easily applied by professionals who normally use that particular measure with that kind of participant in that setting. Many research consumers, however, are interested in broadening the generality of research findings and will, therefore, be more interested in the implications of replication for the extension of external validity.

Unfortunately, replication has not always been as common a practice in behavioral research as it has been in biological, medical, or physical sciences. But in recent years, more and more replication studies have appeared in the literature, perhaps indicating more sensitivity to the need for replications to extend the external validity of behavioral research findings. Smith (1970) identifies several reasons why researchers do not often replicate studies, including such factors as lack of time, funds, or available participants; reluctance of some journals to publish replications of previous work; and development of new research interests by the investigator. In commenting on many of these reasons, Smith (1970, p. 971) states that

> if the goal of scientific research is to render established truths, then the neglect of replication must be reviewed as scientific irresponsibility.

Smith further suggests that many of these barriers to replication can be overcome by obtaining replication data when the original study is conducted. A section on replication can then be added to the original article. Muma (1993) issues a call for more replication research in communicative disorders. He surveyed research journals in the field over a ten-year period and found relatively few replications published, raising the possibility that there may be some unreplicable findings in the research literature.

Many combined experimental–descriptive studies involve a form of systematic replication because they compare experimental effects for different kinds of participants. The examples cited in Chapter 2 in the section entitled Combined Experimental and Descriptive Research show how the experimental effect on one type of participant may be compared with the experimental effect on another type of participant.

There are some excellent examples of replications that extend external validity in the communicative disorders literature. Guitar (1976) includes a direct replication in his correlational study of pretreatment factors associated with improvement in stuttering treatment and Monsen (1978) includes a direct replication in his regression analysis of acoustic variables used to predict the intelligibility of deaf speakers. In both cases the direct replications show results that are quite consistent with the results of the original studies, thus strengthening the generality of the original results within the limits of the same type of participants, settings, and measures.

Systematic replications have also appeared as follow-up articles or have been included in an article reporting the replication along with the original results. Silverman (1976) provides an excellent example of a systematic replication in which an experiment on listener reactions to lisping was replicated with a different kind of participant used as listeners in order to extend generality regarding other participants. Costello and Bosler (1976) evaluated generality to four other settings in their study of the efficacy of articulation treatment. Cottrell, Montague, Farb, and Throne (1980) examined generality to other measurements in their study of operant conditioning for improvement of vocabulary definition of developmentally delayed children by testing the degree to which their original results generalized to untrained vocabulary words within the same semantic classes. Courtright and Courtright (1979) examined external validity in regard to other treatments. They extended their earlier findings regarding imitative modeling as a language intervention strategy by replicating an earlier study of modeling versus mimicry and examining two other treatment variables associated with modeling—reinforcement and origin of the model—to determine their influence on the effectiveness of modeling.

The importance of replication for confirming the generality of results was recently highlighted in an exchange of letters to the editor in the *Journal of Speech, Language, and Hearing Research* concerning the efficacy of treatment for voice disorders. Roy, Weinrich, Tanner, Corbin-Lewis, and Stemple (2004) vigorously defended the results of an earlier article concerning a randomized clinical trial of voice treatment on the basis of the agreement of its results with a subsequent replication study. As Roy et al. (2004, p. 358) stated in their defense:

> We welcome the opportunity to respond to the recent letter to *JSLHR* from Dworkin, Abkarian, Stachler, Culatta, and Meleca (2004) wherein they questioned the strength of our evidence to support the effectiveness of voice amplification for teachers with voice disorders (as shown in Roy et al., 2002). Our first response is to make Dworkin and coauthors aware of another recently published randomized clinical trial by our group wherein the significant treatment results obtained with voice amplification (VA) in this study were replicated using a larger and entirely different group of teachers with voice disorders (Roy et al., 2003). In brief, we enrolled another 87 teachers with voice disorders, then randomly assigned them to one of three treatment groups: voice amplification (VA), resonance therapy (RT), and respiratory muscle training (RMT). Inspection of the results revealed that only the VA and RT groups reported significant reductions in mean Voice Handicap Index (VHI; Jacobson et al., 1997) scores and in voice severity self-ratings following treatment. Furthermore, results from the identical posttreatment questionnaire regarding the perceived benefits of treatment showed that compared to the other two treatment groups, teachers in the amplification group reported significantly more overall improvement, greater vocal clarity, and greater ease of speaking and singing. When one compares the results from our original investigation with the subsequent replication study, the similarity of the results observed for

the VA group in these two studies is both striking and confirmatory. Indeed, many of the concerns expressed by Dworkin et al. regarding the robustness, repeatability, and validity of the positive results obtained for the VA group in the first study are answered by this replication study. Muma (1993) suggested that "replicated results not only become factual but constitute substantiation and verification functions for research that extend external validity" (p. 927). Thus, in light of this replication, we find it highly unlikely that the positive treatment outcomes demonstrated by the VA group in the original study were somehow spurious or related to any of the measurement or methodological issues raised by Dworkin and colleagues in their critique. The more likely, and reasonable, conclusion is that the results from both studies are valid and reflect actual treatment gains made by each of these groups of voice-disordered teachers. In short, we feel secure in responding to Dworkin and colleagues' title question, "Is voice amplification for teachers with dysphonia really beneficial?" with an unequivocal "Yes."[3]

In addition to the obvious practical value of replication in affirming research results in this manner described by Roy et al. (2004), replication adds value to theoretical explanation of phenomena by the accumulation of consistent results across participants, settings, measurements, and treatments to extend external validity. Replication, then, is a critical step in the development of the nomothetic network. As Reynolds (1975, p. 14) concluded:

No single piece of research is sufficient to formulate a general principle; rather, each experiment contributes, either by repeating and verifying what is believed or by extending the generality of the principle.

Cohen (1997, p. 32) commented on the role of replication in the process of induction:

Induction has long been a problem in the philosophy of science. Meehl (1990a) attributed to the distinguished philosopher Morris Raphael Cohen the saying "All logic texts are divided into two parts. In the first part, on deductive logic, the fallacies are explained; in the second part, on inductive logic, they are committed" (p. 110). We appeal to inductive logic to move from the particular results in hand to a theoretically useful generalization. As I have noted, we have a body of statistical techniques, that, used intelligently, can facilitate our efforts. But given the problems of statistical induction, we must finally rely, as have the older sciences, on replication.

In summary, external validity, or generality of results, is usually limited in any single research article. Random sampling and direct replication can help to improve generalization within the limits of type of participant, setting, measurement, and treatment. Systematic replication can help extend generalization to other kinds of participants, settings, measurements, or treatments. As Hunter and Schmidt (1990, p. 13) state:

Scientists have known for centuries that a single study will not resolve a major issue. Indeed, a small sample study will not even resolve a minor issue. Thus, the foundation of

---

[3]From "Replication, Randomization, and Clinical Relevance: A Response to Dworkin and Colleagues (2004)," by N. Roy, B. Weinrich, K. Tanner, K. Corbin-Lewis, and J. Stemple, 2004; *Journal of Speech, Language, and Hearing Research, 47,* p. 358. Copyright 2004 by the American Speech-Language-Hearing Association. Reprinted by permission.

science is the cumulation of knowledge from the results of many studies. There are two steps to the cumulation of knowledge: (1) the cumulation of results across studies to establish facts and (2) the formation of theories to place the facts into a coherent and useful form.

Hunter and Schmidt (1990), then, emphasize not only the empirical importance of external validity but also its theoretical importance, which is in consonance with Stevens's (1968) reminder of the schemapiric view of science. In other words, external validity is important not only in research design but also in the integration of rational and empirical evidence in the explanation of the laws of behavior.

## Study Questions

**1.** Read the following article:

Bedore, L. M., & Leonard, L. B. (2000). The effects of inflectional variation on fast mapping of verbs in English and Spanish. *Journal of Speech, Language, and Hearing Research, 43,* 21–33.

  **a.** Describe the between-subjects and within-subjects components of this study.
  **b.** Identify which independent variables are manipulable and which are not.

**2.** Read the following article:

Jacobs, B. J., & Thompson, C. K. (2000). Cross-modal generalization effects of training noncanonical sentence comprehension and production in agrammatic aphasia. *Journal of Speech, Language, and Hearing Research, 43,* 5–20.

  **a.** What research design is used in this study?
  **b.** What are the various conditions used in this design?
  **c.** Examine Figures 2, 3, 4, and 5 and describe the effects of the independent variables on the dependent variables for these participants.

**3.** Read the following article:

Swanson, L. A., Leonard, L. B., & Gandour, J. (1992). Vowel duration in mothers' speech to young children. *Journal of Speech and Hearing Research, 35,* 617–625.

  **a.** Did this study use a between-subjects or within-subjects design to study changes in mothers' speech?
  **b.** What steps did the authors take to strengthen internal validity in this design?

**4.** Read the following article:

Stevens, L. J., & Bliss, L. S. (1995). Conflict resolution abilities of children with specific language impairment and children with normal language. *Journal of Speech and Hearing Research, 38,* 599–611.

   **a.** Did this study use a between-subjects or within-subjects design to study conflict resolution abilities in these children?
   **b.** What steps did the authors take to strengthen internal validity in this design?

5. Read the following article:

   Windsor, J. (2000). The role of phonological opacity in reading achievement. *Journal of Speech, Language, and Hearing Research, 43,* 50–61.

   **a.** How are between-subjects and within-subjects research designs mixed in this study?
   **b.** Identify the active and attribute independent variables that are used.
   **c.** Which of these variables is examined between-subjects and which within-subjects?

6. Read the following article:

   Gordon-Salant, S., & Fitzgibbons, P. J. (1995). Comparing recognition of distorted speech using an equivalent signal-to-noise ratio index. *Journal of Speech and Hearing Research, 36,* 706–713.

   **a.** How are between-subjects and within-subjects research designs mixed in this study?
   **b.** Identify the active and attribute independent variables that are used.
   **c.** Which of these variables is examined between-subjects and which within-subjects?

7. Read the following article:

   Blood, G. W. (1994). Efficacy of a computer-assisted voice treatment protocol. *American Journal of Speech-Language Pathology, 3,* 57–66.

   **a.** What kind of research design did the author employ?
   **b.** Identify the steps taken to improve internal validity.

8. Read the following article:

   Guitar, B. (1976). Pretreatment factors associated with the outcome of stuttering therapy. *Journal of Speech and Hearing Research, 19,* 590–600.

   **a.** What steps did the author take to improve external validity?
   **b.** Did this improve generalization *to* or *across* populations?

9. Read the following article:

   Muma J. (1993). The need for replication. *Journal of Speech and Hearing Research, 36,* 927–930.

   **a.** What are the results of Muma's survey of replications in a decade of published studies?
   **b.** According to Muma, how would replication improve research in communicative disorders?

# REFERENCES

Barlow, D. H., & Hersen, M. (1984). *Single case experimental designs.* Boston: Allyn & Bacon.

Bordens, K. S., & Abbott, B. B. (2002). *Research design and methods: A process approach* (5th ed.). New York: McGraw-Hill.

Campbell, D. T., & Stanley, J. C. (1966). *Experimental and quasi-experimental designs for research.* Chicago: Rand-McNally.

Christensen, L. B. (2004). *Experimental methodology* (9th ed.). Boston: Allyn & Bacon.

Cohen, J. (1988). *Statistical power analysis for the behavioral sciences* (2nd ed.). Mahwah, NJ: Lawrence Erlbaum Associates.

Cohen, J. (1997). The earth is round ($p < .05$). In L. L. Harlow, S. A. Mulaik, & J. H. Steiger (Eds.). *What if there were no significance tests?* (pp. 21–35). Mahwah, NJ: Lawrence Erlbaum Associates.

Costello, J., & Bosler, S. (1976). Generalization and articulation instruction. *Journal of Speech and Hearing Disorders, 41,* 359–373.

Cottrell, A. W., Montague, J., Farb, J., & Throne, J. M. (1980). An operant procedure for improving vocabulary definition performances in developmentally delayed children. *Journal of Speech and Hearing Disorders, 45,* 90–102.

Courtright, J. A., & Courtright, I. C. (1979). Imitative modeling as a language intervention strategy: The effects of two mediating variables. *Journal of Speech and Hearing Research, 22,* 389–402.

Ferguson, G. A., & Takane, Y. (1989). *Statistical analysis in psychology and education* (6th ed.). New York: McGraw-Hill.

Guitar, B. (1976). Pretreatment factors associated with the outcome of stuttering therapy. *Journal of Speech and Hearing Research, 19,* 590–600.

Hunter, J. E., & Schmidt, F. L. (1990). *Methods of meta-analysis: Correcting error and bias in research findings.* Thousand Oaks, CA: Sage Publications.

Ingham, J. C., & Riley, G. (1998). Guidelines for documentation of treatment efficacy for young children who stutter. *Journal of Speech, Language, and Hearing Research, 41,* 753–770.

Kerlinger, F. (1979). *Behavioral research: A conceptual approach.* New York: Holt, Rinehart and Winston.

Kerlinger, F., & Lee, H. B. (2000). *Foundations of behavioral research* (4th ed.). New York: Harcourt Brace.

Kratochwill, T. R., & Levin, J. R. (Eds.). (1992). *Single-case research design and analysis: New directions for psychology and education.* Mahwah, NJ: Lawrence Erlbaum Associates.

McReynolds, L. V., & Kearns, K. P. (1983). *Single-subject experimental designs in communicative disorders.* Baltimore: University Park Press.

Monsen, R. B. (1978). Toward measuring how well hearing-impaired children speak. *Journal of Speech and Hearing Research, 21,* 197–219.

Muma, J. (1993). The need for replication. *Journal of Speech and Hearing Research, 36,* 927–930.

Pedhazur, E. J., & Schmelkin, L. P. (1991). *Measurement, design, and analysis.* Mahwah, NJ: Lawrence Erlbaum Associates.

Prins, D. (1993). Models for treatment efficacy studies of adult stutterers. *Journal of Fluency Disorders, 18,* 333–349.

Reynolds, G. S. (1975). *A primer of operant conditioning.* Glenview, IL: Scott Foresman.

Robey R. R. (1999). Speaking out: Single-subject versus randomized group design. *Asha, 41(6),* 14–15.

Roy, N., Weinrich, B., Tanner, K., Corbin-Lewis, K., & Stemple, J. (2004). Replication, randomization, and clinical relevance: A response to Dworkin and colleagues (2004). *Journal of Speech, Language, and Hearing Research, 47,* 358–365.

Sidman, M. (1960). *Tactics of scientific research.* New York: Basic Books.

Silverman, E. M. (1976). Listeners' impressions of speakers with lateral lisps. *Journal of Speech and Hearing Disorders, 41,* 547–552.

Smith, N. C. (1970). Replication studies: A neglected aspect of psychological research. *American Psychologist, 25,* 970–975.

Stevens, S. S. (1968). Measurement, statistics, and the schemapiric view. *Science, 161,* 849–856.

Underwood, B. J., & Shaughnessy, J. J. (1975). *Experimentation in psychology.* New York: John Wiley & Sons.

Van Dalen, D. B. (1966). *Understanding educational research.* New York: McGraw-Hill.

Wambaugh, J. (1999). Speaking out: Single-subject versus randomized group design. *Asha, 41(6),* 14–15.

# CHAPTER 4

# Measurement Issues in Communicative Disorders Research

This chapter considers some general issues regarding behavioral and instrumental measures of speech, language, and hearing used in communicative disorders research. The topics to be discussed are (1) definition of measurement, (2) levels of measurement, (3) quality of measurement, (4) reliability of measurements, and (5) validity of measurements.

Measurement in communicative disorders research takes many forms. We may classify these measures generally as (a) instrumental measures of physical variables and (b) observer measures of behavioral variables. For example, electronic instrumentation is used for measurement of physiological variables, such as airflow, or acoustical variables, such as formant frequency. Behavioral observation is used for measurement of language variables, such as mean length of utterance, or speech variables, such as frequency of nonfluency. In many cases there are clear correlations between physical and behavioral variables, such as between vocal fundamental frequency and perceived vocal pitch. In many other instances, there are no clear correlations between physical and behavioral variables.

Measurement of many speech, language, and hearing behaviors depends on human observation of behavior in the form of self-reports (e.g., questionnaires or interviews), perceptual judgments of speech samples, transcription and analysis of language samples, auditory tests (e.g., SRT and speech discrimination), and formal language and speech tests. Baken and Orlikoff (2000, p. 1) state that

> Ever since the birth of their discipline, speech pathologists have relied heavily... on their highly trained ears for judgments of speech acceptability.

Gerratt, Kreiman, Antonanzas-Barroso, and Berke (1993, p. 14) also raise this issue in their discussion of voice quality measurement:

> Voices can be objectively measured in many ways (see, e.g., Baken, 1987; Hirano, 1981). However, voice *quality* is fundamentally perceptual in nature. Patients seek treatment for voice disorders because they do not sound normal, and they often decide on whether treatment has been successful based on whether they sound better or not. For this and other reasons, speech clinicians use and value perceptual measures of voice and speech far more than instrumental measures (Gerratt, Till, Rosenbek, Wertz, and Boysen, 1991). Further,

listeners' judgments are usually the standard against which other measures of voice (acoustic, aerodynamic and so on) are evaluated.

On the other hand, the importance of instrumental analysis in communicative disorders cannot be denied. As Baken and Orlikoff (2000, p. 2) point out: "objective observation and measurement of the speech signal and of its physiologic bases is a sine qua non of effective practice," and argue further that technological advances have led to a number of speech and voice measurement improvements including

- Increased precision of diagnosis, with more valid specification of abnormal functions that require modification.
- More positive identification and documentation of therapeutic efficacy, both for short-term . . . and long-term monitoring. . . .
- Expansion of options for therapeutic modalities. Most measurement techniques offer a means of demonstrating to patients exactly what is wrong, and they can often provide feedback that is therapeutically useful.

Advances in technology and our understanding of basic underlying physiologic and acoustic aspects of speech production have greatly improved instrumental measurements over the past few years. But, arguably, the personal computer has been the major driving force in the increased *use* of instrumental measurement procedures. Baken and Orlikoff (2000, p. 3) state that

Thanks to the proliferation of commercially available computer systems it has suddenly become easy to get measures, to generate numbers, to derive indices of function. In fact, it has become the "in" thing to do.

Sophisticated instruments coupled with high-performance computer systems are not, in and of themselves, an unmitigated solution to all measurement issues in communicative disorders. Baken and Orlikoff (2000, p. 3) offer the following caveat:

. . . the proliferation of plots, tabulation of ratios, elaboration of quotients, and extraction of indices does not inevitably indicate better diagnosis, deeper insight, or improved intervention. Data are valuable only to the extent that they are relevant to the problem at hand, are valid and reliable, and interpretable.

Clinicians must be cognizant of the principles, or rules, of instrumental measurement. Baken and Orlikoff (2000, p. 3) discuss several instrumental measurement principles and conclude their remarks on the subject with the following overriding principle:

Because the sole value of a measurement is in its interpretation, measurements can be no better than the knowledge and skills of the clinician who chooses and obtains them.

It should be obvious from the foregoing that *both* instrumental and behavioral measurements play an important role in clinical and research activity in communicative disorders. The main issue here for consumers of research is the importance of evaluating the quality of any measurements used in communicative disorders research. Regardless of whether measurements are instrumental or behavioral, accurate quantification of communication variables can be achieved only through careful measurement procedures that are designed to yield valid and reliable results.

## Definition of Measurement

We must first define *measurement* and identify some important properties of measurement that are required for valid quantification of communication variables. Stevens (1946, p. 677) presents a succinct definition of measurement when he states that

> . . . measurement, in the broadest sense, is defined as the assignment of numerals to objects or events according to rules. The fact that numerals can be assigned under different rules leads to different kinds of scales and different kinds of measurement. The problem then becomes that of making explicit (a) the various rules for the assignment of numerals, (b) the mathematical properties (or group structure) of the resulting scales, and (c) the statistical operations applicable to measurements made with each type of scale.

Nunnally (1978, p. 3) reinforces Stevens's definition with a similar statement:

> Although tomes have been written on the nature of measurement, in the end it boils down to something rather simple: *measurement consists of rules for assigning numbers to objects in such a way as to represent quantities of attributes.* The term *rules* indicates that the procedures for assigning numbers must be explicitly stated. In some instances the rules are so obvious that detailed formulations are not required. . . . Such examples are, however, the exception rather than the usual in science. . . . Certainly the rules for measuring most psychological attributes are not intuitively obvious.

Nunnally further states that measurement is a process of abstraction about an object or event because we measure its various *attributes* or *features*. In behavioral science, the objects that we measure are people who have many different attributes, and the events that we measure are their behaviors that have many attributes. Nunnally, and more recently, Graziano and Raulin (2004) emphasize the importance of careful consideration of the nature of each attribute before trying to measure it and careful attention to the rules of measurement to be sure that they are clear, are practical to apply, and do not require different kinds and amounts of skills by persons who use the measurement procedure. When different people employ the measuring instrument, or supposedly, alternate measures of the same attribute, they should obtain similar results.

Thus, an important goal in communicative disorders research is the measurement of speech, language, and hearing variables with a clear and practical set of rules. Nunnally (1978, p. 5) summarizes the process of development of measurement rules succinctly:

> In establishing rules for the employment of a particular measure, the crucial consideration is that the set of rules must be unambiguous. The rules may be developed from an elaborate deductive model, they may be based on much previous experience, they may flow from

common sense, or they may spring from only hunches; but the proof of the pudding is in how well the measurement serves to explain important phenomena. Consequently, *any* set of rules that unambiguously quantifies properties of objects constitutes a *legitimate* measurement method and has a right to compete with other measures for scientific usefulness.

# Levels of Measurement

In addressing the issue of explicit measurement rules, Stevens (1946, 1951) specifies four scales or levels of measurement on the basis of the operations performed in assigning numerals to objects or events. Although there is some debate among statisticians (Haber, Runyon, & Badia, 1970) regarding the number, characteristics, and appropriateness of Stevens's scales, his original measurement scheme has remained influential in modern statistical treatment of data (Kerlinger & Lee, 2000; Siegel, 1956) and will be used in this discussion. Knowing what level of measurement has been used to assign numerals to objects or events is an important step in ascertaining the appropriateness of procedures used to organize and analyze the results of a study.

The four levels of measurement outlined by Stevens are *nominal, ordinal, interval,* and *ratio* levels arranged from simplest to most complex. Table 4.1 shows defining characteristics and examples of each of the four levels of measurement. As Stevens (1951) points out, these scales reflect various degrees of correspondence between the properties of the number scale and the empirical operations performed to assign numbers to attributes of objects and events. Graziano and Raulin (2004) discuss four characteristics of the abstract number system that match empirical operations used in measurement of an attribute: identity, magnitude, equality of interval, and a true zero (or absence of the attribute measured). The four characteristics may be used to define the four levels of measurement and are cumulative in their application from nominal to ordinal to interval to ratio.

## Nominal Level of Measurement

The nominal level is the simplest level of measurement. The word *nominal* is derived from the Latin word for *name,* and the process of nominal measurement is essentially the naming of attributes of objects or events. At the nominal level of measurement, attributes of objects or events are classified into mutually exclusive categories by determination of the equality of the attribute measured for the members of each category. The only mathematical property applied to nominal measurements is identity: each member of a named class is identical in the attribute measured. "**Identity** means that each number has a particular meaning" (Graziano & Raulin, 2004, p. 77). Examples include the assignment of numbers to gender (female = 1 versus male = 2) or to a screening test result (pass = 1 versus fail = 0) or to a diagnostic category (stutterer = 1 versus nonstutterer = 2). In the three examples, each member of each category is considered identical for purposes of nominal measurement. Thus, all males are identical as a group and all females are identical as a group with respect to measurement of gender. All passes are identical as a group and all failures are identical as a group with respect to performance on the screening test. All stutterers are identical as a group and all nonstutterers are identical as a group with respect to diagnostic category.

**TABLE 4.1   Levels of Measurement**

| Scale | Defining Characteristics | Examples |
|---|---|---|
| Nominal | Mutually exclusive categories or named groupings | Pass/fail criterion on screening test<br>Type of nonfluency (prolongation vs. repetition)<br>Type of hearing loss (conductive, sensorineural, or mixed)<br>Stimulus categories (meaningful vs. meaningless syllables)<br>Diagnostic category (stutterer vs. nonstutterer)<br>Phoneme production (correct vs. incorrect) |
| Ordinal | 1. Mutually exclusive categories or named groupings<br>2. Ranks or ordered levels | Ranked severity groups (mild, moderate, severe)<br>Stimulus complexity (easy, moderate, difficult)<br>Socioeconomic status (low-, middle-, upper class)<br>Rank in class (e.g., first, second, third, etc.)<br>Ranking of members of a group by rated degree of any subject attribute (e.g., perceived degree of vocal hoarseness) |
| Interval | 1. Mutually exclusive categories or named groupings<br>2. Ranks or ordered levels<br>3. Equivalence of units throughout scale or constant distance between adjacent intervals | Standard scores on behavioral tests (e.g., PPVT-R, TOLD, CELF)<br>Ratings obtained with many equal-appearing interval scales<br>Fahrenheit and Celsius temperatures |
| Ratio | 1. Mutually exclusive categories or named groupings<br>2. Ranks or ordered levels<br>3. Equivalence of units throughout scale or constant distance between adjacent intervals<br>4. Equivalence of ratios among scale values can be determined<br>5. A true zero point exists on the scale | Vowel duration<br>Voice onset time<br>Sound frequency<br>Sound intensity<br>Air pressure<br>Air flow<br>Stuttering frequency<br>Number of misarticulations<br>Diadochokinetic rate<br>Speech intelligibility score |

The only mathematical operation accomplished with nominal level measurements is counting the frequency of occurrence of members of each category. Sometimes the categories are assigned numbers (e.g., pass = 1 and fail = 0; female = 1 and male = 2), but these numbers are just labels used for identification purposes and do not specify magnitude. Telephone numbers, Social Security numbers, or numbers on football players' jerseys are good examples of the use of numbers for identification at the nominal level. You cannot perform meaningful mathematical manipulations of these identification numbers other than counting frequency of occurrence of items in each category. For example, you cannot add two telephone numbers together, dial the result, and reach both parties. You cannot state that a football player numbered 19 is better than a player numbered 12 because his number is higher. A person with a higher Social Security number does not pay a higher premium or receive a higher benefit because of the higher social security number.

## Ordinal Level of Measurement

The ordinal level of measurement considers not only the identity of members of a category but also the magnitude of the attributes of objects or events by allowing us to rank these magnitudes from least to most. "**Magnitude** means that numbers have an inherent order from smaller to larger; for example, 5 is larger than 3" (Graziano & Raulin, 2004, p. 77). At the ordinal level of measurement, objects or events are put into a relative ranking by determination of a greater or lesser value of the attribute to be measured. An ordinal scale of height, for example, can be constructed by visually arranging a group of children from shortest to tallest without actually using a ruler to determine the height of each child. Attributes such as vocal hoarseness or stuttering severity can be ordered from least to most severe using a listener judgment procedure. With an ordinal scale, we know how the objects or events line up with respect to the attribute, but we do not know the size of the differences between each object measured. Class rank is a good example: the difference between the first and second student is not necessarily the same as the difference between the second and third student in their actual grade-point averages, which might be 95, 94, and 90. They rank 1, 2, and 3, but the difference between 1 and 2 is one point whereas the difference between 2 and 3 is four points.

## Interval Level of Measurement

The interval level of measurement includes identity and magnitude and allows us to specify the equality of the intervals between adjacent examples of the attribute measured. The interval level of measurement involves the determination of the equality of the distance, or equal intervals, between the objects or events on the attribute to be measured, but does not include a true zero point that indicates the absence of the attribute. "**Equal intervals** means that the difference between units is the same anywhere on the scale; for example, the difference between 2 and 3 is the same as the difference between 99 and 100." (Graziano & Raulin, 2004, pp. 77–78). The most common example of an interval scale is temperature measurement with the Celsius or Fahrenheit scales: the temperature markings on the thermometer are equal interval distances painted on the glass surface to represent changes in the volume of mercury as temperature rises and falls. However, the zero point is arbitrary and does not represent the absence of temperature. We can say that the difference between sixty and seventy degrees is the same as the difference between seventy and eighty degrees, but we cannot specify equality of ratios between temperatures. Some variables in communicative disorders (e.g., speech naturalness; see Martin, Haroldson, and Triden, 1984) can be measured with equal-appearing interval scales (say, for example, a one- to nine-point scale). Many standardized behavioral test scores are measured at the interval level, including psychological tests of intelligence, personality, and achievement that have scores based on deviation away from the average but that do not have a true zero. Many language tests have standard scores that are constructed in this way and result in interval level measurements (e.g., standard scores on PPVT-R, TOLD, or CELF).

### Ratio Level of Measurement

Ratio level measurements include identity, magnitude, and equality of intervals and allow for specification of ratios between numbers. The ratio level of measurement requires the establishment of a true zero and the determination of the equality of ratios between the objects or events in the attribute to be measured. "The zero on the abstract number scale is a **true zero,** which means that zero represents none of the variable" (Graziano & Raulin, 2004, p. 78). True zero represents an absence of the attribute being measured. Most physical measures are ratio level measurements (e.g., length, height, weight, pressure, velocity). Many behavioral attributes can also be measured at the ratio level, especially those that are based on summing the number of occurrences of a specific behavior. Stuttering frequency, for example, can be counted in a speech sample. It is possible to have zero nonfluencies (absence of stuttering behavior), and twenty nonfluencies in a sample represent twice the stuttering frequency as ten nonfluencies. In another example, speech intelligibility can be measured with a word-recognition test by counting the number of words spoken by a speaker that are heard correctly by a listener. A speaker can have an intelligibility score of zero, indicating that none of his or her words can be recognized correctly; and a listener can recognize twice as many words spoken by a speaker who is 80 percent intelligible as by a speaker who is 40 percent intelligible.

When a choice of levels is available, the preferred order is ratio, interval, ordinal, and nominal. Stevens (1951) argues for this order of preference because more statistical operations are permissible with the ratio than with the interval, with the interval than with the ordinal, and with the ordinal than with the nominal level (Stevens, 1951; see especially Table 6, p. 25). As Stevens (1958, p. 384) has said:

> Each of these scales has its uses, but it is the more powerful ratio scale that serves us best in the search for nature's regularities. . . . Why, it may be asked, do we bother with the other types of scales? Mostly we use the weaker forms of measurement only *faute de mieux.* When stronger forms are discovered we are quick to seize them.

Although researchers try to reach the highest level of measurement available (i.e., ratio), practical limitations or the lack of a suitable higher level measurement may force the use of a lower level of measurement. The statistical operations permissible with each level of measurement will be discussed in Chapter 6.

## Factors That Affect Quality of Measurement

A number of factors can affect the quality of measurements made in communicative disorders research. As Campbell and Stanley (1966) point out, instrumentation is one of the most important factors that can jeopardize the internal validity of treatment efficacy research. An exhaustive discussion of factors that can affect the quality of measurements in communicative disorders research is beyond the scope of this book, but mention of a few key factors can provide an important guide for consumers of research to follow in evaluating the quality of measurements made in research studies they read. Several sources are available that review specific factors to be considered in speech, language, and hearing measurements (see Baken & Orlikoff, 2000; Haynes & Pindzola, 2000; Katz, 1994). We will first consider some specific factors that need to be controlled in making measurements in communicative disorders research and then discuss the two general qualities of reliability and validity that are fundamental requirements in any behavioral or instrumental measurements.

## Test Environment

A poor test environment can easily jeopardize any behavioral or instrumental measurement of speech, language, or hearing. For example, research data may be contaminated by distractions, noise, interruptions, poor lighting, or inappropriate stimuli in a test environment. The degree to which the test environment affects a measure will vary depending on the measure, but several obvious examples come to mind immediately. Measures of auditory threshold may be affected by background noise, a problem in educational settings or industry, but one that is capable of much better control in research conducted in laboratories or clinics. Research measurements for children may be more prone to problems of distraction in an environment that is new, colorful, or filled with stimuli that can attract their attention. Any measurements that require adequate visual perception for correct responses must be made in an environment that has adequate lighting. Thermal comfort is necessary for participants to pay attention to tasks that require vigilant responses. In addition, it is important to keep such factors, as those mentioned, constant across participants so as not to differentially affect the performances of different participants. In short, the test environment must be appropriate to the task and kept constant across participants to avoid contamination of measurements.

## Instrument Calibration

Electronic and mechanical instruments must be kept in good working order and meet current calibration standards. For example, audiometers should be calibrated according to the current standard (ANSI, 1996). Calibration should not be faulty because of malfunction nor should it drift during the course of an experiment. Therefore, it is important for a researcher to check the calibration of instrumentation periodically during the course of a study. Instrumentation should not be changed during a study because measurements taken with one instrument may not necessarily match those from another (Read, Buder, & Kent, 1990; 1992). The method section of a research article should contain sufficient information for the consumer of research to ascertain the adequacy of the instrumentation and its calibration.

## Instructions to Participants

Instructions to participants for the completion of their tasks must be clear and appropriate for the population being measured. Cronbach (1984, pp. 56–57), for example, outlines several effective techniques for giving directions to formal test takers, stressing the need to be firm, audible, and polite in standardizing the instructions given to all participants. He stresses that directions should be "complete and free from ambiguity" and that testers should attempt to "standardize the state of examinees." Much like the test environment, instructions should remain constant across participants. Of great concern in recent years have been the issues of measurement with multicultural populations and individuals with disabilities (see Thorndike, Cunningham, Thorndike, & Hagen, 1991, pp. 16–17 and Chapters 14 and 15). The implication of linguistic differences and differential abilities for clarity of instructions is obvious in both issues. For example, measurements with deaf children whose first language is ASL should include instructions in ASL, not in signed English.

## Observer Bias

When human beings are judges, there is ample opportunity for their judgments to be confounded by bias in observing or rating samples of behavior of different participants or of participants participating in different experimental conditions. For example, judges' standards may change from one experimental session to another, raters may be influenced by knowledge of the purpose of the investigation, or observers may make judgments based partially on their expectations about the behavior of participants in different groups (e.g., children with and without cleft palate).

Rosenthal (1966) has written extensively about the effects on research results of the human experimenter as part of the measurement system and many writers now call the problem of biased human observations the "Rosenthal Effect." Rosenthal and Rosnow (1991, pp. 125–129) categorize these experimenter effects as "interactional" versus "noninteractional" observer biases based on whether the experimenter actually affects the participant's behavior or simply errs in observing it. A *noninteractional* effect occurs when the observer does not actually affect the participant's performance but does affect the *recording* of the participant's behavior. This class of experimenter effect includes *observer effects* (i.e., systematic errors in observation of behavior), *interpreter effects* (i.e., systematic errors in interpretation of behavior), and *intentional effects* (i.e., dishonesty or carelessness in recording data). As an example of noninteractional observer bias, consider what might happen if judges were asked to rate hypernasality in speech samples of children with cleft palate recorded before and after pharyngeal flap surgery. Observers might expect less hypernasality after surgery and thereby unknowingly rate the postsurgery tape recordings with lower hypernasality ratings: This will have no effect on the *actual* hypernasality in the children's speech but will affect the *reported* data. An *interactional* effect occurs when the observer's interaction with the participant actually changes the participant's behavior during the experiment. Rosenthal and Rosnow (1991) summarize five factors associated with human observers that may actually influence the behavior of research participants: *biosocial* attributes of experimenters (e.g., gender, age, race, bodily activity, etc.), *psychosocial* attributes of experimenters (e.g., personality characteristics such as anxiety, hostility, authoritarianism, etc.), *situational* variables (e.g., experimenter's experience in prior experiments or on earlier trials of the same experiment, familiarity with subjects, etc.), *modeling effects* (i.e. participants may behave as the experimenter does), and *self-fulfilling prophecies* (i.e., the experimenter's expectations and consequent treatment of participants may influence the participants' behavior). Rosenthal and Rosnow (1991, pp. 130–133) outline a number of techniques for controlling observer bias, including using multiple observers, minimizing observer–participant contact, and making observers "blind" regarding the nature of participants.

It is obvious from the foregoing that a number of specific factors can affect the quality of measurements made in communicative disorders research. The specific constellation of factors that needs careful attention will depend on the nature of the specific measurement to be made. Consumers of research will need to depend somewhat on their measurement experience in evaluating the quality of measurements made in the research articles they read. We now turn to two particularly important and general topics concerning what Thorndike et al. (1991) have termed "qualities desired in any measurement procedure"— reliability and validity.

## Reliability of Measurements

Reliability is an integral part of any research undertaking; it generally refers to the degree to which we can depend on a measurement. Two definitions of reliability are currently used in behavioral research. First, reliability means measurement *precision* (Kerlinger, 1979; Thorndike et al. 1991; Pedhazur and Schmelkin, 1991). A precise measure can be expected to remain reasonably stable if the measurement procedure is repeated with the same participant. An imprecise measure will show more fluctuation with remeasurement over time. Cordes (1994, p. 265) states that the most common use of the term *reliability* in communicative disorders research is related to the "general trustworthiness of obtained data," that common synonyms for reliability include "dependability, consistency, predictability, and stability," and that this view of reliability concerns the question of whether the observed "data could be reproduced if the same subjects were tested again under similar circumstances."

A second definition of reliability refers to measurement *accuracy* and stems from the mathematical *true score* model (also called *classical test theory*). Cordes (1994, p. 265) suggests that this second definition is a "subtype of the more general reliability, when that term is defined as consistency, dependability, reproducibility, or stability." In classical test theory, reliability of measurement is defined as the ratio of true-score variance to observed-score variance. As Pedhazur and Schmelkin (1991, p. 83) state:

> According to the true-score model, an observed score is conceived of as consisting of two components—a true component and an error component. In symbols:
>
> $$X = T + E$$
>
> where X is the fallible, observed score; T is the true score; and E is random error.

They further explain that

> Conceptually, the true score can be thought of as the score that would be obtained under ideal or perfect conditions of measurement. Because such conditions never exist, the observed score always contains a certain amount of error (Pedhazur & Schmelkin, 1991, p. 84).

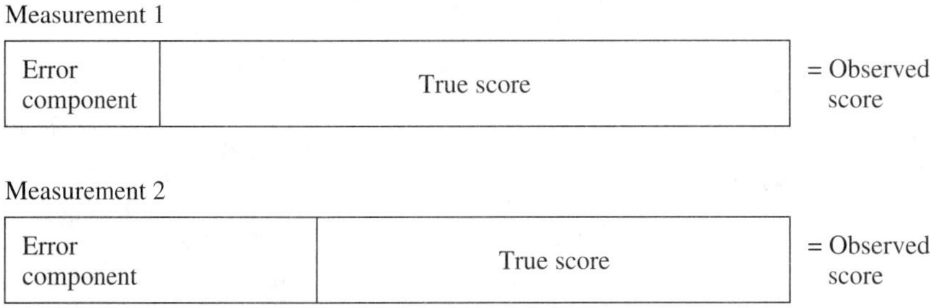

Measurement 1

| Error component | True score | = Observed score |
|---|---|---|

Measurement 2

| Error component | True score | = Observed score |
|---|---|---|

**FIGURE 4.1   Schematic Illustration of the Relationship of True Score and Error Component to Observed Score for Two Different Measurements.**

The concept of true scores and random (measurement) errors is illustrated schematically in the two hypothetical measurements shown in Figure 4.1. This illustration shows the partitioning of an observed score into a true score and measurement error and indicates the relative contribution of each to the observed score. One can see that the first measurement procedure has less error than the second. Observed scores obtained from the first measurement procedure will clearly be closer to the individual's true score than those obtained from the second measurement procedure. In classical test theory, then, the measurement with less error is more reliable because its observed score provides a more accurate (i.e., less error-prone) approximation of the true score.

Pedhazur and Schmelkin (1991) discuss two types of errors that may influence the reliability of the measurement process. The first type of measurement error is systematic. Systematic errors recur consistently with every repeated measurement. An example of systematic measurement error is an improperly calibrated audiometer that consistently produces an output of 20 dB HTL when the intensity dial is set at 10 dB HTL. The second type of measurement error is unsystematic error that occurs in unpredictable ways during repeated measurements. We can use the audiometer once again as an example of unsystematic measurement error. Suppose that this audiometer has an intermittent malfunction in the circuitry that controls the frequency of the sound being produced. When the frequency dial is set at 1,000 Hz the malfunction intermittently results in frequency outputs that vary anywhere between 900 Hz and 1,100 Hz unbeknownst to the examiner. In this situation the examiner would not know exactly what the actual output frequency is without monitoring each presentation with a frequency meter.

Measurement error emanates from many different sources and various authors have described potential reliability influencing factors from different perspectives. Lyman (1978) lists five general sources of measurement error that may affect reliability: (1) characteristics of the examinee, (2) behavior of the examiner-scorer, (3) aspects of the test content, (4) time factors, and (5) situation factors. Thorndike and Hagen (1977) identify three important classes of reasons for poor measurement reliability: (1) the person who is being measured may actually change from day to day; (2) the task may be different in two forms of the same measure or in different parts of one measure; and (3) the measure may provide a limited sample of behavior that may not yield dependable characterizations

**TABLE 4.2    Categories of Reliability and Methods of Assessment**

| Categories of Reliability | | |
| --- | --- | --- |
| *Stability* | *Equivalence* | *Internal Consistency* |
| Test-retest | Alternate or parallel forms | Split-half |
| | | Cronbach's alpha |
| | | Kuder-Richardson 20 |

of the behavior over the long run. Isaac and Michael (1971, p. 88) present a table that categorizes sources of measurement error as general versus specific, and temporary versus lasting characteristics of the persons who are measured. Ebel (1965) discusses six ways of improving test characteristics in order to reduce measurement error associated with the instrument itself. Kerlinger and Lee (2000) list a number of factors reflecting the influence of temporal changes in the participant such as mood, memory, and fatigue; the influence of changes in the measurement situation; and the influence of a very important source of measurement error: *unknown causes.*

Several different methods have been used to estimate the reliability of measurements in behavioral research, and these methods can be considered within three broad categories of reliability estimation: (a) *stability* (b) *equivalence,* and (c) *internal consistency.* The specific method chosen will depend largely on the specific sources of error being considered (Pedhazur & Schmelkin, 1991). Each of these approaches has certain advantages and disadvantages, and Cordes (1994) provides an excellent discussion of the limitations of each approach to reliability estimation in communicative disorders research. The different methods for estimating measurement reliability within each of the three broad categories are summarized in Table 4.2.

## Stability

The primary method for estimating the stability of measurement is known as the test-retest method. Pedhazur and Schmelkin (1991, p. 88) state that the test-retest method most closely relates to the "view of reliability as consistency or repeatability of measurement." This approach involves performing a complete repetition of the exact measurement and correlating the results of the two measurements. The resultant correlation coefficient, sometimes called the *coefficient of stability,* is taken as an estimate of measurement reliability. Cordes (1994) and Pedhazur and Schmelkin (1991) contend that the test-retest method of reliability estimation is particularly vulnerable to carry-over effects that may lead to overestimation of reliability.

## Equivalence

The primary method for estimating the equivalence of measurement is called the *alternate* or *parallel forms* method. This method of reliability estimation is sometimes used to avoid the potential carry-over effects associated with the test-retest method. Reliability estimation using equivalent forms is accomplished by correlating the scores of two different forms of a measure of the same attribute. The resultant correlation coefficient, sometimes called the *coefficient of equivalence* or *alternate form reliability,* is taken as an estimate of reliability. The principal limitation of using equivalent forms for the estimation of reliability is the difficulty associated with construction of equivalent forms and in the determination of the actual equivalence of measurements (Pedhazur & Schmelkin, 1991; Thorndike et al., 1991).

## Internal Consistency

One common method for estimating the internal consistency of measurement is known as the *split-half* method. This approach to measurement reliability was developed out of the confluence of theoretical limitations of the test-retest and equivalent forms methods and of certain practical limitations that dictate a single administration of measurements. Split-half reliability is, in a sense, a variation on alternate form reliability in which the two halves of a measure may be seen as constituting two alternate forms. The split-half approach requires that the items that constitute a given measure be split in half (e.g., even- versus odd-numbered questions of a test); each half is then correlated with the other for the measurement of the reliability coefficient (Pedhazur & Schmelkin, 1991).

A correlation coefficient used frequently with split-half data to express internal consistency reliability is derived from the Spearman-Brown formula (Thorndike et al., 1991). Using the split-half method to estimate the reliability of a one hundred–item test will result in a correlation coefficient that is based on only fifty item pairs; the effective length of the test is cut in half. The Spearman-Brown formula is based on the assumption that increasing the length of a test will, in turn, increase its reliability because larger samples of behavior permit more adequate and consistent measurements (Anastasi & Urbina, 1997). In essence, the Spearman-Brown formula mathematically corrects for the split-half reduction in test items and yields an estimate of the correlation coefficient that would be expected for the correlation of two versions of the whole one hundred–item test. For this reason, the Spearman-Brown formula is sometimes referred to as the Spearman-Brown *prophecy formula.*

Two other methods for internal consistency estimation of reliability are Cronbach's alpha and the related Kuder-Richardson #20 Formula (KR-20), which provide reliability coefficients that estimate the average of all possible split-half correlations among the items of a measure (Cronbach, 1990, pp. 202–206). Cronbach's alpha procedure is used for test items that are scored with multiple answers (e.g., multiple-choice items, answer ensembles such as "always, sometimes, never" or "strongly agree, agree, neutral, disagree, strongly disagree," or five-point rating scales). The KR-20 is conceptually and computationally similar to Cronbach's alpha but is used for dichotomously scored items (e.g., "correct-incorrect" such as the word-recognition scores of speech audiometry). Both methods provide indications of the homogeneity of test items relative to overall performance on a measure as an index of reliability.

The three categories of reliability estimation methods discussed previously are concerned with measurement error associated with temporal fluctuations (i.e., stability), differences between parallel forms (i.e., equivalence), and interitem consistency (i.e., internal consistency). These three methods, however, do not account for measurement errors that may emanate from the observer or observers who are making the measurements. A method that has become quite common in behavioral research for the estimation of measurement error associated with the observer is called "*inter*observer" or "interrater" agreement. Kearns (1990, p. 79) describes the interobserver method of estimating measurement error as follows:

> Interobserver agreement coefficients are used to evaluate the level of variability or inconsistency among observers who score the same behaviors. An acceptable level of agreement between observers is generally taken as an indication that changes in the observed behavior are true changes and not a result of variability in the way that target behaviors were scored.

Graziano and Raulin (2004, p. 88) discuss another way to conceptualize interrater reliability by stating

> If the measure involves behavior ratings made by observers, there should be at least two independent observers to rate the same sample of behavior. To rate independently, both raters must be **blind** to the ratings of the other; that is, they must be unaware of other observer's ratings.... If two raters always agree with one another, then the interrater reliability is perfect. If their ratings are unrelated to one another, then the interrater reliability is zero. However, the actual level of reliability is likely to be somewhere in between.

Interobserver agreement coefficients are typically derived from measurements made by two or more observers measuring the same event. In some instances, however, it is important to know how stable one observer is in measuring the same event on two different occasions. In that case, the measures made by one observer at two different times are compared and an "*intra*observer" agreement coefficient is calculated.

It is tempting to consider observer agreement coefficients in light of the categories of measurement listed in Table 4.2. In this regard, interobserver agreement would be placed under the general category of equivalence and intraobserver agreement under the category of stability. Despite the intuitive appeal for such categorization, it is conceptually unwise to do so. As Kearns (1990, p. 79) suggests, "Although the terms reliability and interobserver agreement have been used interchangeably in the applied literature, these terms actually differ in their conceptual and statistical properties."

Similarly, Cordes (1994, p. 270) points out that interobserver agreement methods of reliability estimation do not use the conceptual underpinnings of the true-score model and that they do not address reliability in terms of "dependability or reproducibility." Rather, interjudge agreement reliability estimates address only measurement consistency, or lack thereof, that can be attributed to "differences among observers." Cordes (1994, p. 276) issues a caveat regarding observer agreements that should be heeded by the prudent consumer of research:

> The reliability of observational data is more complex than reporting that some vaguely described observer agreement statistic fell at some certain numeric level.

Intraobserver and interobserver agreement measures, then, are important only because they tell us that the observer(s) measured the same thing. They do not, however, tell us if the measure itself is accurate in a "true-score" sense. Two observers can be in perfect agreement in providing an inaccurate measure. Intraobserver and interobserver agreement can, therefore, be considered an important first step in establishing reliability because they show that observers are consistent with each other, but more information about the accuracy and precision of the measure itself must accompany any observer agreement index.

A question frequently asked is "How high should the reliability coefficient be? Is 0.6 a sufficient reliability coefficient or should it be higher before I put my faith in the measurement?" Pedhazur and Schmelkin (1991) suggest that various researchers have used guidelines regarding minimally acceptable levels of reliability that tolerate low coefficients in the early stages of research but require high reliabilities when measurements are used for making important selection and placement decisions about individuals. Questioning the wisdom of such formulations, Pedhazur and Schmelkin (1991, p. 110) point out that an acceptable reliability coefficient cannot be achieved by decree, but, rather, "it is for the user to determine what amount of error he or she is willing to tolerate, given the specific circumstances of the study (e.g., what the scores are to be used for, cost of the study)."

The interpretation of reliability data is sometimes facilitated by the computation of the *standard error of measurement.* Thorndike et al. (1991, p. 102) define the standard error of measurement as "the standard deviation that would be obtained for a series of measurements of the same individual." In practice, the standard error of measurement is an estimate of the standard deviation of observed scores (Pedhazur & Schmelkin, 1991) that is used to assess the precision of a given measurement. Estimates of the standard error of measurement give an indication of the variability that might be expected in the score of any individual if the measurement were to be repeated a number of times. In general, small standard errors of measurement are associated with higher measurement reliability. Thorndike et al. (1991) have provided an excellent discussion regarding the computation and the interpretation of the standard error of measurement.

In evaluating the reliability of a measure, then, the consumer of research should look for both reliability coefficients and standard errors of measurement. A measure with good reliability will have a high reliability coefficient and a low standard error of measurement. A measure with poor reliability will have a lower reliability coefficient and a higher standard error of measurement.

As discussed previously, measurement errors may arise from a variety of sources. Cordes (1994, p. 273) points out that traditional reliability estimation methods that appear frequently in communicative disorders research are not comprehensive and may fail to capture and differentiate among these sources of error. Cronbach, Gleser, Nanda, and Rajaratnam (1972) advance the notion of generalizability theory that has been described as the most comprehensive method available for estimating measurement reliability (Cordes, 1994). Generalizability theory extends classical test theory by enabling the examiner to simultaneously "identify and distinguish among several sources of error (e.g., subjects, occasions, raters, items, time)" in a measurement (Pedhazur & Schmelkin, 1991, p. 115). Cordes (1994) and Pedhazur and Schmelkin (1991) point out that generalizability theory has been used fairly infrequently, probably because of its computational complexities. A readable discussion of generalizability theory and its applications is provided by Shavelson, Webb, and Rowley (1989). Notable uses of generalizability theory in communicative disorders research are the studies by Demorest and Bernstein (1992) and Demorest, Bernstein, and DeHaven (1996) regarding speechreading skills assessment. The introduction of more generalizability theory studies in our literature will advance our understanding of the reliability of measurements commonly used in communicative disorders research and will ultimately lead to improvement in the form of more reliable measures. For example, Scarsellone (1998) demonstrates how generalizability theory can be used for estimating multiple sources of error in the collection of observational data in speech and language research.

The conceptual and statistical underpinnings of generalizability theory have also been discussed by O'Brian, O'Brian, Packman, and Onslow (2003). Additionally, in a companion article these authors provide a practical application of generalizability theory by calculating various sources of measurement error in speech naturalness ratings (O'Brian, Packman, Onslow, & O'Brian, 2003). The discussion in the companion article clearly illustrates the utility of this method of analysis when one is examining observational data.

# Validity of Measurements

The validity of a measurement generally refers to the "truthfulness" of the measurement (Shaughnessy, Zechmeister, & Zechmeister, 2000). The validity of a measurement, then, can be defined as the degree to which it measures what it purports to measure (Kerlinger & Lee, 2000; Thorndike et al., 1991). Whereas reliability is the consistency or precision or accuracy of measurement, validity is truthfulness or correctness or reality of measurement. A reliable measure may be quite repeatable or precise but may not be true or correct. For example, a scale in a butcher shop may consistently and precisely weigh the meat put on it at a half-pound over the true or correct weight. Such a scale would be reliable but not valid, and customers of this shop would consistently and repeatedly pay the price of an extra half-pound for all of the meat they purchase. Reliability, then, does not ensure validity, but it is a necessary prerequisite for validity. That is to say, to be valid, a measure must first be reliable. Once reliability has been established, then the validity of a measure can be assessed.

As Kerlinger and Lee (2000) point out, if the measure in question is a physical one (e.g., measuring the sound pressure level of a pure tone), there is usually little difficulty in determining its validity. Physical measures generally present a more or less direct analogue of the property that the researcher wishes to measure. The validity of behavioral or cognitive measures, however, is often more difficult to determine. In some cases, it may be so difficult to directly measure certain human behaviors or characteristics that researchers may have to resort to indirect measures to make inferences about them. This has often occurred, for instance, in language research when data concerning linguistic performance has been used to make inferences about linguistic competence or language-processing strategies. The validity of such indirect measures may be difficult or even impossible to establish.

There are basically three ways in which to examine the validity of a measurement: (a) content validity; (b) criterion validity; and (c) construct validity (Anastasi & Urbina, 1997; Kerlinger & Lee, 2000; Thorndike et al., 1991).

## Content Validity

The content validity of a measurement may be established by logical examination of the content of test items to see how well they sample the behavior or characteristic to be measured. The various parts of the measure should be representative of the behaviors or characteristics that it is supposed to measure. This is usually determined by first describing all of the behaviors or characteristics to be measured and then checking the measure to see how well it samples these behaviors or characteristics. Suppose, for example, that researchers want to measure the language performance of a group of children. First, the researchers will have to outline all of the behaviors that will constitute those aspects of language performance they wish to sample (e.g., use of past and future tense of certain verbs or comprehension of grammatical relation between subject and object). Then they will have to determine how well their measure samples this universe of possible behaviors.

Content validation, then, is basically a subjective procedure for logically or rationally evaluating the measurements to see how well they reflect what the researcher wishes to measure. This analysis is usually done by the researcher or by a panel of judges assembled by the researcher for this task. As such, the analysis is not a strictly empirical measure of validity, but more a rational one, and it may be subject to error arising from the particular bias of the judges. There are many situations, however, in which content validity is the only type of validity that can be established.

Occasionally, the term *face validity* is confused or used interchangeably with *content validity*. Anastasi and Urbina (1997, p. 117) make the distinction between the two very clear by stating that face validity

> . . . is not validity in the technical sense; it refers, not to what the test actually measures, but to what it appears superficially to measure. Face validity pertains to whether the test "looks valid" to the examinees who take it, the administrative personnel who decide on its use. . . . Fundamentally, the question of face validity concerns rapport and public relations.

The fact that the face validity of a measurement is not considered validity in a technical sense in no way implies that it is a trivial concern. Anastasi and Urbina (1997, p. 117) point out that face validity is a desirable feature of a particular measurement in that "if test content appears irrelevant, inappropriate, silly, or childish, the result will be poor cooperation, regardless of the actual validity of the test."

## Criterion Validity

The criterion validity of a measurement may be established by empirical examination of how well the measure correlates with some outside validating criterion. The degree to which the measure correlates with a known indicator of the behavior or characteristic it is supposed to measure gives an indication of its criterion validity. There are two types of criterion validity that differ from one another only with respect to the time of administration of the outside criterion.

The first is *concurrent validity*. Concurrent validity is assessed when a measure and an outside validating criterion are administered at the same time. It might be important, for example, to develop a measure that is less time-consuming, cumbersome, and expensive than an existing one. The concurrent validity of the shorter version will be established by examining how well it correlates with the longer version. Concurrent validity may also be important in determining how well a measure is related to some concomitant occurrence in the real world outside the testing situation. For example, the concurrent validity of selected acoustic measurements of voice production could be established by examining them in relationship to listener judgments of voice quality.

The second type of criterion validity is *predictive validity*. Predictive validity is assessed when a measure is used to predict some future behavior. In such a case, the measure is administered first, time elapses, and then the criterion measure is administered. For example, college admissions officers may use college board scores to predict how well high school students might be expected to do in college. A treatment study may involve the use of certain pretreatment measures to predict how much patients might be expected to improve during the course of treatment.

The greatest difficulty in determining criterion validity lies in the selection of an appropriate outside validating criterion. There may be none in existence or it may be very difficult to measure one. The outside criterion itself needs to be valid and reliable and available for measurement. Many measures have never been subjected to examination of their criterion validity simply because no suitable outside criteria are available for measurement.

## Construct Validity

The construct validity of a measurement may be established by means of both empirical and rational examination of the degree to which the measure reflects some theoretical construct or explanation of the behavior or characteristic being measured. Kerlinger and Lee (2000, p. 670) call construct validity "one of the most significant advances of modern measurement theory and practice" because it brings both empirical and theoretical considerations together in examining *why* a measure is valid. As we emphasized in Chapter 1, a theory is an explanation of empirical knowledge of some phenomenon. If such an explanation exists, then the results of a measure should confirm the theory if the measure is valid *and* the theory is correct.

Construct validity can be established in several ways. For instance, a theory might predict that a particular behavior should increase with age. The measure can be administered to persons of different ages, and if the measured behaviors are found to increase with age, the construct validity of the measure with respect to the age aspect of the theory will be established. The theory might also predict that different kinds of people (e.g., pathological versus normal) should score in certain ways. If empirical testing with the measure confirms this, then the measure will have construct validity with respect to that aspect of the theory. The theory might also state that certain experimental manipulations should affect the measure; for example, drug administrations should reduce scores, whereas reinforcement should increase scores on the measure. If experiments are carried out that confirm these effects, the measure will have construct validity with respect to this aspect of the theory. Factor analysis, a statistical technique for reducing a large number of variables to a smaller number of clusters of common variables that identify common traits, might also be used to establish construct validity. This will involve the determination of how much the measure has in common with other measures known to fit certain theoretical constructs. Also, the internal consistency of the measure might be assessed by item analysis, a statistical technique for correlating each item in the measure with the overall score to see if each item measures the construct as well as the overall measure does.

The greatest problem in establishing construct validity lies in the validity or the correctness of the theoretical constructs used to predict performance. This is analogous to the problem finding a suitable outside validating criterion in predictive and concurrent validity. As Thorndike et al. (1991) point out, the construct validity of a test or measure is borne out if measurements agree with the theoretical prediction, but if the prediction is not verified, it may be the result of an invalid measure *or* an incorrect theory *or* both. A variety of sources are available to those interested in test validity and reliability, test development and standardization, and similar topics (Anastasi & Urbina, 1997; Cronbach, 1990; Thorndike et al., 1991). The reader is urged to consult these sources.

An excellent review of the reliability and validity of language and articulation tests was published by McCauley and Swisher (1984). They applied ten psychometric criteria to thirty articulation and language tests for preschool children and found many of the tests lacking in specificity regarding the ten criteria. The criteria included aspects of test construction such as description of the normative sample, sample size, evidence of test-retest reliability, information about criterion validity, and so on. Their results were not particularly encouraging and they (pp. 40–41) conclude that

> the reviewed tests failed to provide compelling evidence that they can reliably and validly be used to provide information concerning the existence of language or articulation impairment. These findings suggest important limitations on the use of such tests that must be considered by investigators and by speech-language clinicians.

McCauley and Swisher suggest that test authors and publishers should be encouraged to gather empirical evidence of test reliability and validity as an integral part of test development and that test users can wield considerable influence as consumers by evaluating the adequacy of tests before purchasing them. Sturner, Layton, Evans, Heller, Funk, and Machon (1994) conducted a psychometric examination of speech and language screening tests and drew conclusions similar to those of McCauley and Swisher regarding diagnostic tests.

## Study Questions

1. Read the following article:

   Klee, T., Carson, D. K., Gavion, W. J., Hall, L., Kent, A., & Reece, S. (1998). Concurrent and predictive validity of an early language screening program. *Journal of Speech, Language, and Hearing Research, 41,* 627–641.

   a. How are concurrent and predictive validity established for the Language Development Survey?
   b. What conclusions are drawn regarding the concurrent and predictive validity of the Language Development Survey?

2. Read the following article:

   Stuart, A., Allen, R., Downs, C. R., & Carpenter, M. (1999). The effects of venting on in-the-ear, in-the-canal, and completely-in-the-canal hearing aid shell frequency responses: Real ear measures. *Journal of Speech, Language, and Hearing Research, 42,* 804–813.

    **a.** What kind of reliability procedure is used in this investigation?

    **b.** Explain the reliability figure on page 807.

**3.** Read pages 21–30 in Chapter 3 of Siegel, S. (1956). *Nonparametric statistics for the behavioral sciences.* New York: McGraw-Hill.

    **a.** Write a brief summary of Siegel's discussion of each level of measurement.

    **b.** Siegel's examples of each level of measurement come from psychology and sociology. Find examples of each level of measurement in communicative disorders.

**4.** Read the following article:

McCauley, R. J., & Swisher, L. (1984). Psychometric review of language and articulation tests for preschool children. *Journal of Speech and Hearing Disorders, 49,* 34–42.

    **a.** What are the ten criteria suggested for reviewing language and articulation tests?

    **b.** Identify the consequences of each unmet criterion.

**5.** Read the following article:

Sturner, R. A., Layton, T. L., Evans, A. W., Heller, J. H., Funk, S. G., & Machon, M. W. (1994). Preschool speech and language screening: A review of currently available tests. *American Journal of Speech-Language Pathology, 3,* 25–36.

    **a.** What psychometric characteristics of screening tests do the authors review?

    **b.** Which of the tests reviewed meet the criteria for first level screening outlined by the authors?

**6.** Read the following article:

Punch, J., & Rakerd, B. (1993). Loudness matching of signals spectrally shaped by a simulated hearing aid. *Journal of Speech and Hearing Research, 36,* 357–364.

    **a.** How do the authors simulate a monaural hearing aid with multiple frequency response?

    **b.** What steps did the authors take to ensure proper calibration of this listening system?

**7.** Read the following article:

Kreiman, J., Gerratt, B. R., Kempster, G. B., Erman, A., & Berke, G. S. (1993). Perceptual evaluation of voice quality: Review, tutorial, and a framework for future research. *Journal of Speech and Hearing Research, 36,* 21–40.

    **a.** What problems with voice quality ratings are raised by the authors?

    **b.** What suggestions for improving the reliability of perceptual measures of voice quality are outlined by the authors?

**8.** Read the following articles:

Preminger, J. E., & Van Tasell, D. J. (1995). Quantifying the relation between speech quality and speech intelligibility. *Journal of Speech and Hearing Research, 38,* 714–725.

Preminger, J. E., & Van Tasell, D. J. (1995). Measurement of speech quality as a tool to optimize the fitting of a hearing aid. *Journal of Speech and Hearing Research, 38,* 726–736.

**a.** What procedures do the authors use to measure intrasubject and intersubject reliability?

**b.** What practical implications of their reliability results do they discuss?

**9.** Read the following article:

Nicholas, L. A., & Brookshire, R. H. (1995). Presence, completeness, and accuracy of main concepts in the connected speech of non-brain-damaged adults and adults with aphasia. *Journal of Speech and Hearing Research, 38,* 145–156.

**a.** How did the authors validate the main concepts?

**b.** What different measures of reliability and agreement were used by the authors?

# REFERENCES

American National Standards Institute. (1996). *American National Standard specifications for audiometers (ANSI s3.6–1996).* New York: American National Standards Institute.

Anastasi, A., & Urbina, S. (1997). *Psychological testing* (7th ed.). Upper Saddle River, NJ: Prentice Hall.

Baken, R. J., & Orlikoff, R. F. (2000). *Clinical measurement of speech and voice* (2nd ed.). San Diego, CA: Singular.

Campbell, D. T., & Stanley, J. C. (1966). *Experimental and quasi-experimental designs for research.* Chicago, IL: Rand-McNally.

Cordes, A. K. (1994). The reliability of observational data: I. Theories and methods for speech-language pathology. *Journal of Speech and Hearing Research, 37,* 264–278.

Cronbach, L. J. (1984). *Essentials of psychological testing* (4th ed.). New York: Harper & Row.

Cronbach, L. J. (1990). *Essentials of psychological testing* (5th ed.). New York: HarperCollins.

Cronbach, L. J., Gleser, G., Nanda, H., & Rajaratnam, N. (1972). *The dependability of behavioral measurements: Theory of generalizability of scores and profiles.* New York: John Wiley & Sons.

Demorest, M. E., & Bernstein, L. E. (1992). Sources of variability in speechreading sentences: A generalizability analysis. *Journal of Speech and Hearing Research, 35,* 876–891.

Demorest, M. E., Bernstein, L. E., & DeHaven, G. P. (1996). Generalizability of speechreading performance on nonsense syllables, words, and sentences: Subjects with normal hearing. *Journal of Speech, Language, and Hearing Research, 39,* 697–713.

Ebel, R. L. (1965). *Measuring educational achievement.* Upper Saddle River, NJ: Prentice Hall.

Gerratt, B. R., Kreiman, J., Antonanzas-Barroso, N., & Berke, G. S. (1993). Comparing internal and external standards in voice quality judgments. *Journal of Speech and Hearing Research, 36,* 14–20.

Graziano, A. M., & Raulin, M. L. (2004). *Research methods: A process approach* (5th ed.). Boston: Allyn & Bacon.

Haber, A., Runyon, R. P., & Badia, P. (Eds.). (1970). *Readings in statistics.* Reading, MA: Addison-Wesley.

Haynes, W. O., & Pindzola, R. H. (2000). *Diagnosis and evaluation in speech pathology* (5th ed.). Boston: Allyn & Bacon.

Isaac, S., & Michael, W. B. (1971). *Handbook in research and evaluation.* San Diego, CA: Edits.

Katz, J. (1994). *Handbook of clinical audiology* (4th ed.). Baltimore: Williams & Wilkins.

Kearns, K. (1990). Reliability of procedures and measures. In L. B. Olswang, C. K. Thompson, S. F. Warren, & N. J. Minghetti (Eds.), *Treatment efficacy research in communicative disorders.* Rockville, MD: American Speech-Language-Hearing Foundation.

Kerlinger, F. (1979). *Behavioral research: A conceptual approach.* New York: Holt, Rinehart and Winston.

Kerlinger, F. N., & Lee, H. B. (2000). *Foundations of behavioral research* (4th ed.). New York: Harcourt Brace.

Lyman, H. B. (1978). *Test scores and what they mean* (3rd ed.). Upper Saddle River, NJ: Prentice Hall.

Martin, R. R., Haroldson, S. K., & Triden, K. A. (1984). Stuttering and speech naturalness. *Journal of Speech and Hearing Disorders, 49,* 53–58.

McCauley, R. J., & Swisher, L. (1984). Psychometric review of language and articulation tests for preschool children. *Journal of Speech and Hearing Disorders, 49,* 34–42.

Nunnally, J. C. (1978). *Psychometric theory.* New York: McGraw-Hill.

O'Brian, N., O'Brian, S., Packman, A., & Onslow, M. (2003). Generaliziability theory I: Assessing reliability of observational data in the communication sciences. *Journal of Speech, Language, and Hearing Research, 46,* 711–717.

O'Brian, S., Packman, A., Onslow, M., & O'Brian, N. (2003). Generaliziability theory II: Application to perceptual scaling of speech naturalness in adults who stutter. *Journal of Speech, Language, and Hearing Research, 46,* 718–723.

Pedhazur, E. J., & Schmelkin, L. P. (1991). *Measurement, design, and analysis.* Mahwah, NJ: Lawrence Erlbaum Associates.

Read, C., Buder, E. H., & Kent, R. D. (1990). Speech analysis systems: A survey. *Journal of Speech and Hearing Research, 33,* 363–374.

Read, C., Buder, E. H., & Kent, R. D. (1992). Speech analysis systems: An evaluation. *Journal of Speech and Hearing Research, 35,* 314–332.

Rosenthal, R. (1966). *Experimenter effects in behavioral research.* New York: Appleton-Century-Crofts.

Rosenthal, R., & Rosnow, R. L. (1991). *Essentials of behavioral research* (2nd ed.). New York: McGraw-Hill.

Scarsellone, J. M. (1998). Analysis of observational data in speech and language research using generalizability theory. *Journal of Speech, Language, and Hearing Research, 41,* 1341–1347.

Shaughnessy, J. J., Zechmeister, E. B., & Zechmeister, J. S. (2000). *Research methods in psychology* (5th ed.). New York: McGraw-Hill.

Shavelson, R. J., Webb, N. M., & Rowley, G. L. (1989). Generalizability theory. *American Psychologist, 44,* 922–932.

Siegel, S. (1956). *Nonparametric statistics for the behavioral sciences.* New York: McGraw-Hill.

Stevens, S. S. (1946). On the theory of scales of measurement. *Science, 103,* 677–680.

Stevens, S. S. (1951). Mathematics, measurement, and psychophysics. In S. S. Stevens (Ed.), *Handbook of experimental psychology* (pp. 1–49). New York: John Wiley & Sons.

Stevens, S. S. (1958). Measurement and man. *Science, 127,* 383–389.

Sturner, R. A., Layton, T. L., Evans, A. W., Heller, J. H., Funk, S. G., & Machon, M. W. (1994). Preschool speech and language screening: A review of currently available tests. *American Journal of Speech-Language Pathology, 3,* 25–36.

Thorndike, R. L., & Hagen, E. P. (1977). *Measurement and evaluation in psychology and education* (3rd ed.). New York: John Wiley & Sons.

Thorndike, R. M., Cunningham, G. K., Thorndike, R. L., & Hagen, E. P. (1991). *Measurement and evaluation in psychology and education* (5th ed.). New York: Macmillan.

# Evaluating Treatment Efficacy Research

The purposes of this chapter are (1) to review factors that jeopardize the internal and external validity of research designs and (2) to analyze the internal and external validity of selected treatment efficacy research designs.

Although reports of treatment efficacy research in communicative disorders have appeared in the research literature for many years, recent attention has focused on efficacy research as an important component of "evidence-based practice" (Apel & Self, 2003). The concept of evidence-based practice originated in internal medicine with the work of Sackett and his colleagues in Canada (Sackett, Straus, Richardson, Rosenberg, & Haynes, 2000), and Ingham (2003) has discussed the history of the importation of this concept from medicine into our discipline. The often-quoted basic definition of *evidence-based practice,* published in an editorial on evidence-based medicine in the *British Journal of Medicine* by Sackett, Rosenberg, Gray, Haynes, and Richardson (1996, p. 71), is

> ...the conscientious, explicit, and judicious use of current best evidence in making decisions about the care of individual patients. The practice of evidence based medicine means integrating individual clinical expertise with the best available external clinical evidence from systematic research.

According to Ochsner (2003, p. 27):

> Evidence-based practice and its components of treatment efficacy and treatment effectiveness are receiving a growing emphasis. This increase is due, in part, to the requests of payers for proof that reimbursed services are likely to produce improvement. The growing trend of referencing research evidence to support clinical decision making also furthers our goal of providing the highest quality services to individuals with hearing, speech, and language disorders.

Robey and Schultz (1998) have discussed the source of pressures from government regulatory agencies and third-party payers for evidence of aphasia treatment efficacy and suggested a model that meets the research standards of accepted clinical research disciplines.

A recent flurry of publications on the importance of evidence-based practice in communicative disorders has appeared, including the special section of the Autumn 2003 issue of the *Journal of Fluency Disorders,* which contained five articles on evidence-based treatment of stuttering; a book and an article by Schlosser (2003, 2004) on evidence-based practice in augmentative and alternative communication; and the initiation of a series of articles on evidence-based practice by *The ASHA Leader* that began with a description of the myths and realities of applying the notion of evidence-based practice in communicative disorders (Dollaghan, 2004); and an ASHA Research Symposium published in the 2004 (vol. 37, no. 5) *Journal of Communication Disorders.* This chapter will not consider all of the broad issues that evidence-based practice comprises, but rather will focus specifically on the evaluation of treatment efficacy research as an important core component of evidence-based practice.

Olswang (1998) classifies *treatment efficacy research* along with *treatment outcomes research* as two subcategories of *clinical research.* Olswang defines clinical research as (1998, pp. 134–135) "that type of research that follows guidelines and principles of science to provide an understanding of human experience and behavior change" and specifies that in communicative disorders it is a "clinically relevant science" that attempts to understand the assessment and treatment of disorders by combining "scientific/methodological rigor and ecological validity." She differentiates treatment efficacy research that *proves treatment benefits* from treatment outcomes research that *identifies treatment benefits,* and states that "Efficacy research provides evidence that treatment works by ruling out possible alternative explanations for client change" (1998, p. 135). This chapter will focus on the concept of treatment efficacy from this point of view rather than on the broader areas of outcomes research or outcomes measures, which are covered in more detail by Fratelli (1998) than can be accommodated in this chapter.

Treatment efficacy research has been fundamental to the field of communicative disorders as witnessed by such publications as one sponsored by the American Speech-Language-Hearing Foundation (Olswang, Thompson, Warren, & Minghetti, 1990) and another sponsored by the National Institute on Deafness and Other Communication Disorders, which was published in its entirety in the combined June and September 1993 issue of the *Journal of Fluency Disorders.* In the latter volume, Olswang (1993, p. 126) states:

> In our discipline, the focus is on discovering the ways in which biological/organismic variables and environmental variables interact to define normal and disordered (typical or atypical) communication behaviors; the way these behaviors are acquired, lost, and restored. Accordingly, treatment efficacy research is an investigatory tool for examining the effects of environmental variables (i.e., treatment) on organismic variables (i.e., communication behaviors). As such, efficacy research is not limited to solely being a category of research designed to answer clinical questions regarding whether or not a treatment is effective. Rather, efficacy research is viewed more broadly as part of an armament for furthering scientific knowledge, for investigating phenomena with both theoretical and clinical application.

The Academy of Rehabilitative Audiology includes in its 1994 monograph *Research in Audiological Rehabilitation: Current Trends and Future Directions* a chapter on treatment efficacy by Montgomery that reviews the federal government definitions of treatment efficacy and effectiveness and discusses the use of outcomes measures in establishing treatment efficacy. Montgomery (1994, p. 318) cites the language used in the federal Office of Technology Assessment guidelines and states that the government defines efficacy as the "probability of benefit . . . under ideal conditions of use," whereas it defines effectiveness as the "probability of benefit . . . under ordinary conditions." Montgomery summarizes the relationship between treatment efficacy and effectiveness by stating (1994, p. 318)

> Thus, efficacy is an idealized concept—what one can expect of a particular clinical proce-dure at its best, whereas effectiveness refers to the results of the procedure applied in every-day practice. Most attention, not surprisingly, has been on establishing efficacy, because if a clinical procedure is not efficacious, it cannot be effective in routine use.

The American Speech-Language-Hearing Association published two supplements on treatment efficacy, one in the October 1996 issue of the *Journal of Speech and Hearing Research* and one in the February 1998 issue of the *Journal of Speech, Language, and Hearing Research*. The history of these articles, as traced by the editor of the supplements (Carney, 1996, pp. S3–S4), indicates the importance of and broad interest in this topic. In 1993 the American Speech-Language-Hearing Association, the National Institute on Deaf-ness and Other Communication Disorders, and the American Speech-Language-Hearing Foundation invited a group of researchers and clinicians to write technical articles regard-ing treatment efficacy for several different communicative disorders. The articles were originally designed to be used in contract negotiations with health care networks and for health care lobbying and advocacy activities. Although the articles were used for such pur-poses, an ASHA task force concluded that wider dissemination of the information would be useful to both researchers and clinicians. Following peer review, the articles were pub-lished in the two treatment efficacy supplements cited previously covering eight different communicative disorders including

- Traumatic brain injury in adults
- Stuttering
- Aphasia
- Hearing aids in the management of hearing loss in adults
- Dysarthria
- Hearing loss in children
- Phonological disorders in children
- Voice disorders

The coordinating editor of the two supplements highlighted the significance of the articles by stating (Carney, 1998, p. S60):

> Taken together, the articles in Parts I and II underscore the reality that each disorder has unique problems and solutions. More significantly, the articles demonstrate the efficacy of treatments that clinicians deliver to affected individuals in an effort to improve their ability to communicate. Implicit in all this is the contribution that communication scientists and re-searchers make to clinical intervention.

The broad concept of treatment efficacy is also related to the issue of outcomes mea-sures, and, therefore, should be an important part of the infrastructure of the National Out-comes Measurement System (NOMS) developed by the American Speech-Language-Hearing Association (Schooling, 2000). Montgomery (1994) states that the definition of efficacy implies several things, including the implication that benefit must be carefully defined with an "outcome measure that identifies and quantifies the presence and extent of the benefit" and he uses this concept in his working definition of treatment efficacy in adult aural rehabilitation (1994, p. 318):

> Treatment efficacy is the probability that individuals with hearing impairment in a carefully-defined diagnostic category will benefit from the application of a specific audiological rehabilitation procedure as determined by performance above a predetermined level on an outcome measure that meets stated standards for reliability and for validity of inferences that are typically drawn from it.

Montgomery's definition fits squarely with the measurement concepts just discussed in Chapter 4 and sets the stage for the analysis of research designs for the evaluation of treatment efficacy to be presented in this chapter.

In considering how outcomes are measured, Fratelli (1998, p. 16) discussed a range of measures and a range of methodologies used for measurement including the three-class system used for classifying outcomes measurements by the U.S. Department of Health and Human Services Agency for Health Care Policy and Research, as well as by the American Academy of Neurology. *Class I* includes Well-controlled studies, such as randomized treatment and control-group studies and time-series single-subject designs; *Class II* includes studies such as nonrandom group assignment research, program evaluations, and quality improvement studies; and *Class III* includes projects, such as case studies and historical reports. In this chapter, we are interested in outcomes measurement and methodology only within the context of the design of group and single-subject (primarily Class I and to some extent Class II) research studies for demonstration of treatment efficacy. Holland, Fromm, DeRuyter, and Stein (1996) apply the three-class system to the evaluation of treatment efficacy in aphasia, and a number of chapters in Fratelli (1998) consider many other aspects of Class II and III evidence.

More recently, Robey (2004) has presented an overview of classes of evidence applicable to evidence-based practice, highlighting the importance of inventorying the literature for relevance, quality, number, and consistency of findings to examine outcomes. He indicated that many hierarchies exist for classifying level or strength of evidence in addition to the three-class system cited by Fratelli (1998). Robey's brief report is so important and specific to the principles of evaluation of treatment efficacy research that we reprint it in its entirety here in Excerpt 5.1.

Olswang states (1998, p. 138) that treatment efficacy research employs many different designs because so many different research questions may be asked and that the independent variables include the treatment conditions and participant characteristics. Using our scheme outlined in Chapter 2, the treatment conditions will be manipulable (active) independent variables examined for cause–effect relations, and participant characteristics will be nonmanipulable (attribute) independent variables examined to assess the generalization of the effect of treatment conditions across populations. Olswang also states (1998, p. 140) that research questions drive the selection of dependent variables because the "... questions determine what data are needed to answer them..." and she discusses several different types of dependent variable measures that might be used for different purposes, such as measuring

## Levels of Evidence

### by Randall R. Robey

The evidence in evidence-based practice (EBP) may take many forms ranging from expert opinion to meta-analysis. Each form of evidence, though, is not equally persuasive in making the case that a certain clinical procedure should become an aspect of recommended care for members of a certain clinical population. The greater the scientific rigor in producing clinical evidence, the more potent is that evidence for influencing the formation of policies affecting clinical practice.

The literature bearing on a certain clinical procedure is inventoried for: the *relevance* of findings, the *quality* of findings, the *number* of findings, and the *consistency* of findings for establishing a clear and singular linkage between a certain clinical outcome and a certain clinical procedure applied to members of a certain clinical population.

The terms "levels of evidence" or "strength of evidence" refer to systems for classifying the evidence in a body of literature through a hierarchy of scientific rigor and quality. Several dozen of these hierarchies exist (Agency for Healthcare Research and Quality [AHRQ], 2002b). Some systems comprise three levels and others eight or more. The gradations in some hierarchies are based on randomization and experimental controls. The organizing focus for others may center on magnitude of effect sizes, confidence intervals, number of results, consistency of results, sample size, or Type I and Type II error rates (AHRQ, 2002a). In each application of EBP process, reviewers must select the most relevant levels-of-evidence system for the type of procedure being assessed (e.g., measurement technologies, diagnosis, prognosis, safety, efficacy, and effectiveness).

In the United States, the recognized authority regarding the assessment of scientific clinical research as AHRQ and the system in the "Example Levels of Evidence" table below is one used by AHRQ (2001). Some international organizations adapt AHRQ systems (e.g., Scottish Intercollegiate Guidelines Network); others use wholly different systems (e.g., World Health Organization).

### Example Levels of Evidence

| Sources of Evidence | Classification |
| --- | --- |
| Meta-analysis of multiple well-designed controlled studies | 1A |
| Well-designed randomized controlled trials | 1 |
| Well-designed non-randomized controlled trial (quasi-experiments) | 2 |
| Observational studies with controls (retrospective studies, interrupted time-series studies, case-control studies, cohort studies with controls) | 3 |
| Observational studies without controls (cohort studies without controls and case series) | 4 |

### References

Agency for Healthcare Research and Quality. (2001). *Making health care safer: A critical analysis of patient safety practices.* Evidence Report/Technology Assessment: Number 43. AHRQ Publication No. 01-EO58. Rockville, MD: Agency for Healthcare Research and Quality (www.ahrq.gov/clinic/ptsafety/).

*(continued)*

**E X C E R P T   5.1   Continued**

Agency for Healthcare Research and Quality. (2002a). *Rating the strength of scientific research findings.* AHRQ Publication No. 02-P022. Rockville, MD: Agency for Healthcare Research and Quality (www.ahrq.gov/clinic/epcsums/strenfact.htm).

Agency for Healthcare Research and Quality. (2002b). *Systems to rate the strength of scientific evidence. Summary, evi-*

*dence report/technology assessment: Number 47.* AHRQ Publication No. 02-E015. Rockville, MD: Agency for Healthcare Research and Quality (www.ahrq.gov/clinic/epcsums/strengthsum.htm).

impairment versus disability versus handicap, or measuring behavior change during treatment versus behavior change during a separate probe situation for assessing generalization. In addition, Olswang (1998) reviews the documentation of treatment efficacy through systematic analysis and interpretation of change in behavioral, physiological, and subjective dependent variables that reflect the different constructs of interest to investigators. In answer to the question "Why bother to conduct efficacy research?" Olswang (1998, p. 147) concludes that the need for treatment efficacy research "goes beyond calls for accountability" and embraces the notion that treatment efficacy research contributes to our understanding of the process of communication and its attendant disorders.

The federal government has long viewed treatment efficacy research within the context of experimental epidemiological designs for clinical trials of disease treatment, especially with regard to pharmacology research as administered by the U.S. Food and Drug Administration (FDA). Pocock (1983, p. 1) amplified this historical context in his statement:

> The evaluation of possible improvements in the treatment of disease has historically been an inefficient and haphazard process. Only in recent years has it become widely recognized that properly conducted clinical trials, which follow the principles of scientific experimentation, provide the only reliable basis for evaluating the efficacy and safety of new treatments.

How are clinical trials defined and what specific principles of scientific experimentation need to be applied? According to Pocock (1983, p. 1),

> Firstly, we need to define exactly what is meant by a "clinical trial": briefly the term may be applied to any form of *planned experiment* which involves patients and is designed to elucidate the most appropriate treatment of future patients with a given medical condition. Perhaps the essential characteristic of a clinical trial is that one uses results based on a limited *sample* of patients to make inferences about how treatment should be conducted in the general *population* of patients who will require treatment in the future. (author's italics)

Pocock (1983) outlined and described the classification, rationale, and scientific principles of clinical trials for various types of treatments, not only with particular attention to what is necessary for pharmacological studies but also with regard to other forms of treatment in addition to drug therapy. In discussing these other types of nonpharmacological treatments, he stated (Pocock, 1983, p. 2):

> Unfortunately, there has generally been inadequate use of well-designed clinical trials to evaluate these other non-pharmaceutical aspects of patient treatment and care....

Since the time of that writing, much attention has been devoted to improving the design of clinical trial research in many areas of behavioral treatment. According to Moscicki (1993, p. 183)

> The basic design in such research is the randomized controlled clinical trial, in which subjects are randomly assigned to experimental and control groups, and conditions of masking, or blindness, are maintained. This general design has been used most often in the pharmacotherapy trials; it is also applicable to trials of behavioral therapies.

These randomized clinical trials are often set within a more general research program that may be sponsored by the federal government or various private health groups. An overview of the administrative and funding issues of clinical research trials can be found on the FDA website (www.fda.gov/cder/handbook).

Moscicki reviewed the steps in the development of such research programs and stated (1993, p. 183):

> Development of such tests must follow an organized, systematic research program, in which treatment research progresses in several phases, with each phase building on the previous one.... Because of the complexity inherent in well-designed controlled clinical trials, conducting one or more pilot studies is essential to resolving difficult design and other issues prior to initiation of the full-scale experimental study.

Typically such research programs comprise five phases, as described in a number of important recent publications such as the following: the FDA website, the Moscicki (1993) article, the Pocock (1983) book on clinical trials for disease treatment, a background paper published by the U.S. government (Office of Technology Assessment, 1983), a project introduction paper by the Ad Hoc Practice Guidelines Coordinating Committee of the Academy of Neurologic Communication Disorders and Sciences (2001), an article on aphasia treatment (Robey & Schultz, 1998), an article on stuttering treatment (Jones, Gebski, Onslow, & Packman, 2001), and two editorials in the *American Journal of Speech-Language Pathology* (Peach, 2003, 2004). The five phases have been variously titled and defined in these references but basically they are described as the following:

- Phase I—research concerned with hypothesis development, safety issues, and risk factors
- Phase II—development of treatment methods and outcomes measures, and pilot studies of potential treatment effects
- Phase III—randomized clinical trials for evaluating treatment efficacy
- Phase IV—post marketing studies of long-term effectiveness and safety of treatment
- Phase V—follow-up studies of cost-effectiveness and consumer satisfaction

Robey and Schultz (1998) have adapted the five-phase model to research programs for evaluating the efficacy and effectiveness of aphasia treatment, pointing out where this health care model applies to aphasia and identifying which parts of it do not fit as well with behavioral treatments, such as issues of toxicity and safety. They summarized many of the aphasia treatment research activities that would fit under the general descriptions of the five phases listed and made a number of specific suggestions for the design of controlled clinical trials in Phase III aphasia treatment efficacy research. Robey and Schultz (1998, p. 795) captured the evolution from efficacy to effectiveness when they stated in their overview of the model,

> ...this broadly accepted model of clinical outcome research begins in Phase I with an insightful experimental treatment of some few individuals and culminates in Phase V with the assessment of the consequences of that treatment, perhaps as it has evolved, in terms of public health and the general economy.

The August 2001 issue of the *American Journal of Speech-Language Pathology* (vol. 10, no. 3) included a "Special Forum on Fast ForWord," which presented seven articles reviewing evidence concerning this treatment procedure within the context of these five phases of systematic research for determining the efficacy and effectiveness of treatment. The research reported in this forum was predominantly Phases I and II and the introduction to the forum stated that these studies set the stage for much needed Phases III, IV, and V studies to determine the efficacy and effectiveness of the Fast ForWord treatment. It is within this same context of research development stages that we will consider the design of treatment efficacy research, and our emphasis in this chapter will be on the validity of Phase III studies of randomized clinical trials for the evaluation of treatment efficacy.

Much of the material in this chapter is based on the survey of research designs in educational psychology research by Campbell and Stanley (1966) entitled *Experimental and Quasi-Experimental Designs for Research*. Their classification of research designs and of the factors that threaten the internal and external validity of these designs has had a strong impact on behavioral research. The popularity of their classification is evident in the many textbooks on behavioral research that have adopted it (e.g., Bordens & Abbott, 2002; Kerlinger & Lee, 2000; Pedhazur & Schmelkin, 1991).

The Campbell and Stanley classification comprises experimental and quasi-experimental designs commonly used in educational psychology, especially in research on teaching. Because we are dealing with research in communicative disorders that includes some other designs and that excludes some of the designs they use, some modification of their classification is necessary. Our discussion, however, is mainly based on their system, and we wish to express our debt to them for the influence that their work has had in shaping our thinking about the evaluation of research designs.

The next two sections of this chapter will be concerned with the two major criteria of internal and external validity formulated by Campbell and Stanley (1966) for evaluation of research designs on the effects of teaching methods and with the factors that jeopardize internal and external validity. These criteria are intended to be used for the evaluation of both experimental designs, in which the independent variable can be manipulated easily and extraneous variables can be well controlled, and quasi-experimental designs, in which the independent variable cannot be manipulated easily and extraneous variables cannot be well controlled. The latter designs are compromise attempts to approximate experiments in situations that will not allow for the easy manipulation of the independent variable and control of extraneous variables. These criteria are easily applied to treatment efficacy research in communicative disorders.

Campbell and Stanley (1966, p. 5) state that internal validity concerns the question: "Did in fact the experimental treatments make a difference in this specific experimental instance?" If an experiment has internal validity, the experimenter can conclude that manipulation of the independent variable (experimental treatment) caused the change in the dependent variable and competing explanations from lack of control of extraneous variables are minimized within the confines of the specific experiment. Christensen (2004, p. 198) defines internal validity as "...the extent to which we can accurately infer that the independent variable caused the effect observed on the dependent variable." If, indeed, a study has internal validity, the next concern is the degree to which the results of the experiment can be generalized. External validity according to Campbell and Stanley (1966, p. 5) "...asks the question of generalizability: To what populations, settings, treatment variables, and measurement variables can this effect be generalized?" Christensen (2004, p. 217) defines external validity as "...the extent to which the results of an experiment can be generalized across variations in people, settings, treatments, outcomes, and times." Campbell and Stanley formulate a list of twelve factors, of which eight jeopardize internal validity and four jeopardize external validity. An examination of the degree to which an experimental design minimizes these twelve factors indicates the degree to which the experiment has internal and external validity. In summarizing these important criteria, Campbell and Stanley (1966, p. 5) state:

> Both types of criteria are obviously important, even though they are frequently at odds in that features increasing one may jeopardize the other. While *internal validity* is the sine qua non, and while the question of *external validity,* like the question of inductive inference, is never completely answerable, the selection of designs strong in both types of validity is obviously our ideal.

Examination of many research designs reveals that primary emphasis is often put on internal validity and secondary emphasis on external validity. As Cohen (1997, p. 31) states: "... even before we... seek to generalize from our data, we must seek to understand and improve them."

## Internal Validity and Factors That Affect It

A major consideration in the evaluation of research designs is whether the researcher has controlled or accounted for the variety of factors that can have a significant effect on the validity of the data collected. The experimenter (and the consumer) needs to be certain that the change in the dependent variable is, in fact, caused by the experimental treatment and *not* by factors that can mimic the effect of the treatment. That is, the experimenter needs to eliminate alternate explanations that might account for the treatment effect. The fewer the alternate explanations, the greater the internal validity of the experiment. It is to the factors that can affect internal validity in both experimental and descriptive studies that we now turn.

## History

The first factor that can have an effect on internal validity is *history*. History, in an experimental context, is defined as events occurring between the first and second (or more) measurements in *addition* to the experimental variable. In other words: Has some event occurred to a participant or group of participants between measurements to confound the effect of the experimental variable or treatment? In such an instance, the experimenter cannot determine whether the result is a function of the extraneous events alone, the extraneous events interacting with the experimental treatment, or the experimental treatment alone.

An example should help clarify the impact that history can have on validity. Assume that an experimenter is evaluating a particular treatment approach for a group of young children who stutter. Unbeknownst to the experimenter, several of the participants are receiving treatment in their local schools. The experimenter evaluates fluency before and after treatment and concludes that the particular treatment produces increased fluency. The conclusion is suspect because an equally plausible explanation for the improved fluency is that the treatment received in school, rather than the experimental treatment, accounted for the decreased stuttering or, even more likely, the two treatment approaches (one in school, the other given by the experimenter) interacted to produce the observed result.

Some types of experimental designs are more prone to the contaminating effects of history than others. Long-term studies are more likely to be contaminated by history effects than are studies in which data are collected over a short time. In such cases, the longer the interval between the pretest and the posttest, the greater the likelihood that history will serve to contaminate the results.

## Maturation

The effect of maturation is similar to the effect associated with history. History refers to events that occur outside the experimental setting and, thus, outside the control of the experimenter. Maturation, on the other hand, refers to changes in participants themselves that cannot be controlled by the experimenter, changes that may cause effects that are attributed, incorrectly, to the experimental treatment. Examples of maturational factors are age changes, changes in biological or psychological processes that take place over time, and the like.

Obviously, maturation effects can play an important role in long-term treatment research. Take, for example, a language-stimulation program designed to improve expressive language in young children. The program might be introduced to two-year-old children whose language performance is evaluated before the initiation of the program. Then, the effects of the treatment program might be evaluated when the group of children reaches three years of age. Because of changes that occur in language performance (pretest at two years versus posttest at three years), the experimenter concludes that the language-stimulation program was successful in enhancing language development for young children. It is hardly likely, although not impossible, that such a study would appear in print because it is obvious that maturational processes—neurological, physiological, psychological—could have a role in changes in language performance. Furthermore, the interaction between maturational factors and the experimental treatment could have produced the improved performance rather than either maturational processes or the treatment operating singly.

Maturation has served to confuse certain types of research in communicative disorders or, at the very least, has made these kinds of research difficult to perform. A good illustration deals with the efficacy of early treatment for aphasia. There is still controversy over whether early intervention for aphasia produces benefits over and above what might be expected merely as the result of spontaneous recovery. The major difficulty confronting the researcher is to isolate or eliminate the effects of maturation (spontaneous recovery) so that changes in language performance can be attributed to the treatment program.

## Reactive Pretest

A third factor that can affect internal validity is the effect that merely taking a test may have on scores achieved on subsequent administrations of the same test. In other words, participants may react to a pretest when taking a subsequent test. This effect may be due to the practice afforded by the first test, familiarity with the test items or format, reduction of test anxiety, and so on. By their very nature, pretest–posttest designs are especially vulnerable to test-sensitizing effects or test-practice effects. As a simple illustration, take the measurement of speech discrimination in the audiology clinic. Let us assume that the investigator wishes to determine if auditory training will improve speech discrimination. The participant is tested for the first time with a standard discrimination test and then retested after treatment. The participant's score improves significantly and the investigator concludes that the treatment is beneficial. An equally plausible alternate hypothesis, however, is that the improvement in discrimination is simply a function of testing or practice with the discrimination test and that some improvement might have been observed if the participant had been merely retested without the treatment. It may also be, of course, that a portion of the change was due to the treatment. Obviously, in these circumstances, it would be extremely difficult to know which was which. Any time pretreatment tests are used, the reader must ask whether posttreatment changes are due to treatment effects, testing effects, or a combination of the two.

Brief mention should be given here to reactive versus nonreactive measures. Huck, Cormier, and Bounds (1974), among others, note that tests, inventories, and rating scales are referred to as *reactive* measures. They are reactive because they may change the phenomenon that the researcher is investigating. Huck et al. (1974, p. 235) emphasize that

> . . . any measure is reactive if it has the potential for modifying the variables under study, it may focus attention on the experiment, if it is not part of the normal environment, or if it exercises the process under study.

As Campbell and Stanley (1966, p. 9) point out, "the more novel and motivating the test device, the more reactive one can expect it to be." Videotapes and tape recordings may also be reactive measures. As a result, special care must be taken by the investigator to reduce the reactive effects of these recording devices.

A *nonreactive* measure, on the other hand, does not change what is being measured. Isaac and Michael (1971) put nonreactive measures into three categories: (1) *physical traces*—for instance, examining the condition of library books to determine their actual use rather than giving students a questionnaire on book usage; (2) *archives and records*—such as clinic folders, attendance records, and school grades; and (3) *unobtrusive observation*—in which the participant may not know that a particular behavior is being observed.[1] Although Isaac and Michael emphasize that nonreactive measures are not impervious to sampling bias and other kinds of distortion, Campbell and Stanley (1966) urge the use of such measures whenever possible.

## Instrumentation

Campbell and Stanley (1966, p. 5) define the instrumentation threat to internal validity as one "...in which changes in the calibration of a measuring instrument or changes in the observers or scorers used may produce changes in the obtained measurements." It should be clear from the following discussion that this threat to validity transcends types of research in communicative disorders. Instrumentation effects can be a threat to the internal validity of any research study.

The most obvious instrumentation threat to the validity of studies in communicative disorders is faulty, inadequate, or changing calibration of the equipment used in the research. Because all students in communicative disorders are taught about the importance of calibration in their clinical work, there is no need to belabor the point here. Appropriate calibration and ongoing monitoring of calibration are absolutely essential ingredients in the collection of valid data, whether the data are for research purposes *or* for clinical purposes.

How does the reader of a research article determine whether the equipment was calibrated or maintained in calibration throughout the duration of the study? In many instances, the researcher provides a detailed description of the equipment employed and the calibration techniques used. Provided that the reader has some knowledge of instrumentation and calibration procedures, the adequacy of the instrumental array can be assessed by a careful reading of the method section. Often, however, only sketchy information is available on the instrumentation used and the calibration procedures employed. Because journal space is at a premium, editors have a tendency to prune procedures to a bare minimum. As a result, we may run across such statements as, "the equipment was calibrated and remained in calibration throughout the study" or "calibration checks were conducted periodically during the course of the investigation."

Although it is readily apparent that mechanical and electrical instruments can be sources of error that pose threats to validity, it may be less obvious that such devices as rating scales, questionnaires, attitude inventories, and standardized language tests are also instruments and that their use or misuse can have a profound influence on the adequacy of the data

---

[1]For the interested reader, unobtrusive measures are discussed at length by Webb, Campbell, Schwartz, and Sechrest (1966), and Bordens and Abbott (2002).

collected in either experimental or descriptive research. A poor pencil-and-paper test, one that has not been standardized, one that has inadequate reliability, or one that was standardized on a sample different from that under investigation can have serious consequences for internal validity. For communicative disorders and other behavioral disciplines as well, considerable attention and research effort have been given to the development and evaluation of rating scales. These efforts have been made in recognition of the need to develop valid and reliable rating scale instruments to reduce the chances that the rating scale itself would pose an instrumentation threat to validity.

## Statistical Regression

Statistical regression is a phenomenon in which participants who are selected on the basis of atypically low or high scores change on a subsequent test so that their scores are now somewhat better (in the case of the low scorer) or somewhat poorer (in the case of the high scorer) than they were originally. The investigator may conclude that the treatment produced the change when, in reality, the scores have simply moved or regressed toward a more typical, mean score—that is, the scores have become less atypical. This occurs primarily because of measurement errors associated with the test instrument used in selecting and evaluating the participants. The more deviant or atypical the score, the larger the error of measurement it probably contains (Campbell & Stanley, 1966).

To illustrate, let us say that an experimenter is interested in assessing the value of an articulation treatment program in a school setting. After screening all the children with an articulation screening test, the experimenter selects for study those ten children who performed the poorest on the test; that is, had the lowest scores. The treatment program is initiated for the children, and a month later, the children are retested. An improvement is noted and the experimenter concludes that the treatment program is a success. The conclusion may be unwarranted if changes could have been caused by the extreme, atypical performance becoming less atypical (regressing toward the mean). If no intervention had been provided, the retest scores might still have shown some improvement without treatment.

To give another example, a group of hearing-impaired people might be evaluated and chosen to participate in a counseling study on the basis of their high scores on the Hearing Handicap Scale (HHS). In this case, a high score represents considerable handicap and a low score represents little handicap. A counseling program is initiated and after four counseling sessions, the participants are retested with the HHS. The investigator finds that after counseling the scores are lower than they were before counseling and concludes, again erroneously, that the counseling program was successful in reducing self-assessed hearing handicap. An equally plausible explanation is that the improved scores simply represent statistical regression and that the atypical scores would have become more typical scores even without counseling. It should be emphasized that statistical regression is not always a concomitant of extreme scores. As Campbell and Stanley (1966) point out, if a group selected for independent reasons turns out to have extreme scores, there is less likelihood that the data will be contaminated by regression effects. Zhang and Tomblin (2003) have published a tutorial on regression in longitudinal studies of clinical populations, and Tomblin, Zhang, Buckwalter, and O'Brien (2003) have analyzed regression in measures of language disorders four years after kindergarten diagnosis.

## Differential Subject-Selection[2]

The selection of persons to form experimental and control groups in experimental research can affect internal validity if selection is not done properly. Internal validity may be threatened because differences between participants in the experimental and control groups may account for the treatment effects rather than the treatment itself. In most experimental research, one important requirement is that the participants should be equal, on important dimensions, before experimental treatment or manipulation. The experimenter attempts to ensure equality by random assignment of participants to experimental and control groups. The absence of equality prior to treatment poses a subject-selection threat to the internal validity of experimental research.

To further explain, let us use an example dealing with an experimental study of phonological processing treatment. Assume that a researcher wishes to conduct an experiment to evaluate the efficacy of a new method of phonological processing treatment with young children. The researcher selects a sample of children with phonological processing deficits and assigns participants *randomly* to one of three groups: (1) a nontreatment group, (2) a standard-treatment group, and (3) a new-treatment group. Through random assignment, the researcher attempts to reduce the effects of any pretreatment differences among participants by distributing these differences randomly among the three groups. In this way, the effects of differences between experimental and control participants on treatment outcomes are minimized and differential selection of participants poses little threat to internal validity.

## Mortality

Mortality refers to the differential loss of participants between experimental and control groups or between other comparison groups that can threaten the internal validity of treatment efficacy research. The threat occurs because the participants who fail to complete the research procedure may be quite different in important respects from those participants who continue to participate in the study, and it is difficult to know how dropouts may differ from those participants who remain. For example, it might be possible that the participants who dropped out were the ones who might have benefited the least (or the most) from an experimental treatment. Follow-up studies are especially prone to the problems of mortality in studying the long-term results of treatment programs, because of the difficulty in locating the participants after the treatment has ceased.

Roy, Weinrich, Gray, Tanner, Stemple, and Sapienza (2003) addressed the issue of dealing with mortality in their study of three different treatments for eighty-seven teachers with voice disorders in which sixty-four participants completed all treatment and measurement aspects of the investigation. Roy et al. (2003, pp. 676–677) discussed two approaches to including participants in the final analysis of the results of the experiment: "intention-to-treat" versus "as-treated" analysis. In the intention-to-treat analysis, all of the participants are included in the final data analysis regardless of whether they completed the treatment.

---

[2]Although the current terminology identifies persons who participate in research as "participants" rather than as "subjects," we will continue to use the traditional term for the "differential subject-selection" threat to internal validity in order to be consistent with the terminology found in the extant body of research literature.

This assumes, of course, that the investigator can find all of the dropouts at the end of the study for posttest measurement. It often happens that not all can be found, but the investigator tries to include as many of the dropouts as possible. In the as-treated analysis, only those participants who completed all phases of the treatment are included in the final data analysis as a subset of participants representing those who stayed in the experiment. Then the researcher compares the as-treated participant group data to the intention-to-treat participant group data to determine if there are any substantial differences between the pretest–posttest outcomes for the two groups that would point to a specific effect that mortality had on the results. Roy et al. (2003) were not able to acquire data from all of the dropouts, but the intention-to-treat and the as-treated participant group comparisons yielded very similar results. Nevertheless, they exerted several cautions in their interpretation of the results because of the mortality problem. For example, they speculated that it might have been possible that the dropouts in one of the treatment groups had withdrawn because they did not perceive sufficient benefit from treatment, which would have inflated the average improvement results. Roy et al. also pointed out that analysis of the as-treated participants reflects what would be expected from the population that does finish treatment. It could be argued that this is really the population of interest in treatment efficacy research, that is, treatment under ideal conditions. In any case, mortality is a difficult issue to confront and Roy et al. (2003) dealt with it in as forthright a manner as could be expected.

## Interaction of Factors

The final threat to internal validity deals with the possible interaction effects among two or more of the previously described jeopardizing factors. Although these factors have been treated singly in this discussion, there is little question that they can interact with one another to cause an effect greater than each operating independently and, more importantly, greater than the experimental effect under investigation. As noted earlier, each of the jeopardizing factors or a combination of factors may also interact with the experimental variable to produce an effect that can be mistaken for the experimental effect alone. Oftentimes, however, it is the interaction between subject-selection and some other factor, especially maturation, that confounds the interpretation of the data.

One example may suffice. Let us say that we have an experimental group composed of second graders with specific language impairment on whom we wish to assess the efficacy of an experimental language treatment program. We use third-grade children with specific language impairment as the control group. The treatment program is initiated, and significantly greater gains are noted for the experimental group than are noted for the control group. We conclude that our experimental treatment program is a success. Note, however, that maturational influences may operate differentially for the two groups so that more rapid maturation and change in language development may occur for the younger children. Thus, the effect of the treatment program can be in large part due to subject-selection-maturation interactions rather than to the program itself. The picture is further clouded if a history threat has also occurred so that a significant portion, or perhaps any portion, of the experimental group receives treatment outside school. Instrumentation can interact with maturation and history if the language tests used to evaluate performance had low reliability, especially for second-grade children.

The major point is that the factors that can jeopardize internal validity can act singly or in concert to produce changes in performance or behavior that can be mistaken for the effect of the experimental treatment.

## External Validity and Factors That Affect It

As noted earlier in this chapter, external validity, as defined by Campbell and Stanley (1966), simply refers to the generalizability of the data; that is, the extent to which the results of a research study can be generalized to other people, settings, measurements, and treatments. Each of these four ways of generalizing results will be considered in this section. Four threats to external validity that are identified by Campbell and Stanley (1966) are outlined here. Each of these four threats provides an example of a problem in generalizing in one of these four ways: to other people, settings, measurements, or treatments.

Bracht and Glass (1968) extend Campbell and Stanley's (1966) discussion of external validity to include twelve threats to generalization that they classify under the rubrics of population validity and ecological validity. Population validity factors concern the populations to which results can be generalized. Ecological validity factors concern the environments to which results can be generalized (i.e., settings, measures, treatments). Consideration of all twelve factors is beyond the scope of this chapter, and we have chosen to review the four Campbell and Stanley threats as examples of threats to each of the main areas of generalization: people, settings, measures, and treatments. Interested readers are referred to the Bracht and Glass (1968) article for a fuller treatment of external validity.

It should also be pointed out that threats to external validity are qualitatively different from threats to internal validity. Serious threats to internal validity render results meaningless and uninterpretable and preclude the drawing of valid conclusions about the relations among the variables studied. Threats to external validity, however, only *limit* the degree to which internally valid results can be generalized. No single research study is expected to have wide-ranging generalizability to many different kinds of people, settings, measures, or treatments. Generalizations grow from cumulative research centered on a given topic. Researchers build a case for generalization from comparison of the results of many studies. Also, efforts to control threats to internal validity often reduce external validity by introducing greater specificity to the population and environment of the research design. Therefore, the accumulation of several internally valid research studies is necessary to overcome limitations to external validity. Christensen (2004, p. 217) states that "External validity is an inferential process because it involves making broad statements based only on limited information."

### Subject-Selection[3]

The first threat to external validity presents a problem in generalizing to other people. This threat concerns the degree to which the participants chosen for the study are representative

---

[3]Although the current terminology identifies persons who participate in research as "participants" rather than as "subjects," we will continue to use the traditional term for the "subject-selection" threat to external validity in order to be consistent with the terminology found in the extant body of research literature.

of the population to which the researcher wishes to generalize. If there are important differences between the two (and these differences may not always be apparent to the experimenter), then meaningful generalizations will be limited. We have emphasized earlier the importance of subject-selection to internal validity. It should be clear that subject-selection procedures can pose an equally important threat to external validity, especially because subject-selection may interact with the experimental variable to produce positive results only for certain people and not for others. Brookshire (1983, p. 342) discusses the problems of generalization of results of aphasia experiments and states:

> In any experiment, the population to which experimental findings can be generalized is determined by the characteristics of the subjects who participate in the experiment. In order for the results of an experiment to be generalizable to a given population, the sample of subjects which participates in the experiment must be representative of the population. That is, the sample must resemble the population with regard to those variables which are likely to affect the relationship between the independent and dependent variable(s).

Brookshire further states that investigators should report both the relevant variables used to select people and the characteristics of the people on these variables in order to make legitimate generalizations to a specific population. He discussed eighteen specific characteristics (e.g., age, severity of aphasia, handedness, visual acuity, time post onset) that could be relevant in specifying an intended target population for generalization.

The important point is that generalization should be limited to people who have characteristics in common with the participants studied. In other words, the participants must be representative of the population to which the researcher wishes to generalize and the relevant characteristics of the participants that determine their degree of representativeness should be specified in the article to allow readers to evaluate the generality of results to other people.

## Interactive Pretest

The second threat to external validity presents a problem in generalizing to other measures. This threat concerns the degree to which a reactive pretest may interact with an independent variable in determining the participants' performance on the dependent variable. In other words, participants who are exposed to a reactive pretest may react to an experimental treatment in a way that is different from people who have not been exposed to the pretest. The effect of the treatment may be demonstrated only for participants who are tested just before treatment and not for the population at large who might receive the treatment without the specific pretest.

Suppose a researcher is interested in assessing a particular aspect of stuttering treatment designed to reduce fear of speaking situations. The pretest involves an interview in which various measures of speaking fear are taken. The treatment program is initiated and following its completion, the participant is again required to answer questions about fear or to demonstrate his or her mastery of fear. The experimenter notes a significant decrease in fear of speaking situations and concludes that the program is successful. Although it may be true for the participants in the experiment, it may very well be that the treatment program would not be successful or would be less successful if administered to individuals who have not had the pretest experience. In this example, external validity is in jeopardy because of the interaction of the pretest and the experimental treatment.

## Reactive Arrangements

The third threat to external validity presents a problem in generalizing to other settings. Christensen (2004, p. 220) defines ecological validity as "the generalizability of the results of the study across settings or from one set of environmental conditions to another" and reactive arrangements limit this generalization. This threat concerns the degree to which the setting of the research is reactive or interacts with the independent variable in determining the participants' performance on the dependent variable. Campbell and Stanley (1966, p. 6) note that the "reactive effects of experimental arrangements" are such that they "would preclude generalization about the effect of the experimental variable upon persons being exposed to it in nonexperimental settings." For example, a child is taken from the classroom to the speech clinician's office to be given an experimental language-stimulation program. Is the effect of that language-stimulation program specific to the experimental setting of the clinician's office or can the language-stimulation program be equally effective in the normal classroom environment? How does the experimental arrangement interact with the treatment to produce the observed effect? If there is an interaction, then the treatment effects cannot be generalized to people who have not experienced the experimental arrangement. In this example, the experimental language-stimulation program might be modified so that it could be administered in the classroom and its effect there directly evaluated. If the treatment program is designed specifically to be administered by the speech clinician working in an office and no claims are made about the efficacy of the program in the classroom, then the experimenter would be justified in generalizing the treatment to all similar "experimental arrangements"; that is, *limiting* the generalization to similar settings rather than trying to extend it to a large variety of settings without sufficient evidence.

Some texts refer to a particular reactive arrangement as the "Hawthorne effect." Rosenthal and Rosnow (1991, p. 620) defined the Hawthorne effect as "the notion that the mere fact of being observed experimentally can influence the behavior of those being observed." The Hawthorne effect is basically a reactive arrangement in which changes in a participant's behavior occur simply because the participant knows that he or she is participating in a research study. The increased attention that the participant receives, the change in routine, the experimental setting itself may all act to cause a performance change that may mimic or accompany the change attributed to the independent variable alone. This effect was first noticed in studies of worker performance at a Hawthorne, Illinois, Western Electric Company telephone-assembly plant in the 1920s, hence, the name, Hawthorne effect. Parsons (1974) completed an exhaustive reanalysis of the Hawthorne research and concluded that the key elements of the Hawthorne effect are feedback to participants about their performance and reinforcement of performance. Parsons (1974, p. 930) concluded by defining the Hawthorne effect as "the confounding that occurs if experimenters fail to realize how the consequences of subjects' performance affect what subjects do." In other words, the Hawthorne effect is not just the simple problem of participants' awareness that they are participating in a research study but is related to how they perceive the consequences of their behavior during the course of the research. The control of the Hawthorne effect is best accomplished by ensuring comparability of treatment between groups in their knowledge of the nature of experimental treatments.

## Multiple-Treatment Interference

The fourth threat to external validity presents a problem in generalizing to other treatments. This threat concerns the degree to which various parts of a multiple treatment interact with each other in determining participants' performance on the dependent variable. This effect is likely to occur when more than one experimental treatment is administered to the same participants or when a treatment consists of a carefully sequenced set of steps. The threat to external validity lies in the fact that the results of a multiple-treatment study can be generalized only to people who would receive the same sequence and number of treatments.

An example might be a study in which fluency is reinforced and nonfluency is punished during a conditioning segment of an experiment on stuttering. It would be difficult to ferret out the individual effects of the punishment and the reinforcement in examining any reduction in nonfluency because of the multiple-treatment effect. Separate studies would be needed of the individual effects of punishment of nonfluency, reinforcement of fluency, and the combined punishment of nonfluency and reinforcement of fluency. In other words, the treatment must be representative of the kind of treatment to which the results can be generalized.

# Evaluation of Some Experimental Designs for Studying Treatment Efficacy

In this section, much of the material discussed previously will be applied to the evaluation of experimental designs for studying treatment efficacy. Many individuals express an interest in the analysis of treatment efficacy research because of the direct applicability of such research to clinical work. Also, much has been written about the validity of these designs (e.g., Campbell & Stanley, 1966). These designs incorporate within-subjects, between-subjects, or mixed comparisons and, therefore, serve to illustrate many of the concepts advanced in the earlier sections of this book.

In outlining the paradigms of the experimental designs to follow, we will adopt Campbell and Stanley's notation system (1966). The left-to-right orientation will indicate the progression of time from before to after treatment, and the vertical orientation will indicate simultaneous occurrences. *X* will be the symbol for the administration of the experimental treatment, and *O* will refer to the observation and measurement of the dependent variable. When participants are randomly assigned to groups, *R* will precede the appropriate groups. When participants are matched on known extraneous variables and subsequently assigned to groups at random, *MR* will precede the appropriate groups. When there are no formal means for certifying either of these attempts to equate groups in an experiment, dashed lines (- - - - - - - -) will separate the groups.

## Weak Designs

Campbell and Stanley (1966) identify several weak designs in educational research that may be applicable to the investigation of treatment efficacy in communicative disorders.

These experimental designs are weak in both internal and external validity. They are presented here to help the consumer of research to identify weak treatment research. They also may serve as a frame of reference for understanding the manner in which the stronger designs represent improvements on the weaker designs.

*The One-Shot Case Study.*    The first weak design is what Campbell and Stanley call the one-shot case study, and it can be diagrammed as follows:

X  O

In such a study, a single group is observed only once, after having been exposed to some treatment. For example, children with articulation disorders might be given an articulation test after treatment has been administered and their scores on this measure (dependent variable) used as an indication of the success of the treatment (independent variable). The major problem is that there is no reference point for comparison of the posttreatment scores on the articulation test; no pretest was administered and no control group was used. The *effects* of the articulation treatment cannot be evaluated because no comparison can be made to either pretreatment articulation performance or the performance of some group that does not receive treatment. Even if the articulation test scores are compared to existing norms, there is no basis for the conclusion that treatment affects the scores without pretreatment or control-group comparisons because no evidence is shown to indicate that articulation is better after treatment than it was before treatment. Campbell and Stanley also point out that this design may suffer from the "error of misplaced precision" because careful data collection represents a wasted effort without the opportunity for comparison of the posttest scores with control-group or pretest scores. The one-shot case study is fraught with threats to both internal and external validity when used as an experimental design for studying treatment efficacy. It is extremely difficult, if not impossible, to draw valid conclusions from the results of a one-shot case study.

*One-Group Pretest–Posttest Design.*    A second weak design discussed by Campbell and Stanley is the one-group pretest–posttest design, which may be diagrammed as follows:

$O_1$  X  $O_2$

In such a design, one group is assembled, pretested, exposed to the experimental treatment, and posttested. This is a within-subjects design because all participants are tested under two conditions: before and after treatment. For example, a group of children might be pretested on a language test and then tested again after treatment on the language test. This design is more commonly found in the research literature and represents some improvement over the one-shot case study. However, there are still numerous drawbacks to this design because of the threats to its internal and external validity.

The first problem concerns the effects of history because many events that could affect the posttest outcome may have occurred during the course of the experiment in addition to the experimental treatment. A child may participate in language activities in school that influence his or her performance after treatment. Maturation is also a threat because growth and development during the course of a study might affect the posttest, regardless of the application of the experimental treatment. Testing represents still a third threat because the pretest may increase the participants' ability to perform well on the posttest.

Instrumentation could be a threat if care is not taken to be sure that the pretest and posttest measures are equivalent. This is especially important when judgments of human observers are used in the pretest and posttest. For instance, the Rosenthal Effect could operate if the human observers are biased in their observations by the belief that a change should have taken place as a result of the experimental treatment.

Statistical regression is a threat to internal validity when groups with extreme scores are retested. This will be important when participants are selected because they have extremely poor pretest scores and are thereby considered good candidates for treatment. In such a case, regression toward the mean on a second test would be expected and could be a competing explanation for any performance gains after treatment. Threats to external validity are primarily the interaction of selection or pretesting with the experimental variable, factors that are better controlled in the stronger designs to follow. Therefore, even though this design appears to be an improvement over the one-shot case study, it is still a weak design with many threats to both internal and external validity.

**The Static-Group Comparison.**    Another weak design is called the static-group comparison and can be diagrammed as follows:

$$\frac{X \quad O_1}{O_2}$$

In such a study, a group that has been exposed to the experimental treatment is compared to another group that has not, but no attempt is made to pretest the groups or to equate them by randomization or matching. This is a between-subjects design because two different groups are compared to each other. For example, children exposed to language treatment might be compared with children not exposed to such treatment to study the effects of treatment on their language performance.

There are two major problems with such a design. First, there is no pretest against which to compare posttest scores. Second, there is no formal means of certifying the equivalence of the groups on relevant extraneous variables, so any differences between the two groups may not be a result of the treatment program alone. Differential subject-selection in the two groups would, therefore, be the greatest threat to internal validity because of lack of knowledge about extraneous variables in both groups. Also, any experimental mortality would seriously affect the internal validity of this design because there would be no way of certifying extraneous variables associated with mortality or what effect such variables would have on the dependent variable in addition to the experimental treatment. Interaction of selection and mortality with the other factors would also threaten internal validity. The interaction of selection with the experimental variable would be the greatest threat to external validity, again because of the lack of knowledge about extraneous variables.

***Nonequivalent Control-Group Design.***   A fourth weak design is the nonequivalent control-group design, which can be diagrammed as follows:

$$\begin{array}{c} O_1 \quad X \quad O_2 \\ \hline O_3 \qquad O_4 \end{array}$$

In such a study, one group is formed, pretested, exposed to the experimental treatment, and posttested, whereas another group is formed, pretested, not exposed to the experimental treatment, and posttested. This is a mixed design because it has both a within-subjects component (pretest versus posttest) and a between-subjects component (experimental versus control group). A difference between the two groups in the *improvement from pretest to posttest* is an index of the effect of the experimental treatment. This type of study might be done with naturally assembled groups because of the convenience of using one group intact as the experimental group and the other group intact as the control group. For instance, groups of participants in two different clinics or schools might be compared. The participants in one school will be exposed to the experimental treatment, whereas the participants at the other school will be the control group receiving no treatment to compare the effect of treatment to no treatment. Sometimes this design is seen with the control group receiving a regularly scheduled treatment to compare the effect of a new treatment against the effect of an old treatment. Some studies also use two control groups, one without treatment and another with the older treatment in order to make both comparisons.

This design may eliminate contamination of internal validity by the effects of history, maturation, and pretesting because of the introduction of a control group and may appear, therefore, to be a better design than the previous three, especially if the two groups perform similarly on the pretest. But there are problems involving the subject-selection factor and its interaction with the other factors that jeopardize internal validity. Because the groups have been selected on the basis of convenience rather than assembled on the basis of randomization or matching, it is possible that certain biases may arise from group composition that the experimenter cannot account for or measure. For example, if patients from a private clinic constitute one group and patients from a public clinic constitute the other, there might be important differences that relate to their decision to attend a private versus a public clinic. More affluent patients might attend the private clinic so that socioeconomic status would not be controlled as an extraneous variable. Private patients might be more motivated in therapy because they pay more for services rendered by the private clinic than do those patients in the public clinic. On the other hand, less affluent patients in a public clinic might be more motivated because they are striving to achieve better financial conditions and believe that better communication will help them to obtain better jobs. The effects of these possible threats to internal validity as a result of differential subject-selection are unknown. In addition, interaction of subject-selection and other factors, such as history, maturation, or mortality, could also jeopardize internal validity.

Even though this design represents an obvious improvement over the previous three designs, it is not as strong in either internal or external validity as the designs in the next section. Unfortunately, the nonequivalent control-group design will probably find continued use in the literature because of its convenience, and readers should, therefore, be aware of the limitations inherent in this design.

## Stronger Designs

Now that we have examined the pitfalls of some weak designs for studying treatment efficacy, let us turn to the evaluation of stronger designs that illustrate some methods of reducing threats to internal and external validity.

***Randomized Pretest–Posttest Control-Group Designs.*** Campbell and Stanley (1966) outline designs that include steps to ensure that (1) experimental and control groups are equivalent at the outset and (2) experimental and control groups are tested at equivalent time intervals to reduce threats to internal validity arising from factors such as maturation or regression.

The basic randomized pretest–posttest control-group design may be diagrammed as follows:

$$R \quad O_1 \quad X \quad O_2$$
$$R \quad O_3 \qquad O_4$$

In this mixed design, two groups are formed by randomly assigning half of the participants to the experimental group and half to the control group. Both groups are pretested and posttested in the same manner at the same times. The factors that could jeopardize internal validity are well controlled in this design as the following discussion indicates.

History should be controlled because general historical events should theoretically have as much effect on the $O_1$–$O_2$ difference as on the $O_3$–$O_4$ difference because the groups are randomly assembled at the same time. There may be the possibility, however, of specific historical events differentially affecting one group and not the other (e.g., participants in the experimental group meet for coffee between experimental sessions and influence each other's attitudes toward the experiment). Careful monitoring of such events can often preclude their threats to internal validity. Maturation and pretesting effects should be equivalent in both groups and affect the $O_2$ and $O_4$ scores by approximately the same amounts if randomization is used. Regression is not a threat, even if both groups have extreme scores on the pretest because both groups should evidence the same amount of regression as a result of random assignment. Differential subject-selection is controlled because the groups have been randomly assembled and, therefore, extraneous variables should be randomly distributed among the participants.

Attention must be paid to instrumentation and mortality, of course. Instrumentation problems are minimized if careful calibration of equipment is achieved and if human observers are carefully employed by the researcher to preclude bias in their use of measurements. If mortality exists in any experiment, it poses a threat to internal validity. In this design, mortality should not generally affect one group more than the other because it should be present to the same extent in both groups if it is related to any extraneous variable (e.g., motivation). If, however, the researcher notes that the mortality rate is high or, perhaps, that it is unevenly distributed between groups, he or she should undertake a replication of the experiment and also try to determine if any participant characteristics are related to mortality. Whenever mortality rates are high or unevenly distributed among groups in this or any research design, a serious threat may be posed to internal validity.

But differential mortality is much less likely to occur with random assignment to experimental and control groups because the potential for attrition is randomly distributed.

In general, then, this design is strong in internal validity. There are also several variations on the randomized pretest–posttest control-group design that may be considered. For example, matching may be used in conjunction with randomization to assemble the groups if there are certain extraneous variables that experimenters know should be controlled. The experimental and control groups would be formed by matching pairs of participants on the known extraneous variables and, then, randomly assigning one member of each pair to the experimental group and the other member to the control group. Such a design can be diagrammed as follows:

$$\text{MR} \quad O_1 \quad X \quad O_2$$
$$\text{MR} \quad O_3 \qquad O_4$$

The matching would equate pair members on extraneous variables known to correlate with the dependent variable, and the random assignment of pair members to experimental and control groups should ensure that overlooked extraneous variables would be randomly distributed.

The randomized control-group design has been conceptualized by some researchers as a mixed design with a between-subjects independent variable (experimental versus control groups) and a within-subjects independent variable (pretesting versus posttesting). In this case, the *score* on whatever behavior is tested in the pretests and posttests will be the dependent variable. It has also been suggested (Campbell & Stanley, 1966) that the *gain in score* from pretest to posttest be considered the dependent variable. In that case, the *gain* of the control group will be compared to the *gain* of the experimental group, and the experiment can be considered a simple bivalent experiment with just a between-subjects comparison of the control-group gain to the experimental-group gain as an index of the effectiveness of treatment. The bivalent independent variable is treatment and assumes two values: presence versus absence of treatment.

Using the pretest-to-posttest gain as the dependent variable, this design can be extended to a multivalent experiment by assembling groups that receive different values or different amounts of the experimental treatment (independent variable). For example, if the treatment involves training a certain behavior, several groups can each receive different amounts of training. Rather than simply comparing practice drills to no practice drills, the experimenter will be able to demonstrate changes in the dependent variable as a function of amount of practice drill. Such a design can be diagrammed as follows:

$$\text{Group 1} \quad R \quad O_1 \quad X_1 \quad O_2$$
$$\text{Group 2} \quad R \quad O_3 \quad X_2 \quad O_4$$
$$\text{Group 3} \quad R \quad O_5 \quad X_3 \quad O_6$$
$$\text{Group 4} \quad R \quad O_7 \qquad O_8$$

In this case, Group 1 might receive a certain amount of practice, Group 2 twice as much practice, Group 3 three times as much practice, and Group 4 would receive no practice and serve as the control group.

The design could be extended to a parametric design by studying the effects of two types of practice drills with varying amounts of each. For example, massed practice versus distributed practice (Bordens & Abbott, 2002, pp. 290–292; Willingham, 2002) in three different amounts could be studied in the following paradigm:

$$
\begin{array}{lll}
\text{Group 1} & \text{R} \quad O_1 \; X_{\text{Massed 1}} & O_2 \\
\text{Group 2} & \text{R} \quad O_3 \; X_{\text{Massed 2}} & O_4 \\
\text{Group 3} & \text{R} \quad O_5 \; X_{\text{Massed 3}} & O_6 \\
\text{Group 4} & \text{R} \quad O_7 \; X_{\text{Distributed 1}} & O_8 \\
\text{Group 5} & \text{R} \quad O_9 \; X_{\text{Distributed 2}} & O_{10} \\
\text{Group 6} & \text{R} \quad O_{11} X_{\text{Distributed 3}} & O_{12} \\
\text{Group 7} & \text{R} \quad O_{13} & O_{14}
\end{array}
$$

The first three groups would receive massed practice, with Group 1 receiving a certain amount, Group 2 twice as much, and Group 3 three times as much. Groups 4 through 6 would receive distributed practice, with Group 4 receiving the same amount of practice as Group 1 did, Group 5 receiving twice as much, and Group 6 receiving three times as much. Group 7 would receive no practice and would act as the control group. These designs may be expensive and difficult to administer, but they can be worth the effort because of the advantages of multivalent and parametric experiments discussed in Chapter 2.

Although these equivalent pretest–posttest control-group designs are strong in internal validity, there are some restrictions on their external validity, mainly because of the interactions of some jeopardizing factors with the experimental treatment. The first problem with external validity involves the interaction of subject-selection with the experimental variable. Although the simple main effect of subject-selection as a threat to internal validity is minimized by random assignment of participants to the experimental and control groups, it is possible that any demonstrated treatment effect may be valid only for the particular people studied in the investigation. For example, the results of a treatment study done with adult, male college students who stutter attending a university clinic may be generalizable only to persons who stutter and are males, adults, college students, and attending a university clinic. Attempts to generalize to females, to children, to persons with less than a college education, or to persons attending other types of clinics may be unwarranted. There is no guarantee, then, that generalization across people who are different from those studied in the original experiment will be valid. This does not mean that generalization never occurs; it simply means that it cannot be assumed until it has been proven. The possibility of the interaction of subject-selection and the experimental treatment *limits* the generalizability to people who are equivalent to those in the original study until subsequent research demonstrates broader generalizability of the results.

One way to overcome this limitation and thereby extend generalization across people is to perform replications with other types of people. Replication of the experiment with different types of people would help to delineate the extent to which subject-selection and the experimental treatment interact by demonstrating the relative effectiveness of the treatment with various types of people.

Readers should recognize that such replication could be considered a combination of descriptive and experimental research because the experimental treatment would be manipulated by the experimentor but the participant classification would not. The experiment would be replicated with people who differed in some classification variables such as age, gender, socioeconomic status, or type of pathology.

Such a replication of a randomized pretest–posttest control-group design can be diagrammed as follows:

| | | | | |
|---|---|---|---|---|
| *Initial experiment:* | R | $O_1$ | X | $O_2$ |
| *Adults* | R | $O_3$ | | $O_4$ |
| *Replication:* | R | $O_5$ | X | $O_6$ |
| *Children* | R | $O_7$ | | $O_8$ |

In such a replication, the $O_1 - O_2$ difference would be compared with the $O_3 - O_4$ difference in the first experiment to examine the effect of the experimental treatment for the adult subjects. The replication with children would then be run and the $O_5 - O_6$ difference compared to the $O_7 - O_8$ difference to examine the effect of the experimental treatment for the children. The replication would then be compared with the initial experiment to see whether the same effect that was obtained with the adults could be generalized to children. Such systematic replication is the most promising method of reducing the threat to external validity posed by the interaction of participant selection and the experimental treatment. Otherwise, experimental results remain applicable only to participants with essentially the same characteristics as those who participate in the original investigation.

A second threat to the external validity of the preceding designs is posed by the reactive effect of experimental arrangements. Experiments are usually novel events in the lives of participants who participate in them, and experimental settings or situations are usually somewhat artificial. Participants are often aware that they are participating in experiments, and they may differ in their attempts to discern the purpose of the experiment and in their conclusions regarding what the purpose is. The Hawthorne effect has always been thought to operate in experiments on human participants as a threat to external validity. Government agencies now insist on protection of the rights of experimental participants, and researchers must obtain informed consent from participants before the experiment begins. Even if participants agree to wait until after the experiment to be informed of its true purpose, they may have a preconceived notion of the purpose of the experiment and behave according to what they think the experimenter wants them to do (or does *not* want them to do).

In many cases, it is not possible to control such reactive arrangements entirely, but they may be somewhat attenuated. For example, some studies may compare a placebo group to both the experimental and control groups to examine the effect of the suggestion to participants that they are participating in an experiment. If the placebo group shows more improvement than the control group, a reactive arrangement may have accentuated improvement in the experimental group. Reactive arrangements are probably present in most experiments to the extent that participants behave differently than they would if they did not know or believe they were in an experiment and the degree to which the experimental setting can be made more "natural" is important in reducing this threat to external validity. Systematic replication of the experiment in more "natural" settings may also help to extend the generalization of the results.

Still a third threat to external validity of the designs we have discussed so far is the interaction of pretesting with the experimental variable. It is possible that the pretest itself may sensitize the participants to the possible effects that can be caused by the independent variable and make them more likely to show improvement. If the pretest sensitizes participants to respond more to the experimental variable than would people who were not pretested, then the results cannot be generalized to people who have not had the same pretest. If the experimenter wishes to generalize only to people who will always have the same pretest, there is little problem with this factor. But suppose that someone in another clinic that does not use the same pretest wishes to use the treatment of an experiment. Can it be assumed that the same results will be obtained without using the same pretest? Such generalization from any of the previous designs cannot be made and only the next design is able to deal with the interaction of pretesting with the experimental treatment.

***The Solomon Randomized Four-Group Design.***    Campbell and Stanley (1966, pp. 24–25) discuss a design first used by Solomon in 1949 that not only is strong in internal validity but also makes a successful attempt to control one factor affecting external validity—the interaction between pretesting and the experimental treatment. The Solomon Randomized Four-Group Design may be diagrammed as follows:

Group 1   R   $O_1$   X   $O_2$
Group 2   R   $O_3$        $O_4$
Group 3   R        X   $O_5$
Group 4   R            $O_6$

In the Solomon design, the participants are randomly assigned to one of four groups. Group 1 receives the pretest, the experimental treatment, and the posttest. Group 2 is pretested, is *not* exposed to the experimental treatment, and is posttested (i.e., Group 2 acts as a traditional control group). Group 3 is *not* pretested, *does* receive the experimental treatment, and *is* posttested. Group 4 is *not* pretested, is *not* exposed to the experimental treatment, but is posttested. Because this design is an extension of the randomized pretest–posttest control-group design, comparison of Groups 1 and 2 is used to show the effect of the experimental treatment and has the same internal validity as the randomized pretest–posttest control-group design. In addition, by paralleling Groups 1 and 2 with Groups 3 and 4 (groups that are not pretested), the interaction of pretesting and the experimental treatment can be evaluated.

The statistical analysis of the results of the pretests and posttests of a Solomon design is complex and controversial because of the asymmetry caused by removing the pretest for Groups 3 and 4. It is assumed that randomization should have resulted in essentially equivalent pretest scores (or *potential* pretest scores for the unpretested groups). Campbell and Stanley (1966, p. 25) suggest examining posttest scores only. Comparing the average scores on $O_2$ and $O_5$ to the average scores on $O_4$ and $O_6$ gives an index of the effectiveness of treatment. Comparing the average scores on $O_2$ and $O_4$ to the average scores on $O_5$ and $O_6$ gives an index of the influence of the pretest as a threat to internal validity. Comparing all four scores will indicate whether there is an interaction between the pretest and the experimental treatment that threatens external validity. If the $O_2 - O_4$ difference is greater than the $O_5 - O_6$ difference, this indicates that pretesting interacts with the experimental treatment, thereby precluding generalization to unpretested groups.

The Solomon design has been used in a number of investigations in educational psychology and it was used in an investigation of self-assessed sign language skills among beginning signers (Lodge-Miller & Elfenbein, 1994). We hope that the Solomon design will find more application in the communicative disorders literature in the future because it will pay off handsomely in improving treatment research.

***Time-Series Designs.***      A great deal of interest in the use of time-series designs in treatment efficacy research has developed in recent years. Rather than using a single pretest and a single posttest with a large number of participants, time-series designs employ repeated measurements of the dependent variable over an extended period of time with a single participant or a small number of participants. The designs have found wide application in behavior modification research, and a number of examples of these designs can now be found in the communicative disorders literature.

In describing the time-series design as a quasi-experiment, Campbell and Stanley (1966, p. 37) state:

> The essence of the time-series design is the presence of a periodic measurement process on some group or individual and the introduction of an experimental change into this time series of measurements, the results of which are indicated by a discontinuity in the measurements recorded in the time series.

The simplest time-series design is the AB design, which may be diagrammed as follows:

$$O_1 \quad O_2 \quad O_3 \quad O_4 \quad X \quad O_5 \quad O_6 \quad O_7 \quad O_8$$

$$\underbrace{\hphantom{O_1 \quad O_2 \quad O_3 \quad O_4}}_{\text{A segment}} \qquad \underbrace{\hphantom{O_5 \quad O_6 \quad O_7 \quad O_8}}_{\text{B segment}}$$

In this design, repeated measurements of the dependent variable are made in the A segment ("baseline") before the experimental treatment is introduced. In the B segment ("experimental segment"), the experimental treatment is introduced and several more repeated measurements of the dependent variable are made. This is a within-subjects design because each person participates in two conditions—baseline and experimental segments. Comparison of performance in the baseline with performance in the experimental segment indicates the effect of the experimental treatment on the dependent variable.

This design has many strengths. It also has a few weaknesses that may be overcome with simple modifications. The strengths center on the fact that the repeated measurements of the dependent variable in the baseline provide relatively good control over the threats to internal validity posed by maturation, pretesting, regression, and instrumentation. In a sense, the participants act as their own control group during the A (or baseline) segment of the design because the experimenter can examine their performances on the repeated measurements without an experimental intervention. If these baseline data are stable, maturation, pretesting, regression, and instrumentation should not threaten internal validity. Although this time-series design may appear, on the surface, to be similar to the one-group pretest–posttest design, the repeated measurements in the baseline make it a substantially stronger design by reducing these threats to internal validity.

The AB time-series design, however, does have a few weaknesses that merit attention. Even with a stable baseline, history may pose a threat because a historical event that does not occur during baseline but that does occur during the experimental segment may compete with the experimental treatment in affecting the dependent variable. Maturation could also pose a possible threat because it may not always start to affect performance at the outset of the A segment and progress in a linear fashion throughout the course of the experiment. Delayed maturation could, perhaps, begin toward the initiation of the B segment and mimic the effect of the experimental treatment on the independent variable.

Campbell and Stanley (1966) suggest that the addition of control participants to a time-series design is one possible method for improving its internal validity. An AB randomized control design may be diagrammed as follows:

$$R \quad O_1 \quad O_2 \quad O_3 \quad O_4 \quad X \quad O_5 \quad O_6 \quad O_7 \quad O_8$$
$$R \quad O_9 \quad O_{10} \quad O_{11} \quad O_{12} \quad\quad O_{13} \quad O_{14} \quad O_{15} \quad O_{16}$$

$$\underbrace{\phantom{R \quad O_1 \quad O_2 \quad O_3 \quad O_4}}_{\text{A segments}} \qquad \underbrace{\phantom{O_5 \quad O_6 \quad O_7 \quad O_8}}_{\text{B segments}}$$

In this AB randomized control design, participants are randomly assigned to participate as experimental or control participants. This design will now be a mixed design because it has both within-subjects and between-subjects components. The experimental participants are observed several times in the baseline (A segment), and the experimental treatment will be applied in conjunction with more repeated measurements of the dependent variable in the B segment. The control participants will be observed in baseline and also observed during a "pseudo-B segment" with no experimental treatment applied. In essence, they will be observed in two baseline segments. If the experimental participants show performance change in the B segment, but the control participants do not, the possibility of history or delayed maturation affecting the behavior of one group of participants and not the other will be greatly reduced.

The AB design may also be strengthened by its extension to an ABA design that incorporates another baseline segment after the experimental treatment. As mentioned in Chapter 3, the ABA design is often called a "reversal design" because of the reversal to baseline after completion of the experimental segment. An ABA design may be diagrammed as follows:

$$\underbrace{O_1 \quad O_2 \quad O_3 \quad O_4}_{\text{A segment}} \quad \underbrace{X \quad O_5 \quad O_6 \quad O_7 \quad O_8}_{\text{B segment}} \quad (\text{X Removed}) \quad \underbrace{O_9 \quad O_{10} \quad O_{11} \quad O_{12}}_{\text{A segment}}$$

In this design the A segment is followed by the B segment and then another baseline is introduced for observation of the participant's performance without the presence of the experimental treatment. This is a within-subjects design because all participants participate in all conditions. A reversal design is often used to study a dependent variable that may be temporarily affected by the experimental treatment. If the treatment causes a temporary change in the dependent variable, removal of the treatment should cause performance to return to baseline level. Some dependent variables, on the other hand, are permanently affected by the experimental treatment and do not return to baseline levels in the second A segment. In treatment studies, it is desirable to produce a performance change that is maintained after the experimental treatment is removed so that improved behavior is continued beyond the treat-ment setting (Barlow & Hersen, 1984). Sometimes multiple-segment time-series designs are employed (e.g., ABABAB, ..., AB) to study long-term changes in behavior following exper-imental treatment. Performance on the dependent variable may return to baseline level in the first few reversals and then carry-over effects may be evident in improved performance during subsequent baseline segments. Such multiple-segment designs may be costly or time-consuming, but are worthwhile efforts because short-term ABA studies may often obtain dra-matic treatment effects with little or no carryover.

Baseline instability may threaten the internal validity of time-series designs. Insta-bility can be the result of history, maturation, pretesting, regression, or instrumentation problems or of interactions among these factors. Also, the effects of these factors on the dependent variable may not be uniform with time and can, therefore, cause irregularities in the data that may be difficult to interpret. Of course, absolute stability of human behavior in a baseline segment can never be expected, so the real difficulty centers on determining how much variability should be tolerated in the baseline segment.

The external validity of time-series designs is sometimes cited as a problem by expo-nents of more traditional large-sample designs because of the small number of participants used and the complications that may arise if multiple treatments are applied to participants. Because time-series designs involve an in-depth analysis of behavior that is quite time-consuming, it is difficult to run them with large numbers of participants. Critics of time-series designs believe that this may accentuate problems of the interaction of subject-selection with the experimental treatment. Direct and systematic replications can often help to alleviate the external validity problem of subject-selection. The problem of multiple-treatment interfer-ence is best alleviated by replications in which different treatments and treatment combina-tions are applied to individual participants to assess their relative effectiveness.

The repeated testing done in time-series designs may be a reactive arrangement (Christensen, 2004, p. 344) or may accentuate the interaction of pretesting with the experi-mental treatment, thereby limiting generalization to participants who would normally un-dergo such repeated testing. This would not be a serious problem, however, if generalization were limited to people who were enrolled in relatively intensive or long-term treatment pro-grams that would incorporate multiple testing as an integral part of treatment.

Time-series designs may be extended to include numerous combinations of experi-mental treatments and baseline segments that may become quite complicated. Readers who are interested in a more detailed discussion of these designs than could be presented within the limitations of this book are referred to Barlow and Hersen (1984), Shadish, Cook, and Campbell (2002), McReynolds and Kearns (1983), and Kratochwill and Levin (1992) for reviews of various time-series designs and comparisons of the relative merits of time-series and traditional experimental designs.

## Meta-Analysis of Treatment Efficacy Research

In recent years, interest has developed in the possibilities for comparing treatment effi-cacy across various studies that have been published. The technique of cumulating re-search findings across various studies is called *meta-analysis* (Hunter & Schmidt, 1990), and it has been applied to a number of different kinds of research, including studies of treatment efficacy. In explaining the rationale for meta-analysis, Hunter and Schmidt (1990, pp. 34–35) state:

> What is needed are methods that will integrate results from existing studies to reveal patterns of relatively invariant underlying relations and causalities, the establishment of which will constitute general principles and cumulative knowledge.... At one time in the history of psychology and the social sciences, the pressing need was for more empirical studies examining the problem in question. In many areas of research, the need today is not additional empirical data but some means of making sense of the vast amounts of data that have been accumulated. Given the increasing number of areas within psychology and the other social sciences in which the number of available studies is quite large and the importance to theory development and practical problem solving of integrating conflicting findings to establish general knowledge, it is likely that methods for doing this will attain increasing importance in the future.

Hunter and Schmidt (1990) review several different methods of meta-analysis, ranging from narrative review of studies to complex statistical comparison of the results of different studies that incorporate analyses of study characteristics, statistical corrections for factors such as test reliability, and weighting of the results of various studies according to their sample sizes. One important technique in meta-analysis of treatment studies is the evaluation of *effect size,* a method of standardizing across studies the measurement of the amount of pretreatment to posttreatment improvement. Effect size is often measured as the average pre–post difference in a dependent variable divided by the standard deviation of the pretreatment scores on the dependent variable. Calculating effect size in this way results in a reasonably comparable measure of improvement for all the studies that are compared because effect size allows the improvement results of all the studies to be expressed as a standard deviation relative to the pretreatment results.

Andrews, Guitar, and Howie (1980) published a meta-analysis of studies concerned with the effects of stuttering treatment. They analyzed effect sizes for 116 dependent variables that had been examined in forty-two studies of stuttering treatment that had included a total of 756 participants. The overall mean effect size for the 116 dependent variables indicated that participants had improved by 1.3 standard deviations relative to pretreatment measures on the average. Prolonged speech and gentle onset were the two treatment techniques that emerged with the best effect sizes from the meta-analysis.

Robey (1998) conducted a meta-analysis of 55 studies concerned with the effects of treatment for aphasia and found that the average effect size for treatment begun in the acute period was 1.83 times greater than the effect size for untreated persons and the average effect size for treatment begun in the post-acute period was 1.68 times greater than the effect size for untreated persons. A detailed analysis was presented of factors such as amount of treatment applied, type of treatment, and severity and type of aphasia. In general, it was found that magnitude of improvement was greater for longer treatment duration, greatest benefits were found with treatments following Wepman-Schuell-Darley multimodality principles, and treatment gains were largest with more severe aphasia, especially when treatment was begun in the acute period.

There are a number of methodological problems in meta-analysis that must be assessed. First, there is the manner in which the author selects the studies for inclusion in the meta-analysis. Consideration must be given to factors such as the author's attempts to judge the internal and external validity of the original studies, the sample sizes used in the studies, whether the studies were published in refereed journals or in less-selective media, and the types of dependent variables used to measure improvement. Second, there are complex statistical issues that must be dealt with in trying to weigh the equivalence of different studies. Consideration must also be given to different study characteristics such as sample size, method of measurement of dependent variables, kinds of statistics used to report results, type and length of treatments, and selection criteria for including participants in the studies. Hunter and Schmidt (1990) have given extensive attention to a number of these and other problems in meta-analysis and provide an extensive bibliography of material relevant to meta-analysis. Andrews et al. (1980) discuss some of these issues in relation to research on treatment efficacy in communicative disorders. Robey and Dalebout (1998) have published a tutorial on the use of meta-analysis in communicative disorders research that discusses many of these issues and explains in detail the procedures for meta-analysis and the calculation of various effect sizes. More of this kind of attention to meta-analysis in the future of our research literature would be desirable, for, as Cohen (1997, p. 29) has said, "Meta-analysis, with its emphasis on effect sizes, is a bright spot in the contemporary scene."

## Ethics of Using Control Groups in Treatment Efficacy Research

In concluding this discussion of research designs for studying treatment efficacy, some comments are in order on the ethics of using control groups in therapy research. Some professionals have serious reservations about the ethics of withholding treatment from persons with speech, language, or hearing problems, whereas other professionals believe that control groups should be used to confirm treatment efficacy. Kimmel (1996, p. 175) discusses the potential ethical dilemma of using untreated control groups in the following manner:

> When preventive intervention studies are experimental in nature, ethical issues are likely to emerge regarding the use of untreated control groups and other comparison groups. These issues tend to revolve around questions of fairness in terms of who from among a population of individuals is to receive an experimental treatment when all would stand to benefit from it.

An exchange of letters in the *Journal of Speech and Hearing Disorders* illustrates this controversy. Kushnirecky and Weber (1978, p. 106), in commenting on the validity of evidence in a study of treatment efficacy, stated:

> Since matched control subjects were not used, the data have limited interpretive value. It is possible that a control group may have shown that these children may have improved without intervention. Even if the children's rate of gain of language development equaled that of nonlanguage-delayed children, in the absence of controls, any conclusions concerning the effectiveness of the method are at best conjectures.

Lee, Koenigsnecht, and Mulhern (1978, pp. 107–108) replied that, in their opinion, the use of control groups

. . . is impossible on ethical grounds. Kushnirecky and Weber should be strongly advised not to embark on research that withholds treatment from children who need it. . . . It would be unconscionable to withhold clinical training for any period of time from any child who needs it and would be likely to gain from it. This precludes designs in which one group of children receives treatment while treatment is withheld from a comparable group in order to show that the treatment produced results.

An editor's note appended to these two letters indicated that communicative disorders specialists have an ethical obligation to provide treatment when possible but that they also have an ethical obligation to provide treatment that rests on "sound evidence" of its effectiveness. The editor's note also pointed out that control does not always mean withholding of treatment to a control group, as control can sometimes be accomplished with the use of multiple baselines (as in our discussion of time-series designs earlier in this chapter).

The major point illustrated by this exchange of letters is that a potential conflict of interest exists in our ethical obligations both to provide treatment and to demonstrate treatment efficacy when the latter obligation may sometimes require the withholding of treatment to a control group.

Many years have passed since the publication of these letters, but the issue is still controversial. It has been argued, for example, that stuttering treatment efficacy with preschool children has not been scientifically established due in large part to the absence of untreated control groups in treatment efficacy research. Curlee and Yairi (1997, p. 14) stated:

> The use of randomly assigned, untreated control groups has long been viewed as essential for evaluating treatment effectiveness. Treatment outcome findings obtained without such controls have not been accepted as scientific evidence but only as data from uncontrolled pilot studies.

Kimmel (1996, p. 176) offers some general considerations for the ethical use of control groups in treatment efficacy research:

> The use of untreated controls is likely to be viewed as ethically appropriate, even though the . . . intervention is expected to be strong, in research situations where the beneficial treatment could not reasonably be offered to everyone in need because of limited resources.

Kimmel (1996, p. 178) goes on to say:

> Another case in which untreated control groups would be acceptable is that in which participants can experience a successful treatment once the research is completed, or as soon as the effectiveness of the treatment becomes evident. . .

Many clinics have large caseloads; therefore, staff clinicians often cannot accommodate all applicants immediately. Applicants for treatment could be randomly assigned to immediate treatment or to the waiting list and all applicants could be pretested at the time of application for treatment. At the end of the experiment, then, the control group on the waiting list could be used as the new experimental group in a direct or systematic replication of the study. This would be especially suitable when the experimental treatment can be accomplished in a relatively short time.

The use of time-series designs is another obvious approach, and its potential for resolving the control group problem may be one of the reasons for the increased use of time-series designs. The ethics of withholding treatment from a control group remains controversial in a number of disciplines, and we expect that it will be some time before such issues are resolved. Nonetheless, treatment efficacy research must continue and expand. As Curlee and Yairi (1997, p. 16) state:

> ... there must be a strong and widespread commitment to obtain the scientific data needed to demonstrate that only those procedures that are necessary and effective will be provided.... We believe that such a commitment ought to be seen as this profession's ethical responsibility to the clinical populations it seeks to serve.

Ethical standards in behavioral research have been described in more detail in *Ethical Principles in the Conduct of Research with Human Participants* (American Psychological Association, 2002). This document is reprinted in a book of readings edited by Bersoff (2003) along with a number of articles covering topics such as ethical principles and the protection of confidentiality and privacy in treatment, research, and teaching.

## Protection of Human Participants in Research

A broader issue than the ethics of using control groups in treatment research also needs to be addressed: the protection of human participants who participate in any research studies in communicative disorders. In recent decades, the scientific community and various governmental agencies have taken steps to safeguard the rights of human participants in any kind of research. Past abuse of human research participants is one reason for this concern, but even in the absence of actual abuse of human participants, researchers and consumers of research need to be aware of the potential for physical or psychological harm to human participants and of the need to protect the dignity and privacy of research participants. Maloney (1984) provides a detailed account of the federal laws and regulations regarding the protection of human participants in research.

The issue of protection of research participants is complex, and federal regulations have been established to provide safeguards for human research participants. These regulations are quite detailed, and a comprehensive coverage of them goes beyond the scope of this text. The consumer of research, however, should be aware of the general history of these regulations and how they are applied to human participants in communicative disorders research.

The National Research Act of 1974 (Public Law 93-348) created the National Commission for the Protection of Human Subjects in Biomedical and Behavioral Research. This commission was given the responsibility to develop the basic principles that underlie participant protection in biomedical and behavioral research and the methods to ensure compliance with those principles. After seven years of development, the final code of federal regulations was published in the *Federal Register* in 1981 under the title "Protection of Human Subjects," Title 45, Code of Federal Regulations, Part 46.

Since their introduction in 1981, the federal regulations for protection of human research participants has undergone several revisions. For example, in 1983, Subpart D was added to the code, extending protection for children used in research, and in 1991 Subpart A of the code was amended to include all government agencies that conduct or sponsor research. This latter addition is known as the "Final Common Rule for Protection of Human Subjects." Also, on a regular basis the Office for Protection from Research Risks (OPRR), a division of the Department of Health and Human Services, issues recommendations to institutions conducting research that need to be considered in conjunction with the federal code of regulations.

The local Institutional Review Board (IRB) is the major component of the federal regulations for protection of human research participants. Members of a local IRB are appointed by top officials of the administration at the institution. IRBs at institutions such as universities, hospitals, or school districts applying for federal research funding must provide written assurance that they will comply with the regulations. Federal funding will not be granted without these assurances. Each IRB must have a minimum of five members, and federal regulations require that one person on the board must have a nonscientific background (e.g., lawyers or members of the clergy) and one person must not be affiliated with the institution.

Local IRBs can reject research proposals if the potential benefits of the study in relation to the potential risks to the participant are great. IRBs must also ensure that potential participants have been adequately informed about their participation in the study and that the participants have signed informed consent documents. The informed consent document must include (a) statements about the purpose of the study, (b) description of potential benefits and risks to the participant, (c) disclosures of alternate procedures or treatments, if any, and (d) statements regarding how participant confidentiality will be maintained.

An important issue in informed consent that affects all individuals concerned with research in communicative disorders and sciences is the concern for vulnerable populations who need special informed consent protections. The U.S. Department of Health and Human Services (HHS) Office for Human Research Protections (OHRP) has a "Special Issues" section on its website (www.hhs.gov/ohrp) dealing with protection of populations such as children in research. In addition, an article in *The ASHA Leader* by Maher (2002) discussed the issue of securing informed consent from persons with aphasia because of the potential effect of language impairment on informed decision-making ability. She stressed the need to examine each person individually rather than make broad assumptions about the ability of individuals with aphasia to comprehend the information and decision-making process, a caution that could be taken into account in considering informed consent procedures for all persons with speech, language, and hearing disabilities.

It should be pointed out that both the topics of ethics of using control groups and the protection of human participants in research are part of the overarching issue of research integrity that has been addressed in a number of publications of interest to all individuals concerned with research in communicative disorders and sciences. Professionals in the field became painfully aware of the general issue of research integrity with the recent publication of a report concerning an experiment in 1939 that allegedly attempted to make normal speakers stutter (Annett, 2001). The importance of the general issue of research integrity has been highlighted in many professional activities and publications, including ASHA's addition of new material on research to its Code of Ethics (ASHA, 2003), an

ASHA conference on promoting research integrity (ASHA, 2001), a "Focus on Ethics" piece in *The ASHA Leader* (Costello & Horner, 2004), and a federal grant to ASHA to conduct a survey to determine how students are exposed in the curriculum to knowledge of research ethics and scientific integrity (Lansing & Moss, 2003).

Research on human beings is a dynamic enterprise, changing constantly and expanding our knowledge base at an astonishing rate. As such, the federal code of regulations that protects human participants from research risks must be equally dynamic and modified in accordance with the expanded knowledge base and new research directions. Changes to the federal code of regulations are being made as we write this edition of the book and will continue to be made as you read it. Individuals interested in the federal code of regulations and current modifications can visit either the OHRP website (www.hhs.gov/ohrp/) or the National Institutes of Health Office of Extramural Research website (www.grants.nih.gov/grants/oer.htm). In addition, animals are sometimes used in research that relates to communicative disorders and strict federal regulations govern the use of these animals. The current regulations for the humane care and use of laboratory animals can be obtained by visiting the website of the National Institutes of Health Office of Laboratory Animal Welfare (www.grants. nih.gov/grants/olaw/olaw.htm).

Metz and Folkins (1985) have provided a historical review of the federal regulations for protection of human research participants as they relate specifically to communicative disorders research. In addition, ASHA has become a signatory to the proclamation on human participants in research written by the Association of American Medical Colleges and the National Health Council that is reprinted in the Appendix. An online training course on protection of human participants in research is available for researchers from the National Institutes of Health at its website (http://69.5.4.33/c01/nih_intro_01.htm).

## Study Questions

1. Visit the Office for Human Research Protections (OHRP) website (www.hhs.gov/ohrp).

   a. Click on "Regulations" and examine the current regulations and new additions to the federal code.
   b. While you are on the OHRP website, click on "Regulations," then on "Informed Consent," and examine the "Informed Consent Tips" and "Informed Consent Checklist."

2. Visit the website of the National Institutes of Health Office of Extramural Research (www.grants.nih.gov/grants/oer.htm).

   a. Click on the "Funding Opportunities" icon, then enter the "Search" entry form and type in a topic that interests you (e.g., speech, voice, language, hearing, etc.). What are the funding opportunities related to treatment efficacy in your area of interest?
   b. What other funding opportunities are available?

**3.** Read the following article:

Riley G. D., & Ingham, J. C. (2000). Acoustic duration changes associated with two types of treatment for children who stutter. *Journal of Speech, Language, and Hearing Research, 43,* 965–978.

   **a.** Identify the experimental treatments and dependent variables used in this treatment efficacy study.
   **b.** What differences were found among the different groups that were treated?

**4.** Read the following article:

Roy, N., Gray, S. D., Simon, M., Dove, H., Corbin-Lewis, K., & Stemple, J. (2001). An evaluation of the effects of two treatment approaches for teachers with voice disorders: A prospective randomized clinical trial. *Journal of Speech, Language, and Hearing Research, 44,* 286–296.

   **a.** Identify the experimental treatments and dependent variables used in this treatment efficacy study.
   **b.** What differences were found among the different groups that were treated?

**5.** Read the following article:

Katz, R. C., & Wertz, R. T. (1997). The efficacy of computer-provided reading treatment for chronic aphasic adults. *Journal of Speech, Language, and Hearing Research, 40,* 493–507.

   **a.** How is treatment efficacy defined?
   **b.** What research design for evaluating treatment efficiency is used in this study?
   **c.** What did the authors conclude about treatment efficacy?

**6.** Read the following article:

Gierut, J. A. (1998). Treatment efficacy: Functional phonological disorders in children. *Journal of Speech, Language, and Hearing Research, 41,* S85–S100.

   **a.** How are phonological disorders defined?
   **b.** What evidence is used to support the notion that treatment is beneficial?

**7.** Read the following article:

Conture, E. G. (1996). Treatment efficacy: Stuttering. *Journal of Speech and Hearing Research, 39,* S18–S26.

   **a.** How is stuttering defined?
   **b.** What evidence is used to support the notion that treatment is beneficial?

**8.** Read the following article:

Weinstein, B. E. (1996). Treatment efficacy: Hearing aids in the management of hearing loss in adults. *Journal of Speech and Hearing Research, 39,* S37–S45.

**a.** How is a hearing disability defined?

**b.** What evidence is used to support the notion that hearing aid use is beneficial?

**9.** Read the following article:

Boberg, E., & Kully, D. (1994). Long-term results of an intensive treatment program for adults and adolescents who stutter. *Journal of Speech and Hearing Research, 37,* 1050–1059.

**a.** What measures are taken to strengthen the potential internal validity threat of instrumentation?

**b.** To what groups can you generalize these findings?

**10.** Discuss the reasons for the following points made by Campbell and Stanley (1966):

**a.** efforts to increase internal validity may jeopardize external validity and vice versa;

**b.** internal validity is the *sine qua non* of research; and

**c.** the question of external validity can never be completely answered.

**11.** Read the following article:

Lodge-Miller, K. A., & Elfenbein, J. L. (1994). Beginning signers' self-assessment of sign language skills. *Journal of Communication Disorders, 27,* 281–292.

**a.** What internal validity threats do the authors claim are controlled by the Solomon Randomized Four-Group Design?

**b.** How does the design also control external validity threats?

# REFERENCES

Ad Hoc Practice Guidelines Coordinating Committee. (2001). *Evidence-based practice guidelines for the management of communication disorders in neurologically impaired individuals: Project introduction.* Washington, DC: Academy of Neurologic Communication Disorders and Sciences. Retrieved June 29, 2004, from www.ancds.duq.edu/PracticeGuidelines.pdf

American Psychological Association. (2002). *Ethical principles of psychologists and code of conduct.* Washington, DC: American Psychological Association. Retrieved June 17, 2004, from www.apa.org/ethics/code2002.html

American Speech-Language-Hearing Association. (2001). *Promoting research integrity in communication sciences and disorders and related disciplines.* Rockville, MD: Author.

American Speech-Language-Hearing Association. (2003). Code of ethics (revised). *ASHA Supplement, 23,* 13–15.

Andrews, G., Guitar, B., & Howie, P. (1980). Meta-analysis of the effects of stuttering treatment. *Journal of Speech and Hearing Disorders, 45,* 287–307.

Annett, M. M. (2001). Article alleges 1939 study taught children to stutter. *The ASHA Leader, 6(13),* 1, 17.

Apel, K., & Self, T. (2003). Evidence-based practice: The marriage of research and clinical services. *The ASHA Leader, 8(16),* 6–7.

Barlow, D. H., & Herson, M. (1984). *Single case experimental designs.* Boston: Allyn & Bacon.

Bersoff, D. N. (2003). *Ethical conflicts in psychology* (3rd ed.). Washington, DC: American Psychological Association.

Bordens, K. S., & Abbott, B. B. (2002). *Research design and method: A process approach* (5th ed.). New York: McGraw-Hill.

Bracht, G. H., & Glass, G. V. (1968). The external validity of experiments. *American Educational Research Journal, 5,* 437–474.

Brookshire, R. H. (1983). Subject description and generality of results in experiments with aphasic adults. *Journal of Speech and Hearing Disorders, 48,* 342–346.

Campbell, D. T., & Stanley, J. C. (1966). *Experimental and quasi-experimental designs for research.* Chicago, IL: Rand-McNally.

Carney, A. E. (1996). Introduction to supplement on treatment efficacy: Part I. *Journal of Speech and Hearing Research, 39,* S3–S4.

Carney, A. E. (1998). Introduction to supplement on treatment efficacy: Part II. *Journal of Speech, Language, and Hearing Research, 41,* S60.

Christensen, L. B. (2004). *Experimental methodology* (9th ed.). Boston: Allyn & Bacon.

Cohen, J. (1997). The earth is round (*p* < .05). In L. L. Harlow, S. A. Mulaik, & J. H. Steiger (Eds.), *What if there were no significance tests?* (pp. 21–35). Mahwah, NJ: Lawrence Erlbaum Associates.

Curlee, R. F., & Yairi, E. (1997). Early intervention with early childhood stuttering: A critical examination of the data. *American Journal of Speech–Language Pathology, 6(2),* 8–18

Dollaghan, C. (2004). Evidence-based practice: Myths and realities. *The ASHA Leader, 9(7),* 4–5, 12.

Fratelli, C. M. (1998). Outcomes measurement: Definitions, dimensions, and perspectives. In C. M. Fratelli (Ed.), *Measuring outcomes in speech-language pathology.* New York: Thieme.

Holland, A. L., Fromm, D. S., DeRuyter, F., & Stein, M. (1996). Treatment efficacy: Aphasia. *Journal of Speech and Hearing Research, 39,* S27–S36.

Huck, S. W., Cormier, W. H., & Bounds, W. G. (1974). *Reading statistics and research.* New York: Harper & Row.

Hunter, J. E., & Schmidt, F. L. (1990). *Methods of meta-analysis: Correcting error and bias in research findings.* Thousand Oaks, CA: Sage.

Ingham, J. C. (2003). Evidence-based treatment of stuttering: I. Definition and application. *Journal of Fluency Disorders, 28,* 197–207.

Ingham, J. C., & Horner, J. (2004). Ethics and research. *The ASHA Leader, 9(5),* 10–11, 24–25.

Isaac, S., & Michael, W. B. (1971). *Handbook in research and evaluation.* San Diego, CA: Edits.

Jones, M., Gebski, V., Onslow, M., & Packman, A. (2001). Design of randomized controlled trials: Principles and methods applied to a treatment for early stuttering. *Journal of Fluency Disorders, 26,* 247–267.

Kerlinger, F., & Lee, H. B. (2000). *Foundations of behavioral research* (4th ed.). New York: Harcourt Brace.

Kimmel, A. J. (1996). *Ethical issues in behavioral research: A survey.* Oxford: Blackwell.

Kratochwill, T. R., & Levin, J. R. (Eds.). (1992). *Single-case research design and analysis: New directions for psychology and education.* Hillsdale, NJ: Lawrence Erlbaum Associates.

Kushnirecky, W., & Weber, J. (1978). Comment on Lee's reply to Simon. *Journal of Speech and Hearing Disorders, 43,* 106–107.

Lansing, C., & Moss, S. (2003). Survey to determine knowledge of research ethics. *The ASHA Leader, 8(22),* 18.

Lee, L. L., Koenigsnecht, R. A., & Mulhern, S. T. (1978). Reply to Kushnirecky and Weber. *Journal of Speech and Hearing Disorders, 43,* 107–108.

Lodge-Miller, K. A., & Elfenbein, J. L. (1994). Beginning signers' self-assessment of sign language skills. *Journal of Communication Disorders, 27,* 281–292.

Maher, L. M. (2002). Informed consent for research in aphasia. *The ASHA Leader, 7(22),* 12.

Maloney, D. M. (1984). *Protection of human research subjects: A practical guide to federal laws and regulations.* New York: Plenum Press.

McReynolds, L. V., & Kearns, K. P. (1983). *Single-subject experimental designs in communicative disorders.* Baltimore: University Park Press.

Metz, D. E., & Folkins, J. W. (1985). Protection of human subjects in speech and hearing research. *ASHA, 27,* 25–29.

Montgomery, A. A. (1994). Treatment efficacy in adult audiological rehabilitation. *Journal of the Academy of Rehabilitative Audiology, 27,* 317–336.

Moscicki, E. K. (1993). Fundamental methodological considerations in controlled clinical trials. *Journal of Fluency Disorders, 18,* 183–196.

Ochsner, G. (2003). Evidence-based practice. *The ASHA Leader, 8(8),* 27.

Office of Technology Assessment (1983). *The impact of clinical trials on health policy and medical practice: Background paper.* Washington, DC: U.S. Congress, Office of Technology Assessment OTA-BP-H-22, August 1983.

Olswang, L. B. (1993). Treatment efficacy research: A paradigm for investigating clinical practice and theory. *Journal of Fluency Disorders, 18,* 125–134.

Olswang, L. B. (1998). Treatment efficacy research. In C. M. Fratelli (Ed.), *Measuring outcomes in speech-language pathology.* New York: Thieme.

Olswang, L. B., Thompson, C. K., Warren, S. F., & Minghetti, N. J. (Eds.). (1990). *Treatment efficacy in communication disorders.* Rockville Pike, MD: American Speech-Language-Hearing Foundation.

Parsons, H. M. (1974). What happened at Hawthorne? *Science, 183,* 922–932.

Peach, R. K. (2003). From the editor. *American Journal of Speech-Language Pathology, 12,* 2.

Peach, R. K. (2004). From the editor. *American Journal of Speech-Language Pathology, 13,* 2.

Pedhazur, E. J., & Schmelkin, L. P. (1991). *Measurement, design, and analysis.* Mahwah, NJ: Lawrence Erlbaum Associates.

Pocock, S. J., (1983). *Clinical trials: A practical approach.* Chichester, UK: Wiley.

Robey, R. R. (1998). A meta-analysis of clinical outcomes in the treatment of aphasia. *Journal of Speech, Language, and Hearing Research, 41,* 172–187.

Robey, R. R. (2004). Levels of evidence. *The ASHA Leader, 9(7),* 5.

Robey, R. R., & Dalebout, S. D. (1998). A tutorial on conducting meta-analyses of clinical outcome research. *Journal of Speech, Language, and Hearing Research, 41,* 1227–1241.

Robey, R. R., & Schultz, M. C. (1998). A model for conducting clinical-outcome research: An adaptation of the standard protocol for use in aphasiology. *Aphasiology, 12,* 787–810.

Rosenthal, R., & Rosnow, R. L. (1991). *Essentials of behavioral research* (2nd ed.). New York: McGraw-Hill.

Roy, N., Weinrich, B., Gray, S. D., Tanner, K., Stemple, J., & Sapienza, C. M. (2003). Three treatments for teachers with voice disorders: A randomized clinical trial. *Journal of Speech, Language, and Hearing Research, 46,* 670–688.

Sackett D. L., Rosenberg, W. M. C., Gray, J. A. M., Haynes, R. B., & Richardson, W. S. (1996). Evidence based medicine: What it is and what it isn't. *British Medical Journal, 312,* 71–72.

Sackett D. L., Straus, S. E., Richardson, W. S., Rosenberg, W. M. C., & Haynes, R. B. (2000). *Evidence-based medicine: How to practise and teach EBM* (2nd ed.). Edinburgh: Churchill Livingstone.

Schlosser, R. W. (2003). *The efficacy of augmentative and alternative communication: Toward evidence-based practice.* New York: Elsevier Academic Press.

Schlosser, R. W. (2004). Evidence-based practice in AAC. *The ASHA Leader, 9(12),* 6–7, 10.

Schooling, T. (2000). NOMS bears fruit. *The ASHA Leader, 5(10),* 4–5.

Shadish, W. R., Cook, T. D., & Campbell, D. T. (2002). *Experimental and quasi-experimental designs for generalized causal inference.* Boston: Houghton Mifflin.

Tomblin, J. B., Zhang, X., Buckwalter, P., & O'Brien, M. (2003). The stability of primary language disorder: Four years after kindergarten diagnosis. *Journal of Speech, Language, and Hearing Research, 46,* 1283–1296.

Webb, E. J., Campbell, D. T., Schwartz, R. D., & Sechrest, L. (1966). *Unobtrusive measures: Nonreactive research in the social sciences.* Chicago, IL: Rand-McNally.

Willingham, D. T. (2002). Allocating student study time: "Massed" versus "distributed" practice. *American Educator, 6(2),* 37–39, 47.

Zhang, X., & Tomblin, J. B. (2003). Explaining and controlling regression to the mean in longitudinal research designs. *Journal of Speech, Language, and Hearing Research, 46,* 1340–1351.

# CHAPTER 6

# Organization and Analysis of Data

The purpose of this chapter is to describe some basic terms, concepts, and procedures used in the organization and analysis of data derived from communicative disorders research. Our intention is to explain some basic considerations that will help consumers of research to understand the meaning of research results. This chapter will *not* be concerned with extensive details about derivations, formulae, calculations, or other aspects of data analysis that are necessary for the producer of research. For more detailed treatments of statistical methods, consumers are referred to statistical textbooks such as those by Ferguson and Takane (1989), Guilford (1965), Hays (1994), Kirk (1999), Kranzler and Moursund (1999), Pedhazur and Schmelkin (1991), and Siegel (1956) included in the reference list at the end of this chapter. Also, readers are reminded that Chapter 9 provides many examples of data organization and analysis that have been excerpted from communicative disorders research articles.

Data organization and analysis techniques are statistical tools that assist the researcher in drawing conclusions and making inferences from a study. Experimental and descriptive studies both employ data organization or analysis procedures to aid in answering research questions by indicating how plausible certain conclusions are in light of the obtained data. Because many of the same statistical techniques may be used to analyze either experimental or descriptive data, the type of data organization or analysis used does not indicate whether a study is experimental or descriptive.

The organization and analysis techniques for empirical research are commonly referred to as *statistics* because they are derived from a branch of mathematics by that name. However, the term *statistics* also refers to the numeric descriptors of a *sample,* as opposed to the companion term *parameter,* which refers to the numeric descriptors of the *population* from which a sample is drawn. In this usage, then, the term *statistics* may be defined as computed estimates of parameters because it is only rarely that an entire population can be studied directly.

To illustrate, suppose that we wish to know the average number of articulation errors made by children at age five years. The average number of errors made by all five-year-old children (i.e., the population of interest) will be a parameter. We could never test all of the five-year-olds who speak English to get a direct measure of this population characteristic. So, we would select a sample of five-year-old speakers of English, say two hundred, and determine their average number of articulation errors. The average number of articulation errors made by this sample of five-year-olds would be a statistic and could be used in estimating the parameter. In other words, a statistic is a number describing a sample characteristic, and a parameter is a number describing a population characteristic.

# Data Organization

Completion of data collection results in the amassing of a body of *raw* data. These unprocessed data have not been arranged or organized for viewing. The data need to be organized so that they can be interpreted in regard to the structure of the research design.

## Data Distributions

Whenever measures on one or more variables are obtained in a research study, the obtained values form a *distribution*. The distribution is the frequency count of attributes of objects or events that fall into different categories for a nominal level measurement or the arrangement of relative attribute values in a rank order for an ordinal level measurement. For interval or ratio level measurements, the distribution will include a listing of the number of cases that occurred at each score value on the interval or ratio level measurement. The distributions of nominal and ordinal level measurements are relatively straightforward and usually are demonstrated in a table or figure that shows the category frequencies or the relative rankings. However, the distributions of interval and ratio level measurements often require more attention to determine their characteristics. Most of the following discussion, then, will concern the distribution of interval and ratio level measurements; for the most part, the issues in describing the distributions of interval and ratio level measurements are the same.

The distributions of interval and ratio level measurements have four characteristics that are usually described: *central tendency, variability, skewness,* and *kurtosis.* Before proceeding with the analysis of research results, the researcher usually ascertains these characteristics and presents information on at least the first two so that readers may examine the organized data to see the overall pattern of results. There are two ways to provide this information that we will discuss in the next two sections: (1) through tabular or graphic presentation and (2) through calculation of summary statistics.

## Tabular and Graphic Presentation

Many researchers present the distribution of data in the form of a table or a figure for inspection before performing further data analysis. Tabular or graphic presentations have the advantage of showing the overall contour of the distribution so that the four characteristics of the distribution can be seen visually. Frequency tables, histograms, polygons, and cumulative frequency distributions are some of the more common means of tabular and graphic presentations.

To illustrate some of these basic data-organization techniques, a set of hypothetical data is shown in Table 6.1. The data for eighty participants are first presented in raw form, just as they might appear in the researcher's notes. The data are then *grouped* in a frequency table so that, for each score value, the number of cases obtaining that score is shown in the frequency ( $f$ ) column. The cumulative frequency (cum $f$ ) column shows, for each score value, the number of cases that obtained scores *at* or *below* that value. Thus, looking at the score of six, we note that sixteen participants received scores of six and forty-nine participants received scores at or below six.

In some instances, when the researcher is working with a fairly small number of values and wishes to keep individual participant data on a number of variables together, the use of

**TABLE 6.1  Hypothetical Example of Conversion of Raw Scores into a Frequency and Cumulative Frequency Table Using Grouped Data**

| | | | | | | | | Grouped Scores | Frequency | Cumulative Frequency |
| --- | --- | --- | --- | --- | --- | --- | --- | --- | --- | --- |
| | | | Raw Scores | | | | | Score | f | cum f |
| 4 | 4 | 3 | 6 | 8 | 8 | 2 | 5 | 10 | 5 | 80 |
| 7 | 9 | 2 | 7 | 4 | 5 | 6 | 6 | 9 | 6 | 75 |
| 3 | 8 | 3 | 6 | 3 | 4 | 5 | 9 | 8 | 9 | 69 |
| 6 | 5 | 4 | 1 | 4 | 7 | 8 | 4 | 7 | 11 | 60 |
| 2 | 4 | 2 | 10 | 1 | 2 | 5 | 3 | 6 | 16 | 49 |
| 5 | 8 | 6 | 7 | 5 | 6 | 5 | 7 | 5 | 13 | 33 |
| 7 | 9 | 5 | 7 | 6 | 9 | 5 | 6 | 4 | 8 | 20 |
| 5 | 6 | 8 | 9 | 8 | 7 | 5 | 5 | 3 | 5 | 12 |
| 6 | 7 | 6 | 9 | 10 | 6 | 7 | 8 | 2 | 5 | 7 |
| 6 | 8 | 6 | 7 | 10 | 10 | 10 | 6 | 1 | 2 | 2 |
| | | | | | | | | | $N = 80$ | |

*ungrouped* data is feasible. This type of organization simply shows the score values listed in order rather than showing the *f* and cum *f* columns. In addition, the mechanics of calculating some of the indices to be shown later will be altered somewhat from the examples given in this chapter.

Figure 6.1 shows how this hypothetical set of scores can be presented graphically. Figure 6.1a shows a histogram, or bar graph, of the scores. Note that the midpoint of each bar is directly above the score value on the horizontal axis of the graph. If we take these midpoints, record them on a graph, and connect these points with straight lines, the results will be the frequency polygon shown in Figure 6.1b. Figure 6.1c shows a cumulative frequency polygon. This is a graphic representation of the cumulative frequency (cum *f*) column rather than the frequency (*f*) column in Table 6.1. One distinctive characteristic of cumulative frequency polygons is that the graph is always ascending or stable; it never descends because it always represents the cumulation of scores so far in the distribution. In contrast, the frequency polygon ascends or descends to show the frequency with which cases occur at each possible score point.

The overall shape of the distribution and the four characteristics of data distributions listed can be visualized graphically through inspection of figures. Figure 6.2 shows three distributions with different shapes. Figure 6.2a is a rectangular-shaped distribution indicating the same frequency of occurrence of each score in the distribution. The distribution shown in Figure 6.2b is bell-shaped (the so-called normal distribution), indicating the higher frequency of occurrence of middle scores and lower frequency of both higher and lower scores in the distribution. The distribution shown in Figure 6.2c is bimodal, indicating two clusterings of high frequency of occurrence of scores within the distribution toward the high and low ends, rather than a single clustering of scores in the middle. The next four figures will graphically illustrate each of the four characteristics of data distributions listed previously.

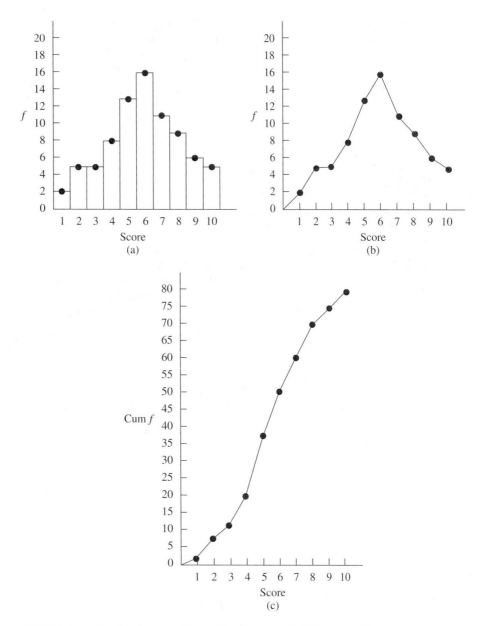

**FIGURE 6.1    Graphic Presentation of Test Scores: (a) Histogram of Scores, (b) Frequency Polygon of Scores, (c) Cumulative Frequency Polygon.**

Figure 6.3 illustrates three distributions with different *central tendencies.* The central tendency, or average, can be seen graphically by examining the concentration of scores toward the middle of the distribution. Figure 6.3a is the distribution with the lowest average, Figure 6.3c is the distribution with the highest average, and Figure 6.3b has an average

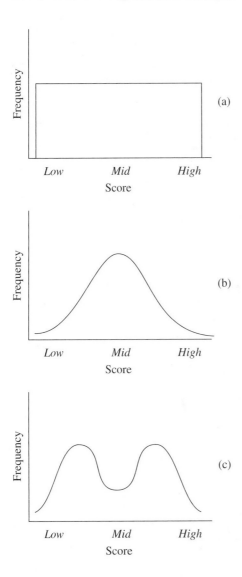

**FIGURE 6.2  Three Distributions with Different Shapes: (a) Rectangular, (b) Normal, (c) Bimodal.**

between the other two. Calculation of various measures of central tendency is shown in Table 6.2 and discussed in the next section.

Figure 6.4 illustrates three distributions with different *variabilities.* The variability, or degree to which the scores spread out from the center of the distribution, can be seen graphically by examining the width of the distribution. Figure 6.4a is the distribution with the lowest variability, Figure 6.4c has the highest variability, and Figure 6.4b has a variability

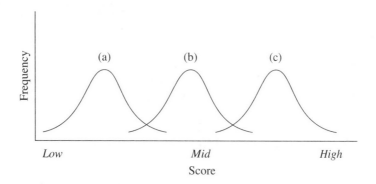

**FIGURE 6.3   Three Distributions with Different Central Tendencies: (a) Low, (b) Medium, (c) High.**

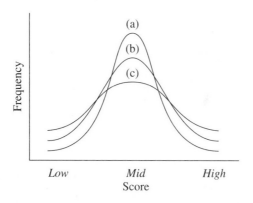

**FIGURE 6.4   Three Distributions with Different Variabilities: (a) Low, (b) Medium, (c) High.**

between the other two. Calculation of various measures of variability is shown in Table 6.3 and discussed in the next section.

Figure 6.5 illustrates three distributions with different *skewness*. The skewness, or lack of symmetry of the distribution, can also be visualized graphically by examining the form of the distribution. A symmetrical distribution (Figure 6.5a) looks the same on right and left sides; therefore, it is not skewed in one direction or the other. A negatively skewed distribution (Figure 6.5b) is one in which most scores cluster around a high value but a small number of scores spread out (or skew) into the very low score end at the left of the distribution. A positively skewed distribution (Figure 6.5c) is one in which most scores

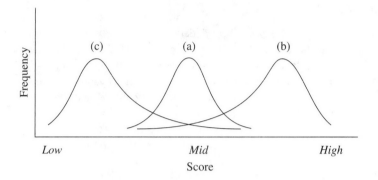

**FIGURE 6.5    Three Distributions with Different Skewness:
(a) Symmetrical, (b) Negatively Skewed, (c) Positively Skewed.**

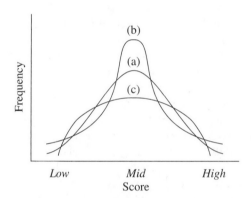

**FIGURE 6.6    Three Distributions with
Different Kurtosis: (a) Normal Mesokurtic,
(b) Leptokurtic, (c) Platykurtic.**

cluster around a low value but a small number of scores spread out (or skew) into the very high score end at the right of the distribution.

Figure 6.6 illustrates three distributions with different *kurtosis.* The kurtosis, or general form of concentration of scores around the center of the distribution, can be seen graphically by examining the center of the distribution to see if it is flat or peaked in shape. Kurtosis also affects the shape of the bend at the tails of the distribution. Kurtosis is often evaluated relative to the bell-shaped normal distribution (Figure 6.6a), which is called *mesokurtic* because of its medium shape between flat and peaked. A *leptokurtic* distribution (Figure 6.6b) is more peaked than normal and a *platykurtic* distribution (Figure 6.6c) is flatter than normal.

## Summary Statistics

The second way to organize research data is to summarize them in numerical form. Because summary statistics are the foundation on which most data-analysis techniques rest, the selection of appropriate summary statistics is critical to the clear reporting of research findings. These statistics describe the characteristics of the data by answering the following questions: "What is the average or typical value in the distribution?" and "How much variety or dispersion is there in the values represented by the distribution?" Although graphs and tables can provide a pictorial presentation of answers to these questions, the summary statistics present more precise quantitative information that is amenable to further data analysis. Summary statistics include measures of central tendency, variability, skewness, and kurtosis.

*Measures of Central Tendency.*    There are three common measures of central tendency—the mode, the median, and the mean. The *mode* is the most frequently occurring score in a distribution. The *median,* or middlemost score, can be determined as long as the data can be ranked. The median describes the point in the distribution that separates the upper half of the data from the lower half. It is determined by counting how many scores there are and finding out which score is in the middle of the distribution. If the median is 40, then you know that one-half the scores in the distribution are below 40 and one-half are above 40. The last index of central tendency is the *mean,* or arithmetic average, of the values in a set of data. It is found by adding up all the values and dividing by the number of values there are in a set of data. Table 6.2 illustrates the calculation of these three measures of central tendency for the hypothetical set of grouped data presented in Table 6.1.

Readers will note that Table 6.2 and other tables in this chapter contain statistical formulae and notation. These are presented for illustrative purposes for those readers who wish to examine the calculation of these statistics, and they are derived from two basic statistics texts (Guilford, 1965; Siegel, 1956). There are numerous alternate formulae and notation

**TABLE 6.2   Determining Measures of Central Tendency**

| Scores | | | | | | |
|---|---|---|---|---|---|---|
| X | f | cum f | fX | Mean | $= \bar{X} = \dfrac{\Sigma f(X)}{N} = \dfrac{473}{80} = 5.91$ | |
| 10 | 5 | 80 | 50 | Mode | = The most frequently occurring score is 6.0. | |
| 9 | 6 | 75 | 54 | Median = | The score separating the upper half of the cases ($\frac{1}{2}N$) from the lower half of the cases. | |
| 8 | 9 | 69 | 72 | | | |
| 7 | 11 | 60 | 77 | | In this instance, it is the point separating the upper 40 cases from the lower 40 cases. | |
| 6 | 16 | 49 | 96 | | | |
| 5 | 13 | 33 | 65 | | | |
| 4 | 8 | 20 | 32 | | Inspection of the cum f column shows that this point is somewhere between a score of 5 and 6. | |
| 3 | 5 | 12 | 15 | | | |
| 2 | 5 | 7 | 10 | | The exact value, by interpolation, is 5.43. | |
| 1 | 2 | 2 | 2 | | | |
| | | | $\Sigma fX = 473$ | | | |

conventions for most statistical calculations; readers should not feel that one type of notation or one formula is inherently superior to other techniques for obtaining the same information.

***Measures of Variability.***    The other major category of summary statistics includes those that indicate the amount of dispersion, spread, or variability in a set of data. Known as indices of variability, the major statistics in this category include the range, the variance ($\sigma^2$), the standard deviation (SD or $\sigma$), and the semi-interquartile range *(Q).*

The *range* is simply the spread from the lowest value to the highest value in a distribution of data. It can be expressed in several ways, including the following: "scores ranged from _____ to _____" and "the range was _____ points." The smaller the range, the less variability there is in a distribution; conversely, the larger the range, the more variability there is in a distribution.

The *variance* is determined by finding the mean of the values in a distribution and determining how far each value in the distribution deviates from the mean. Then these deviation scores are each squared to deal with the fact that half of the deviation is negative (i.e., below the mean) and half is positive (i.e., above the mean). If these deviation scores are not squared, their sum will always be zero and, therefore, useless. Then the squared deviation scores are summed and averaged to compute the variance. The variance cannot be presented in the original units of measurement because of the squaring, so it is not usually used as an absolute index of how the data spread out from the mean. But, the variance has two particularly important uses in data organization and analysis.

First, the variance is a most important number that represents variability and is used in the calculation of some statistics that will be described later in this chapter. These statistics include the correlation coefficient for analyzing relationships among variables and the analysis of variance for analyzing differences between groups of participants. Second, the square root of the variance is a useful measure of the average amount by which all of the scores deviate from the mean of a distribution, and it is presented in the original units of measurement. This average amount of dispersion of the scores in a distribution is called the *standard deviation* (SD) and is a most important statistic for organizing the data of a study. A small SD indicates that the scores in the distribution do not spread out from the mean very much; that is, the group is relatively homogeneous. A large SD, on the other hand, indicates a wide dispersion of scores from the mean of the distribution; that is, the group is more heterogeneous.

The interpretation of the SD depends on what statisticians call the normal curve model and assumes that the values in the distribution are symmetrically arranged on either side of the mean. The normal curve model and its uses will be discussed later. The last measure of variability, the *semi-interquartile range,* is used if the values in a distribution are *not* symmetrically arranged around the central tendency and it indicates one-half the range of the middle 50 percent of the scores in the distribution. Table 6.3 illustrates calculation of some measures of variability for the set of grouped data presented in Tables 6.1 and 6.2.

In general, if the SD is about one-fourth to one-sixth as large as the range, the sample is typical of that usually found in most statistical work. Likewise, if the SD is about one-and-one-half times as large as the semi-interquartile range, the distribution is not significantly skewed (Guilford, 1965).

**TABLE 6.3    Determining Measures of Variability**

| $X$ | $f$ | cum $f$ | $fX$ | $X - \bar{X}$ | $(X - \bar{X})^2$ | $f(X - \bar{X})^2$ |
|-----|-----|---------|------|---------------|-------------------|--------------------|
| 10 | 5 | 80 | 50 | +4 | 16 | 80 |
| 9 | 6 | 75 | 54 | +3 | 9 | 54 |
| 8 | 9 | 69 | 72 | +2 | 4 | 36 |
| 7 | 11 | 60 | 77 | +1 | 1 | 11 |
| 6 | 16 | 49 | 96 | 0 | 0 | 0 |
| 5 | 13 | 33 | 65 | −1 | 1 | 13 |
| 4 | 8 | 20 | 32 | −2 | 4 | 32 |
| 3 | 5 | 12 | 15 | −3 | 9 | 45 |
| 2 | 5 | 7 | 10 | −4 | 16 | 80 |
| 1 | 2 | 2 | 2 | −5 | 25 | 50 |
| | | | $\Sigma fX = 473$ | | | $\Sigma f(X - \bar{X})^2 = 401$ |

$\bar{X}$ (from Table 6.2) = 5.91     median = 5.43     mode = 6.0
Statement of range = "the scores ranged from 1 to 10."

$$\text{Standard deviation}^a = \text{SD} = \sigma = \sqrt{\frac{\Sigma f(X - \bar{X})^2}{N}} = \sqrt{\frac{401}{80}}$$

$$= \sqrt{5.01} = 2.23$$

$$\text{Semi-interquartile range} = Q = \frac{P75 - P25}{2}$$

P75 = (calculation not shown) the point separating the upper 25% of the cases from the lower 75% of the cases. For these data, P75 is 7.0.

P25 = (calculation not shown) the point separating the upper 75% of the cases from the lower 25% of the cases. For these data, P25 is 4.0.

$Q$ = one-half the range of the middle 50% of scores

$$\frac{7.0 - 4.0}{2} = \frac{3.0}{2} = 1.5$$

---

$^a$For convenience sake, the mean has been rounded to 6.0 for calculation of the deviation scores $(X - \bar{X})$.

*Measures of Skewness.*    A skewness statistic (called *Sk*) is sometimes computed to indicate the degree of asymmetry of a distribution (Kirk, 1999, pp. 129–131). The Sk statistic is calculated from the third power of the deviations above and below the mean (rather than from the square of deviations as in the variance): an Sk of zero indicates a symmetrical distribution, a positive Sk indicates a positively skewed distribution, and a negative Sk indicates a negatively skewed distribution. Skewness can also be detected by comparing indices of central tendency, particularly the mean and median. Positive skewness inflates the mean and negative skewness deflates the mean, but neither type of skewness affects the median. Thus, if the mean is greater than the median, the distribution is positively skewed; if the mean is smaller than the median, the distribution is negatively skewed.

***Measures of Kurtosis.***    A kurtosis statistic (called *Kur*) is sometimes computed to indicate the degree of kurtosis of a distribution (Kirk, 1999, pp. 129–131). The Kur statistic is calculated from the fourth power of the deviations above and below the mean: a Kur of zero indicates a normal or mesokurtic distribution, a positive Kur indicates a leptokurtic distribution, and a negative Kur indicates a platykurtic distribution.

The author of a research article should provide appropriate summary statistics to describe the data distribution. Usually the mean and standard deviation are reported for a normal distribution of interval or ratio level measurements. A distribution is considered normal if it is bell-shaped, mesokurtic, symmetrical on right and left sides (i.e., not skewed in either direction), with a concentration of scores in the middle and progressively fewer cases occurring at score values toward the extremes (tails) of the distribution. If the distribution is not normal, then the median and semi-interquartile range are often reported. Sometimes a comparison of mean and median or the measures of skewness and kurtosis are reported to document the lack of normality. Appropriate data organization is the prelude to data analysis and the characteristics of the data distribution, along with other factors such as the level of measurement and the specific research design employed, determine the type of statistical analysis procedure to be used.

# Data Analysis

## Basic Concepts of Data Analysis

***Appropriate Methods.***    As indicated previously, selection and application of data-analysis techniques beyond summary statistics is determined partly by the research questions of a study and partly by the level of the data yielded by the research. Basically, analysis techniques may be either *correlational* or *inferential,* depending on whether they are used to describe existing *relationships* or *differences* among data. In addition, the choice of the exact analysis procedure also depends on the number of variables being examined, the size and characteristics of the samples used, and the type of research plan in effect. Techniques of data analysis seem to be amenable to classification and description by "families" based on their derivation and their methodological assumptions. Because this is not a statistics text, each member of the procedural "families" will not be discussed at length. Instead, a summary of which procedures fit into the various situations described appears in Table 6.18 (at the end of the chapter).

For our purposes, it is sufficient to indicate that the various families of data-analysis techniques are more or less powerful (able to detect trends or differences in data), more or less well known, and more or less respected. However, each has unique characteristics that set it apart from the others and make it particularly useful in the right circumstances. Later sections of this chapter will describe each of these techniques and give some examples of how they may be used in communicative disorders research.

***The Normal Curve Model.***    We have previously referred to statistical procedures based on assumptions of the normal curve model, and it is appropriate to summarize the basic concepts of the model before proceeding.

The normal curve model is a construct based on the observation that measures of physical or psychological variables, derived from large numbers of people (or animals), tend to form a characteristic type of distribution when graphed. This distribution is the familiar symmetrical, bell-shaped curve that shows a concentration of values in the middle of the distribution with fewer and fewer values as the extremes are approached (Figure 6.7). The generalizability of this curve and its mathematical properties were first described by Gauss, and it is sometimes known as a Gaussian curve. Because it is the kind of distribution that data typically resemble, it also became known as a "normal" curve.

Inspection of Figure 6.7 reveals the symmetry of a normal distribution. It can be seen that most cases fall in the middle of the distribution, with fewer cases seen at the lower and higher score values at the extreme right- and left-hand sides of the distribution. About two-thirds of the cases fall within plus-or-minus 1 SD of the mean; 95 percent of the cases fall within plus-or-minus 2 SDs of the mean; and 99 percent of the cases fall within plus-or-minus 3 SDs of the mean. Although a perfect Gaussian or normal distribution is never attained in practice, there is enough resemblance between it and the actual obtained-data distributions to warrant its adoption as a mathematical model for statistical procedures that are used to analyze relationships and differences. The extent to which actual data resemble the model determines the usefulness of the model and statistical procedures derived from

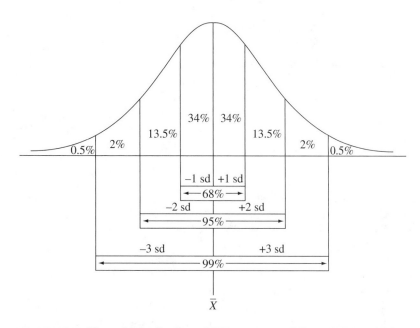

**FIGURE 6.7    Normal Distribution with Percentages of Cases Falling within SD Bands.**

it. If data do not approximate a normal distribution in the way they occur in a sample or population, then the normal curve model and the statistical procedures based on it are simply not applicable. Therein lies the necessity to ascertain whether the assumptions of the model and methods based on it fit the particular set of data to be analyzed. These considerations lead us to a discussion of statistics based on a normal curve model (*parametric statistics*) versus statistics that are not based on a normal curve model (*nonparametric statistics*).

***Parametric and Nonparametric Statistical Procedures.*** Parametric statistics are based on certain assumptions about the population from which the sample data are obtained. Because population quantities are often called parameters and sample quantities are often called statistics in statistical work, the term *parametric statistics* has been applied to data-analysis procedures that rest on certain assumptions about the population.

There are several assumptions about the population, and the sample drawn from it, that underlie the use of parametric statistics:

1. The population parameter should be normally distributed.
2. The level of measurement of the parameter in question should be interval or ratio.
3. When there are two or more distributions of data to be analyzed (e.g., two groups of participants are tested or one group of participants is tested under two different conditions) the *variances* of the data in the two different distributions should be about the same.
4. The sample should be fairly large. There is no agreed-on, absolute definition of "large," but most statisticians consider thirty subjects to be large enough (Hays, 1994).

When all of these assumptions can be met, parametric statistics are appropriate for data analysis. If one or more of these assumptions is seriously violated, parametric statistics may be inappropriate.

When assumptions about the populations cannot be met, researchers use nonparametric statistics. Nonparametric statistics are often called *distribution-free* statistics because they do not rest on assumptions about the distribution of the population parameter. Nonparametric statistics deal with data at the nominal or ordinal level of measurement. When a researcher has interval or ratio level data, but realizes that they are not normally distributed (or fail to meet one of the other assumptions listed), the data can be *transformed* from interval or ratio level to nominal or ordinal level in order to be used in a nonparametric test. For example, interval level scores can be classified as "pass" or "fail" by using a cutoff score on the interval scale. Another alternative is to rank-order all the subjects on the basis of their interval scale scores and then use their ranks as the data for a nonparametric statistical analysis. Of course, if the original data are already nominal or ordinal, then a nonparametric statistical procedure will have to be used instead of a parametric procedure.

Although it may appear that the use of nonparametric alternatives to parametric statistical analysis is always the "safest" way to analyze data, this is not really true. Parametric statistics are more powerful (i.e., more sensitive to differences and relationships) than nonparametric tests; therefore, they are preferred when the assumptions listed can be met. Throughout the rest of this chapter, we generally will describe a parametric procedure for each particular kind of analysis and then consider nonparametric alternatives to each parametric statistic.

***Testing a Null Hypothesis.***    Statistical analysis is concerned with making decisions about the existence versus the nonexistence of differences between groups or relationships among variables. This is usually done by examining the plausibility of a *null hypothesis* in light of obtained data. A null hypothesis is a hypothesis that states that there is no difference between groups or no relationship among variables. A simple null hypothesis may state, for example, that there is no difference between the means of two groups of participants on some dependent variable. The mean of the sample of group one would be compared to the mean of the sample of group two to decide how plausible that null hypothesis is. If the means of the two groups are about the same, then it is plausible that the null hypothesis is true, and the researcher can accept it. If, however, the means of the two groups are quite different, it does not seem plausible that the null hypothesis is true, and the researcher can reject it. The concept of testing a null hypothesis is the basis for *statistical inference* and underlies all of the methods for testing differences to be discussed subsequently in this chapter. Inferential hypothesis testing can also be applied in analyzing relationships, as will be seen later.

***Type I and Type II Errors.***    When a researcher makes a decision about a null hypothesis, one of four things can happen: the hypothesis can be true or false and the researcher can accept or reject it. Figure 6.8 illustrates the contingencies of this situation.

Inspection of Figure 6.8 reveals that there are two possible correct decisions that a researcher can make: accepting a true null hypothesis and rejecting a false null hypothesis. There are two possible incorrect decisions: rejecting a true null hypothesis (called a *Type I error*) and accepting a false null hypothesis (called a *Type II error*).

If a researcher concludes on the basis of the sample data that two groups are different, the decision will either be correct (if the groups are different) or a Type I error (if the groups are not different). If a researcher concludes on the basis of the sample data that the two groups are not different, the decision will either be correct (if the two groups are not different) or a Type II error (if the two groups are different). Statistical analysis helps the researcher to make the decision about a null hypothesis by indicating the probability that a decision to reject a null hypothesis is a Type I error. Statistical analysis can also help a researcher to make a decision to accept a null hypothesis by indicating the probability of making a Type II error. Unfortunately, the probability of making a Type II error is not as easily determined as the probability of making a Type I error. Consumers of research are

|  | Status of null hypothesis | |
| --- | --- | --- |
| Researcher's decision | Null hypothesis is true | Null hypothesis is false |
| Accept null hypothesis | Correct decision | Type II error |
| Reject null hypothesis | Type I error | Correct decision |

**FIGURE 6.8    Contingencies Involved in Making a Decision about a Null Hypothesis.**

more likely to find analyses of the probability of making a Type I error in articles that report group differences and are less likely to find analyses of the probability of committing a Type II error in articles reporting no differences between groups or conditions.

***The Level of Significance.***    The probability of making a Type I error is called the *level of significance.* When a researcher decides to reject a null hypothesis and conclude that there is a difference between two sets of data, he or she does so because the statistical test comparing the two sets of data indicates that the probability of making a Type I error in rejecting the null hypothesis is quite small. This probability is expressed by stating the level of significance (sometimes called *alpha*) associated with the comparison. Stating the level of significance indicates the degree of confidence that the researcher has that the difference seen in the sample data would not have occurred by chance alone. In fact, the level of significance is sometimes called the *level of confidence* for the comparison. The comparison of two data sets may be a between-subjects comparison such as the comparison of the means on some dependent variable between two groups of participants. It may also be a within-subjects comparison such as the comparison of the means on some dependent variable of participants tested under two different experimental conditions.

If the statistical analysis shows that it is highly improbable that an obtained sample difference would have occurred if the null hypothesis were true, then the researcher will reject the null hypothesis because the probability of committing a Type I error is small. If, however, the statistical analysis shows that it is not improbable that an obtained sample difference would have occurred if the null hypothesis were true, the researcher will not reject the null hypothesis because the probability of committing a Type I error is not small enough. How small must the probability of committing a Type I error be for a researcher to reject the null hypothesis? In other words, what must the level of significance be for a comparison of sample groups of data for a researcher to conclude that the groups of data are different?

Although there is no absolute answer to the question of what level of significance should be adopted, there are conventional preferences that have evolved. The most frequently used levels of significance are 0.05 and 0.01. These figures mean that the probability of committing a Type I error is 0.05 (five chances in one hundred) or 0.01 (one chance in one hundred). In other words, if the level of significance yielded by a statistical analysis indicates that the difference between the data sets could have resulted by chance (if null hypothesis were true) only five times out of one hundred, then, the null hypothesis will be rejected and the difference will be called "significant at the 0.05 level." Sometimes the level of significance is indicated by using the letter $p$ (for probability) and then stating the value of the probability of committing the Type I error. For example, a researcher might state: "The difference between the two groups was significant ($p = 0.05$)." Selection of the 0.05 versus the 0.01 level of significance by an investigator is arbitrary. Because the 0.01 level of significance indicates less chance of a Type I error than the 0.05 level, it is stricter or more conservative than the 0.05 level of significance. In other words, other things being equal, a larger difference between two sets of sample data must be found to reach the 0.01 level of significance than to reach the 0.05 level of significance.

The selection of a level of significance is a complicated process, a discussion of which is beyond the scope of this chapter. In general, however, if the study is in a previously unexplored domain or is one in which the researcher is trying to identify possibilities for further study at a later time, then a more lenient level of significance may be reasonable. If, on the other hand, the researcher is examining well-developed hypotheses or replicating a study, a stricter level of significance may be desired.

Two final remarks about significance levels are in order. First, many consumers of research interpret the term *significant* to mean a result that has clinical relevance or theoretical meaning. This is not necessarily true. A very small difference between groups that has little or no clinical relevance or theoretical meaning may be statistically significant in the sense that it is highly improbable to occur if the null hypothesis were true. Perhaps in that sense the term *significant* is inappropriate and the term *level of confidence* is a better one because it simply indicates the confidence that the researcher has that the result did not simply occur by chance. Whether a statistically significant difference between two groups of data also has theoretical or clinical significance is a rational matter that is more often treated by an author in a discussion section of an article than in the results section. Second, it should be pointed out that there are many researchers who prefer not to analyze results with statistical-significance testing procedures. Proponents of this point of view prefer to rely on replication studies and stronger rational examination of the meaning of their research results. Carver (1978) presents this perspective in a lengthy criticism of statistical-significance testing. Consumers of research should realize, then, that not all research articles will include statistical-significance tests and that the absence of such tests does not necessarily mean that the results are not clinically or theoretically significant or that the researcher has been faulty in the data analysis. It may simply mean that the particular researcher is in Carver's camp in opposition to statistical-significance testing. Some recent articles in the communicative disorders research literature (Attanasio, 1994; Meline & Schmitt, 1997; Young, 1993, 1994) raise methodological and statistical points similar to Carver's, emphasizing the importance of measures of effect size, the use of stronger experimental designs, and the routine consideration of replication studies.

Despite these criticisms of statistical-significance testing, this statistical procedure has remained common in many areas of behavioral science, including communicative disorders research. Harlow, Muliak, and Steiger (1997) present a detailed symposium on the pros and cons of null hypothesis significance testing and present a set of eight recommendations for the practice of scientific inference, with a discussion of how their symposium contributors weigh in on each recommendation. With regard to the traditional null hypothesis significance testing approach, Harlow (1997, p. 11) summarizes the symposium participants' overall views by stating:

> The practice of null hypothesis significance testing—making a dichotomous decision to either reject or retain $H_0$—has a long history. From Fisher to the present day, it has offered researchers a quantitative measure of the probability of getting sample results as different or more so than what is hypothesized in $H_0$. When used with well-reasoned and specific hypotheses, and when supplemented with other scientific input, such as effect sizes, power, confidence intervals, and sound judgment, it can be very effective in highlighting hypotheses that are worthy of further investigation, as well as those that do not merit such efforts.

In evaluating the participants' concurrence on statistical inference in her final practical recommendation, Harlow (1997, p. 12) suggests:

There is strong concurrence that statistical inference should include the calculation of effect sizes and power, estimation of appropriate confidence intervals, goodness of approximation indices, and the evaluation of strong theories with critical thinking and sound judgment. The chapter contributors were unanimous in their support of all of these except goodness of approximation, and nearly so for the latter. Thus, researchers should be encouraged to incorporate these methods into their programs of scientific research.

*One- and Two-Tailed Tests.*    Another important consideration in evaluating the results of data analysis is whether the researcher has chosen a one-tailed (directional) test or a two-tailed (nondirectional) test. This decision is made in relation to the questions or hypotheses posed in the study. If the researcher has made a directional hypothesis, he or she applies one-tailed tests. Examples of statements calling for one-tailed tests include "Scores of group $X$ will be higher than scores of group $Y$," "Scores will be significantly below average," and "There will be more persons in the $X$ category than in the $Y$ category." If the researcher is considering questions or hypotheses that are nondirectional, she or he applies two-tailed tests. Examples of statements calling for two-tailed tests include: "There will be a difference in scores between group $X$ and group $Y$," "Scores will be significantly different from the average," and "There will be a different number of persons in the $X$ category than in the $Y$ category."

Consumers of research should be aware that two-tailed tests are more strict or conservative than one-tailed tests. That is to say, a greater difference between groups must be found to call the difference significant when using a two-tailed test. A somewhat smaller difference may not be significant with a two-tailed test but may be significant when analyzed with a one-tailed test. Typically, one-tailed tests are used when the researcher has some reason to suspect in advance that the difference between groups or conditions should be in one direction. There is some controversy about when it is appropriate to select the more liberal one-tailed test, and more conservative statisticians and researchers generally recommend the more stringent two-tailed tests. For example, Cohen (1988) strongly advises researchers to avoid one-tailed tests. Consumers should expect to find both one-tailed and two-tailed tests in the literature, however, and they should realize that significant differences found with two-tailed tests are, in a sense, more significant than those found with one-tailed tests.

*Degrees of Freedom.*    The importance of sample size in the selection and application of a particular analysis procedure is highlighted by the concept of degrees of freedom. To interpret the results of a given statistical procedure, the researcher must know the degrees of freedom ($df$) in the data before tables of statistical significance can be used. In a most basic sense, $df$ indicate the number of values in a set of data that are free to vary once certain characteristics of the data are known. Generally, if the mean or the sum of a set of scores is known, then the $df$ are equal to the number of scores in each distribution minus 1 ($df = n - 1$).

The formula for determining the number of the $df$ varies according to the procedure employed for analysis, and the number of the $df$ should always be reported when analyses are described and interpreted. In a table or in the text of the results section of an article, the $df$ are usually listed as an accompaniment to the outcome of the particular data analysis procedure that is used. A discussion of the techniques for calculating $df$ for all the various analysis procedures is beyond the scope of this text. Consumers of research, however, should be aware that each analysis procedure must take into account the correct number of *df* in determining statistical significance. Authors usually show *df* in the results section to demonstrate to the editors and to readers more familiar with statistical analysis that the *df* are correctly accounted for in the analysis.

The following sections will examine how some of the commonly used parametric and nonparametric analysis procedures are used in communicative disorders studies. Procedures are grouped under two major headings: (1) methods for analyzing relationships and (2) methods for describing differences. The reader will find it useful to refer frequently to Table 6.18 while reading these sections because this table summarizes these analysis procedures regarding (1) the level of measurement for which each is appropriate, (2) whether the procedure analyzes differences or relationships, and (3) whether the procedure is parametric or nonparametric. Although this table is not a complete list of all statistical methods used in communicative disorders research, it does give an organized overview of those common procedures considered in this chapter.

## Methods for Analyzing Relationships

Often the researcher wishes to determine the strength and direction of relationships that exist in a set of data or simply whether some overall association occurs among variables in a given sample or population. To do this, two or more sets of scores or ranks or classifications are derived from a particular sample and subjected to analysis.

The relationship between two variables can be described graphically using a scattergram or scatterplot. Each participant has a pair of scores or ranks on the variables, and these are plotted on a bivariate graph with the axes representing the variables under study. Table 6.4 shows three sets of score pairs for ten participants. The corresponding scatterplots for these data sets appear in Figure 6.9.

Examination of the scatterplot will reveal the *direction* of the relationship. If the scores on one variable tend to *increase* as the other variable *increases,* the relationship is *positive* (Figure 6.9a). If one variable *decreases* as the other variable *increases,* the relationship is *negative* (Figure 6.9b). These relationships are shown by the direction in which the plot moves across the graph as in Figure 6.9(a–c). Moreover, the density with which the data points on the plot are clustered together reveals the *strength* of the relationship. Figures 6.9a and b show points tightly clustered, indicating a strong relationship, whereas Figure 6.9c shows a wide dispersal of points, indicating a weak relationship.

Although scatterplots are useful, they do not give a precise index of association between variables. For this reason, most relationships are reported as *correlation coefficients.* Many types of coefficients exist, depending on the methods used to obtain them, but the two most common ones are the *Pearson Product-Moment Correlation Coefficient* (a parametric index) and the *Spearman Rank-Order Correlation Coefficient* (a nonparametric index). Occasionally, a partial, multiple, biserial, point biserial, tetrachoric, or phi correlation may be cited, but these indices are interpreted in essentially the same way as the Pearson and Spearman indices.

Correlation coefficients have two components: a sign and a numeric value. The sign indicates the *direction* of the relationship (– is a negative or inverse relationship; + is a pos-

**TABLE 6.4 Score Pairs for Three Sets of Ten Participants**

| | Illustration A | | | Illustration B | | | Illustration C | |
|---|---|---|---|---|---|---|---|---|
| _Participants' Initials_ | _Score on First Variable_ | _Score on Second Variable_ | _Participants' Initials_ | _Score on First Variable_ | _Score on Second Variable_ | _Participants' Initials_ | _Score on First Variable_ | _Score on Second Variable_ |
| RB | 4 | 16 | CJ | 21 | 8 | DS | 21 | 2 |
| CS | 6 | 14 | DD | 53 | 5 | BC | 83 | 1 |
| JD | 8 | 17 | NS | 14 | 9 | WD | 45 | 7 |
| WM | 3 | 13 | IV | 67 | 6 | MC | 17 | 4 |
| SV | 2 | 11 | TY | 82 | 4 | HC | 62 | 8 |
| BP | 7 | 18 | BH | 98 | 1 | DR | 91 | 3 |
| BD | 1 | 12 | GS | 34 | 10 | AT | 37 | 9 |
| TM | 5 | 15 | JF | 47 | 7 | JN | 99 | 6 |
| FD | 10 | 19 | RF | 94 | 2 | RP | 72 | 5 |
| MC | 9 | 20 | TD | 76 | 3 | JF | 56 | 10 |

itive relationship). The numeric value indicates the strength of the relationship and may take on an absolute value ranging from 0.00 (no relationship) to 1.00 (a perfect relationship). Thus correlation coefficients can range from –1.00 (a perfect negative relationship) to +1.00 (a perfect positive relationship), as shown in the interpretive guide in Figure 6.10.

One point of confusion in interpreting these indices lies in the fact that the strength and direction of the coefficient are independent. Commonly, we think of negative numbers as being less desirable or significant than positive numbers; this is not true of correlation. For instance, if we were given the two correlation coefficients

$$r_{ab} = -0.79$$
$$r_{ac} = +0.63$$

and ask which describes a _stronger_ relationship, the answer is $r_{ab} = -0.79$, even though it is a negative coefficient. Incidentally, the subscripts _ab_ and _ac_ are a statistical convention for telling the reader which variables are being correlated; in this case $r_{ab}$ is the correlation between two variables, _a_ and _b_, whereas $r_{ac}$ is the correlation between two variables, _a_ and _c._

Moreover, the coefficients

$$r_{ad} = -0.43$$
$$r_{bc} = +0.43$$

indicate relationships of the _same_ strength, even though the relationship between variables _a_ and _d_ is inverse and the relationship between variables _b_ and _c_ is positive.

The Pearson Product-Moment Correlation Coefficient uses actual scores in the calculation, whereas the Spearman Rank-Order Correlation Coefficient requires that ranks or

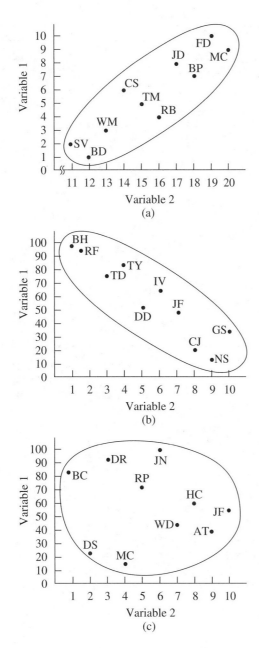

**FIGURE 6.9    Graphic Presentation of Relationships: (a) Scatterplot for Data in Illustration A (Table 6.4), (b) Scatterplot for Data in Illustration B (Table 6.4), (c) Scatterplot for Data in Illustration C (Table 6.4).**

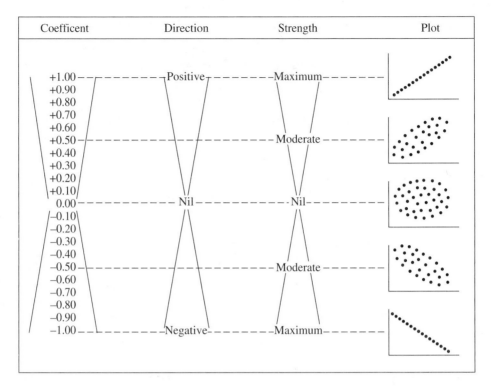

**FIGURE 6.10    Interpretive Guide for Correlation Coefficients.**

scores converted to ranks be used in the calculation. Generally, the Pearson coefficient applies to sample sizes of twenty-five or more with data at the interval or ratio levels, whereas the Spearman is used for ordinal data or when the sample size is less than twenty-five. No matter which of these or the other methods listed earlier is used, the researcher should clearly specify the procedure selected for analyzing particular sets of data. For purpose of illustration, both the Pearson and Spearman indices have been computed (Table 6.5) for the illustrative data sets in Table 6.4.

Rather than reporting entire lists of correlation coefficients showing relationships between variable pairs in a multivariate study, many experimenters present these data in a *table of intercorrelations* or in a *correlation matrix*. This way, the reader can, by locating the desired variable pairs in the row and column headings, find the correlation between those two variables. Table 6.6 shows a correlation matrix for five variables. By consulting the table, the reader can see that the correlation of variable *b* with variable *d* is −0.60, and so forth. Note that the entries in the table are duplicated below the underlined diagonal values. For that reason, the shaded portion often does not appear in research reports. In addition, the underlined diagonal values represent the correlation of each variable with itself and, therefore, equal +1.00, a perfect positive correlation.

When correlation coefficients are reported, the researcher may accompany this with some statement of the *statistical* significance of the index, that is, whether the correlation

**TABLE 6.5    Correlation Coefficients for Data of Illustrations A, B, and C Listed in Table 6.4 and Graphed in Figure 6.9**

| Data Set | Pearson $r$ | Spearman Rho |
|:---:|:---:|:---:|
| A | +0.91 | +0.92 (Very strong positive correlation) |
| B | −0.93 | −0.93 (Very strong negative correlation) |
| C | −0.10 | −0.13 (Very weak correlation) |

**TABLE 6.6    A Hypothetical Correlation Matrix**

| Variable | $a$ | $b$ | $c$ | $d$ | $e$ |
|:---:|:---:|:---:|:---:|:---:|:---:|
| $a$ | 1.00 | 0.64 | 0.14 | −0.39 | 0.04 |
| $b$ | 0.64 | 1.00 | 0.79 | −0.60 | 0.43 |
| $c$ | 0.14 | 0.79 | 1.00 | 0.98 | 0.16 |
| $d$ | −0.39 | −0.60 | 0.98 | 1.00 | −0.37 |
| $e$ | 0.04 | 0.43 | 0.16 | −0.37 | 1.00 |

coefficient is *significantly different from zero.* Because statistical significance may be obtained for very small correlations if the sample is large enough, small correlation coefficients should be interpreted cautiously. For example, for a sample size of two hundred, a correlation of plus or minus 0.14 is considered statistically significant (Guilford, 1965, p. 581). However, the *practical* usefulness of this index is limited because it is, at best, a modest correlation.

To evaluate the practical meaning of a correlation coefficient of a given magnitude, a statistic known as the Index of Determination is often used. This index, commonly known as $r^2$, is the square of the correlation coefficient, and it gives an indication of the actual amount of overlap between two variables in terms of shared variance. For example, a correlation, $r_{de} = +0.50$, indicates that there is actually only a 25 percent ($0.50^2$) overlap between the variables $d$ and $e$ in terms of variance accounted for. This is illustrated by Figure 6.11, which shows two variable domains—domain $G$ and domain $H$. If the correlation between the two variables ($G$ and $H$) is $r_{gh} = +0.60$, then this indicates that 36 percent ($0.60^2$) of the two domains actually overlap, leaving a full 64 percent of the domain variability unaccounted for. Figure 6.11 also illustrates the Indices of Determination for correlations of −0.30 and +0.20. The shaded areas represent the amount of variance that overlaps or is shared by the two variables; the white areas with question marks indicate the variance that is not accounted for by the correlation. The reader can readily see that the statistical significance of a correlation is only one indication of its quality and that the $r^2$ value can be a more pragmatically useful index for judging the meaning of the correlation.

Another consideration necessary for proper interpretation of correlation coefficients is that correlation does *not* imply that a cause–effect relationship exists between the variables being correlated. Thus, if variable *a* and variable *b* are correlated, this should be interpreted to mean that they *co*-relate, or vary together in some describable way so that as one variable moves in one direction, the other *tends* to move in the same direction (for a

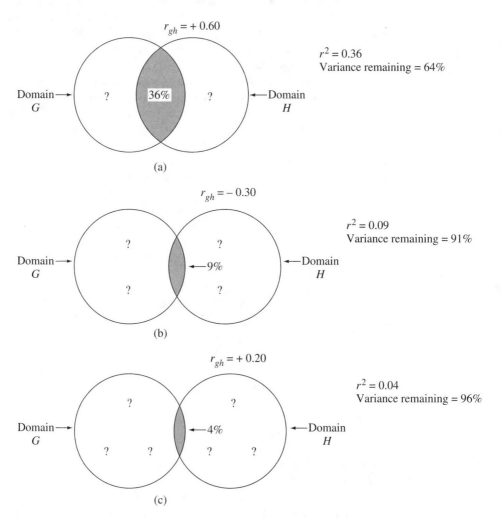

FIGURE 6.11 **The Index of Determination as an Indication of the Variance Shared by Two Variables.**

positive relationship) or the opposite direction (for a negative relationship). One does not necessarily *cause* the other to vary.

In addition to ascribing causality to correlations, there exists another common *misinterpretation* of correlation coefficients. This is the direct translation of a coefficient into a percentage or proportion. Often, students tend to think that if we know the correlation between two variables is +0.58 and have data for one of these variables, we will correctly predict what the data for the other will be 58 percent of the time. This is *not* correct, and researchers who make these kinds of statements are being inaccurate. Instead, a +0.58 correlation indicates that there is a moderately positive relationship between two variables so that, in general, the individuals who have high scores or rankings on one variable will probably tend to have high scores or rankings on the other. Note the qualifiers: "in general," "probably," and "tend to" in the preceding statement. These indicate the tentative nature of interpretation of correlation coefficients and the possibility that, unless the relationship is *perfect,* there will be some cases in any sample or population that do not behave in the same way as the majority.

In addition to allowing researchers to understand the relationships among variables, correlational analysis allows researchers to make predictions of the value of one variable from knowledge of the values of other variables. For example, a research study may be concerned with prediction of some criterion performance such as degree of success in a treatment program (designated a dependent variable) from knowledge of factors such as pretreatment test scores, prognostic indicators, or severity of disorder (designated as independent variables). To accomplish this, the researcher assembles data for a sample of participants and correlates all of the independent variables with the dependent variables. Often, the independent variables are termed *predictor* variables and the dependent variables are termed *predicted* variables because of the direction of the prediction. The relationships, expressed as correlation coefficients, can be presented in tables of intercorrelations showing how each variable relates to each other variable and to the criterion. In rare instances, a single factor emerges as having such a strong relationship with the criterion that it can be used as the sole predictor in a regression equation. Most of the time, however, the array of correlations indicates that several variables should be used in combination to predict the criterion more closely than any single variable can.

The researcher then sets out to find the best linear combination of predictors, that is, one that acknowledges the unique relationship of each predictor with the criterion, minimizes the overlap (correlation) among predictors, and maximizes the combined strength of the predictors. Rather than attempt this task of finding the optimal combination of predictors through trial and error, the researcher uses a statistical technique known as multiple-regression analysis. In brief, this technique mathematically enables the researcher to determine the *order* in which predictor variables should be entered in a prediction equation to maximize prediction; assigns a *weight* to each predictor variable entered into the equation; and (in a stepwise multiple regression) indicates the *contribution* of each new added variable to the predictive validity of the equation. By the use of these methods, the researcher may initially examine the relationships among each of twenty variables themselves. The researcher may then conclude the analysis by specifying three or four variables that can be combined in a given order and with given weights in a regression equation to best predict the criterion.

The success and meaning of multiple-regression analysis depends on a number of factors the researcher must consider. These factors include (1) care in selection of the initial variables for the analysis, (2) the reliability and validity with which the variables are measured, (3) the size and representativeness of the sample used for study, (4) the reliability and validity of the criterion measure, and (5) the practicality of gathering all of the predictor data appearing in the equation. Multiple-regression analysis is a popular and appealing data-manipulation procedure. Unfortunately, the attractiveness of this procedure often results in its misuse.

The correlation and regression methods discussed previously give quantitative descriptions of the strength and direction of association among variables that can be assigned ranks or score values. Occasionally, however, the researcher is faced with the task of ascertaining whether there is an association between two or more variables when at least one of them is a nominal variable. This is especially pertinent to studies using questionnaire or demographic data that can be reported as frequencies in categories but cannot satisfactorily be expressed in ordinal or interval scales.

To organize such nominal-level data, the researcher may present them in *contingency tables*. The categories used for one variable are listed across one axis of the table, whereas those for a second variable are listed along the other axis. Contingency tables can also be generated for more than two variables, but they are somewhat awkward and are not found as often in the research literature. The entries in the table are the frequencies with which participants had that particular combination of values. Table 6.7 shows a contingency table having two rows and two columns, which is therefore known as a 2 × 2 contingency table. Hypothetical data on pass–fail performance of speakers with normal palate and cleft palate are entered in the cells of Table 6.7.

Although contingency tables are useful on their own, they are usually accompanied by further data analysis that enables the researcher to determine whether significant relationships exist among the variables. Two common analysis techniques that may be applied to such data are the chi square ($\chi^2$) and the contingency coefficient ($C$).

Application of chi square to the data in the contingency table discussed previously yields a value of 9.39. Consulting a table of chi square values required for the 0.01 level of statistical significance shows that the required value for this set of data having 1 *df* is 6.64 (Siegel, 1956, p. 249). Thus, this chi square will be statistically significant beyond the 0.01

**TABLE 6.7  A 2 × 2 Contingency Table Illustrating Data from Hypothetical Performance of Speakers with and without Cleft Palate on Some Categorical Performance Measure**

|  | Cleft Palate | Normal Palate |
|---|---|---|
| Passed | 3 | 17 |
| Failed | 13 | 6 |

$$\chi^2 = 9.39$$
$$C = 0.44$$

level, indicating that there is a relationship between the two categorical variables that can have occurred only by chance less than one time in one hundred.

Briefly, a chi square analysis requires that the actual observed ($O$) frequencies listed in the contingency table be compared to expected ($E$) frequencies generated during the analysis or postulated by the researcher earlier on the basis of some theory or prior experience with similar data. If the discrepancy between what was actually observed in the study and the estimates given by the expected values is large enough, the resulting chi square value will reach statistical significance. The reader will note that the outcome of the analysis must be evaluated by consulting statistical tables of significance using the *df* determined from the data. These significance tables give the minimal values of the chi square statistic needed with various *df* to permit the conclusion that there is a statistically significant relationship between or among the variables in question. The chi square analysis does *not* indicate the strength of any relationship that exists nor the direction of that relationship. Chi square indicates only the extent to which the relationship is outside the realm of chance or normal probability. The contingency coefficient is used to measure the extent or strength of the relationship and can be computed by a formula that employs the chi square value. The contingency coefficient for the data in Table 6.7 is $C = 0.44$ and this coefficient would be interpreted in much the same way as the other correlation coefficients discussed earlier except that the upper limit for $C$ for a 2 × 2 table is 0.707, not 1.0.

The upper limit of $C$ is a function of the number of categories under examination in the contingency table (Siegel, 1956). When the number of rows ($r$) and columns ($c$) of the contingency table are the same (as in Table 6.7), the upper limit of $C$ is computed as follows:

$$C = \sqrt{\frac{r-1}{c}}$$

Thus, for the 2 × 2 contingency table, the upper limit of $C$ is $\sqrt{1/2} = 0.707$. For a 3 × 3 contingency table, the upper limit of $C$ is $\sqrt{2/3} = 0.816$.

Although chi square is often used for ascertaining the presence of significant bivariate relationships, it can be extended to multivariate situations as long as a participant's data can be classified within one value or category in each variable. Thus, chi square can be used for a 2 × 3 × 5 contingency table or a 3 × 6 × 2 × 7 contingency table. The only difficulties lie in finding a way to present these data and interpret the meaning of three-way and four-way relationships.

Although chi square is used to determine the presence of relationships in nominal-level data, it is an extremely flexible procedure that can also be used as a method for analyzing *differences* in groups. In this sense, the method provides a link between procedures that show relationships and those that describe differences. The major difference among the applications of this procedure lies in the nature of the questions or hypotheses examined, as we will see in the next section.

## Methods for Analyzing Differences

Many research problems in communicative disorders concern differences between (or among) groups of participants. For example, a researcher might ask if there is a difference between normal-hearing and hearing-impaired children on a particular language measure. Other problems concern differences between (or among) conditions for the same group of participants. For example, a researcher might ask if there is a difference between hearing-impaired participants' speech-discrimination scores before and after auditory training. In other words, researchers are concerned about the analysis of between-subjects differences and within-subjects differences. In analyzing the between-subjects and within-subjects differences, researchers want to determine whether the differences are large enough in the sample data to rule out the probability that they could be attributed to chance or sampling error. The procedures of statistical inference are used to make such an analysis for determining the statistical significance of differences between-subjects and within subjects. In other words, the researcher will examine the probability of making a Type I error in concluding that there is a between-subjects or a within-subjects difference.

Table 6.18 (at the end of this chapter) summarizes many of the common analysis procedures and the situations in which they are applicable. The table indicates the level of measurement for which each procedure is applicable and shows which procedures are parametric and which are nonparametric. Also indicated is whether the procedure is applicable to between-subjects comparisons (i.e., independent samples tests) or within-subjects comparisons (i.e., related samples tests). Some of the statistical tests are also identified as appropriate for comparing only two samples or for comparing more than two samples of data.

We will first consider statistical methods that are used to ascertain the significance of the difference between *two groups of data* on a *single dependent variable.* These procedures can be used to compare two different groups of participants or to compare one group of participants under two different conditions, such as speaking in quiet versus noise. In other words, these procedures can be used to make between-subjects comparisons (i.e., to compare independent or uncorrelated samples) or to make within-subjects comparisons (i.e., to compare related or correlated samples).

In the two-group one-variable analysis situation described previously, the basic parametric procedures for determining the significance of differences are the *z*-ratio and the *t*-test. The *z*-ratio is used when the samples are large (thirty or more) and the *t*-test is applicable for smaller samples. Basically, both of these methods (and their various subroutines) examine a theoretical distribution of *differences* in means to determine how the observed differences derived from a particular study compare to the average differences in a theoretical distribution. If the observed difference departs markedly from the average difference in the theoretical distribution, it is judged significant at a given level of significance (usually the 0.05 or 0.01 level, as described earlier). This is accomplished through the use of established formulae and tables available in statistical texts.

In the case of the *z*-ratio, the values required for statistical significance are 1.96 (0.05 level) and 2.58 (0.01 level) for two-tailed tests and 1.65 (0.05 level) and 2.33 (0.01 level) for one-tailed tests. With the *t*-test, the values required for statistical significance vary according to the number of degrees of freedom available for the data and require the consultation of a table showing significant *t*-values for different degrees of freedom. The researcher who uses these procedures should cite both the *z*-ratio or *t*-value obtained for the data in the study and the statistical significance at the level chosen for the study.

Table 6.8 shows examples of the application of the *z*-ratio to compare means from two different groups and to compare the pretreatment and posttreatment means from a

**TABLE 6.8  Summary Table for $z$-Ratio**

| | Illustration Different Groups | | | | Illustration Same (Correlated) Groups | | |
|---|---|---|---|---|---|---|---|

<table>
<tr><td colspan="3">Illustration<br>Different Groups<br>$H_0: M_1 = M_2$<br>$H_1: M_1 \neq M_2$</td><td></td><td colspan="3">Illustration<br>Same (Correlated) Groups<br>$H_0: M_1 = M_2$<br>$H_1: M_1 \neq M_2$</td></tr>
<tr><td></td><td>Group 1</td><td>Group 2</td><td></td><td></td><td>Testing 1</td><td>Testing 2</td></tr>
<tr><td>N</td><td>35</td><td>41</td><td></td><td>N</td><td>40</td><td>40</td></tr>
<tr><td>$M$*</td><td>29.5</td><td>31.2</td><td></td><td>M</td><td>53.1</td><td>55.4</td></tr>
<tr><td>$\sigma$</td><td>5.3</td><td>4.8</td><td></td><td>$\sigma$</td><td>7.9</td><td>8.1</td></tr>
<tr><td>$\sigma_M$</td><td>0.91</td><td>1.76</td><td></td><td>$r_{M_1 M_2}$†</td><td>—    0.80</td><td>—</td></tr>
<tr><td>$\sigma_{D_M}$</td><td>—</td><td>1.18    —</td><td></td><td>$\sigma_M$</td><td>1.3</td><td>1.3</td></tr>
<tr><td></td><td></td><td></td><td></td><td>$\sigma_{D_M}$</td><td>—    0.83</td><td>—</td></tr>
</table>

Formula for $z$-ratio:  $z = \dfrac{D_M}{\sigma_{D_M}}$

(where $D_M = M_2 - M_1$) $= \dfrac{31.2 - 29.5}{1.18}$

$= 1.44$

The $z$-ratio of 1.44 is less than that required for statistical significance at the 0.05 level (1.96) for a two-tailed test. Therefore, the difference in the two means is not significant and could have occurred by chance more than 5 times in 100.

Decision: accept $H_0$.

Formula for $z$-ratio:  $z = \dfrac{D_M}{\sigma_{D_M}}$

(where $D_M = M_2 - M_1$) $= \dfrac{55.4 - 53.1}{0.83}$

$= 2.77$

The $z$-ratio of 2.77 exceeds that required for statistical significance at the 0.01 level for the two-tailed test (2.58). Therefore, the difference in means between the two testings is statistically significant and could have occurred by chance less than 1 time in 100.

Decision: reject $H_0$; accept $H_1$.

*Either $M$ or $\overline{X}$ can be used to represent the mean score.
†Correlation between testing 1 and testing 2 derived during prior analysis and used in calculating $\sigma_{D_M}$.

single group. Similar examples for the $t$-test appear in Tables 6.9 and 6.10. In the examples in Tables 6.8 and 6.9, it is the *mean* of the group or groups that is examined rather than individual values. The $t$-test for correlated groups shown in Table 6.10 uses mean pair differences and deviations of pair differences in the calculations.

Also listed in these tables are the null hypotheses ($H_0$) and their alternates ($H_1$, $H_2$, and so on) that are tested with each statistical procedure. Each statistical procedure considers the probability of the hypothesis ($H_0$) that there are no differences between the groups of scores. If the obtained statistic indicates that this null hypothesis is highly improbable (i.e., the statistic reaches the significance level), then the $H_0$ is rejected in favor of one of the alternate hypotheses listed.

**TABLE 6.9** **Summary Table for *t*-Test (*Uncorrelated Groups*)**

$$H_0 = \bar{X}_1 = \bar{X}_2$$
$$H_1 = \bar{X}_1 > \bar{X}_2$$

Directional hypotheses; call for one-tailed test.

|  | Group 1 |  | Group 2 |
|---|---|---|---|
| N | 21 |  | 23 |
| $\bar{X}$ | 15.7 |  | 13.5 |
| $\sigma$ | 3.7 |  | 3.9 |
| *$\Sigma x^2$ | 287 |  | 349 |
| $X_1 - X_2$ | — | 2.2 | — |

Formula for *t* (difference between uncorrelated means):
$$\frac{\bar{X}_1 - \bar{X}_2}{\sqrt{\left(\dfrac{\Sigma x^2{}_1 + \Sigma x^2{}_2}{N_1 + N_2 - 2}\right)\left(\dfrac{N_1 + N_2}{N_1 N_2}\right)}}$$

*t* for these data = 1.88 *df* for these data = 42

*t* required for 42 *df* one-tailed test = 1.68 (0.05 level)

The *t*-value of 1.88 exceeds that required for statistical significance at the 0.05 level for a one-tailed test with 42 *df*. Therefore, the difference in means between the two groups is statistically significant and would have occurred by chance fewer than 5 times in 100. The mean of Group 1 is significantly larger than the mean of Group 2.

Decision: reject $H_0$; accept $H_1$.

*Information derived during analysis; calculations not shown.

When the assumptions required for the use of parametric methods cannot be met (e.g., the data are not in interval or ratio scales or sample sizes are extremely small), the researcher applies analogous nonparametric procedures to the data. Among them are the Wilcoxon Matched-Pairs Signed-Ranks Test for changes within a group over time and the Mann–Whitney *U* Test that examines differences between groups. The values reached by use of these procedures must be compared with values in appropriate tables. Examples of the Wilcoxon and the Mann–Whitney procedures are found in Tables 6.11 and 6.12. A more detailed description of nonparametric methods for describing differences is found in Siegel (1956).

We will now consider situations in which there are *more than two groups* for comparison and *more than two conditions* under which each group is tested. The parametric statistical procedure used for these situations in most studies is the *analysis of variance* (usually abbreviated ANOVA). The statistic calculated in ANOVA is called the *F-ratio,* and the outcome of the analysis is usually reported in the form of a summary table. Interpretation of an

**TABLE 6.10 Summary Table for *t*-Test (*Correlated Groups*)**

$$H_0 = \bar{X}_1 = \bar{X}_2$$
$$H_1 = \bar{X}_1 \neq \bar{X}_2$$

*Note:* This procedure tests for differences in score pairs rather than means.

*Raw Data for 18 Participants*

| | Subject | Pretest | Posttest | Subject | Pretest | Posttest |
|---|---|---|---|---|---|---|
| $N = 18\ X_1 = 21.8\ X_2 = 22.7$ | a | 23 | 28 | j | 28 | 27 |
| | b | 24 | 22 | k | 27 | 27 |
| | c | 16 | 18 | l | 18 | 15 |
| | d | 15 | 16 | m | 21 | 23 |
| | e | 18 | 23 | n | 26 | 27 |
| | f | 16 | 18 | o | 19 | 25 |
| | g | 21 | 20 | p | 21 | 19 |
| | h | 25 | 23 | q | 26 | 26 |
| | i | 26 | 28 | r | 23 | 24 |

Information derived from these data during analysis includes:

$$M_d = 1.0 \quad \Sigma x^2_d = 110$$

*t*-test formula: $t = \dfrac{M_d}{\sqrt{\Sigma x_d^2 / N(N-1)}}$

*t* for these data = 1.69

*t* required for statistical significance (two-tailed test; *df* = 17)
  2.1 (at the 0.05 level);
  2.9 (at the 0.01 level).

The *t*-value of 1.69 is less than that required for statistical significance with 17 *df* at the 0.05 level for a two-tailed test. Therefore, the difference in the scores received on pretest and posttest is not statistically significant and could have occurred by chance variation more than 5 times in 100.

Decision: accept $H_0$.

---

*F*-ratio requires consultation of special significance tables. However, the summary table should present the value of *F* required for significance (or the *p* value of each reported *F*) and the appropriate number of *df* for each comparison.

We cannot provide a detailed explanation of the assumptions underlying ANOVA and the procedures for calculating *F*-ratios. However, we will try to present the overall logic of ANOVA as a test for differences among several means. If there is a difference

**TABLE 6.11   Summary of Wilcoxon Matched-Pairs Signed-Ranks Test ($T$)**

$$H_0 = \Sigma Ranks_1 = \Sigma Ranks_2$$
$$H_1 = \Sigma Ranks_1 \neq \Sigma Ranks_2$$

Hypothetical raw data for seven participants measured before and after treatment.

| Participant | Score before Treatment | Score after Treatment | Difference $d$ | Rank of $d$ | Rank with Less Frequent Sign |
|---|---|---|---|---|---|
| a | 17 | 19 | + 2 | 2 | |
| b | 17 | 16 | − 1 | 1 | 1 |
| c | 20 | 14 | − 6 | 5 | 5 |
| d | 13 | 21 | + 8 | 7 | |
| e | 16 | 19 | + 3 | 3 | |
| f | 14 | 21 | + 7 | 6 | |
| g | 19 | 14 | − 5 | 4 | 4 |

$T = 10$

This procedure determines the statistic $T$ for the data, which is the sum of the ranks with the less frequent sign, and compares this value to those required for statistical significance that are tabulated in the appendices in Siegel (1956). The value of $T$ for these data is 10 and the $T$ required at alpha = 0.05 is 2 and at alpha = 0.01 is 0 for $N = 7$ participants.

*Note:* In this procedure observed $T$ must be *smaller* than the required value to be significant.

The observed $T$ is larger than that required for statistical significance at the 0.05 level. Therefore, the shift in scores between pretesting and posttesting is not significant and could have occurred by chance more than 5 times in 100.

Decision: accept $H_0$.

The Wilcoxon $T$ can also be converted to a $z$-score with the formula:

$$z = \frac{T - u_T}{SD_T}$$

The $z$-score for these data is 0.11, which is not significant at the alpha = 0.05 level. This conversion is required for large samples ($N > 25$), but Siegel (1956, p. 79) has indicated that conversion to a $z$-score may also be used for small samples and he provides the formulae for calculation of $u_T$ and $SD_T$. The $z$ has a mean of zero and a standard deviation of one with the opposite direction of the $T$ for significance. A large $T$ would result in a $z$ approaching zero and a small $T$ would increase the $z$ to a more significant value (i.e., lower probability of Type I error).

**TABLE 6.12    Summary of Mann–Whitney $U$ Test ($U$)**

$$H_0 = \text{Ranks}_1 = \text{Ranks}_2$$
$$H_1 = \text{Ranks}_1 \neq \text{Ranks}_2$$

Hypothetical raw data for two samples of ten participants on a vocabulary test.

| Group 1 Score | Rank | Group 2 Score | Rank |
|:---:|:---:|:---:|:---:|
| 20 | 7 | 23 | 9 |
| 15 | 4 | 16 | 5 |
| 18 | 6 | 13 | 3 |
| 25 | 10 | 12 | 2 |
| 10 | 1 | 22 | 8 |
| $R_1 = 28$ | | $R_2 = 27$ | |

The Mann–Whitney procedure determines the statistic $U$ for these data and compares this value to those required for statistical significance that are tabulated in the appendices in Siegel (1956). The value of $U$ for these data is 12 and the $U$ required at alpha = 0.05 is 4 and at alpha = 0.01 is 2 for $N$ = 5 participants per group.

*Note:* The observed value of $U$ must be *smaller* than the required value to be statistically significant at that level.

The observed $U$ is larger than that required for statistical significance at the 0.05 level. Therefore, the difference between Groups 1 and 2 is not statistically significant and may have occurred by chance more than 5 times in 100.

Decision: accept $H_0$.

---

among a set of group means, the variance *between the groups* will be significantly larger than the variance *within each of the groups.* The variance between the groups can be thought of as the variance of the group means around the *grand mean* of all the scores.

For instance, a researcher might ask if children of different ages differ in their performance on some language task. Using a cross-sectional developmental approach, the researcher assembles four age groups (five-, six-, seven-, and eight-year-olds), with one hundred children in each group, and assesses the performance of these four hundred children using a one-way ANOVA design (see Table 6.13). This ANOVA is called a one-way ANOVA because there is only one independent (classification) variable. In other words, the structure of an ANOVA, or the number of "ways" it tests for mean differences, is determined by the structure of the independent variables in the research study.

Within each age group, there will be some variation among the one hundred children tested so that there will be an age-group mean and an age-group variance for each of

**TABLE 6.13   Representation of a One-Way ANOVA Design for Comparing the Means of Four Age Groups**

| | *Independent (Classification) Variable = Age* | | | |
| --- | --- | --- | --- | --- |
| | **Group A (5-year-olds)** | **Group B (6-year-olds)** | **Group C (7-year-olds)** | **Group D (8-year-olds)** |
| Dependent (criterion) variable | $\bar{X}_a$ | $\bar{X}_b$ | $\bar{X}_c$ | $\bar{X}_d$ |
| | $\sigma_a$ | $\sigma_b$ | $\sigma_c$ | $\sigma_d$ |
| | $N_a = 100$ | $N_b = 100$ | $N_c = 100$ | $N_d = 100$ |

$H_0$ = there are no differences in the means of the four groups.
$H_1$ = there is a difference among the means of the four groups.

the four age groups. If the variance *between the age-group means* (relative to the grand mean) is much larger than the variance *within each age group,* then there will be a significant difference among the age groups as shown by the *F*-ratio. The *F*-ratio that results from such an ANOVA is the ratio of the between-groups variance (called Mean Square between groups or MS between) to the within-groups variance (called MS within). When the between-groups variance is much larger than the within-groups variance, the *F*-ratio is large and reaches statistical significance when it is large enough for the appropriate number of *df* and alpha level. When the between-groups variance is not larger than the within-groups variance, the *F*-ratio is small and does not reach statistical significance. A table summarizing a possible ANOVA for the hypothetical cross-sectional study discussed previously is shown in Table 6.14.

If there is only one independent or classification variable in a study (i.e., age or clinical diagnosis), then the data form a one-way classification problem, and a one-way ANOVA is performed with the resulting *F*-ratio reported, as in the example in Table 6.14. The *F*-ratio is the ratio of a between-groups value called the mean square (MS between) to the within-groups mean-square (MS within) value, which are calculated during the analysis.

Let us now proceed to a more complex situation that takes the basic problem outlined previously one step further. Suppose our researcher felt that the children's gender was also a factor involved in language performance. The research design would then be constructed so that in addition to the four age categories, each age group would be divided into a group of males and a group of females. The researcher now has a 4 by 2 design (often abbreviated 4 × 2), and the resulting data would be analyzed using a two-way ANOVA in which one variable of interest is age and the other is gender. Hypothetical data for a 4 × 2 design are shown in Table 6.15 with a list of the statistical hypotheses that would be evaluated. The researcher is, then, asking more than one question in the analysis, namely:

1. Is there a difference in language performance among children of different ages?
2. Is there a difference in language performance among children of different genders?

**TABLE 6.14   Summary Table for One-Way ANOVA (Using Example from Text)**

| Components | Sum of Squares | Degrees of Freedom (*df*) | Mean Squares | *F*-Ratio |
|---|---|---|---|---|
| Between groups (ages) | 53.19 | 3 | 17.73 | 3.1 |
| Within groups | 2265.12 | 396 | 5.72 | |
| Total | 2318.31 | 399 | | |

$$F = \frac{\text{MS between}}{\text{MS within}} = \frac{17.73}{5.72} = 3.1$$

$F_{\text{required}} \ (3/396 \ df) = 2.62 \ (p = 0.05)$
$\qquad\qquad\qquad\quad 3.83 \ (p = 0.01)$

The observed *F*-ratio of 3.1 falls between that required at the 0.05 level and that required at the 0.01 level. Therefore, there is a statistically significant difference among the four groups. This difference could occur by chance fewer than 5 times in 100 but more than 1 time in 100.

Decision: reject $H_0$; accept $H_1$.

Both of these questions concern so-called *main effects* in the ANOVA. In addition, another question has been implicitly introduced: Is there an *interaction* of age and gender with respect to language performance? Thus, might males and females show a different pattern of language performance across ages? Therefore, ANOVA has to examine three sources of variance in this problem—variance across age (MS age), variance across genders (MS gender), and variance owing to the interaction of age and gender (MS age × gender)—and compare each of these three sources of variance with the variance within the eight groups (MS within groups). There will then be three *F*-ratios calculated: the *F*-ratio for age, the *F*-ratio for gender, and the *F*-ratio for the interaction. Any, all, or none of these might be statistically significant. The summary table for the example we have discussed is shown in Table 6.16. The information in the table that is most pertinent to the consumer of research is in the far-right column in which the *F*-ratios appear. These can be compared with the required values given below the body of the table to determine their statistical significance. In addition, a frequent notation for indicating level of significance appears in the table: the use of the single asterisk (*) to denote statistical significance at the 0.05 level, and the use of the double asterisk (**) to denote statistical significance at the 0.01 level.

We should now return to the notion of interaction and deal with it in a bit more detail. We have seen that once the researcher moves away from designs having a single independent or classification variable to designs having several independent or classification variables, concern for the main effects of each of these variables is supplemented by consideration of the interaction between or among the variables. These interactions are aptly named because interaction variations are not attributable to any of the main effects acting *alone* but rather to the *joint action* of two or more variables. Sometimes, interactions are called crossover effects because of the way they show up in graphic representations of data. In the hypothetical example used earlier, gender and age showed a significant interac-

**TABLE 6.15   Representation of a 4 × 2 Design Suitable for a Two-Way ANOVA**

|  | *Independent (Classification) Variable Age of Participants* | | | |
|---|---|---|---|---|
|  | **Group A (5-year-olds)** | **Group B (6-year-olds)** | **Group C (7-year-olds)** | **Group D (8-year-olds)** |
| Males | $\bar{X}_{ma}$ $\sigma_{ma}$ $N_{ma} = 50$ | $\bar{X}_{mb}$ $\sigma_{mb}$ $N_{mb} = 50$ | $\bar{X}_{mc}$ $\sigma_{mc}$ $N_{mc} = 50$ | $\bar{X}_{md}$ $\sigma_{md}$ $N_{md} = 50$ |
| Females | $\bar{X}_{fa}$ $\sigma_{fa}$ $N_{fa} = 50$ | $\bar{X}_{fb}$ $\sigma_{fb}$ $N_{fb} = 50$ | $\bar{X}_{fc}$ $\sigma_{fc}$ $N_{fc} = 50$ | $\bar{X}_{fd}$ $\sigma_{fd}$ $N_{fd} = 50$ |

$H_0$ (for main effect of gender): there are no differences between the means of the male and female groups.

$H_1$ (for main effect of gender): there are differences between the means of the male and female groups.

$H_0$ and $H_1$ for main effect of age take the same form as above.

$H_0$ (for age by gender interaction): there are no differences between the means of various ages by gender groups.

$H_1$ (for age by gender interaction): there are differences between the means of various ages by gender groups.

tion. This is illustrated in Table 6.17 and Figure 6.12, which show the performances for the various ages and genders. Note that the plots for gender and age are *not* parallel; although females *generally* have a higher performance than males, the female performance advantage is not the same at each age, and by age eight, male and female scores are essentially equivalent. That is to say, the performance difference between males and females decreases as their ages increase to eight years when males catch up to females.

Every field of research has identified and studied variables that tend to interact. In our hypothetical example we have considered a so-called two-way interaction. In a design using three variables, both two-way and three-way interactions must be examined. For instance, a communicative disorders study might look at the effects of gender, clinical classification, and length of time in treatment on some outcome variable. The ANOVA for this situation considers the following main effects and interactions:

1. Gender ($G$)
2. Clinical classification ($C$)
3. Length of time in treatment ($T$)
4. $G \times C$ interaction

**TABLE 6.16   Summary Table for Two-Way ANOVA (Using Example from Text)**

| Components | Sum of Squares | Degrees of Freedom (*df*) | Mean Squares | *F*-Ratios |
|---|---|---|---|---|
| Between groups (ages) | 54.00 | 3 | 18 | 5.8** |
| Between groups (genders) | 12.10 | 1 | 12.1 | 3.9* |
| Interaction of age × gender | 38.10 | 3 | 12.7 | 4.1** |
| Within groups | 1215.20 | 392 | 3.1 | |
| Total | 1319.40 | 399 | | |

*$p < .05$
**$p < .01$

| Calculation of *F*-Ratios | | Required *F*-Ratios for Significance | | |
|---|---|---|---|---|
| *F* for age | $= \dfrac{18.0}{3.1} = 5.8$ | 2.62 | 3.83 | ($df = 3,392$) |
| *F* for gender | $= \dfrac{12.1}{3.1} = 3.9$ | 3.86 | 6.70 | ($df = 1,392$) |
| *F* for age × gender interaction | $= \dfrac{12.7}{3.1} = 4.1$ | 2.62 | 3.83 | ($df = 3,392$) |
| | | 0.05 | 0.01 | |
| | | Level of significance | | |

The obtained *F*-ratios can be evaluated as follows:
   *F* for main effect of age indicates significant differences among ages
   *F* for main effect of gender indicates significant differences between genders
   *F* for interaction of age and gender indicates significant interaction effect

    **5.** $G \times T$ interaction
    **6.** $C \times T$ interaction
    **7.** $G \times C \times T$ interaction

From a practical standpoint, most studies do not involve interactions of more than three variables. Not only are more complex interactions difficult to interpret but the sample size and other design considerations required for such studies present difficulties for the researcher. Moreover, interaction effects should be carefully evaluated when reporting research results. In fact, in some research studies, interaction effects may be more important than main effects. Often ANOVA will show both significant main effects and significant interaction effects.

    Once a researcher has, through application of ANOVA procedures, shown that a significant difference occurs among the groups in the study, further analyses may be con-

**TABLE 6.17   Hypothetical Row and Column Means Illustrating Main Effects of Age and Gender on Language Performance and Interaction of Age and Gender**

| Gender of Participants | Age of Participants | | | | |
| --- | --- | --- | --- | --- | --- |
| | Group A (5-year-olds) | Group B (6-year-olds) | Group C (7-year-olds) | Group D (8-year-olds) | Ages Combined |
| Males | 12.0 | 16.0 | 21.0 | 24.0 | 18.25 |
| Females | 17.0 | 20.0 | 23.0 | 23.0 | 20.75 |
| Genders combined | 14.50 | 18.00 | 22.00 | 23.50 | |

ducted to ascertain the location of the significant differences among the groups. Historically, *t*-tests are used to compare pairs of means following determination of a significant *F*-ratio. However, newer procedures are often used instead of *t*-tests for various mathematical and logical reasons. Among these are the Tukey, Duncan, Newman-Keuls, and Sheffé procedures. The reader may often find that research reports contain references to these analyses following ANOVA in order to identify specific significant differences.

The application of nonparametric methods to designs that lend themselves to ANOVA procedures is found in communicative disorders research when data are in the form of nominal or ordinal scales, making use of such methods imperative. As noted in Table 6.18, the nonparametric procedures that more or less parallel the parametric ANOVA

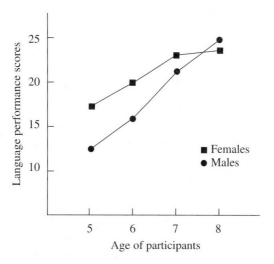

**FIGURE 6.12   Graphic Plot for Visualizing Interaction of Two Independent (Classification) Variables in a Hypothetical Two-Way (4 × 2) ANOVA Problem.**

**TABLE 6.18   Summary of Selected Analysis Procedures**

| Level of Measurement | Methods for Analyzing Relationships | Methods for Analyzing Differences | | |
|---|---|---|---|---|
| | | WS **Related Samples** | | **Independent** BS **Samples** |
| Nominal | *Nonparametric methods* — Contingency Coefficient ($C$) Chi Square ($\chi^2$) | Cochran $Q$ Test | | Chi Square Test for Independent Samples ($\chi^2$) |
| Ordinal | Spearman Rank-Order Correlation Coefficient (Rho) | Two Samples | Wilcoxon Matched-Pairs Signed-Ranks Test ($T$) | Mann–Whitney $U$ Test |
| | | More than Two Samples | Friedman Two-Way ANOVA | Kruskal-Wallis One-Way ANOVA |
| Interval or ratio | *Parametric methods* — Pearson Product-Moment Correlation Coefficient ($r$) | Two Samples | $t$-Test for Correlated Groups $z$-Ratio | $t$-Test for Independent Groups $z$-Ratio |
| | Multiple-Regression Analysis | More than Two Samples | ANOVA ($F$) ANCOVA ($F$) MANOVA ($T^2, \Lambda, F$) | ANOVA ($F$) ANCOVA ($F$) MANOVA ($T^2, \Lambda, F$) |

are the Kruskal-Wallis One-Way ANOVA by Ranks (H), the Friedman Two-Way ANOVA by Ranks ($X_r^2$), the Cochran $Q$ Test, and a chi square test for independent samples. Discussion of each of these methods can be found in Siegel (1956). H and $X_r^2$ both test the hypothesis that a number of samples (groups) have been drawn from the same population and, hence, have similar average values in rank. Cochran's $Q$ tests whether frequencies or proportions from correlated groups (or repeated measures on a single set of participants) differ across occasions. The chi square test for independent samples tests the hypothesis that different samples come from the same population; it is useful for data that can be presented as frequencies.

This overview for describing differences will close with a very brief description of two other varieties of analyses included here because they may be mistakenly confused with ANOVA. They are (a) multivariate analysis of variance (MANOVA), and (b) analysis of covariance (ANCOVA). In contrast to the ANOVA, which examines the effects one or more independent variables have on a *single* dependent variable, the MANOVA examines the effects of one or more independent variables on *multiple dependent* variables. Bordens & Abbott (2002) suggest two potential advantages of using a MANOVA: (1) the MANOVA treats the dependent variables as a correlated set revealing relationships among the independent and dependent variables that may otherwise be missed by the ANOVA, and (2) using a MANOVA rather than two or more ANOVAs reduces the chance of committing a Type I error. The statistics that may be computed for a MANOVA include Hotelling's $T^2$, Wilks' Lambda ($\Lambda$), and various $F$-ratios (Huck, Cormier, & Bounds, 1974; Monge & Cappella, 1980; Tabachnick & Fidell, 2001; Winer, Brown, & Michels, 1991). Analysis of *co*variance (ANCOVA) is used in studies in which one of the independent or classification variables is related inextricably to the dependent variable. The analysis itself controls for the *co*-relation of the two variables by virtue of the method used to compute the $F$-ratios and the outcome is interpreted in the same manner as ANOVA results. An example of a situation requiring the use of ANCOVA would be one in which verbal aptitude is an independent classification variable and vocabulary scores are a dependent variable in a study of the effects of different language treatment programs. Because verbal aptitude is significantly related to vocabulary scores, the ANCOVA would control for this relationship in determining whether significant differences in vocabulary scores existed as a function of the programs independent of verbal aptitude.

## Effect Size and the Power of Statistical Tests (Power Analysis)

Consumers of research are likely to encounter two related statistical procedures that have not appeared widely in past extant communicative disorders literature: *effect size* and *power analysis.* The recent increased use of effect size estimates is partially attributable to a recommendation in the fifth edition of the *Publication Manual of the American Psychological Association* (American Psychological Association, 2001, p. 25), advising authors of journal articles thus:

> For the reader to fully understand the importance of your findings, it is almost always necessary to include some index of effect size or strength of relationship in your Results section.

The manual lists several different statistical procedures that may be used to indicate effect size and further advises authors (American Psychological Association, 2001, p. 26) that

> The general principle to be followed, however, is to provide the reader not only with information about statistical significance but also with enough information to assess the magnitude of the observed effect or relationship.

Thus, reporting of effect size estimates is becoming an increasingly common procedure for indicating not only the statistical significance of results but also the practical significance of the data (Huck, 2004). Huck's assertion is consistent with recent findings regarding the use of effect size estimators in communicative disorders quantitative research. Meline and Wang (2004) conducted a census of effect size reporting practices in the four journals published by the American Speech-Language-Hearing Association (i.e., *American Journal of Audiology, American Journal of Speech-Language Pathology, Journal of Speech, Language, and Hearing Research,* and *Language, Speech, and Hearing Services in Schools*). They reported (p. 202):

> Inclusion of effect size in quantitative research reports increased from 5 reports with effect size in 1990 to 1994 to 120 reports in 1999 to 2003.

Meline and Wang point out, however, that effect size estimates were reported less than 30 percent of the time when inferential statistics were reported during the epoch of 1999 to 2003. Meline and Wang (2004, p. 207) concluded their census report with the following:

> Researchers should routinely (a) include estimates of effect size and (b) interpret effect size metrics within the context of their experiment.

What are effect size estimates? Effect size estimates are standardized values (similar to a *z*-score) and they are scale free (Robey, 2004). Effect sizes are not interpreted as being statistically significant or insignificant; they are estimates of how much a dependent variable is explained by an independent variable. As such, they provide a means for interpreting a statistical result that is independent of statistical significance.

As Robey (2004) explains, effect size estimates provide an independent index of the plausibility of a null hypothesis. When experimental data are completely consistent with the null hypothesis, the effect size estimate is zero. When experimental data are inconsistent with the null hypothesis, the effect size estimate differs from zero. For example, two commonly used effect size estimators in communicative disorders research are eta-square ($\eta^2$) and Cohen's *d*. Generally, eta-square is the ratio of the sum of squares of the effect to the sum of squares of the effect plus the sum of squares of the error, or

$$\eta^2 = (SS_{effect}/SS_{effect} + SS_{error})$$

Eta-square is interpreted in exactly the same way that $r^2$ is interpreted. For example, $\eta^2 = 0.90$ means that 90 percent of the variability in the dependent variable can be explained or accounted for by the independent variable. As such, $\eta^2 = 0.20$, $\eta^2 = 0.50$, and $\eta^2 = 0.80$ can be interpreted as small, medium, and large effect sizes, respectively.

Cohen's *d* is generally defined as the difference between two group means, $M_1 - M_2$, divided by the standard deviation, *s,* of either group, or

$$d = M_1 - M_2/s$$

Cohen (1988) suggests that one can interpret $d = 0.20$, $d = 0.50$, and $d = 0.80$ as small, medium, and large effect sizes, respectively.

Different computational formulae are used to compute effect size estimates for different research design strategies and statistical procedures. As such, the actual magnitude of effect size estimators varies and must be interpreted accordingly. Tables regarding the interpretation of various effect size estimators have been developed by Cohen (1988).

Power analysis has two general uses: (1) a priori, to determine the participant sample size required to reach a given alpha level, and (2) post hoc, to further evaluate research that has been completed to determine if a failure to reject a null hypothesis was related to the use of a too small participant sample size (Rosenthal & Rosnow, 1991). The power of a study is the probability of rejecting a null hypothesis when the null hypothesis is, in fact, false (Jones, Gebski, Onslow, & Packman, 2002; Rosenthal & Rosnow, 1991). Power is equal to the complement of the probability of making a Type II error, or Power = 1 – Type II (beta). As explained by Jones et al. (2002, p. 244):

> This is because a Type II error occurs when a statistically significant difference is not detected when it is present, and power is the probability to detect a statistically significant difference if it exists. Cohen (1969) recommends minimum power of .80, and this has become accepted as a benchmark, just as .05 has been accepted as a benchmark for the probability of a Type I error in a study.

Computational formulae for calculating power can be found in statistics and research books such as Cohen (1988) and Rosenthal and Rosnow (1991). Also, commercial software used for such computations is readily available and as Jones et al. (2002) point out, much of it is available on the Internet as shareware.

## Study Questions

1. Read pages 18–22, 30–34 in Chapter 3 of Siegel, S. (1956). *Nonparametric statistics for the behavioral sciences.* New York: McGraw-Hill.

   Write a brief summary of Siegel's discussion of statistical models and parametric and nonparametric statistical tests.

2. **a.** Which measures of central tendency and variability are usually reported when the distribution of data is normal?
   **b.** Which measures are usually reported when the distribution is skewed?

3. Examine the data in each of the following tables:

   Table 1 in: Gravel, J. S., & Wallace, I. F. (1992). Listening and language at 4 years of age: Effects of early otitis media. *Journal of Speech and Hearing Research, 35,* 588–595.

   Table 1 in: DePaul, R., & Brooks, B. R. (1993). Multiple orofacial indices in amyotrophic lateral sclerosis. *Journal of Speech and Hearing Research, 36,* 1158–1167.

   Which measures of central tendency and variability are used in each table to summarize the distribution of the data?

4. Examine the data in each of the following figures:

   Figure 4 in: Ellis Weismer, S., Murray-Branch, J., & Miller, J. F. (1994). A prospective longitudinal study of language development in late talkers. *Journal of Speech and Hearing Research, 37,* 852–867.

   Figure 1 in: Onslow, M., Hayes, B., Hutchins, L., & Newman, D. (1992). Speech naturalness and prolonged speech treatments for stuttering: Further variables and data. *Journal of Speech and Hearing Research, 35,* 274–282.

   **a.** How are the means displayed in each of these figures?
   **b.** Summarize, in your own words, what differences among the means are displayed in these figures.

5. **a.** Describe what is meant by the strength and direction of a relationship between two variables.
   **b.** How are these two aspects of a relationship demonstrated in a scattergram?
   **c.** How are they demonstrated in a correlation coefficient?

6. Examine the data in the following table:

   Table 7 in: Shriberg, L. D., Gruber, F. A., & Kwiatkowski, J. (1994). Developmental phonological disorders III: Long-term speech sound normalization. *Journal of Speech and Hearing Research, 37,* 1151–1177.

   **a.** Which correlation coefficient is used to analyze the relationships among the variables listed in this table?
   **b.** Which correlations are significantly different from zero at the 0.05 level? At the 0.01 level?
   **c.** Which pair of variables show the strongest relationship? Which pair show the weakest relationship?

7. Examine the data in Tables 5 and 6 and the analysis in the paragraphs "Changes in Stuttering" in: Riley, G. D., & Ingham, J. C. (2000). Acoustic duration changes associated with two types of treatment for children who stutter. *Journal of Speech, Language, and Hearing Research, 43,* 965–978.

   **a.** What statistical technique is used to analyze the pre- and posttreatment differences in acoustic variables for the two groups of participants?
   **b.** What statistical technique is used to analyze the pre- and posttreatment differences in stuttering frequency for the two groups of participants?
   **c.** Why did the authors use two different techniques for analyzing these differences?

8. Examine the data in Table 1 and the analysis in the accompanying paragraphs in: Dollaghan, C. A., Campbell, T. F., Paradise, J. L., Feldman, H. M., Janosky, J. E., Pitcairn, D. N., & Kurs-Lasky, M. (1999). Maternal education and measures of early speech and language. *Journal of Speech, Language, and Hearing Research, 42,* 1432–1443.

   **a.** What statistical technique is used to analyze the differences between the three groups of mothers?
   **b.** Why did the authors use this statistical technique for analyzing these differences?
   **c.** Which dependent variables show significant differences among the mothers and which did not?

9. Read the following article:

   Jones, M., Gebski, V., Onslow, M., & Packman, A. (2002). Statistical power in stuttering research: A tutorial. *Journal of Speech, Language, and Hearing Research, 45,* 243–255.

   **a.** Discuss why one needs to consider power analysis prior to conducting an investigation.
   **b.** Discuss the parameters that can influence the power of a given investigation.

10. Read the following article:

   Roy, N., Merrill, R. M., Thibeault, S., Gray, S. D., and Smith, E. M. (2004). Voice disorders in teachers and the general population: Effects on work performance, attendance, and future career choices. *Journal of Speech, Language, and Hearing Research, 47,* 542–551.

   **a.** What was the nonparametric statistic that was used in this study?
   **b.** Why was the nonparametric statistic used?

# REFERENCES

American Psychological Association. (2001). *Publication manual of the American Psychological Association* (5th ed.). Washington, DC: American Psychological Association.

Attanasio, J. S. (1994). Inferential statistics and treatment efficacy studies in communication disorders. *Journal of Speech and Hearing Research, 37,* 755–759.

Bordens, K. S., & Abbott, B. B. (2002). *Research design and method: A process approach* (5th ed.). New York: McGraw-Hill.

Carver, R. P. (1978). The case against statistical significance testing. *Harvard Educational Review, 48,* 378–399.

Cohen, J. (1988). *Statistical power analysis for the behavioral sciences* (2nd ed.). Mahwah, NJ: Lawrence Erlbaum Associates.

Ferguson, G. A., & Takane, Y. (1989). *Statistical analysis in psychology and education* (6th ed.). New York: McGraw-Hill.

Guilford, J. P. (1965). *Fundamental statistics in psychology and education.* New York: McGraw-Hill.

Harlow, L. L. (1997). Significance testing introduction and overview. In L. L. Harlow, S. A. Mulaik, & J. H. Steiger (Eds.), *What if there were no significance tests?* Mahwah, NJ: Lawrence Erlbaum Associates.

Harlow, L. L., Mulaik, S. A., & Steiger, J. H. (Eds.). (1997). *What if there were no significance tests?* Mahwah, NJ: Lawrence Erlbaum Associates.

Hays, W. L. (1994). *Statistics* (5th ed.). New York: Harcourt Brace.

Huck, S. W. (2004). *Reading statistics and research* (4th ed.). Boston: Allyn & Bacon.

Huck, S. W., Cormier, W. H., & Bounds, W. G. (1974). *Reading statistics and research.* New York: Harper & Row.

Jones, M., Gebski, V., Onslow, M., & Packman, A. (2002). Statistical power in stuttering research: A tutorial. *Journal of Speech, Language, and Hearing Research, 45,* 243–255.

Kirk, R. E. (1999). *Statistics: An introduction* (4th ed.). New York: Harcourt Brace.

Kranzler, G., & Moursund, J. (1999). *Statistics for the terrified.* Upper Saddle River, NJ: Prentice Hall.

Meline, T., & Schmitt, J. F. (1997). Case studies for evaluating statistical significance in group designs. *American Journal of Speech-Language Pathology, 6(1)* 33–41.

Meline, T., & Wang, B. (2004). Effect-size reporting practices in *AJSLP* and other ASHA journals, 1999–2003. *American Journal of Speech-Language Pathology, 13,* 202–207.

Monge, P. R., & Cappella, J. N. (1980). *Multivariate techniques in human communication research.* New York: Academic Press.

Pedhazur, E. J., & Schmelkin, L. P. (1991). *Measurement, design, and analysis.* Mahwah, NJ: Lawrence Erlbaum Associates.

Robey, R. (2004). Reporting point and interval estimates of effect size for planned contrasts: Fixed within effects analyses of variance. *Journal of Fluency Disorders, 29,* 307–341.

Rosenthal, R., & Rosnow, R. L. (1991). *Essentials of behavioral research* (2nd ed.). New York: McGraw-Hill.

Siegel, S. (1956). *Nonparametric statistics for the behavioral sciences.* New York: McGraw-Hill.

Tabachnick, B. G., & Fidell, L. S. (2001). *Using multivariate statistics* (4th ed.). Boston: Allyn & Bacon.

Winer, B. J., Brown, D. R., & Michels, K. M. (1991). *Statistical principles in experimental design* (3rd ed.). New York: McGraw-Hill.

Young, M. A. (1993). Supplementing tests of statistical significance: Variation accounted for. *Journal of Speech and Hearing Research, 36,* 644–656.

Young, M. A. (1994). Evaluating differences between stuttering and nonstuttering speakers: The group difference design. *Journal of Speech and Hearing Research, 37,* 522–534.

# Evaluation of the Components of a Research Article

## Overview

The main purpose of Part II is to show how the principles discussed in Part I can be applied to the evaluation of research. Part II provides specific guidelines for analyzing and critically evaluating the four basic parts of the research article.

The four chapters of Part II cover the Introduction, Method, Results, and Discussion sections of a research article. The journals published by the American Speech-Language-Hearing Association (ASHA)—as well as many other journals of interest in communicative disorders—follow the style specified in the current edition of the *Publication Manual of the American Psychological Association.* The manual states (American Psychological Association, 2001, p. 7):

> Journal articles are usually reports of empirical studies, review articles, or theoretical articles. Reports of empirical studies are reports of original research. They typically consist of distinct sections that reflect the stages in the research process and that appear in the sequence of these stages:
>
> - *introduction:* development of the problem under investigation and statement of the purpose of investigation;
> - *method:* description of the method used to conduct the investigation;
> - *results:* report of the results that were found; and
> - *discussion:* interpretation and discussion of the implications of the results.

Thus, we will follow the APA style suggestions in outlining the various parts of a research article in this part of the book.

Although much has been written about methods and statistical analyses in a number of texts, relatively little attention has been devoted to the evaluation of the research problem itself. Chapter 7 presents some guidelines for evaluating the introductory part of the research article. Emphasis here is placed on assessing the adequacy of the rationale for the study, on deciding if the literature citations support the need for the study, and on evaluating the research questions or hypotheses. Numerous examples, drawn from the communicative disorders literature, are used throughout this chapter and the chapters that follow. The chapter concludes, as do the other chapters in this part, with an Evaluation Checklist.

A brief word is necessary here about the Evaluation Checklists. Our intention in presenting the Checklists is to help the reader *focus* on those *key* elements of an article that deserve careful attention. We recognize that it is unlikely that most consumers of research will conduct the type of intensive analysis suggested by the Checklists, at least not in ordinary circumstances. We also recognize that because of the variety of research designs found in the literature, not all items on the Checklists will be applicable to all research reports. This is especially true for the Method Checklist. Nevertheless, the Checklists represent a didactic device that should be useful to the consumer, the would-be researcher, the researcher preparing a report of his or her study, and editorial consultants.

Chapter 8 deals with the Method section of the research article. It is in this section of the article that threats to internal and external validity are identified; thus, the Method section is of vital importance to the critical evaluator. Chapter 8 is divided into the three typical components of a Method section: participants, materials, and procedures. The reader is urged to pay careful heed to how participants are selected, how they are assigned to treatment groups, the reliability and validity of measurements used in the research, the research design employed, and whether the design reduces confounding threats to internal and external validity.

The next chapter is concerned with the Results section of an article. Nothing is introduced in Chapter 9 that has not already been treated in Chapter 6. The whole point of this chapter is simply to illustrate the concepts and principles detailed earlier. The chapter deals with the adequacy of figures and tables, with the appropriateness of the statistical treatment, and with the interpretation of the data analysis.

The final chapter of Part II outlines criteria to be used in evaluating the Discussion and Conclusions section of the research article. Here, as in the Introduction section of an article, remarkably few guidelines are available to the critical evaluator. Yet, the Discussion and Conclusions section represents the culmination of a particular research effort and frequently is of considerable interest to the practitioner because of the possible implications for clinical practice. Some of the questions that are addressed in this chapter include Are the conclusions fairly and accurately drawn from the results? Are the limitations of the study identified? Are there implications for future research, theory, or application and do these implications stem from the data? Are comparisons with previous research fair and objective?

# REFERENCE

American Psychological Association. (2001). *Publication manual of the American Psychological Association* (5th ed.). Washington, DC: American Psychological Association.

# The Introduction Section of the Research Article

We have previously emphasized the importance of the problem in initiating and designing a research study. The Introduction section of the research article is of the utmost importance to the critical reader of the research literature. It is in this section that the researcher presents the rationale for doing the research. If the author fails in this task, the remainder of the article may founder as well. It cannot be emphasized too strongly that the research problem, as described in the introduction to the article, is the thread that ties together the Method, the Results, and the Discussion sections. In essence, the good introduction is very much like a legal brief. Just as a legal brief is designed to convince the judge or jury, so, too, is the introduction designed to convince the reader of the need and the value of the study being proposed.

The various components of the introduction to a research article are the following:

1. Title
2. Abstract
3. General statement of the problem
4. Rationale for the study
5. Review of the literature
6. Specific purposes, research questions, or hypotheses

These six components do not always appear as separate entities in this order in every research article. Different authors have different writing styles and preferences for the organization of the introduction. Each of these components is identified in one form or another in the *APA Publication Manual* (APA, 2001, pp. 10–17) as a key part in writing the introduction to a research article. Therefore, we will identify, describe, and exemplify each of these six components of the introduction in this chapter.

## Title of the Article

The introduction to a research article actually begins with the title of the article. The title is important because it is the first thing the reader sees. It alerts the reader to an article that may be of professional interest. The title should identify the general problem area, including the specification of independent and dependent variables and the target population.

The *APA Publication Manual* (APA, 2001, p. 10–11) states that the "title should summarize the main idea of the paper" and that it should be "fully explanatory when standing alone" because a title has two main functions. The title informs readers about the article and is used as the basis for indexing the article in the journal's index and in the various abstracting services and journals.

Three examples of research article titles are shown in Excerpts 7.1, 7.2, and 7.3.

---

**E X C E R P T  7.1**

Effect of compression ratio on speech recognition and speech-quality ratings with wide dynamic range compression amplification.

From K. T. Boike and P. E. Souza, 2000, *Journal of Speech, Language, and Hearing Research, 43,* p. 456. Copyright 2000 by the American Speech-Language-Hearing Association. Reprinted with permission.

---

The title shown in Excerpt 7.1 is long, but complete. It identifies the independent variable (compression ratio), the dependent variables (speech recognition and speech-quality ratings), and the type of amplification that is being investigated (wide dynamic range compression). The reader should have no difficulty in knowing what the article is about, and the article can be indexed quite well from the title alone.

---

**E X C E R P T  7.2**

Speaking fundamental frequency changes over time in women: A longitudinal study.

From A. Russell, L. Penny, and C. Pemberton, 1995, *Journal of Speech and Hearing Research, 38,* p. 101. Copyright 1995 by the American Speech-Language-Hearing Association. Reprinted with permission.

---

The title shown in Excerpt 7.2 is shorter, but it still conveys the essence of the study. The article examines changes in women's vocal fundamental frequency over time. The title also clearly states that the research design is longitudinal.

---

**E X C E R P T  7.3**

Speech synthesis using damped sinusoids.

From J. M. Hillenbrand and R. A. Houde, 2002, *Journal of Speech, Language, and Hearing Research, 43,* p. 926. Copyright 2002 by the American Speech-Language-Hearing Association.

---

Even a very short title can fully inform the reader about the nature of a study. In the five words of the title of Excerpt 7.3, the authors have told us what their study is about. A reader will know immediately if the article is of interest, and an abstracting service can do a reasonable job of indexing the article from the title.

In summary, the title of an article should capture the essence of the topic that is investigated. It should be concise and well written, and should identify the variables studied and the target population.

## The Abstract

Many journals require a short abstract that briefly summarizes the major points of the article. The *APA Publication Manual* (APA, 2001, pp. 12–15) suggests that an empirical research article should contain an abstract of no more than 120 words that describes the problem, the participants, the method, the findings, and the conclusions. The manual further states that the abstract should be accurate, self-contained, concise, specific, comprehensive, and readable. It should be aimed at increasing the audience and the future retrievability of the article. Abstracts are not easy to write. Important, precise information must be packed into a small space. But the importance of the abstract is highlighted by the following statement (APA, 2001, p. 12):

> A well-prepared abstract can be the most important paragraph in your article. . . . Readers frequently decide on the basis of the abstract whether to read the entire article; this is true whether the reader is at a computer or is thumbing through a journal. The abstract needs to be dense with information but also readable, well organized, brief, and self-contained.

The abstract shown in Excerpt 7.4 is an example of an abstract that covers considerable ground in a small space. The first sentence states the purpose and identifies the participants. The next few sentences describe the method and results; the last sentence deals with implications of the findings and the need for further research.

---

### EXCERPT 7.4

The purpose of this study was to determine the psychophysical character and validity of auditory-perceptual ratings of naturalness and overall severity for tracheoesophageal (TE) speech. This was achieved through use of direct magnitude estimation (DME) and equal-appearing interval (EAI) scaling procedures. Twenty adult listeners judged speech naturalness and overall severity from connected speech samples produced by 20 adult male TE speakers. A comparison of DME- and EAI-scaled judgments yielded a metathetic continuum for naturalness and a prothetic continuum for overall severity. These data provide support for the use of either DME or EAI scales in auditory-perceptual ratings of naturalness, but they provide support only for DME scales in judging overall severity for TE speech. The present results suggest that the nature of perceptual phenomena (prothetic vs. metathetic) for TE speakers is consistent with findings for the same dimensions produced by normal laryngeal speakers. These data also support a need for further study of perceptual dimensions associated with TE voice and speech in order to avoid the inappropriate and invalid use of EAI scales frequently found in diagnosis, assessment, and evaluation of this clinical population.

**EXCERPT  7.5**

The purpose of this study was to evaluate the effectiveness of several acoustic measures in predicting breathiness ratings. Recordings were made of eight normal men and seven normal women producing normally phonated, moderately breathy, and very breathy sustained vowels. Twenty listeners rated the degree of breathiness using a direct magnitude estimation procedure. Acoustic measures were made of: (a) signal periodicity, (b) first harmonic amplitude, and (c) spectral tilt. Periodicity measures provided the most accurate predictions of perceived breathiness, accounting for approximately 80% of the variance in breathiness ratings. The relative amplitude of the first harmonic correlated moderately with breathiness ratings, and two measures of spectral tilt correlated weakly with perceived breathiness.

The abstract shown in Excerpt 7.5 also deals concisely and clearly with the study reported thereafter. The purpose of the study is described, participants and method are briefly treated, and the results are summarized.

A word of caution: the adequacy of a research article cannot be evaluated simply by reading the abstract. The purpose of the abstract is to provide an overview of the article so that the reader can determine quickly if the article should be read. What may seem on the basis of the abstract to be an exciting and original contribution to the literature may on closer inspection of the article itself turn out to be a poor study, both conceptually and methodologically. The only way to determine the quality of a research study is to read the whole article.

## General Statement of the Problem

We have identified four major components in the text of the introduction to a research article. Although these components are frequently woven together in the introduction and may not receive separate subheadings to help the reader identify them, the evaluation process is facilitated if the reader can identify these components for the purpose of analysis.

The first component is the general statement of the problem. Here the author sets forth the topic of the article, including the major variables and the target population. The problem can be described in a variety of ways and different authors have different preferences and styles.

The general statement of the problem lends perspective to the specific empirical operations of a research article. It provides a context for the specific purpose, method, and results to make the conclusions meaningful. The general problem statement may be a short first paragraph or it may run through a few initial paragraphs, including references to previous research, to help establish the context of the research.

A simple, straightforward general problem statement is shown in Excerpt 7.6. In a short paragraph, the author clearly states what general issues will be addressed. The use of temporal information by older listeners was examined under the conditions of compression-amplified speech and linearly amplified speech. The author discusses an important methodological issue

## EXCERPT 7.6

In this study, use of temporal information by older listeners was assessed in compression-amplified speech, as well as linearly amplified speech in which the amplitude envelope was preserved. Because the availability of spectral cues may obscure or confound the use of temporal information, recognition scores were also obtained for speech that had been processed digitally to minimize spectral cues. To control for the effect of decreased audibility, younger and older listeners were matched carefully for hearing sensitivity. The primary goals were to determine whether an age effect existed and, if so, to compare the effect of age on recognition for linearly amplified versus compression-amplified speech.

From "Older Listeners' Use of Temporal Cues Altered by Compression Amplification," by P. E. Souza, 2000, *Journal of Speech, Language, and Hearing Research, 43,* p. 662. Copyright 2000 by the American Speech-Language-Hearing Association. Reprinted with permission.

regarding the control of spectral cues that may confound the listeners' use of temporal cues and clearly states the primary goals of the study in the last sentence of the paragraph.

The example shown in Excerpt 7.7 regards the external validity issue of generalizability. The general problem statement includes a concise rationale for the replication of a previous research study. The concluding sentence of Excerpt 7.7 states what the authors hope to accomplish through such a replication.

Excerpt 7.8 shows the statement of the problem of a study designed to investigate the influence of utterance length and syntactic complexity on childhood stuttering. The first three sentences of the paragraph state that although there is evidence suggesting relationships among utterance length, syntactic complexity and childhood stuttering, the exact

## EXCERPT 7.7

The veracity of a self-assessment inventory is enhanced when its psychometric properties can be replicated across a variety of settings beyond the one in which it was developed. The sources and magnitude of measurement error can vary from one facility to another because of differences, for instance, in demographic composition and clinical operating procedures (Demorest & Walden, 1984). Cox and Gilmore (1990) developed a self-report questionnaire to quantify the performance of hearing aid users in communicative and environmental situations typically encountered in daily life. These researchers designated their inventory the Profile of Hearing Aid Performance (PHAP), and a salient feature of their study was to establish test-retest reliability and critical difference values for the PHAP scales and subscales. The purpose of the present study was to replicate the test-retest reliability and critical difference components of the Cox and Gilmore (1990) investigation. Repeating the Cox and Gilmore (1990) study with a different group of subjects in a different setting would serve to assess the generalizability of the PHAP test-retest reliability data and critical difference values reported by the original investigators.

From "Test-Retest Reliability of the Profile of Hearing Aid Performance," by C. T. Nelson and C. V. Palmer, 1994, *Journal of Speech and Hearing Research, 37,* p. 1212. Copyright 1994 by the American Speech-Language-Hearing Association. Reprinted with permission.

**EXCERPT 7.8**

In sum, there are compelling clinical and theoretical reasons to examine relationships among utterance length, syntactic complexity, and fluency. The studies conducted to date have confirmed that disfluent utterances are likely to be longer and more complex, on average, than fluent utterances. Still, the fact that utterance length and syntactic complexity appear to be strongly related to one another, combined with the fact that prior studies have used unitary measures of complexity and averaged data across utterances or across subjects, suggests that further research will be needed to more fully explore these issues. Accordingly, the purposes of this study were (a) to examine the independent influences of utterance length and syntactic complexity on children's speech fluency; (b) to assess several different aspects of syntactic complexity, such as clause-level or phrase-level complexity; and (c) to determine whether relationships among utterance length, syntactic complexity, and speech fluency observed in group-averaged data are also present in individual speech samples produced by children who stutter.

From "Utterance Length, Syntactic Complexity, and Childhood Stuttering," by J. S. Yaruss, 1999, *Journal of Speech, Language, and Hearing Research, 42,* p. 332. Copyright 1999 by the American Speech-Language-Hearing Association. Reprinted with permission.

---

nature of this relationship is not well understood. In the remaining sentences of the paragraph, the author details explicitly how he intends to delineate these relationships.

In all of these introductory statements, the essence of the general problem area is defined along with an implicit or explicit statement of the importance of the problem. Literature citations are used, if necessary, to buttress the authors' position. As we will see later, the reader's substantive background in the area investigated plays a critical role in the evaluation of the introductory section. Familiarity with the theory and data concerning a particular topic is necessary for the reader to evaluate the arguments developed in an introduction. Even the novice reader, however, should be able to follow the *logic* of the arguments presented and should understand the importance of the general problem.

## The Rationale for the Study

The rationale for the study constitutes the second component of the text of the introduction and should stem from the general statement of the problem. The rationale presents the reasons for doing the particular study. It is here that the author justifies the selection of the particular independent and dependent variables studied with the specific population. Because it is impossible to investigate all aspects of the general problem in one research study, the rationale presents the case for studying selected aspects of the problem and may identify limitations imposed on the study.

The major question that the critical reader needs to ask about the rationale is whether the reasons for doing the study are clearly and explicitly stated and documented with literature citations. A variety of reasons are offered by investigators to support the importance and need for the study. The author may cite and attempt to document the inadequacy of previous research in the area under investigation. Another reason for doing the research is to follow up on previous research or to resolve conflicting or inconclusive results reported by other investigators. Still another reason offered by researchers is to provide empirical data related to theoretical aspects of the phenomenon under question. Finally, the rationale may be based on the paucity or absence of previous research in a given area. Any one or combination of these reasons might be used to develop a need for the study.

Excerpt 7.9 is from a study concerning the potential causes underlying the difficulty some elderly persons experience understanding speech in noise. The authors speculate that impaired central binaural auditory processing could potentially contribute to such speech understanding difficulties. The authors further point out, however, that degraded information from the periphery can contribute to diminished binaural processing. To rule out the

---

**EXCERPT  7.9**

Many elderly listeners experience some difficulty understanding speech in noise. Age-related, or presbycusic, changes of the auditory system include both a reduced speech understanding in noise and a high-frequency sensorineural hearing loss (cf. Marshall, 1981; Working Group on Speech Understanding and Aging, 1988). Both aspects of hearing impairment tend to worsen with advancing age (Davis, 1989; Gilad & Glorig, 1979; van Rooij, Plomp, & Orlebeke, 1989). It is therefore not surprising that the reduction in speech understanding appears to be largely attributed to a loss in sensitivity (Humes & Roberts, 1990). However, it is likely that factors other than sensitivity loss also contribute to speech understanding difficulties in noise among the elderly (Abel, Krever, & Alberti, 1990; Bergman, 1971; Helfer & Wilber, 1990; Jerger 1992; Lutman, 1991; Marshall, 1981, 1985; Noble, 1978; Plomp, 1986; Ventry & Weinstein, 1983).

One factor that could potentially contribute to speech understanding difficulties in noise is impaired binaural auditory processing. In typical competitive listening situations, listeners with normal hearing are able to use binaural cues to their advantage in facilitating speech understanding in noise. The binaural cues are based largely on the interaural time and level differences arising from the spatial separations of the target speech and competing noise sources (Durlach, Thompson, & Colburn, 1981; Green & Yost, 1976).

Impaired binaural processing would be expected to result in a diminished binaural advantage for distinguishing between spatially separated target speech and noise sources (Warren, Wagner, & Herman, 1978). It is the intent of this study to examine the status of binaural processing in elderly listeners.

Reduced binaural processing in the elderly might be due to a combination of two factors. First, the "binaural processor" itself might be impaired. Physiological and anatomical studies have highlighted changes due to aging throughout the auditory system (Bredberg, 1990; Hinchcliffe, 1991; Marshall, 1981; von Wedel, von Wedel, & Streppel, 1991). It is reasonable, therefore, to expect some change in the central aspects of auditory processing in elderly listeners. The second factor that might contribute to reduced binaural processing in the elderly listener is a degradation of the input to the "binaural processor" from the auditory periphery (Roush, 1985). Corruptions in the coding of time and level cues in the periphery would be expected to diminish binaural performance. In an effort to distinguish between these two factors, the present study examined binaural processing in elderly listeners whose peripheral sensitivity was normal, or near-normal. By measuring binaural effects in elderly listeners in the absence of presbycusic sensitivity loss, any changes in binaural processing that might be observed could be more strongly attributed to changes at a central level.

**EXCERPT  7.10**

Despite a long history in the psychophysical literature (cf. Stevens, 1975) for the application of direct magnitude estimation (DME), the DME method is re-emerging in relation to perceptual judgments of various parameters of voice and speech. DME scales permit listeners to make perceptual judgments in relation to a "standard" that is designed to represent the approximate midpoint of any given set of stimuli in a perceptual continuum (Schiavetti, 1984). This standard is termed a "modulus" and is usually given a value of 100. For example, in an auditory-perceptual task, listeners are asked to judge the voice or speech of a group of speakers (e.g., individuals with dysphonia or dysarthria) for a given perceptual attribute (e.g., roughness or intelligibility). Then speech samples are judged (i.e., a numerical rating value is given) for the specified perceptual attribute. Individual samples with a voice or speech attribute that is judged to be twice as good as the modulus are assigned a value of 200, whereas speaker samples judged to have a voice or speech attribute only half as good as the modulus are assigned a value of 50. As such, the endpoints of the DME continua are unspecified, as perceptual phenomena are scaled relative to the modulus.

In contrast, equal-appearing interval (EAI) scales require listeners to provide perceptual ratings based on a fixed, predefined scale that suggests implied "equality" of perceptual distance, weight, or magnitude between numeric components. In the voice literature, most EAI scales are 7 points (i.e., 7 pt-EAI), with "1" (e.g., normal voice quality) representing one end of the scale and "7" (e.g., severely impaired voice quality) representing the other extreme (Kreiman, Gerratt, Kempster, Erman, & Berke, 1993). Other common EAI scales used in the literature include 5-point and 9-point EAI scales (Kreiman et al., 1993). Unlike DME, the endpoints of EAI scales are fixed, and scaling is performed using whole number representatives (i.e., any whole number between "1" and "n").

Stevens (1975) has indicated that there are basically two types of perceptual continua that can be scaled: *prothetic* and *metathetic*. A prothetic continuum is additive and *quantitative* in nature. It is best scaled using DME because observers cannot subdi-

vide a prothetic continuum into equal intervals. In contrast, a metathetic continuum is a substitutive, *qualitative* continuum that can be scaled using either DME or EAI scaling procedures. The prototypical example for a prothetic continuum is loudness, whereas pitch best exemplifies a metathetic continuum. Stevens (1975) outlined a method for determining whether a given dimension falls along a metathetic or prothetic continuum. In this procedure, the arithmetic means of the EAI ratings of a scale are plotted against the geometric means of the DME scores. If the relationship between these means is linear, then the scale is considered metathetic in nature, implying equal perceptual space between the intervals of the scale. Metathetic dimensions, therefore, may be scaled using either DME or EAI scales. However, if the relationship between the EAI scores and DME scores is nonlinear, it is suggestive of a prothetic continuum, for which only the DME method is appropriate.

Researchers in communication sciences and disorders have tested a variety of psychophysical attributes of voice and speech using Stevens' (1975) procedure. Perceptual dimensions commonly scaled in voice and speech often have revealed prothetic continua, suggesting that for these dimensions, DME rating scales are most appropriate. Using the methodology of Stevens (1975) and others (e.g., Barry & Kidd, 1981), the speech intelligibility of speakers with hearing loss (Schiavetti, Metz, & Sitler, 1981), stuttering severity (Schiavetti, Sacco, Metz, & Sitler, 1983), judgments of roughness for sustained vowels (Toner & Emanuel, 1989), ratings of nasality for synthesized vowels (Zraick & Liss, 2000), and ratings of hypernasality in connected speech samples of individuals with repaired cleft palate (Whitehill, Lee, & Chun, 2002) have been found to be prothetic. However, in examining the acoustic and psychophysical dimensions of perceived speech naturalness of nonstutterers and posttreatment stutterers, Metz, Schiavetti, and Sacco (1990) found that speech naturalness behaves like a metathetic continuum. Sewall, Weglarski, Metz, Schiavetti, and Whitehead (1999) found that the ratings of breathiness in normal speakers also are metathetic. Because EAI scales abound in the speech-language pathology literature (cf. Kreiman et al., 1993), it is critical that the nature (i.e., prothetic or metathetic) of perceptual dimensions is determined such that appropriate and valid scales are used. The validity of such auditory-perceptual scales has widespread implications for diagnosis and treatment outcomes, as perceptual scales are used most often and valued most highly by clinicians (Gerratt, Till, Rosenbek, Wertz, & Boysen, 1991).

To date, the construct validity of DME versus EAI scaling has only been investigated for dimensions of speech and voice in laryngeal speakers, with only limited work undertaken that concerns the voice/speech of the postlaryngectomy "alaryngeal" speaker. However, due to the unique nature of alaryngeal speech, the relevance of Stevens' (1976) procedures continues to raise questions concerning listener judgments of inherent perceptual dimensions. Such work has the potential to serve as a frame of reference for determining one or more aspect(s) of postlaryngectomy "outcomes" for individuals who use alaryngeal speech (i.e., esophageal, tracheoesophageal, or artificial laryngeal methods of postlaryngectomy communication).[1]

Since its development in 1980, the tracheoesophageal (TE) puncture technique has offered an option for postlaryngectomy voice and speech production (Singer & Blom, 1980). In the TE puncture procedure, a fistula is surgically created so that there is a connection between the trachea and the esophagus (which serves as the vicarious voice source). When air is exhaled and the tracheostoma is occluded, pulmonary air is shunted through a TE voice prosthesis into the esophageal reservoir, where it then creates oscillation of the pharyngoesophageal (PE) sphincter. Oscillation of the PE sphincter then creates the alaryngeal voice source that is used for speech production (Blom, Singer, & Hamaker, 1986). A clear advantage of the TE puncture approach is that there is access to pulmonary air for voice production, thereby permitting higher trans-pseudoglottal airflow values (Moon & Weinberg, 1987). Higher airflow rates subsequently affect pitch (i.e., higher than traditional esophageal speech), with

some researchers finding a nonsignificant difference between normal laryngeal speakers and TE speakers for the acoustic measure of fundamental frequency (Finizia, Dotevall, Lundström, & Lindström, 1999; Hillman, Walsh, Wolf, Fisher, & Hong, 1998; Robbins, Fisher, Blom, & Singer, 1984; Trudeau & Qi, 1990; Van As, Hilgers, Verdonck-de Leeuw, & Koopmans-van Beinum, 1998). Access to pulmonary air also permits a speech rate that is comparable to normal laryngeal speakers (Pindzola & Cain, 1989). When compared to the other methods of alaryngeal voice and speech production, TE speakers are usually judged as being most "intelligible and pleasant" and are among those that exhibit frequency, intensity, and durational values closest to normal when compared with other alaryngeal methods (cf. Hillman et al., 1998; Pindzola & Gain, 1988, 1989; Robbins et al., 1984; Van As et al., 1998; Williams & Watson, 1985; and others).

Although speech acceptability has been shown to be high in TE speakers, it must be emphasized that alaryngeal methods may be judged to be less acceptable and TE speakers have been rated as exhibiting decreased voice quality relative to normal laryngeal speakers, as well as those speakers who have undergone radiation therapy (Finizia et al., 1999; Tardy-Mitzell, Andrews, & Bowman, 1985). These studies illustrate the following principle—although alaryngeal modes of communication have improved in the past few decades, alaryngeal speakers can still be identified as "different" from normal speakers, and variability between speakers within any given alaryngeal group (e.g., TE speakers) will exist. Hence, it may be postulated that more holistic auditory-perceptual judgments of alaryngeal speech in general, and TE speech in specific, may provide the best arbiter of voice and speech performance and, possibly, rehabilitation success. That is, comprehensive perceptual judgments of alaryngeal speech may provide the ultimate index of postlaryngectomy communication effectiveness or success as perceived by the listener in a communication context (Doyle & Eadie, in press).

Given that alaryngeal voice is characterized by a substantial number of parameters, the interaction among these variables must be delineated so that a comprehensive approach to rehabilitation is undertaken. Therefore, auditory-perceptual judgments of "naturalness" and "severity" may provide two meaningful indicators of rehabilitation success because they

---

[1]It is beyond the scope of the present paper to describe each postlaryngectomy voice and speech option. For a more thorough presentation of this information, the reader is referred to texts by Blom, Singer, and Hamaker (1998); Doyle (1994); Keith and Darley (1986, 1994): and Snidecor (1978).

### E X C E R P T   7.10   Continued

represent a multidimensional, overall index of the voice/speech signal. If such auditory-perceptual features hold promise as dimensions that can be assessed in order to better define a given alaryngeal speaker's voice/speech character, we are then required to ascertain what method of auditory-perceptual evaluation is most appropriate. The essential question in this context centers specifically on whether the auditory-perceptual feature under evaluation is prothetic or metathetic. This obliges those interested in alaryngeal voice and speech to first address issues of what type of scaling procedure is most appropriate for each perceptual dimension and then determine the reliability of such measures as a clinical tool. As such, it is important that the validity of scaling multidimensional perceptual phenomena such as naturalness and overall severity be investigated in TE speakers. Consequently, the purpose of the present study was to (a) determine the psychophysical nature of speech naturalness and severity in TE speakers using Stevens' (1975) methods and (b) determine the construct validity of rating scales used for perceptual dimensions in this population of speakers.

From "Direct Magnitude Estimation and Interval Scaling of Naturalness and Severity in Tracheoesophageal (TE) Speakers," by T. L. Eadie and P. C. Doyle, 2002, *Journal of Speech, Language, and Hearing Research, 45,* pp. 1088–1090. Copyright 2002 by the American Speech-Language-Hearing Association. Reprinted with permission.

possibility that degraded information from the periphery is diminishing binaural processing, the authors use elderly persons who have relatively normal audiograms to test their hypothesis.

The introductory paragraphs shown in Excerpt 7.10 present general and specific rationales regarding the need to study the psychophysical attributes of tracheoesophageal speech. The first three paragraphs provide historical and technical considerations regarding two types of continua (prothetic and metathetic) that may be scaled perceptually and the appropriateness of two types of strategies (direct magnitude estimation and equal-appearing interval scales) that are used to scale the two types of perceptual continua. Subsequent paragraphs review relevant literature regarding the underlying psychophysical continua associated with commonly scaled speech and voice dimensions. In the concluding paragraphs, the authors develop a compelling case for determining whether selected dimensions of tracheoesophageal speech lie on a prothetic or metathetic continuum and for determining the construct validity of scaling procedures used to evaluate these dimensions of tracheoesophageal speech.

Excerpt 7.11 is taken from a study designed to examine the effects of reverberation, noise, and their combination on consonant and vowel feature perception by children. In the first paragraph of this excerpt, the author reviews literature regarding some of the acoustic features that adults with normal hearing and with hearing impairment use to identify consonants and vowels. In the second paragraph, she notes that few studies have investigated children's consonant and vowel feature perception in quiet, reverberation, and/or noise environments. In the third paragraph, the author poses three explicit research questions designed to explore, in detail, children's consonant and vowel feature perception.

## EXCERPT 7.11

Bilger and Wang (1976), Reed (1975), and Walden and Montgomery (1975) found that the consonant errors of listeners with flat sensorineural hearing losses could be explained chiefly on the basis of sibilance. However, some studies reported that listeners with normal hearing and hearing impairment used similar features for consonant perception in noise. For example, Danhauer and Lawarre (1979) found that listeners with normal hearing and those with hearing impairment used sibilance, sonorants, plosives, and dental (place) for consonant perception in noise. Similarly, Doyle, Danhauer, and Edgerton (1981) found that listeners with normal hearing and those with hearing impairment used the features of voicing, place, sibilance, and frication. Helfer (1992) found dissimilar error patterns for listeners' perception of consonant features in reverberation versus noise. She found that reverberation affected the perception of low-frequency features more than high-frequency features. For example, a greater binaural advantage was found in reverberation for voicing and manner of articulation than for place of articulation. Furthermore, listeners made many errors in the perception of nasals in reverberation that masks F2 transitions that are critical for correct identification. However, listeners' perception of initial plosives was resistant to reverberation.

Few studies have investigated children's use of consonant feature perception by children in quiet, reverberation, and/or noise. Danhauer, Abdala, Johnson, and Asp (1986) found that children with normal hearing and

hearing impairment showed similar performance patterns and used the features of voicing, nasality, sonorancy, sibilance, and place of articulation in noise. In contrast, Johnson, Stein, Broadway, and Markwalter (1996) reported that adults' performance reflected a greater amount of information transmitted, both overall and for individual features, than the performance of children with normal hearing and minimal amounts of high-frequency sensorineural hearing loss. In addition, the children with normal hearing had a greater amount of information transmitted (both overall and for consonant features) in reverberation than the children with minimal amounts of high-frequency sensorineural hearing loss. However, when noise was added to reverberation, both groups of listeners had similar amounts of information transmitted both overall and for individual features.

This study was designed to answer three questions. First, at what SL do young listeners (i.e., aged six years through young adult) achieve maximum consonant and vowel identification performance in reverberation, noise, and combined conditions? Second, how do children's consonant and vowel identification scores compare to those of young adults in optimal (i.e., no reverberation, no noise), reverberation-only, noise-only, and reverberation-plus-noise listening conditions? Third, how does children's identification of voicing, manner, and place of articulation features compare to that of young adults in these listening conditions?

From "Children's Phoneme Identification in Reverberation and Noise," by C. E. Johnson, 2000, *Journal of Speech, Language, and Hearing Research, 43*, pp. 145–146. Copyright 2000 by the American Speech-Language-Hearing Association. Reprinted with permission.

Excerpt 7.12 shows three introductory paragraphs of an article regarding how well children recognize speech features presented on a spectrogram. The author develops the rationale for the study by reporting that there are a limited number of investigations regarding the abilities of children with normal hearing and children with hearing impairments to perceive speech cues in spectrograms. He goes on to point out that there are also conflicting results in the limited extant research regarding the abilities of children with hearing impairments to recognize speech features on a spectrogram.

The rationale shown in Excerpt 7.13 takes a somewhat different approach. This argument is not based so much on a review of discrepant results or the need to compare

EXCERPT 7.12

Few investigations have directly assessed the ability of children with hearing impairments to perceive speech cues in spectrograms. In an early study, Stark (1972) used a prototype of the SD (i.e., the Visual Speech Translator) to teach ten 7–12-year-olds to distinguish between /pa/ and /ba/ based on differences in voice onset time (VOT). After 10–15 min of training, 8 of the children achieved accuracy scores of 90% or higher. The remaining 2 participants reached the 90% level after a single, additional training session. This high success rate and the short duration of training indicate that children can learn to recognize relatively discrete spectrographic cues.

More recently, two 9-year-old children with profound hearing losses judged the correctness of their own vowel productions through spectrographic feedback as part of a multiple-baseline, single-case treatment study (Ertmer et al., 1996). One participant (S1) made relatively rapid improvements in producing /i/, /o/, and /æ/. On average, his judgments of correctness agreed 87% of the time with the clinician's auditory perceptual judgments. The second child (S2) made slower and more limited improvements in the production of /a/, /æ/, and /i/. Her judgments agreed with the clinician's auditory perceptual judgments approximately 67% of the time, a level close to chance performance. These differences in production and perception led the authors to propose a need for further evaluation of children's abilities to discriminate a variety of formant patterns. This need can reasonably be extended to consonants, as there are little or no data regarding children's abilities to perceive cues for manner, place, and voicing features in spectrograms.

The reviewed speech training and visual perception studies strongly suggest that some speech cues are salient and consistent enough to be recognized by children. However, the kinds of spectrographic cues that children can recognize have not been fully ascertained, and the ages at which these cues are recognized is unknown. In addition, it has not been determined whether children with impaired hearing and those who hear normally perceive spectrographic cues with comparable proficiency. There are several compelling reasons for examining visual recognition skills in both groups.

measurements for accuracy. Rather, the authors logically develop a rationale for how a measurement of dynamic motor performance, the spatiotemporal index (STI), can be useful in the investigation of the influence of utterance length and syntactic complexity on stuttering. The authors first point out that empirical evidence, using disfluency counts as the dependent variable, suggests that linguistic factors such as sentence length and syntactic complexity may affect speech fluency. They state further, however, that disfluency counts provide only a limited means for explaining the neurophysiologic nature of interactions between linguistic and motor speech processes. Notice how the authors introduce various measurements of speech motor control performance and then logically develop their notions regarding the superiority of the STI.

As these examples have shown, a major part of the introduction to a research article spells out the reasons for doing the particular study. The rationale describes the need for the research. The logic of the arguments presented, with appropriate citations from the

These experimental results suggest that linguistic factors such as sentence length and syntactic complexity may affect the fluency of speech production, specifically in people who stutter. Previous studies, however, have used counts of disfluency almost exclusively as a dependent variable. Although disfluency counts provide much information concerning the frequency and loci of stuttering, this information provides only limited means for explaining the neurophysiological nature of potential interactions between linguistic and motor speech processes. To address questions concerning such interactions, measurements of speech motor performance can be applied. These techniques include, but are not limited to, EMG, neuroimaging, and kinematic recording. For example, some effects of linguistic factors on speech muscle EMG have been documented (Van Lieshout, Starkweather, Hulstijn, & Peters, 1995). Van Lieshout et al. found that words in sentence-initial position were associated with higher EMG peak amplitudes than words in sentence-final position. Surprisingly, increasing sentence length was associated with a significant decrease in the EMG peak amplitude for the lower lip. Using such techniques, it may be possible to detect linguistically driven changes in the speech motor behavior of people who stutter, even in the absence of overt fluency breakdowns.

Experimental variables that explore stability/instability appear to provide promising new tools for analyzing stuttering (Smith & Kelly, 1997). One potentially useful measure of dynamic motor performance is the spatiotemporal index (STI; Smith, Goffman, Zelaznik, Ying, & McGillem, 1995), which was designed to measure movement stability over repeated performance of a motor task. Traditionally, analyses of physiological signals recorded during speech have involved measuring specific variables at single points in time. For example, measurements for the phrase "buy Bobby a puppy" could include the time of onset of closure for the initial /b/ in "buy" or the point at which the peak velocity for this closing movement occurs. Though measures such as these provide valuable descriptive information concerning speech kinematics, they rest upon the assumption that certain times or moments during production are more significant than others. They are also limited when the hypothesis attempts to link linguistic factors and speech motor performance. It is not clear that lin-

guistic complexity should affect measures at single points in time such as displacement, velocity, and/or timing variables in a predictable way. The STI incorporates the entire signal and may be a useful composite measure of underlying performance dynamics. Because the signals are linearly normalized in time and space for the computation of the STI, the STI does not differentiate between spatial and temporal variability. Instead, the STI measures the overall variability of core patterns of speech movements.

The STI has been utilized effectively to describe speech motor characteristics of typical speakers under varying linguistic demands (Maner, Smith, & Grayson, 2000). These authors applied the STI (Smith et al., 1995) to study the effects of increasing length and syntactic complexity on the speech motor stability of children and adults with typical speech and language skills. Lower lip movements were recorded as the participants produced the phrase "Buy Bobby a puppy" alone, embedded in simple sentences, and embedded in complex sentences. Maner et al. found that linguistic factors such as length and syntactic complexity may affect the speech motor functioning of children. Despite their ability to produce fluent, phonologically accurate speech, children demonstrated increased temporal and spatial variability in their speech movements as linguistic demands were increased. Though mean duration of the phrase did not change across conditions for children, the variability of these measures increased from the baseline condition to the low and high complexity conditions. Further, Maner et al. suggested that the specific effects of linguistic variables on speech motor stability may change with maturation.

In summary, though many studies have suggested a positive correlation between linguistic factors and disfluency, few studies have attempted to describe the neurophysiological interactions that may lead to such speech disruptions. The goal of the present experiment was to describe the relationship between linguistic variables and speech motor output by applying methods used to study motor control. Kinematic changes in the fluent speech of adults who do and do not stutter in response to increasing linguistic demands, specifically, increasing syntactic complexity and/or the length of utterances, were observed and analyzed.

literature, should convince the reader of the value of the investigation. The rationale may take different forms, depending on the nature of the study. Some introductions stress the practical nature of a study, such as the need to assess the accuracy of a measurement. Others stress the need to resolve conflicting results or conclusions from previous studies. Many studies develop their rationales on the basis of the importance of the research for theoretical or practical applications. In any case, the rationale for the study is an important component of the text of the introduction.

There are several important questions for the critical evaluator of research to ask about the review of literature in the introduction to a research article. Most of these questions assume some knowledge of the topic on the part of the reader of the article.

First, how thorough is the literature review? Are there important omissions that might change the nature of the rationale or the perspective of the problem? Space limitations in a journal obviously place some constraints on the scope of any literature review. It is simply impossible to cite all the pertinent literature without running into objections by a journal editor who is interested in conserving valuable space. Nonetheless, the key references should be cited to substantiate the need for the study. Despite the apparent thoroughness of a particular literature review, the reader must still determine if key references have been omitted. It is here that the reader's background and expertise in the particular topic of an article play a crucial role in the evaluation process. It is extremely difficult to judge the thoroughness of the literature review without familiarity with the relevant literature.

How recent are the literature citations? Has the author overlooked recent work in reviewing the literature? This does not mean that older references should not be cited. Some older references are classics in a field and have had such a germinal influence on so many studies since their publication that they are constantly referred to. See, for example, Excerpt 7.10 in which the authors refer to the classic work of Stevens that was published in 1975. It is not surprising that this reference is cited because it is a classic. The point is that the author has an obligation to cite the relevant work, new and old, that is necessary to place the problem in perspective and develop a convincing rationale. It may be that there is no recent literature on a given topic because the article represents renewed interest in a topic that received considerable attention twenty or thirty years ago but little attention in the last five or ten years. Here the researcher may be justified in citing only older studies to make the case for a new study. However, when recent literature on a particular topic exists and is relevant, it should be cited.

A third point is whether the review is critical of previous literature and whether the criticism is objective, unbiased, and justified. Have the data of the previous studies been accurately reported and interpreted? Were the conclusions of the previous research criticized fairly? These are not easy questions to answer because they require the reader to refer to the original studies to determine if the criticisms were justified.

The next question is whether the literature citations are relevant to the purpose and to the need for the study. Once again, the ideal way to evaluate the relevancy of the literature review is to be knowledgeable about the subject matter under investigation. We raise the question of relevancy but we cannot answer it for the reader. There is no easy way of evaluating relevancy without some in-depth familiarity with the topic.

Finally, the careful evaluator of research should be alert to the overuse of unpublished research, citations from obscure references, frequent reference to materials appearing in publications that are inaccessible. The major problem is that the reader cannot consult the original sources to determine whether the researcher has cited them correctly, drawn appropriate conclusions from them, and so forth. The researcher's use of these citations may also suggest research that is out of the mainstream, idiosyncratic, or unimportant.

In summary, the literature review is at the heart of the introduction to the research report. It is of fundamental importance for the critical reader of research to evaluate carefully the adequacy of the literature citations. Special attention should be given to the extent and thoroughness of the review, the recency and relevance of the citations, the objectivity and accuracy of the criticism of previous research. In the final analysis, the reader of the research report must bring expertise, experience, and knowledge to the evaluation of the literature citations. And, if need be, the reader must return to the cited sources to fully appreciate, understand, and evaluate this aspect of the introduction.

# Review of the Literature

The third component of the text of an introduction is the review of literature. The literature review is not really a separate part of an introduction, but it is the fabric from which the statement of the problem and rationale are woven. The literature citations not only serve to document the need for the study, but they also help to put the research into context or historical perspective. Through the use of appropriate references, the researcher identifies how the investigation reported fits into the general theme of research in the same problem area. In a sense, the literature citations pay tribute to those who have gone before. In another sense, the literature citations allow the reader to examine the sources used by the author to make the case for the study. Thus, the reader has an opportunity to evaluate directly the adequacy of the literature citations and to determine whether, in fact, the citations used justify the research reported.

The literature review, then, should be evaluated in regard to (1) the degree to which it helps to place the general problem into perspective and (2) the degree to which it helps to develop the rationale for the study. Different authors have different styles and preferences for the way they use the literature review in relation to the other components of the text of the introduction. For example, the author of Excerpt 7.8 uses the literature review to put the general problem in perspective, whereas the authors of Excerpt 7.13 use the literature to develop their rationale for the use of the STI. The authors of Excerpt 7.10 use the literature review throughout the introduction to develop the general problem and the rationale for the study.

Sometimes the literature review does stand on its own, especially if the author's intent is to review new literature or literature from areas that may be unfamiliar to most readers of a particular journal. An example of this can be seen in Excerpt 7.14 where literature from respiratory physiology is reviewed briefly. This literature is likely to be unfamiliar to most speech-language pathologists and audiologists and needs to be summarized on its own before the development of a general problem statement and rationale.

EXCERPT   7.14

The primary purpose of ventilation is to provide gas exchange for oxygen delivery and maintain blood acid-base homeostasis. Gas exchange for oxygen delivery occurs between the lung alveoli and the blood vessels that surround them. The oxygen ($O_2$), thus exchanged, is transported to the body tissues via blood hemoglobin. After the $O_2$ is utilized by the muscle, the hemoglobin then picks up the metabolic end product, carbon dioxide ($CO_2$), for removal by exhalation through the lungs (Guyton, 1991). Blood acid-base homeostasis is defined as a state of equilibrium in the chemical composition of the blood maintaining a constant pH. This equilibrium is maintained through a balance of metabolic acid production and the elimination of blood acids through the ventilatory system. The relationship between blood acid base and ventilation is defined by the equation $CO_2 + H_2O \Leftrightarrow H_2CO_3 \Leftrightarrow H^+ + HCO_3$ where $H^+$ = hydrogen ion (i.e., metabolic acid); $HCO_3$ = bicarbonate, (i.e., base); and $H_2CO_3$ = carbonic acid (Davenport, 1974). Production of metabolic acid, which would decrease blood pH, is buffered by increasing ventilation, and blowing off $CO_2$ leaving $H_2O$ in the blood. On the other hand, disturbing ventilation sufficiently to prevent the elimination of $CO_2$, even momentarily, results in an increase of blood $H^+$ and a disturbance of blood acid-base homeostasis. A disturbance of normal ventilation, such as speech, will alter the normal mechanisms responsible for maintenance of this homeostasis. The greater the disturbance, the more vigorous is the response to return to homeostasis. Similarly, many tasks, such as breathing, are performed in a manner that minimizes the energy cost and therefore the disturbance (Gesell, 1925). Our hypothesis is that the greater the speech demands (i.e., varied SPL), the greater the potential for the disturbance of homeostasis. Furthermore, we hypothesized that the level of speech chosen by an individual as being comfortable would be the least disturbing to this homeostasis.

The pulmonary system responds to disturbances in ventilation to maintain homeostasis through various adjustments. Planned and artificial perturbations of the respiratory system provide information regarding how ventilation responds to these disturbances (Bouhuys, 1964; Otis & Clark, 1962; Phillipson, McClean, Sullivan, & Zamel, 1978). Challenges to the ventilatory system during speech, such as exercise (Otis & Clark, 1962) or $CO_2$ rebreathing (Bunn & Mead, 1971; Otis & Clark, 1962; Phillipson et al., 1978), stimulate increases in $V_T$ ($V_T$ = the volume of each breath) and breathing frequency ($F_b$ = number of breaths per minute). These alterations in ventilation allow the system to maintain acid-base balance in the blood while maintaining speech production during exercise and $CO_2$ rebreathing (Davenport, 1974; Phillipson et al., 1978). Likewise, disturbances to normal ventilation, such as during speech alone, result in alterations to ventilation that likely alter acid-base homeostasis or metabolic control (Phillipson et al., 1978). In general, $F_b$ is reduced and $V_T$ is increased to accommodate the need for sustained speech-related exhalations with minimal disturbances to fluency (Bunn & Mead, 1971). The effect of speech-induced ventilatory alterations on acid-base homeostasis is not known.

From "Effects of Varied Vocal Intensity on Ventilation and Energy Expenditure in Women and Men," by B. A. Russell, F. J. Cerny, and E. Stathopoulos, 1998, *Journal of Speech, Language, and Hearing Research, 41,* pp. 239–240. Copyright 1998 by the American Speech-Language-Hearing Association. Reprinted with permission.

## Statement of Purpose, Research Questions, and Hypotheses

The introduction of a research article usually concludes with a specific statement of the purpose of the research, with one or more research questions, or with testable hypotheses. Whichever form is used, this section represents the logical culmination of the general

**EXCERPT 7.15**

Four primary research questions were addressed:

1. Can 4-year-old children with typical language development correctly identify the actions associated with manner-of-motion verbs following limited exposure to the verbs? On the basis of the results of the earlier QUIL studies (Oetting, 1999; Oetting et al., 1995; Rice et al., 1990, 1994; Rice & Woodsmall, 1988) and our efforts to reduce the cognitive demands of the QUIL task, we predicted that the children in the experimental group would correctly identify the target words at rates similar to those of the adults and at rates significantly higher than those of the children in the control group.

2. After limited exposure to a new verb, can 4-year-old children correctly reject associations between target actions and inappropriate novel labels? Similarly, can they reject associations between a novel action that differs in semantically important ways from the target and the newly acquired verb? We predicted that the children in the experimental group would perform with a high degree of accuracy on the label mismatch item, on the basis of the results of earlier studies (Golinkoff et al., 1992, 1996) as well as the relatively high number of exposures to the target verb labels that the children in this study received (i.e., 13 exposures per verb). We anticipated that the experimental

group's performance on this item would be significantly more accurate than the age-matched peer group's performance on this item and would be similar to the adult group's performance on this item.

3. Can children correctly generalize recently acquired verb labels to actions in which the manner of motion has been slightly altered in a semantically unimportant way? In other words, will they generalize to similar actions that adults still consider to represent the target label?

4. Can children correctly reject generalizations of recently acquired verb labels to actions in which the manner of motion has been slightly altered in a semantically important way? In other words, will they appropriately refrain from generalizing to similar actions that adults no longer consider to be representative of the spoken label? It was unclear how the children in the experimental group would perform on the items in which the target actions were altered. Forbes and Farrar (1993, 1995) suggested that children generalize action labels to different referents less frequently than adults do. On the basis of this limited evidence, we anticipated that children who presented evidence of learning the target words would generalize the labels to slightly modified actions but that they would do so less consistently than would the group of adults.

From "Quick Incidental Verb Learning in 4-Year-Olds: Identification and Generalization," by T. Brakenbury and M. E. Fey, 2003, *Journal of Speech, Language, and Hearing Research, 46,* p. 316. Copyright 2003 by the American Speech-Language-Hearing Association. Reprinted with permission.

---

problem statement and rationale. As such, the specific purpose, question, or hypothesis should relate directly to what has preceded it. It is important that the statement be clear and precise. If possible, the statement should allow the reader to identify the independent and dependent variables and the type of research strategy used to study them.

Excerpt 7.15 shows the statement of purpose from a study that compared verb learning and generalization skills in two groups of typically developing four-year-old children. One group of children was introduced to selected verbs in an indirect teaching context and the other group (control group) was not. The children's verb learning and generalization

## EXCERPT 7.16

The specific questions under evaluation were as follows:

1. Do young children in syntax-informative input conditions use grammatical information in the assignment of novel words to novel things?
2. Are there differences attributable to the completeness of the child's representation of the linguistic structures such that children with limited grammatical competencies (e.g., SLI children) are less likely to benefit from informative syntax than are children with greater grammatical competencies?
3. Are there developmental differences, both within typically developing groups and SLI groups, such that older children have higher levels of syntax-consistent lexical assignment than younger children?
4. Are there differences in the types of errors made by the three groups which suggest different sources of difficulty?

From "The Use of Syntactic Cues in Lexical Acquisition by Children with SLI," by M. L. Rice, P. L. Cleave, and J. B. Oetting, 2000, *Journal of Speech, Language, and Hearing Research, 43,* p. 584. Copyright 2000 by the American Speech-Language-Hearing Association. Reprinted with permission.

---

skills were also compared to adult verb usage. The statement is broken down into four specific objectives. Three of the objectives contain predictions regarding the children's verb learning and generalization performance that are based on previous research findings.

Excerpt 7.16 shows a statement of purpose from a study of word acquisition skills of children who differ by age and language abilities. The statement is broken down into four specific research questions that address both potential between-group and within-group differences.

The statement of purpose and the specific research questions in Excerpt 7.17 come from a study that is designed to determine whether personality factors play causal, con-

## EXCERPT 7.17

The purpose of this research was to evaluate individual differences in personality and aspects of psychological functioning by comparing a variety of voice-disordered groups on measures of personality and emotional adjustment. Using a superfactor approach to personality description, the following research questions were addressed: (a) Do personality differences exist between voice-disordered groups at the superfactor trait level? (b) If so, are differences consistent with hypotheses derived from the Roy and Bless (2000a) theory describing the dispositional bases of FD and VN? (c) To what extent are these personality differences related to age? (d) Do group differences exist in the presence and degree of self-reported depression and anxiety? If so, are these differences related to the level of vocal handicap and/or the duration of voice symptoms? (e) For clinical purposes, do scales of personality offer useful diagnostic information that would potentially distinguish the groups?

From "Personality and Voice Disorders: A Superfactor Trait Analysis," by N. Roy, D. M. Bless, and D. Heisey, 2000, *Journal of Speech, Language, and Hearing Research, 43,* pp. 749–750. Copyright 2000 by the American Speech-Language-Hearing Association. Reprinted with permission.

comitant, or consequential roles in certain voice disorders. The general statement of purpose in the first sentence is followed by five specific questions that follow logically from a theoretical construct discussed in the first paragraph of the article. The Results section of the article is broken down according to the sequence of research questions, and as such, the reader should have no problem following the presentation of results, given the outlining of the specific research questions.

The example shown in Excerpt 7.18 shows two specific research questions stated in the form of hypotheses. Excerpt 7.18 is from a study that investigated how laryngeal reaction times (LRT) differed (a) when mild and severe stutterers and nonstutterers were given various lengths of time to prepare to respond to a stimulus, and (b) when the complexity of the required response varied. It should be pointed out that this is *not* the null hypothesis tested by a statistical significance test. Although it used to be common for authors to list the various null hypotheses tested, this is relatively uncommon now because the null hypothesis is usually implied by the statement of a specific purpose or question. An investigator may, however, present specific research questions and then relate the research questions to specific hypotheses, as shown in Excerpt 7.19.

The final example, shown in Excerpt 7.20, is from a study of vocal fundamental frequency of speakers with hearing impairment. The author first explains briefly why vocal fundamental frequency ($f_0$) should be compared for oral reading versus spontaneous speech in speakers with hearing impairment and then states what will be studied. Two independent variables will be examined: normal hearing versus hard-of-hearing (classification variable) and oral reading versus spontaneous speech. The dependent variable is fundamental frequency. The results that follow show the means and standard deviations of the fundamental frequencies specifically broken down according to the two independent variables. Again, the author has clearly stated his purpose so that the reader will know exactly what to expect in examining the results of the study.

A number of factors lead researchers to use one form or another to state the specific purpose of a study. The specific manner of stating the purpose or question or hypothesis is not as important as the clarity with which it is stated. The important point is that the author

---

**EXCERPT 7.18**

There were two hypotheses. (a) Stutterers vary as a function of severity in their ability to use a preparation facilitating stimulus presentation condition to reduce LRT. Specifically, nonstutterers and mild stutterers may reduce LRT in a preparation facilitating stimulus condition, whereas severe stutterers are unlikely to do so. (b) All subjects produce shorter LRTs in an isolated vowel response condition than in a VCV condition, but the magnitude of latency difference between response conditions varies as a function of stutterer severity. Specifically, within groups, severe stutterers increase LRT more than mild stutterers or nonstutterers as a function of increased response complexity, with consequently greater between-group differences in the VCV response condition than in the vowel response condition.

E X C E R P T   7.19

## Questions and Hypotheses

The study of adjective definitions should make a valuable contribution to our understanding of language development from childhood to adulthood. As stated earlier, much is currently known about the development of noun definitions, especially for concrete nouns. Research is needed that extends investigation of the development of definition to other grammatical classes, such as adjectives. The specific questions in the present study were: (a) Is the content of adjective definitions influenced by age and word frequency of the word to be defined? (b) Is the form of adjective definitions influenced by age and word frequency of the word to be defined?

The first question represents an examination of differences across age groups of typically developing preadolescents, adolescents, and adults in the content of their definitions of adjectives. The first question also represents an examination of the possible influence of word frequency on the content of adjective definitions for the same age groups. Based on prior research in the content of noun definitions, we hypothesize that the ability to use synonyms, explain a concept, and use superordinate terms will increase with age. Given that adjectives maybe represented in the mental lexicon as antonymous relations, we expect negation or saying what a word does not mean (e.g., "*short* means not tall") to be a frequent response type. The use of negation, however, may decrease with age as an individual acquires more words to express synonymous relations, such as synonyms and superordinate terms.

In terms of word frequency and content, we first hypothesize that language users will know more synonyms for high-frequency words and therefore will use more synonyms in defining such words. High-frequency terms are ones that an individual would encounter often, providing more opportunities for acquiring knowledge of synonyms. A second hypothesis relates to low-frequency words: Because language users have limited knowledge of the meanings of low-frequency words, individuals will give more examples, mention more associated concepts, and make more errors in defining such words. A third hypothesis is that we do not expect word frequency to affect the use of superordinate terms because we believe such terms are more sensitive to age than to frequency of the word to be defined. It is likely that a superordinate category such as "condition" or "quality" may readily have high-frequency members near the center or prototype of the category (e.g., *dark*), as well as low-frequency members toward the fringe of the category (e.g., *defective*).

The second question represents an examination of differences across age groups in the form of definitions of adjectives. This question also represents an examination of the possible influence of word frequency on the form of adjective definitions for the same age groups. Based on prior research, we hypothesize that the use of conventional form to define an adjective (i.e., defining an adjective with another adjective) will increase with age. For word frequency, we first hypothesize that, due to greater knowledge and practice, language users will be more likely to define high-frequency words than low-frequency ones using adjectival form, the conventional form for adjective definitions. Secondly, because language users have limited knowledge of the meanings of low-frequency words, individuals will be more likely to define low- than high-frequency words using noun form—the most familiar form.

should capture the nature of the study in a brief paragraph or so and specify the independent and dependent variables. The reader should move from the statement of specific purpose with a clear idea of what to expect in the Results section of the article. Whichever form is used, the statement should be well written, explicit, and related to the preceding rationale.

Voice characteristics of deaf and hard-of-hearing individuals during spontaneous or impromptu speech need to be investigated because spontaneous speech is a speaking condition of primary interest. In addition, knowledge of differences (or lack of them) in voice characteristics between oral reading and spontaneous speech should be useful in estimating spontaneous oral performance of hard-of-hearing individuals from their oral reading performance. For normal-hearing individuals, there is some evidence that $f_0$ distributional characteristics are different between oral reading and spontaneous speech. Snidecor (1943), for example, found that oral reading conditions produced both greater means and standard deviations of fundamental frequency. It was the purpose of the present study to investigate $f_0$ distributional characteristics of hard-of-hearing individuals during spontaneous speech and oral reading, and to test whether or not $f_0$ relationships, similar to those found in normal-hearing individuals, exist between the two speaking conditions.

## Miscellaneous Considerations

Two final issues need to be addressed with respect to the introduction. First, the reader should be alert to the need for, or the use of, definitions of terms that the author employs throughout the study. Many terms have different meanings for different people. The author has the responsibility of indicating, in the introduction, how those terms are defined in the article. This is accomplished by either defining the term in the introduction or, more commonly, by appropriate citation of other sources that have already defined the term. The reader must remember, however, that the researcher frequently writes for a specific audience, that is, for other researchers working in the same area or for clinicians who presumably are familiar with the subject (and the terminology) under investigation. Thus, terms that the naive reader would like to see defined may not be. Nonetheless, idiosyncratic usage or the use of terms about which there may be differences of opinion as to their meanings requires the specific attention of the author and should be defined in the introduction.

Second, the researcher may spell out some of the limitations of the study about to be reported. There are two types of limitations that might be noted. The first is a limitation that is beyond the investigator's control. An example of this extrinsic limitation is the situation in which a researcher may want to include both males and females in a study but must collect data in a setting in which males predominate. The second type of limitation is an intrinsic one, that is, a limitation self-imposed by the investigator in recognition of the fact that all aspects of a problem area simply cannot be investigated in a single study. Longitudinal studies have to end, despite the researcher's desire to continue to study a child's language development beyond the data-collection period. The investigator who is studying hearing loss in a geriatric population may want to include a number of auditory tests but, because of the nature of the population, limits the study to a selected few procedures.

The limitations of the study, as expressed by the researcher, are important and deserve careful consideration by the reader. Because of the limitations, a study may turn out to be of no consequence. The limitations may suggest that the author should have, at the very least, delayed submitting the research report until the limitations were overcome. The fact that an author recognizes and states the limitations in the introduction does not necessarily relieve the author of the responsibility of dealing with these limitations later in the Discussion section. Because most limitations are, in fact, detailed in the final section of the article, we will have more to say about evaluating author-stated limitations in Chapter 10.

Finally, it goes without saying that the introduction should be well written, clear, and logically organized.

The Evaluation Checklist that follows summarizes the important points made in the chapter and is designed to facilitate the critical evaluation of the Introduction section of the article.

# E V A L U A T I O N   C H E C K L I S T

**Instructions:**   The four-category scale at the end of this checklist may be used to rate the *Introduction* section of an article. The *Evaluation Items* help identify those topics that should be considered in arriving at the rating. Comments on these topics, entered as *Evaluation Notes,* should serve as the basis for the overall rating.

### *Evaluation Items*                                              *Evaluation Notes*

1. Title identified target population and variables under study.

2. Purpose, procedures, important findings, and implications were summarized in the abstract.

3. A clear statement of the general problem was given.

4. There was a logical and convincing rationale.

5. There was a current, thorough, and accurate review of literature.

6. The purpose, questions, or hypotheses were logical extensions of the rationale.

7. The introduction was clearly written and well organized.

8. General Comments.

*Overall Rating (Introduction):*

| Poor | Fair | Good | Excellent |
| --- | --- | --- | --- |

# R E F E R E N C E

American Psychological Association. (2001). *Publication manual of the American Psychological Association* (5th ed.). Washington, DC: American Psychological Association.

CHAPTER 8

# The Method Section

If the Introduction section can be considered the foundation of the research article, then the Method section can be considered its structural framework. Understanding this framework is crucial to the critical evaluation of the Results and Discussion sections that follow. It is in the Method section that the author describes the participants used in the study, the materials employed, and how those materials are used with the participants; that is, the procedures. In addition, the Method section helps the reader to identify the research strategy being reported and the specific research design incorporated in the study. Finally, it is in the Method section that the careful reader can identify how the author dealt with threats to internal and external validity.

The Method section stems directly from the rationale and the purpose of the study stated in the introduction. As such, the first major concern of the critical evaluator is whether the Method section, viewed in its entirety, is related to what has preceded and whether the methods chosen are appropriate to the problem posed in the introduction. The second concern, and one that we seek to answer in this chapter, is whether the methods chosen by the investigator are adequate in and of themselves.

## Participants

We have noted in Part I that participant selection can pose a threat to the internal and external validity of both experimental and descriptive research. The careful reader of a research article must determine, therefore, if the subject-selection procedure reported and the type of participants used compromise the adequacy of the research. Before we present some evaluative guidelines, one general guideline needs to be emphasized with respect to the description of the participants (as well as the description of materials and procedures). This guideline is simply, but importantly, that sufficient description be provided to allow the reader to *replicate* the study reported, at least in its important aspects. Researchers must resist the blue pencil of the cost-conscious editor, and the reader must insist on adequate detail or, at the very least, references to previous research that contain the detailed description of procedures. The important point, again, is that the description of methods must be sufficiently complete to allow for replication.

## Sample Size

The diversity of research in communicative disorders is reflected, in a sense, in the different sample sizes employed in different studies. Sample sizes range from $N = 1$ to $N =$ thousands. Thus, one of the first questions that must be asked by readers (and doers) of research is whether the size of the sample is adequate for the purposes of the study. Unfortunately, there is no simple answer to this question. For example, Pedhazur and Schmelkin (1991, p. 336) state that "decision regarding sample size is a complex one subject to a host of concerns. These include, . . . sampling strategy, types of estimators, practical and economic concerns . . . Type I and Type II errors." Additionally, the purpose of the investigation, previous research, the concern about generalizability, the variability found for the attribute under study, and the research design itself all play a role in deciding whether the number of participants used is appropriate. For instance, in within-subjects designs, in which there are many repeated observations and many data points, small samples have been used and are quite adequate. This type of small sample study is found, for example, in the language-acquisition literature and the psychoacoustic literature. Test standardization and survey research require large samples of participants. Between-subjects designs usually require larger samples than within-subjects designs. If one wishes to generalize data to the majority of children who have articulatory disorders, then, a large number of participants will have to be used. If the experimental treatment is expected to produce only small group differences, large samples may have to be employed to demonstrate statistically significant differences. It has to be acknowledged, of course, that small statistically significant differences obtained on a large sample of participants may have little clinical meaning or value. On the other hand, if large treatment differences are anticipated, on the basis of either pilot data or previous research, then a small sample may be adequate.

Excerpts 8.1 through 8.4 illustrate the broad range of sample sizes found in the communicative disorders literature. The four articles from which the excerpts were selected reflect different purposes, previous sample-size traditions, different research designs, expected variability of the data, and statistical analysis. Each of these considerations may have been more or less responsible for the sample sizes chosen.

Excerpt 8.1 illustrates the use of a large sample of randomly selected participants. We have mentioned previously that consumers of research can have more confidence in the generalization of results when a large number of participants has been randomly selected from the population of interest. Most studies, however, do not incorporate random selection of participants from the total population of interest. The most common reasons are that the universe of participants of interest is not available to the researcher and the cost of such random sampling procedures may be prohibitive. For practical reasons, then, most studies in communicative disorders do not use large random samples of participants.

The exceptions are usually large scale descriptive studies, such as the one shown in Excerpt 8.1, which seeks to identify the prevalence of speech delay and language impairment in six-year-old children living in the United States. The participants described in Excerpt 8.1 are a subsample of 1,328 kindergarten children from an original sample of 7,218 children who were selected randomly on the basis of a technique called stratified cluster sampling. The original sample of 7,218 children was stratified on the basis of residential setting (e.g., urban, suburban, and rural residential strata) across three midwestern popula-

## EXCERPT 8.1

We estimate the prevalence of *speech delay* (L. D. Shriberg, D. Austin, B. A. Lewis, J. L. McSweeny, & D. L. Wilson, 1997b) in the United States on the basis of findings from a demographically representative population subsample of 1,328 monolingual English-speaking 6-year-old children. All children's speech and language had been previously assessed in the "Epidemiology of Specific Language Impairment" project (see J. B. Tomblin et al., 1997), which screened 7,218 children in stratified cluster samples within 3 population centers in the upper Midwest.

From "Prevalence of Speech Delay in 6-Year-Old Children and Comorbidity with Language Delay," by L. D. Shriberg, J. B. Tomblin, and J. L. McSweeny, 1999, *Journal of Speech, Language, and Hearing Research, 42,* p. 1461. Copyright 1999 by the American Speech-Language-Hearing Association. Reprinted with permission.

tion centers. This provided a large sample of children from a variety of demographic conditions. The clusters comprised nine large groups of kindergarten children defined on the basis of geographic region and residential setting. Excerpt 8.1 is from the abstract of the study. Detailed participant selection criteria are given in the Method section of the article. Given the large sample size and sampling method, the external validity of this study should be remarkably good.

The next excerpt (8.2) describes the selection of 80 participants on the basis of chronological age and several other important criteria. Although this sample is not as large as the one reported previously and was not randomly selected, it still represents a relatively large sample of participants. Also, the purpose and design of this study are different from the study shown in Excerpt 8.1. All 80 participants were tested individually in this research. Later in the Method section, it is explained that the various testing conditions were randomized and counterbalanced across the listeners.

In some types of communicative disorders research, listeners or raters are considered participants in the same manner as speakers. Excerpt 8.3 is an example from a study that compared listener ratings of speech naturalness obtained from two different procedures: equal-appearing interval (EAI) ratings and direct magnitude estimation (DME) procedures. In an effort to minimize the effects of extraneous variables, listeners were randomly assigned to use either the EAI or the DME procedure to judge speech naturalness.

In some speech and hearing studies, the sample size and method of participant selection are less important than the instrumentation and procedures and, thus, become almost incidental. This is often true in basic physiologic and psychoacoustic research where the variability of the data is quite small and numerous repeated measurements are made in a within-subjects design. Take, for example, the entire subject-selection section from a study regarding respiratory sinus arrhythmia during speech production shown in Excerpt 8.4. Is this an adequate description of the nine women and nine men participants? Does it matter? Simply put, the nature and purpose of the research were such that any small group of nonsmoking males and females with no history of speech disorders or respiratory, neurological, or cardiovascular disease could probably have been used without significantly affecting the

EXCERPT  8.2

**Listeners**

Eighty listeners with normal hearing participated in the study. Twenty (10 male, 10 female) listeners were selected in each of the following four age groups: (a) 6 years, 0 months to 7 years, 11 months; (b) 10 years, 0 months to 11 years, 11 months; (c) 14 years, 0 months to 15 years, 11 months; and (d) 18 to 30 years of age. Listeners satisfied the following criteria: (a) bilateral puretone air- and bone-conduction thresholds of less than or equal to 15 dB hearing level (HL; ANSI, 1996) for the octave frequencies 250 to 8000 Hz; (b) bilateral speech reception thresholds (SRT) of less than or equal to 15 dB HL; (c) normal bilateral immittance results; (d) no air-bone gaps of more than 10 dB HL; (e) no documented case of otitis media within 6 months prior to participation in the experiment; (f) no apparent artic-ulatory abnormality; (g) native speakers of English; (h) subtest and composite scores of no lower than one standard deviation below the mean for the SCAN: A Screening Test for Auditory Processing Disorders, for children 11 years and under (Keith, 1986) or SCAN–A: A Test for Auditory Processing Disorders in Adolescents and Adults, for listeners ages 12 years and older (Keith, 1994); (i) no history of any language delays and/or disorders; and (j) normal progress in all academic subjects in school. Only native speakers of English were recruited as listeners because the literature has shown that this factor can affect phoneme recognition ability in reverberation and noise (Takata & Nabelek, 1990). Listeners were recruited in the Auburn-Opelika, Alabama area and were recruited through advertisements placed in local newspapers.

From "Children's Phoneme Identification in Reverberation and Noise," by C. E. Johnson, 2000, *Journal of Speech, Language, and Hearing Research, 43,* p. 146. Copyright 2000 by the American Speech-Language-Hearing Association. Reprinted with permission

---

data or modifying the conclusions. In this study, the instrumentation and procedures used were more important than the participants used. Similar examples could easily be cited. Once again the adequacy of the size of the participant sample and the way the participants are selected depend to a very large extent on the basic purpose of the study, the nature of the research design, and the variability of the data.

EXCERPT  8.3

**Raters**

The raters were 40 undergraduate college students enrolled in an introductory course in communication disorders. The raters had no academic or clinical experience with stuttering. None of the raters evidenced a significant speech, language, vision, or hearing problem.

**Procedures**

Half of the raters were randomly assigned to use the EAI rating procedure and the other half to use the DME procedure for the psychophysical scaling of speech naturalness from the audiovisual recordings.

From "Psychophysical Analysis of Audiovisual Judgments of Speech Naturalness of Nonstutterers and Stutterers," by N. Schiavetti, R. R. Martin, S. K. Haroldson, and D. E. Metz, 1994, *Journal of Speech and Hearing Research, 37,* p. 48. Copyright 1994 by the American Speech-Language-Hearing Association. Reprinted with permission.

---

EXCERPT 8.4

## Method

### Participants

Participants included 9 men (age range = 22–37 years; $M$ = 27.9, $SD$ = 5.2) and 9 women (age range = 24–41 years; $M$ = 30.1, $SD$ = 5.1). Participants were non-smokers whose medical histories were negative for speech, respiratory, neurological, or cardiovascular disease. To control for potential changes in baroreceptor responsiveness resulting from the ingestion of caffeine (de Mey, Enterling, Brendel, & Meineke, 1987) or a meal (Mosqueda-Garcia, Tseng, Biaggioni, Robertson, & Robertson, 1990), participants refrained from ingesting caffeine for 4 hr and from eating for 3 hr prior to participation in this experiment.

From "Respiratory Sinus Arrhythmia during Speech Production," by K. J. Reilly and C. A. Moore, 2003, *Journal of Speech, Language, and Hearing Research, 46,* p. 166. Copyright 2003 by the American Speech-Language-Hearing Association. Reprinted with permission.

---

## Criteria for Participant Selection

As we have mentioned throughout, much of the descriptive research in communicative disorders deals with differences and attempts to answer questions such as these: Are people who stutter different from those who don't? Do people with Ménière's disease differ from people with noise-induced hearing loss? Is test A more sensitive than test B in differentiating aphasics from other brain-injured people? In any study involving group differences (between-subjects designs), it is absolutely essential that the experimenter describe and perhaps even defend the criteria used in forming the groups. Inadequate group composition, overlapping groups, and indefensible selection criteria all pose important threats to the internal and external validity of both experimental and descriptive research.

The example shown in Excerpt 8.5 is taken from an article that examined the relationship of language skills and emotion regulation skills to reticent behaviors of children in two age groups (five to eight years and nine to twelve years) who were developing typically and children in two comparable age groups with specific language impairment (SLI). Specific group performance comparisons were also used in this study. The inclusion criteria for the forty-three participants with SLI are listed in detail in the first portion of the article's Method section. The authors then go on to explain that the classroom teacher of each child with SLI provided a list of peers in the same class who were gender and age matched and also met additional stringent inclusion criteria. Participants were randomly selected from these lists of peers to serve as matches for the children with SLI. The detailed list of specific group inclusion criteria, gender and age matching of the groups, and the random selection of the typically developing participants are excellent examples of efforts to control extraneous variables.

Because participant selection procedures are so important in between-group studies in communicative disorders, we have chosen another illustration. Excerpt 8.6 is from a study that was designed to examine potential differences in temperamental characteristics between children who stutter and children who do not stutter. To ensure equivalence

EXCERPT  8.5

## Method

### Participants

The sample consisted of 43 children with SLI and 43 typically developing children matched for gender and chronological age, for a total of 86 participants. Each group is described as follows.

### Participants With SLI

Children were selected from two local school districts. Speech-language pathologists referred children meeting the following criteria from their caseloads.

1. Chronological age between 5 and 8 years or between 9 and 12 years.
2. Nonverbal or performance IQ above 80, to rule out, mental retardation as the basis for language impairment. IQ scores from current school district testing were used when available. Tests used included the Kaufman Assessment Battery for Children (Kaufman & Kaufman, 1983), the Leiter International Performance Scale (Leiter, 1984), the fourth edition of the Stanford–Binet Intelligence Scale (SB; Thorndike, Hagen, Sattler, & Delaney, 1986), the Matrix Analogies Test (Naglieri, 1985), the Woodcock–Johnson Psycho-Educational Battery—Revised (WJ-R; Woodcock & Johnson, 1989), and the Wechsler Intelligence Scale for Children—Third Edition (WISC-III; Wechsler, 1991). In cases where IQ scores were not available, the Test of Nonverbal Intelligence—Second Edition (TONI-2; Brown, Sherbenou, & Johnsen, 1990) was administered. For the 5 children assessed with tests that did not yield a specific measure of nonverbal IQ (SB, WJ-R), a composite IQ score above 80 was considered acceptable (the lowest observed composite score was 86).
3. Diagnosis of language impairment by the school speech-language pathologist and enrollment in speech-language pathology services.
4. Performance at least 1 standard deviation below the mean on a formal measure of receptive and/ or expressive language. The test used by the speech-language pathologist to qualify the child for services was used as a measure of this crite-

rion. Existing tests indicated that the children with SLI demonstrated a range of profiles with regard to expressive and receptive skills. Subsequent testing using the Comprehensive Assessment of Spoken Language (CASL; Carrow-Woodfolk, 1999) confirmed this impression. On the basis of the Syntax Construction subtest (production) and the Paragraph Comprehension subtest (comprehension) of the CASL, 22 participants had better comprehension than production; 17 of these children produced standard scores on the comprehension subtest that were a standard deviation or more higher than scores on the production subtest. Five children scored 7.5 or more points lower in comprehension than production (one half of a standard deviation), and 1 produced a gap larger than a standard deviation. The remaining 16 children had relatively equal production and comprehension scores, with standard scores on the two subtests within 7.5 points of each other. Correlations between the two subtests and the reticence score were not statistically significant.
5. Unremarkable hearing status as indicated by a pure-tone screening performed by school district personnel.
6. No formal diagnosis of emotional or behavioral disorder. This criterion was assessed on the basis of school district records and placement data.

The resulting sample consisted of 11 boys in the younger group (mean age in years;months = 7;6, $SD =$ 9 months) and 12 boys in the older group (mean age =10;9, $SD = 8$ months). There were 10 girls in both the younger and older groups, with mean ages of 6;6 ($SD =$ 12 months) and 10;4 ($SD =10$ months), respectively.

### Participants With Typically Developing Language Skills

For each child with SLI, a classmate of the same gender and age exhibiting typical language skills was selected. The classroom teacher of each child with SLI generated a list of peers in the same class who met the following criteria:

1. Same gender and classroom as the child with SLI.
2. Chronological age within 6 months of the child with SLI. On three occasions it was necessary to use children who were outside of this 6-month guideline to meet the other criteria. These children were within 7, 8, and 11 months of their matches with SLI.
3. No academic, behavioral, or communication problems requiring special services, based on teacher report and placement data.

Children were randomly selected from these lists of peers as matches for the children with SLI. The resulting sample consisted of 11 boys in the younger group (mean age = 7;6, $SD$ = 10 months) and 12 boys in the older group (mean age = 10;9, $SD$ = 8 months). There were 10 girls in both the younger and older groups, with mean ages of 6;7 $(SD$ =13 months) and 10;4 $(SD$ = 11 months), respectively.

**Ethnicity and Socioeconomic Status**

Children in both groups were largely drawn from a White, middle-class population. A measure of socio-economic status for all of the participants was obtained from block group data from the 2000 census (U.S. Census Bureau, 2003). The mean percentage of families with income levels below the poverty level in the neighborhoods surrounding the schools involved in the study was, less than 1% ($M = 0.32, SD = 0.49$). With respect to ethnicity in the group with SLI, 34 of the children were White, 3 were Hispanic, 2 were Asian, 2 were African American, and 2 were of mixed-race background. In the group with typical language skills, 39 children were White, 3 were Hispanic, and 1 was Asian.

---

**EXCERPT 8.6**

## Method

### Participants

Participants were 62 children between the ages of 3;0 (years;months) and 5;4 who are CWS ($n$ = 31; mean age = 48.03 months) and who are CWNS ($n$ = 31; mean age = 48.58 months). The CWS were matched by age (±4 months), gender (6 girls, 25 boys), and race (3 African American, 28 White) to the CWNS. Each participant's socioeconomic status was determined using the Hollingshead Two-Factor Index of Social Position (Myers & Bean, 1968), which involved the assessment of each participant's "head of household" (father in case of dual-parent families, 95.2% of sample; mother in case of single-parent families, 4.8% of sample) occupation and educational level. There were no significant between-talker group differences in terms of social position, $t(52) = 0.12$, $p = .90$, with CWS having a mean social position score of 26.17, $SD = 14.76$ (lower ends of Hollingshead Classification II) and CWNS having a mean social position score of 26.67, $SD = 14.87$ (lower ends of Hollingshead Classification II).

All participants were native speakers of American English with no history of neurological, hearing, psychological, or academic/intellectual problems. All participants (a) scored at the 20th percentile or higher on three standardized speech-language tests (described below), (b) passed a hearing screening (see the *Criteria for Group Classification* section), (c) passed a general/oral motor functioning screening test (the Selected Neuromotor Task Battery [SNTB]; Wolk 1990), and

*(continued)*

## E X C E R P T  8.6  Continued

(d) had received no prior treatment for articulation, language, or stuttering concerns at the time of their participation in this study. All participants were paid volunteers in an ongoing series of studies concerning the relationship between stuttering and language/phonology (e.g., Anderson & Conture, 2000; Melnick, Conture, & Ohde, in press; Pellowski & Conture, 2002). CWS were identified for participation in these studies by their parents, who had heard about them through (a) an advertisement in a free, widely read, monthly parent-oriented magazine (*Nashville Parent,* estimated monthly readership of 230,000); (b) Middle Tennessee area speech-language pathologists, health care providers, daycare centers, and so on; or (c) referral to the Vanderbilt Bill Wilkerson Hearing and Speech Center for the initial assessment of childhood stuttering. Approximately 60% of the CWS were identified through the magazine advertisement, with the remaining 40% being equally divided between professional referral and referral for initial clinical evaluation of stuttering. All children who did not stutter were identified for participation through parental response to the magazine advertisement.

For the CWS, the reported TSO was obtained during the parent interview using a "bracketing" procedure, whereby the interviewer systematically narrows down the time of onset of stuttering (Yairi & Ambrose, 1992). For example, as described by Yairi and Ambrose (1992),

EXAMINER:  When did the child begin stuttering?
PARENT:  Last winter.
EXAMINER:  When during winter?
PARENT:  Around Christmas.
EXAMINER:  Before or after Christmas?
PARENT:  I am sure it was after.
EXAMINER:  Before or after New Year's Day?
PARENT:  After. He did not stutter on New Year's Day.

EXAMINER:  Was it a few days or weeks later?
PARENT:  It was a day or two after we returned from vacation and just before I went back to my job at school. I remember this very clearly.
EXAMINER:  When did you go back to work?
PARENT:  January 5th.
EXAMINER:  So, we are pretty close to pinning it down.
PARENT:  It must have been between January 3rd and 5th. (p. 785)

On the basis of this procedure, the average parent-reported TSO for the 31 CWS used in this study was 12.93 months (range = 4–23 months, $SD$ = 5.12 months), with all CWS having a TSO of 23 months or less.

### Criteria for Group Classification

#### Children Who Stutter (CWS)

A child was assigned to the CWS group if he/she (a) exhibited three or more within-word disfluencies (WWD; i.e., sound/syllable repetitions, sound prolongations, broken words) and/or monosyllabic whole-word repetitions, per 100 words of conversational speech (Bloodstein, 1995; Conture, 2001), and (b) received a total overall score of 11 or higher (i.e., a severity equivalent of at least "mild") on the Stuttering Severity Instrument for Children and Adults—Third Edition (SSI-3; Riley, 1994). Nine CWS were classified as mild, 20 as moderate, and 2 as severe.

#### Children Who Do Not Stutter (CWNS)

A child was assigned to the CWNS group if he/she (a) exhibited two or fewer within-word and/or monosyllabic whole-word repetitions per 100 words of conversational speech (Conture & Kelly, 1991), and (b) received a total overall score of 10 or lower (i.e., a severity equivalent of less than "mild") on the SSI-3.

between the children who stutter and those who do not stutter, the authors carefully paired the participants in the two groups across the dimensions of gender, age, and race. Additionally, the authors determined equivalence of socioeconomic status between the groups by administering the Hollingshead Two-Factor Index of Social Position.

Another aspect of participant selection that directly affects internal validity is whether participants are selected on the basis of extreme scores. We point out in Part I that selecting participants because of their extreme scores may produce regression effects. That is, apparent changes in posttreatment scores may merely reflect the tendency for extreme scores to become less extreme (regress toward the mean) rather than reflecting true treatment effects. The critical reader should be especially alert to regression effects in studies of treatment programs.

Excerpt 8.7 is taken from the Discussion section of a study of regression to the mean in stuttering measures. They measured regression during a pretreatment waiting period and compared their findings to previous studies. Although the amount of regression they found was small, note their suggestions for incorporating a correction for regression in pretest–posttest studies of the effects of stuttering treatment. Note their comments about measures of speech attitude and reaction to speech situations, as well as the actual speech measures of fluency. Similar studies with other speech disorders would help to improve the design of treatment experiments.

The relevant questions about subject-selection criteria that need to be asked for between-group studies can be summarized as follows: (1) Are the criteria for group composition clearly defined and defensible? (2) Is there overlap between groups on the variable that distinguishes the groups? (3) Are exclusion criteria defined and defensible? (4) Are the groups comparable on important extraneous variables? and (5) Have participants been selected on the basis of extreme scores? These questions deal primarily with the issue of internal validity. Regarding external validity, the question is this: Are the participants comparable, on important dimensions, to the population to which the author wishes to generalize?

One final point deserves brief attention. The author of a research article should indicate if participants were volunteers and whether they were paid (or unpaid) to participate in the study. A complete discussion of the effects of the volunteer participant on the outcomes of research is beyond the scope of this book. (The interested reader should consult Rosenthal and Rosnow [1975].) Suffice it to say that volunteer participants, whether paid or unpaid, may be different in important respects from the population to whom the investigator wishes to generalize, thus affecting external validity.

# Materials

The materials part of the research article is a key component of the Method section. The reason for its importance is that it is in this section that researchers identify the materials that have been used to measure or generate the variables under study, and it is here that the critical consumer of research can identify instrumentation threats to internal validity. Underscoring the importance of such threats is the fact emphasized in Chapter 5 that instrumentation threats to internal validity transcend research strategy or design.

There are two basic evaluation questions that need to be asked by the consumer: (1) Was there adequate selection and measurement of the independent (classification, predictor)

## EXCERPT 8.7

The six studies in the literature that have measured stutterers at two or three points in time prior to treatment have all reported a statistically nonsignificant improvement trend. This improvement may be evidence that stutterers come for treatment when their stuttering is worst and spontaneously improve a little with time. Although it is difficult to aggregate data from this small set of studies, examination of the time of the improvement, as reflected by the effect-size statistic, shows that the improvement can be evident as early as three months after initial contact.

The present study of 132 subjects showed that many stutterers waiting for treatment did improve significantly. This may be evidence of regression in the severity of their stuttering to a previously established mean level. Analysis of the present data by the time subjects spent on the waiting list showed that the improvement occurred within the first three months and that no further improvement occurred thereafter.

Regression to the mean appears an effect that could confound estimates of the improvement due to therapy in pre-post treatment outcome designs. There are two ways of allowing for the effect. First, stutterers could be held on a waiting list for three months or until a stable baseline is demonstrated so that the effects of treatment will not be confounded by regression to the mean. Second, if subjects receive treatment immediately after they apply for treatment, a small but definable part of the improvement following treatment will be due to spontaneous regression to the mean, and the treatment results should be corrected accordingly.

Aggregating the data from the six reports in the literature and from the present study suggests that the magnitude of this effect is small; mean effect size = 0.21 (SE 0.04). Subtracting this amount from the pre-post effect size would approximate the actual treatment-related improvement. In practical terms, a group of adult stutterers of mean severity 17%SS when first seen will spontaneously improve to a mean of 14%SS three months later, and improvement beyond this point following treatment is likely to be due to the effects of treatment.

Self-report measures of speech attitude and reaction to speech situations also showed improvement trends, but in both Gregory (1972) and the present study, the changes were of much smaller magnitude than those of speech measures. This improvement trend is so small that it can be disregarded when using self-report measures to calculate the improvement produced by therapy.

From "Regression to the Mean in Pretreatment Measures of Stuttering," by G. Andrews and R. Harvey, 1981, *Journal of Speech and Hearing Disorders, 46,* pp. 206–207. Copyright 1981 by the American Speech-Language-Hearing Association. Reprinted with permission.

variable? and (2) Was there adequate selection and measurement of the dependent (criterion, predicted) variable? Although the researcher's rationale for the selection of variables may appear in either the Introduction or the Method section (and this rationale requires careful scrutiny on the part of the reader), the measurement of variables will almost always be described in either the Materials or the Procedures section. Our purpose here, then, is to lay down some general guidelines that can be used by the critical reader to evaluate possible instrumentation (i.e., materials) threats to the internal validity of both experimental and descriptive research.

## Hardware Instrumentation and Calibration

***Instrumentation.***    Hardware instrumentation plays an important role in research in communicative disorders, especially in speech and hearing science. Much of what we know about normal (and disordered) processes is due, in large part, to technological advances that have made possible the measuring, recording, and analyzing systems that are found in speech and hearing laboratories throughout the country. This is not to say that all research is dependent on or requires sophisticated electronic instrumentation. The exciting advances made in understanding how children acquire language has not required much more than an audiotape recorder or a relatively simple videotape recording system. It is to say, however, that the critical reader of research is often required to read research articles that are heavily weighted in instrumentation. The critical evaluation of such material can be an exceedingly difficult task, especially for the student who has minimal course work or experience in electronics or instrumentation.

Although instrumentation can be complex, the purposes to which the instruments are put are reasonably straightforward. Instruments are used to produce signals (e.g., an audio-frequency oscillator), to measure the signal (e.g., a sound-level meter), to store the signal (e.g., a tape recorder or a computer disk), to control the signal (e.g., an electronic switch), to modify the signal (e.g., a band-pass filter), and to analyze the signal (e.g., a digital sound spectrograph). The reasons for using an instrument are equally straightforward. The researcher (or clinician) uses an instrument to standardize data-acquisition procedures, to help acquire data under known conditions, and to provide a permanent record of the data. Most important, instruments allow the measurement of events that are not directly observable by the senses (Plutchik, 1983). There is nothing inherently mysterious about instrumentation. What is mysterious, perhaps, is why so little attention is paid to laboratory instrumentation in many master's-level communicative disorders training programs. This may very well be the reason that many consumers of research approach the apparatus section of an article with fear and trepidation. Another point to keep in mind is that instruments, like statistics, are tools. The instrument itself, with few exceptions, is not the reason for the research. Thus, again like statistics, a sophisticated instrumental array cannot improve an inadequate research problem and cannot modify a poor research design.

Several guidelines can be used by the practitioner or student while reading the instrumentation section of an article. First, and at the very least, the principal components of the system should be identified by manufacturer and model number. This enables the interested reader to duplicate the system using the same or comparable equipment. It also allows the reader to determine if the components are reasonably standard pieces that have been manufactured by reputable companies. If a new instrument has been developed for a particular study, enough information should be provided to allow the reader to reconstruct the piece. Circuit diagrams, photographs, line drawings, and the like should be included for this purpose. The point here is that there should be sufficient detail for replication purposes and to permit the reader to determine if the components are standard pieces of equipment likely to be found in a well-equipped speech and hearing laboratory. A block diagram showing the interrelationships among components is a useful device for describing the instrumentation array.

Another criterion is whether the same or a similar instrumental array has been used by the investigator in a previously reported study or has been used by other investigators studying the same phenomenon. References to previous research can be of considerable value in assessing the adequacy of instrumentation. The absence of such references, especially when confronted with a custom-built instrument, should alert the reader to the possibility of instrumental error.

Some basic characteristics of the instrumentation used may also be reported in the instrumentation section and may be of value to the reader in helping to assess whether the instrumentation was appropriate to the task at hand. The frequency response characteristics of the earphones, the linearity of attenuators, and the intensity range of an amplifier are just three examples of the kind of descriptive information that might be provided in the instrumentation section.

Excerpt 8.8 provides a detailed description of the equipment used in a study that examined respiratory and laryngeal responses to experimenter-induced changes in intra-oral

## E X C E R P T   8.8

### Equipment

The acoustic signal was transduced with a dynamic, omnidirectional, lavalier microphone (Shure Model SM11). The microphone was placed within a circumferentially vented pneumotachograph mask, through the hole usually used for the mask handle. Thick foam was used to seal the microphone in place and to ensure that no air leaked around the microphone. The mouth-to-microphone distance was held constant at 3.5 cm. Resonances from within the mask were not a concern, as all conditions included the mask. Therefore, any added resonances associated with the mask were the same across all conditions. The signal was stored on a digital audio tape (DAT; Fuji), using a two-channel DAT recorder (Tascam Model DA-P2).

Oral airflow was transduced using the circumferentially vented pneumotachograph mask and a high frequency pressure transducer (Glottal Enterprises, Syracuse, NY; Model PTW-1). Use of this mask was not expected to alter the participants' performance on any of the tasks (Huber, Stathopoulos, Bormann, & Johnson, 1998). Oral pressure was sensed via a 1-mm internal diameter (2-mm external diameter) oral pressure tube placed between the lips just inside the participant's mouth on the left side. The distal end of the oral pressure tube was connected to a low frequency pressure transducer (Glottal Enterprises, Model PTL-1). Respiratory movements were transduced using linearized magnetometers (GMG Scientific Inc., Burlington, MA) using procedures developed by Hixon

and Hoit (i.e., Hixon, Goldman, & Mead, 1973; Hoit & Hixon, 1987). One set was placed at the midpoint of the sternum to track the rib cage movements, and one set was placed just above the umbilicus to track the abdominal movements. Magnetometers were attached to the participants skin using double-sided scotch tape. Signals from the magnetometers were monitored on an x-y oscilloscope (Tektronix Inc., Beaverton, OR; Model 5111A) during data collection.

All signals were digitized on-line to CSpeech SP (Milenkovic, 1997) through an IBM-compatible computer and an A-D/D-A board (Data Translation Inc., Marlboro, MA; Model DT2821). Oral airflow, oral air pressure, and magnetometer signals were low-pass filtered at 4200 Hz for anti-aliasing and digitized at a sampling rate of 10 kHz, using the maximum voltage resolution ($\pm$ 10 volts). The microphone signal was digitized separately from the digital audiotape to the computer after data collection was complete. The microphone signal was low-pass filtered at 8 kHz for anti-aliasing and digitized to the IBM-compatible computer through the A-D/D-A board at a sampling rate of 20 kHz, using the maximum voltage resolution ($\pm$10 volts).

Lung volume was obtained by integrating the airflow signal from the circumferentially vented pneumotachograph mask. This procedure has been found previously to result in a volume signal that is within $\pm$5% of the volume measured from a respirometer (Stathopoulos & Sapienza, 1997).

air pressure. Clearly, the equipment description provided by the authors would permit replication. However, the adequacy of the equipment array could probably be best evaluated by individuals who are familiar with equipment used to measure such respiratory and laryngeal responses.

With the increasing impact of rapid technological developments in the field of communicative disorders, however, consumers of research will find it more and more difficult to evaluate the research in the field without some background in instrumentation. It is obviously beyond the scope of this book to attempt to teach principles of instrumentation to clinicians and students. Many attempts have been made to make professionals aware of the need to understand instrumentation in speech and hearing. Levitt (1983) addressed this issue at the 1983 ASHA National Conference on Undergraduate, Graduate, and Continuing Education. He concisely summarized the problem when he said (Levitt, 1983, p. 88):

> In short, modern technology is transforming virtually every aspect of our profession (and of every other profession as well). It is imperative that a concerted effort be made to train professionals in our field to function effectively in this new environment.

Levitt outlined several issues to be considered in developing guidelines for future incorporation of technological instruction in the education of communicative disorders specialists and made several suggestions to help professionals to understand and use the advancing technology in future clinical and research activities. Levitt (1983, p. 88) emphasized the importance of making technological innovations meaningful and useful to our service-oriented profession, stating:

> It is wholly unrealistic to develop preservice and in-service training programs that will cover all aspects of modern technology. There is a need to be selective. For example, one need not understand the principles of xerography in order to use a Xerox machine effectively. On the other hand, the characteristics and inherent limitations of acoustic amplifiers need to be understood in order to prescribe hearing aids properly.

Students and clinicians must also accept some responsibility for updating their knowledge of technological innovations in the field. Many state and national conventions now offer continuing education activities that deal with the use of technical innovations, computers, and various kinds of instrumentation. Also, many recent articles have appeared in the clinical and research literature that attempt to provide knowledge about instrumentation, computer applications, and measurement techniques that are geared to clinicians. The "Research Notes" of the *Journal of Speech, Language, and Hearing Research* often present information on instrumentation that may help clinicians update their knowledge and skills.

As technological advances progress, communicative disorders specialists need to take advantage of courses and continuing education in instrumentation to keep current in their clinical work and prepare themselves to evaluate the research in the field that relies more and more on electronic instrumentation. The time has come when knowledge of instrumentation is as important a tool to communication disorders specialists as traditional tools such as knowledge of phonetic transcription, anatomy and physiology, or linguistics have been in the past.

The next excerpt (Excerpt 8.9) shows how the authors used block diagrams to complement the narrative description of instruments used in a study that compared two measurement

## EXCERPT 8.9

### Instrumental Assessment of Nasal Resonance

The Model 6200 Nasometer is a microcomputer-based system manufactured by Kay Elemetrics (Figure 1). With this device, oral and nasal components of a subject's speech are sensed by microphones on either side of a sound separator that rests on the upper lip. The signal from each of the microphones is filtered and digitized by custom electronic modules. The data are then processed by an IBM PC computer. The resultant signal is a ratio of nasal to nasal-plus-oral acoustic energy. This ratio is multiplied by 100 and expressed as a "nasalance" score.

Prior to testing, the Nasometer was calibrated and the headgear was adjusted in accordance with instructions provided by the manufacturer. Each subject was then asked to read a standard passage loaded with nasal consonants (see appendix). Those subjects who were unable to read the passage easily were asked to repeat the sentences after the examiner (Rodger Dalston).

### Measurement of Nasal Cross-Sectional Area

Recent advances in respiratory monitoring technology provide the opportunity to define nasal airway impairment objectively. One approach is to measure nasal airway cross-sectional size using a technique developed by Warren for speech research (Warren & DuBois, 1964). The validity of this aerodynamic assessment technique has been substantiated in a number of laboratories (Lubker, 1969; Smith & Weinberg, 1980, 1982, 1983), and a recent study demonstrates that it can be used successfully to define airway impairment (Warren, 1984).

The method used to measure nasal cross-sectional area involves a modification of the theoretical hydraulic principle and assumes that the smallest cross-sectional area of a structure can be determined if the differential pressure across the structure is measured simultaneously with rate of airflow through it. This method, which has been used in speech research by Warren and his associates since 1961 (Warren & DuBois, 1964), was specifically modified for assessing nasal airway patency. The equation employed is

$$\text{Area} = \frac{\text{Rate of nasal airflow}}{k \left[ \frac{2 \times \text{oral} - \text{nasal pressure drop}}{\text{density of air}} \right]^{\frac{1}{2}}}$$

where $k = 0.65$ and the density of air $= 0.001$ gm/cm$^2$. The correction factor $k$ was obtained from analog studies that have been reported previously (Warren, 1984; Warren & DuBois, 1964).

Figure 2 illustrates the aerodynamic assessment technique used in the current study. The oral-nasal pressure drop was measured with pressure transducers connected to two catheters. The first catheter was positioned midway in the subject's mouth, and the

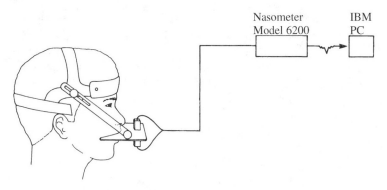

**FIGURE 1    A schematic representation of the instrumentation used to obtain Nasometer measurements.**

second catheter was placed within a nasal mask in front of the nose. Nasal airflow was measured with a heated pneumotachograph connected to the well-adapted nasal mask. Each subject was asked to inhale and exhale as normally as possible through the nose. The resulting pressure and airflow patterns were trans-mitted to the computer, analyzed, and recorded on hard copy. Although nasal areas can be measured during either inspiration or expiration, for the current study they were measured at the peak of expiratory airflow.

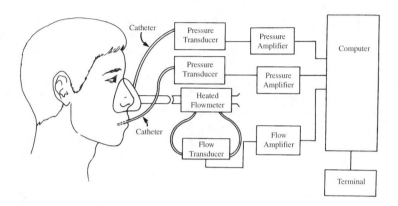

**FIGURE 2    A schematic representation of the instrumentation used to estimate nasal cross-sectional area.**

From "A Preliminary Investigation Concerning the Use of Nasometry in Identifying Patients with Hyponasality and/or Nasal Airway Impairment," by R. M. Dalston, D. G. Warren, and E. T. Dalston, 1991, *Journal of Speech and Hearing Research, 34,* pp. 13–14. Copyright 1991 by the American Speech-Language-Hearing Association. Reprinted with permission.

techniques (measurements of nasal resonance and measurements of nasal cross-sectional area) that can be used to assess hyponasality and/or nasal airway impairment. Calibration and specific measurement procedures are carefully explained in the prose.

*Calibration.*    Adequate calibration of instruments used in a given study is absolutely essential to the reduction of a possible threat to internal validity posed by instrumentation. Faulty calibration must lead to faulty data, either in the laboratory or in the clinic. Unfortunately, calibration procedures are sometimes given short shrift in a journal article. Thus, it is difficult to assess the adequacy of the calibration procedures used. As a result, the reader may have to rely on the integrity and honesty of the researcher in judging the adequacy of calibration.

    The three major questions that the reader must ask about calibration of equipment are (1) What was calibrated? (2) What equipment was used for calibration purposes? and (3) When was calibration performed? Excerpt 8.10 is taken from a study that compared speech intelligibility of nondisabled speakers and speakers with adductor spasmodic dysphonia before and after botulinum toxin injection. In this study, listeners audited audio recordings of all the speakers' utterances by typing what they thought they heard the speaker say into a computer database via a standard keyboard. It was critical that the playback of each

**E X C E R P T   8.10**

The instrumentation setup for this study was composed of two computer terminals. The control system was a 233 MHz Dell Optiplex GXMT 5133 computer equipped with a Soundblaster 16-bit audio output circuit. The output from the control system was input into the left channel of a Crown D-75 preamplifier (Crown Audio, Inc., Elkhart, IN) that was set to approximately 75% of the maximum total output capacity. The preamplifier was interfaced with a Tucker-Davis Technologies PA-4 programmable attenuator (Tucker-Davis Technologies, Alachua, FL), which was set to continuously attenuate the acoustic signal by 25 dB. The acoustic signal was presented inside an Acoustic Systems KE-132-sound-treated booth (Acoustic Systems, Austin, TX) via a Grason-Stadler stereo speaker set 80 cm from the floor of the booth. An AT 486-Sx computer served as a response terminal inside the booth. The response terminal was interfaced with the control system via a serial port. All listener responses were saved to a text file on the control system.

The acoustic output presented via the control system was calibrated prior to each listener session. A ½-inch stand-mounted microphone was placed 1 m away from the output speaker in the sound-treated booth at the approximate height, angle, and location of the ear of an adult seated 1 m away from the speaker. A calibration sound file (a complex tone generated by an electrolarynx) was played over the speaker via the control system. With the Larson-Davis attenuator set at 25 dB, the comfortable listening level of 54–56 dB re: SPL was verified via a Quest 155 sound level meter (Quest Technologies, Inc., Oconomowoc, WI). Calibration of the Quest sound level meter was maintained according to standardized calibration specifications from the manufacturer. This calibration routine assured that there was no drift of the acoustic output from the control system into the sound-treated booth.

From "Speech Intelligibility in Severe Adductor Spasmodic Dysphonia," by B. K. Bender, M. P. Cannito, T. Murry, and G. Woodson, 2004, *Journal of Speech, Language, and Hearing Research, 47,* pp. 24–25. Copyright 2004 by the American Speech-Language-Hearing Association. Reprinted with permission.

speaker's utterances be presented to the listeners at a constant and controlled intensity level. This was accomplished by monitoring the playback levels with a sound level meter, which, as the authors state, was calibrated in accordance with the specifications of the sound level meter's manufacturer. The exact time that these calibration procedures were performed is not specified. But, in the Procedures section of the article, the authors state that each sound file was presented at a listening level that ranged from 54 to 56 dB RMS re: SPL. This statement implies that the calibration procedures were performed individually for each listener prior to the actual auditing of the speaker's utterances.

Another example (Excerpt 8.11) is taken from a study regarding children's abilities to identify sounds in reverberation and noise environments. Instrumentation of both the recording and presentation of the speech stimuli used in the study are presented clearly in the article. In the third paragraph, note the care that was taken to ensure that appropriate sound pressure levels and signal-to-noise ratios were obtained for subsequent presentation to listeners. Another significant aspect of this Method section is the description of interjudge and intrajudge reliability of the listener's responses.

## EXCERPT 8.11

### Instrumentation for the Recording of the Speech Stimuli

The stimuli were played by a stereo cassette tape deck (Optimus, Model No. SCT-88) routed to a stereo receiver (Optimus, STA-825) and loudspeaker (Optimus, Model No. 1050) located in the front and center of the lecture hall. The Auditec of St. Louis multi-talker babble was used as the background noise. The same instrumentation was used to play back the babble, except that the babble was transduced through two loudspeakers (Optimus, Model No. 650) positioned 1.8 m to the right and left of the loudspeaker transducing the speech stimuli.

The speech stimuli were recorded through the Knowles Electronic Mannequin for Acoustics Research (KEMAR). The KEMAR was positioned at a zero degree azimuth to and about 10 m from the diaphragm of the loudspeaker transducing the speech stimuli, which was clearly beyond the critical distance of the lecture hall. The KEMAR was positioned 4.5 m from the left wall, 4.5 m from the right wall, and 2 m from the back wall of the lecture hall. The speech stimuli were recorded through 0.5-inch condenser microphones (Etymotic Research, Model No. ER-11) in the ear canals of KEMAR, which were equipped with preamplifiers that filtered out the ear canal resonances. The output of the microphone in the KEMAR's right ear was sent to Channel 1, and the output of the microphone in the left ear was sent to Channel 2 of a digital audio tape (DAT) deck (Panasonic, Model No. SV-3700).

The sound pressure levels (SPL) of the speech and background noise used in the recordings were measured at the right and left ear canals of the KEMAR. The speech level for the recordings was 92 dB SPL (re: averaged between the peak of the vowel /ei/ in the word "say" in the carrier phrase and the peaks of the consonants in each NST item) resulting in a +52 dB S/N (40-dB sound floor of the lecture hall). For the recording with added background noise, the sound pressure level for the multitalker babble was 79 dB SPL, creating a +13 dB S/N relative to the word "say" in the carrier phrase. This approximates the S/N that teachers try to maintain in the classroom (Pearsons, Bennett, & Fidell, 1977).

### Instrumentation for Experimental Protocol and Presentation of Speech Stimuli

The digital tape recordings of the NST were played through the DAT, routed to a calibrated audiometer (ANSI, 1996), and delivered to listeners through TDH-39 earphones.

Each listener wore a lavalier microphone that was connected to the input of a camcorder, which was positioned at a zero degree azimuth to and 1.5 m away from each listener. The camcorder simultaneously delivered a high-quality audio-visual signal to a 19-inch video monitor to the experimenters in the control room for scoring and recording listeners' responses on videotape for later use in calculating scoring reliability.

. . . . . . . . . . .

### Reliability

All videotapes of listeners' data collection sessions were independently transcribed by one judge twice and two judges once for assessment of intra- and inter-subject reliability using the following equation: [(Agreements + Disagreements)/Agreements] × 100. An agreement was defined as a phoneme being scored as correct or incorrect by the same judge twice (intrajudge) or by two judges independently (interjudge reliability). The one judge's transcription was used for determining listeners' percent-correct consonant and vowel identification scores in each listening condition at each SL. This judge transcribed all listeners' tapes twice. Intrajudge reliability was calculated between those two sets of transcriptions.

Interjudge reliability was calculated between the transcriptions of the other two judges and the judges' transcriptions that were used for determining listeners' percent-correct consonant and vowel identification scores. Intra- and interjudge reliability was 90%.

From "Children's Phoneme Identification in Reverberation and Noise," by C. E. Johnson, 2000, *Journal of Speech, Language, and Hearing Research, 43,* pp. 147–148. Copyright 2000 by the American Speech-Language-Hearing Association. Reprinted with permission.

The last example in this section is Excerpt 8.12. The interesting point here is that not only was there calibration of the instruments used but a physiologic calibration procedure was also employed. The need for this latter calibration procedure is described as well.

## Reliability and Validity of Behavioral Instruments

Under behavioral instruments, we include the enormous array of standardized and non-standardized tests such as paper-and-pencil tests of various types, articulation tests, language tests, speech-discrimination tests, hearing tests, attitude measures, and the like. Any of these kinds of materials may be used by researchers to make measurements of independent or dependent variables. Major problems with such instruments can pose significant threats to internal or external validity. Thus, the critical reader needs to carefully assess the adequacy of behavioral instruments used in research. Most communicative disorders specialists have had a reasonable amount of exposure to behavioral instruments through academic and practicum courses and clinical work. In this section, we will show some examples to illustrate some of the concepts of reliability and validity of measures that were discussed in Part I.

---

### EXCERPT 8.12

**Instrumental Calibration**

Calibration signals for the six physiologic data channels were recorded prior to subject preparation. To calibrate the four EMG channels, a custom-built input simulator was used that generated single pulse signals at 50, 100, 200, and 500 microvolts. The subglottal pressure channel was calibrated using a U-tube manometer, so that pressures from zero to 24 cm of water could be recorded. Calibration of the air-flow channel was conducted using a direct connection between the pneumotachograph and a Brooks flow meter attached to an air supply cylinder. Air-flow rates were recorded in 100 cc/sec steps, from zero to 1000 cc/sec.

**Physiologic Calibration**

No intersubject muscle comparisons could be made from absolute EMG microvolt values, since the magnitude of the EMG signal is a function of the distance between the recording electrodes and their location within the muscle. These positions could not be replicated between subjects; therefore, a physiologic calibration measure was incorporated to normalize the data and permit intersubject comparisons. Immediately before the first experimental task, subjects performed the calibration maneuver of inspiring air, then phonating the vowel /a/ in diatonic steps from the middle to the top of their modal registers. At different points in the performance of this calibration task, high levels of activity were picked up from each of the four muscles. From the EMG data obtained during the calibration maneuver, a metric of muscle activity was established from 100, representing each muscle's maximum activity generated during the calibration maneuver, to zero, the average baseline noise level in that channel.

The VABS adaptive behavior domains have been normed on 3000 individuals from birth through 18 years, 11 months, including 200 subjects in each of 15 age groups. It has undergone extensive reliability assessments and analyses of validity, both of which suggest good performance on these indices (VABS Manual, 1984). In addition, Rescorla and Paul (1990) found that VABS scores in Expressive Communication correlated highly ($r = .85$) with LDS scores. Comparisons of VABS Expressive Communication scores with MLUs at this age level revealed a correlation of .78 for the normal group, suggesting the VABS Expressive score is closely related to direct measures of productive language.

From "Communication and Socialization Skills at Ages 2 and 3 in 'Late-Talking' Young Children," by R. Paul, S. S. Looney, and P. S. Dahm, 1991, *Journal of Speech and Hearing Research, 34,* p. 860. Copyright 1991 by the American Speech-Language-Hearing Association. Reprinted with permission.

***Standardized Instruments.*** Many research articles in communicative disorders report the use of standardized tests for the measurement of variables in their Method section. In some cases, the researcher provides citations to the test manual that contains data on standardization or reference to previous research on the reliability and validity of the instrument used. For example, in an article comparing communication skills of late-talking young children, the authors interviewed the primary caregivers of each child in the study using the Vineland Adaptive Behavior Scales (VABS). Excerpt 8.13 refers to the VABS Manual for normative data and reliability and validity estimates. Additionally, secondary research is reported that attests to the VABS's criterion validity.

Excerpt 8.14 is from the same article. In this example, the authors use previously reported research on the Language Development Survey instrument that establishes its reliability and validity. Use of the checklist format that was used in the study is justified on the basis of previous research.

The Language Development Survey (*LDS*) (Rescorla, 1989) is a checklist of 300 words common to children's early vocabularies. Parent report of expressive vocabulary employing a checklist format such as that used in this study has been shown by Dale, Reznick, Bates, and Morisset (1989) and Reznick and Goldsmith (1989) to be an excellent index of expressive vocabulary size. Rescorla (1989) has reported that the Language Development Survey, using the criteria described above, is highly reliable, valid, sensitive, and specific in identifying language delay, when compared to standardized language measures, in toddlers.

From "Communication and Socialization Skills at Ages 2 and 3 in 'Late-Talking' Young Children," by R. Paul, S. S. Looney, and P. S. Dahm, 1991, *Journal of Speech and Hearing Research, 34,* p. 859. Copyright 1991 by the American Speech-Language-Hearing Association. Reprinted with permission.

Excerpt 8.15 is taken from a study that examined treatment outcomes of persons with severe aphasia who were provided with therapy using a lexical-semantic approach to improve communication skills. In this particular study, various commercially available performance tests were the instruments used to assess therapeutic gains. This section provides adequate information for replication purposes. Additionally, the source of each test is identified by the authors.

Just because a standardized test is well known or widely used does not necessarily mean that its reliability and validity are adequate. McCauley and Swisher (1984) reviewed the psychometric characteristics of thirty language and articulation tests intended for use with preschool children. They applied ten criteria in evaluating the thirty test manuals to assess the documentation of the reliability and validity of the tests, as well as the documentation of other factors such as size and description of the normative samples, description of test procedure, qualifications of examiners, and statistical analysis of test scores of normative sample subgroups. Their analysis found many of the tests lacking in basic documentation of factors, such as reliability and validity, and concluded (McCauley & Swisher, 1984, p. 41):

> Most failures of tests to meet individual criteria occurred as a result of an absence of sought-after information rather than as a result of reported poor performance on them. The tests were not shown to be either well developed or poorly developed. This fact may falsely

---

### E X C E R P T  8.15

**Pre- and Posttreatment Assessment**
Selected subtests from the Psycholinguistic Assessments of Language Processing in Aphasia (PALPA; Kay, Lesser, & Coltheart, 1992) were administered to assess single-word processing abilities before and after treatment. The selected subtests from the PALPA allowed for examination of single-word reading (visual lexical decision and written word-to-picture matching), auditory comprehension (spoken word-to-picture matching); verbal repetition, written naming, and writing to dictation (see Table 2). In addition, the picture version of the Pyramids and Palm Trees Test (Howard & Patterson, 1992) was administered to examine the ability to make semantic associations. This test simply involves matching a target picture to a semantically related picture from a field of two. Peripheral writing processes were assessed using a case conversion task in which participants were asked to write uppercase letters when presented with lowercase letters, and vice versa. Additional information about graphomotor skills was obtained from each participant's performance on direct copying of written words.

Two measures of nonverbal cognitive skills were obtained for each participant: Coloured Progressive Matrices (CPM; Raven, Court, & Raven, 1990), which provides information about visual problem-solving ability, and the Tapping Forward Subtest from the Wechsler Memory Scale—Revised (WMS-R; Wechsler, 1987), which provides an indication of visual memory span. Finally, the oral language portions of the WAB (Kertesz, 1982) were readministered following treatment to examine whether any changes occurred in modalities other than writing (namely, auditory comprehension or verbal expression).

**Proverb Comprehension Task**

The PCT was designed to examine students' comprehension of 20 different proverbs and was a modification of a task that had been used in a previous study (Nippold et al., 1998). Each proverb consisted of a simple declarative sentence of 5 to 7 words that contained one main verb and two nouns. Half the proverbs were classified as "concrete" in that their nouns referred to tangible objects (e.g., "Two *captains* will sink a *ship*," "Scalded *cats* fear even cold *water*"); the other half were classified as "abstract" in that their nouns referred to intangible concepts (e.g., "*Envy* is destroyed by true *friendship*," "*Expectation* is better than *realization*"). The concreteness or abstractness of the nouns had been verified in a previously published study (see Nippold & Haq, 1996, for details concerning the procedures). All proverbs on the PCT were unfamiliar to adolescents and adults as determined in that same investigation (again, see Nippold & Haq, 1996, for details). Each proverb had achieved a mean familiarity rating of less than 2 on a 5-point Likert scale where 1 signified that the proverb had never been heard or read before and 5 signified that it had been heard or read many times before. The two sets of proverbs, concrete and abstract, did not differ in familiarity [$t(18) = .39$, $p > .05$]. Unfamiliar proverbs were used in order to examine students' ability to actively interpret the expressions as opposed to recalling their meanings from past learning experiences.

On the PCT, each proverb was presented in the context of a brief story. The stories focused on topics that would be of interest to American adolescents (e.g., sports, school, dating, automobiles, etc.). Each story consisted of four sentences, and in the final sentence, the proverb was spoken by an individual named in the story. The students read the stories silently and selected the best interpretation of the proverb from a set of four answer choices. Examples of problems from the task are shown in Table 1. The 20 problems were presented in random order.

**Task design.** In designing the PCT, care was taken to ensure that the correct answer to each problem would not be overly obvious. Hence, the four answer choices written to be similar in length, grammatical structure, and relatedness to the story, but only one choice reflected an accurate interpretation of the proverb. To verify that this was indeed the case, a preliminary version of the task was administered to a group of adults ($n = 5$) who were university faculty members or graduate students. This group had a mean age of 36 years (range = 23–52 years). Tested individually, the adults were asked to read each story silently and to circle the answer choice that best explained the meaning of the proverb. They also were asked to indicate if any problems were confusing or otherwise inappropriate. If two or more adults missed a problem or suggested that it could be improved in some way, the problem was revised. As a result of this process, minor revisions were made to five of the original problems.

After the PCT was revised, it was subjected to a validity measure. The purpose of this was to verify that it was indeed necessary for an individual to interpret the proverb in each problem in order to arrive at the correct solution, rather than being able to solve the problem simply by reading the story and the accompanying answer choices. Had the latter situation been possible, the task would have been one of reading comprehension rather than of proverb comprehension. To accomplish this, the PCT was administered to a group of adults ($n = 52$) who were university students (24 undergraduates, 27 graduates). This group had a mean age of 25 years (range = 20–47 years). They were tested in large-group fashion in classrooms at the university. Half of the adults received the task in its complete form and half received it in an incomplete form, with the two versions randomly assigned. For the incomplete form, the proverb was eliminated from each problem, and only the story context and answer choices remained. The adults were asked to read each problem silently and to select the answer choice that offered the best interpretation of the proverb (complete form) or the story (incomplete form).

The adults who took the complete form of the PCT obtained a mean raw score of 18.54 ($SD = 1.56$, range = 14–20, 93% correct). In contrast, those who took the incomplete form obtained a mean raw of 11.27 ($SD = 2.15$, range = 8–15, 56% correct). The maximum was 20 points on both forms. A one-way ANOVA yielded a statistically significant effect for group [$F(1, 50) = 195.62$, $p < .0001$], revealing that the complete form was easier than the incomplete form. This indicated that the proverbs were indeed necessary for university students to perform adequately on the task. Given that these students were, on average, 7 years older than the oldest adolescents participating in the main experiment, it seemed safe to assume that adolescents would be challenged to an even greater degree and that it would be particularly difficult for them to solve the problems simply by reading the stories and the answer choices.

*(continued)*

259

Given the results of this validity measure, no further revisions of the task were deemed necessary. The final version of the PCT was written at the fifth-grade reading level (Fry, 1968).

. . . . . . . . . . .

**Word Knowledge Task**
The WKT was a written multiple-choice task designed to examine students' knowledge of the 20 concrete and 20 abstract nouns contained in the proverbs on the PCT. Word frequency norms from Kucera and Francis (1967) were employed to determine how frequently each word occurred in a corpus of over one million words in printed American English. Frequency values for each noun in the concrete and abstract proverbs were noted, and the values for the two nouns from each proverb were averaged to produce a combined word frequency value for each proverb. For example, for the proverb, "Every horse thinks its own pack heaviest," the values of 117 (*horse*) and 25 (*pack*) were averaged to produce a combined word frequency value of 71. The combined values ranged from 14 to 233 ($M = 63.60$, $SD = 63.73$) for the pairs of concrete nouns and from 10 to 377 ($M = 63.60$, $SD = 113.06$) for the pairs of abstract nouns. A one-way ANOVA indicated that the two sets did not differ in combined word frequency values [$F(1, 18) = 0.00$, $p > .0001$]. This allowed for a clean comparison of abstract and concrete nouns, without the confound of any possible effects of word frequency.

**Task design.** Each noun on the WKT was followed by four possible definitions, one of which best explained its meaning. All answer choices were written in the Aristotelian style, a formal type of definition that includes both the superordinate category term and at least one major characteristic of the word. Aristotelian definitions were employed because this is a literate style that is concise and informative (Watson, 1995). *Webster's Third New International Dictionary* (1987) served as the primary reference for accurate definitions of the words. In designing the task, care was taken to ensure that the correct definition of each word would be applicable to the corresponding proverb in order to determine if students understood the relevant semantic features of the words. For example, the noun *expectation* can assume different meanings de-pending on the context, but on the WKT the correct choice was "a condition of believing something will happen," to be consistent with the proverb, "Expectation is better than realization." The foils for each noun also were written in the Aristotelian style and were similar to the correct choice in length and grammatical structure.

After the task was written, it was administered to a group of adults ($n = 5$) who were university faculty members or students. This group had a mean age of 35 years (range = 19–52 years). Each adult took the task individually and was asked to comment on any items that were confusing. Minor revisions were made in response to their feedback. Table 2 notes examples of problems on the WKT. The words were presented in random order.

. . . . . . . . . . .

**Test-Retest Reliability**
Given that the PCT and the WKT were experimental tools designed for the present investigation, it was important to obtain an estimate of stability on these two measures. To accomplish this, 16 students from the oldest group (7 boys, 9 girls) were randomly selected to take the PCT and the WKT a second time, 5 weeks after the first administration (with scores on the first administration of the PCT and WKT used for the main experiment). The procedures employed for administering the tasks the second time were identical to those that had been used the first time.

**Results**
Test-retest reliability measurements indicated adequate stability for the purposes of reporting group data (Salvia & Ysseldyke, 1981). On the PCT, the 16 students obtained a mean raw score of 15.69 ($SD = 2.63$, range = 10–19) on the first administration and a mean of 15.88 ($SD = 2.66$, range = 10–19) on the second. On the WKT, they obtained a mean raw score of 37.88 ($SD = 1.93$, range = 34–40) on the first administration and a mean of 37.63 ($SD = 1.78$, range = 33–40) on the second. Correlation coefficients between raw scores on the two administrations were statistically significant and strongly positive for the PCT ($r = .87$, $p < .0001$) and the WKT ($r = .72$, $p < .002$).

comfort some readers who may assume that, if collected, the data on their favorite test would be favorable. However, when given no information about a psychometric characteristic, the test user is realistically left to wonder whether or not a test is invalid and unreliable for his or her purposes. Stated differently, no news is bad news.

The lesson for the consumer of research is to look for evidence of reliability and validity of standardized tests used in research and not to assume that a test is reliable and valid just because it is popular.

***Nonstandardized Instruments.*** Many studies make behavioral measurements with instruments that have not been standardized or published commercially. It is important for researchers using such behavioral instruments to indicate the reliability and validity of measurements made with such materials. Excerpt 8.16 illustrates the use of two nonstandardized behavior instruments, the Proverb Comprehension Task and the Word Knowledge Task, for measuring proverb comprehension of adolescents. A careful rationale for the development of the tests precedes their actual description. Notice how the authors

- describe the test development
- establish content validity of both measurements (Task design)
- establish reliability of the measures using a test-retest procedure

Excerpt 8.17 is taken from an article that describes the development and administration of a test used to assess children's production and comprehension of derivational suffixes (morphemes). The production portion of the test required judgments of listeners. To establish the reliability of these judgments, the author calculated two different reliability

---

**EXCERPT 8.17**

## Reliability

Both intra- and interjudge reliability measures were calculated for scoring the children's responses on the production task. As scoring the comprehension task involved only circling responses, no reliability measures were obtained on this task. In order to calculate a measure of intrajudge reliability for production, 12 (20%) randomly selected response sheets were scored twice by the author. The first score was based on online judgments of the children's responses; the second was based on audiotapes of the production task. Across

subjects, a mean of 99.31% agreement was obtained. To calculate interjudge reliability, the same response sheets were scored from the audiotapes by a second, untrained judge. Across subjects, a mean of 87.84% agreement was obtained. Differences between the two judges' scores resulted mainly from like-sounding responses that were not easily differentiated from the audiotape (e.g., "BLID*ed*" versus "BLID*it*," "DAZER-*ous*" versus "DAZER*ess*") and were resolved after listening again to the audiotapes.

From: "Children's Comprehension and Production of Derivational Suffixes," by J. Windsor, 1994, *Journal of Speech and Hearing Research, 37,* p. 411. Copyright 1994 by the American Speech-Language-Hearing Association. Reprinted with permission.

Two male subjects were used, RS and VV, who were able to phonate /a/ at fundamental frequencies as low as 60 Hz. They produced a series of phonations at soft and loud efforts (and for one subject, RS, a medium effort as well). Their VRPs are plotted in Figure 1 for subject RS and in Figure 2 for subject VV. Cases where the clinician read the SPL meter are coded with a /C and cases where microphone re-cordings were made directly into the computer are coded with a /M.

A two-tailed *t*-test of the paired samples was calculated for each subject's effort level. There was no statistical significance at the 5% level at any effort level. Pearson correlation statistics revealed very high correlations between computer-calculated SPL levels and meter-read SPL levels ($r > 0.9$).

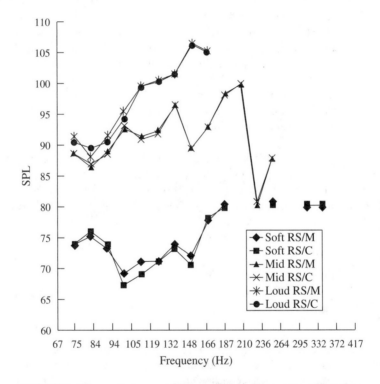

**FIGURE 1    Computer versus SPL meter low-frequency calibration, using human phonation (subject RS). /M is automated computer measurement; /C is clinician measurement using SPL meter.**

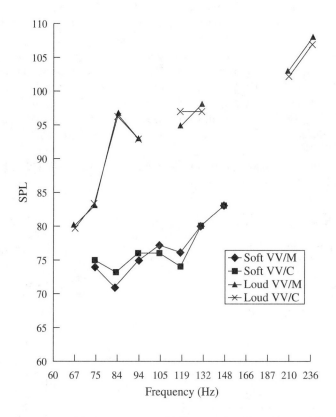

**FIGURE 2   Computer versus SPL meter low-frequency calibration, using human phonation (subject VV). /M is automated computer measurement; /C is clinician measurement using SPL meter.**

From "Comparison between Clinician-Assisted and Fully Automated Procedures for Obtaining Voice Range Profiles," by I. R. Tite, D. Wong, M. A. Milder, S. R. Hensley, and L. O. Ramig, 1995, *Journal of Speech and Hearing Research, 38,* pp. 528–529. Copyright 1995 by the American Speech-Language-Hearing Association. Reprinted with permission.

estimates that are commonly used in communicative disorders literature: intrajudge and interjudge agreements.

Excerpt 8.18 shows a portion of the Method section of a study designed to investigate two different procedures for obtaining a voice range profile (VRP) or, as it is sometimes called, a phonetogram. Standard procedures for obtaining a VRP require a clinician to measure vocal sound pressure levels (SPL) throughout the speaker's fundamental frequency range using a sound level meter. The authors developed a fully automated, computer-based method for obtaining a VRP that used a headmounted microphone directly inputting to a computer rather than the sound level meter used for measuring SPL. Excerpt 8.18 discusses the method used to establish the validity of the computer-based SPL measurements.

To summarize, the basic task in evaluating the adequacy of behavioral instruments in the Method section of a research article is to identify threats to internal validity posed by unreliable or invalid instruments. The task may be simplified if standardized tests are reported because reliability and validity information may be available for these instruments. The task may be more difficult if nonstandardized instruments are used. Here the consumer of research must evaluate the manner in which the instrument was constructed and used in order to determine its adequacy. The description of behavioral instruments used should be clear and comprehensive enough to allow the reader to determine whether the instruments can yield valid and reliable results.

## Other Measurement Considerations

In addition to concern about the calibration of hardware and the reliability and validity of behavioral instruments, several other miscellaneous aspects of the measurement process should be discussed in evaluating the materials described in the Method section. These include the appropriateness of measurements made, the role of the experimenter in making the measurements, the test environment, and the test instructions.

*Appropriateness of Measurements.*    Assuming that the instruments used provide reliable and valid measurements of the variables of interest, the reader should be concerned about the appropriateness of the measurements for fulfilling the specific purpose of the study. In other words, the Method section should be evaluated in light of the purpose and rationale spelled out in the introduction to the article. Excerpt 8.19 includes material from both the Introduction and Method sections of an article on the use of pretreatment measures to predict outcomes of stuttering therapy. The first part of the excerpt shows the author's development of a rationale for the use of measures of stuttering severity, personality, and attitudes toward stuttering as pretreatment predictors of therapy outcome in the introduction to the article. The second part of the excerpt is from the Method section and shows how the author selected instruments for measuring each of these three general variables.

Another aspect of appropriateness is whether the researcher has selected the *most* appropriate kind of measurement from among the various options available. Different kinds of measurements are more or less appropriate for answering different kinds of questions. Many different kinds of measurements may be applied in the study of a particular problem to investigate different aspects of the problem. In Excerpt 8.20 the authors discuss the advantages of using an analytic measurement procedure, the spatiotemporal index (STI), for studying underlying speech motor control processes. Specifically, they argue that measurements of movement trajectories over time are superior to the traditional measurements of movement trajectories taken at selected points in time.

The final concern deals with the appropriateness of the instrument for the participants studied. A test standardized on adults may be ill suited for use with children. A test developed on children from one socioeconomic group may not be valid when administered to children from a different socioeconomic level. Arndt (1977), for instance, criticized the

In all the recent studies, the only high correlation between a pretreatment measure and outcome is the finding by Gregory (1969) that pretreatment severity rating was positively correlated ($r = 0.78$) with change in severity rating from before to immediately after treatment. This result is not surprising, however, since severe stutterers enter therapy with higher levels on the severity scale and thus have a greater range to travel during treatment. Moreover, this correlation is dependent on when outcome is measured. When the nine-month posttreatment changes in severity were correlated with pretreatment severity, the correlation dropped from 0.78 to 0.48.

Changes in stuttering severity from immediately after to many months after treatment, such as shown by Gregory's subjects, are not unusual. Data are now available to support the long-standing clinical impression that many stutterers regress considerably after treatment (Ingham & Andrews, 1973; Perkins, 1973). In fact, those who improve most in treatment may show the greatest regression later (Prins, 1970). Thus, studies which measure stuttering immediately after treatment, such as those of Lanyon (1965, 1966), Prins (1968), and Gregory (1969), may not have assessed the most clinically important outcome of treatment. Long-term outcome is a more accurate assessment of how treatment has affected a stutterer. Of the studies cited here, only Perkins (1973) used longer term outcome in attempting to find predictors of treatment effects.

The lack of useful predictors of long-term outcome of stuttering treatment suggests a need for further investigation. Although personality measures by themselves have not been effective predictors, they might well be combined with overt measures of pretreatment stuttering for prognosis. Besides measures of personality and level of stuttering, some assessment of attitudes might also be helpful in forecasting outcome. This seems particularly possible in light of recent evidence that cognitive variables are important in determining overt behaviors (Kimble, 1973).

The present study was designed to evaluate a combination of pretreatment measures of stuttering, attitudes toward stuttering, and personality factors, as predictors of long-term outcome of treatment.

. . . . . . . . . . .

The basic design of the study was to obtain pretreatment measures from subjects in Group 1 and then evaluate their fluency a year after treatment. Following this, multiple regression analyses were carried out to determine the degree to which pretreatment measures predicted the subjects' outcomes. Equations derived from the regressions were then used to predict the outcomes for subjects in Group 2 on the basis of their pretreatment measures. Correlations between the predicted and actual outcomes for subjects in Group 2 provided cross-validation of the findings for subjects in Group 1.

**Pretreatment Measures**

The pretreatment data, which included measures of personality, attitudes about stuttering, and amount of stuttering, were obtained when subjects entered the hospital.

Personality was assessed by the extroversion and neuroticism scales of the Eysenck Personality Inventory (Eysenck & Eysenck, 1963). Neuroticism and extroversion have been shown previously to be associated with success and failure on stuttering therapy programs (Brandon & Harris, 1967).

Attitudes toward stuttering were measured by the short form of the Erickson Scale of Communication Attitudes (Erickson, 1969; Andrews & Cutler, 1974) and by an abbreviated version of the Stutterer's Self-Rating of Reactions to Speech Situations (Johnson, Darley, & Spriestersbach, 1963; Cutler, 1973). Only the avoidance and reaction responses of the Stutterer's Self-Rating form were used because these appeared to be most related to attitudes. Clinical experience suggested that those stutterers who scored high on the avoidance and reaction parts of this assessment were more likely to be emotionally affected by their stuttering, regardless of their actual level of stuttering.

In addition to the above assessments, amount of stuttering was measured when the subjects entered treatment. Stuttering was measured during conversational speech in percentage syllables stuttered (pre%SS) and syllables per minute (preSPM). These measures have been shown to correlate highly with listener judgments of severity and to be reliable (Young, 1961; Andrews & Ingham, 1971). Stuttering scores used for the multiple regression analyses were %SS and "alpha" score, a measure which combines frequency of stuttering and speech rate. The alpha score was developed because speech rate has been considered an important adjunct in the assessment of fluency (Ingham, 1972; Perkins, 1975).

### Posttreatment Measures

Twelve to 18 months after the subjects completed the three-week treatment program, they were contacted by a management consultant who was unknown to them, and a meeting was arranged in his office in a different part of the city from the place of treatment. A five-minute sample of conversational speech was recorded and later scored by the experimenter. Measures of out-come were percentage of syllables stuttered (post%SS), alpha score (postalpha), and percent change in frequency of stuttering (%change). This last score, %change, was calculated by the following formula:

$$\frac{\text{pre\%SS} - \text{post\%SS}}{\text{pre\%SS}}$$

The majority of studies of speech kinematic output have employed measures at single time points (e.g., Ackermann, Hertrich, & Scharf, 1995; Kent & Moll, 1975; Kuehn & Moll, 1976; Zimmermann 1980a, 1980b) to search for invariant aspects of motor output. In these studies, rather than considering the movement trajectory as a whole, specific points are selected to characterize temporal and spatial aspects of motion. In a smaller number of studies, movement trajectories for single speech movements were analyzed to determine if there is a common pattern in the velocity profile (Adams, Weismer, & Kent, 1993; Ostry et al., 1987; Shaiman, Adams, & Kimelman, 1997). Thus earlier work focused on single points in time to represent fundamental kinematic parameters of movement (e.g., displacement, peak velocity, and duration), and a few investigations attempted to determine if the bell-shaped velocity profile, prevalent in many limb movements, also characterized single speech movements. In 1995, we introduced an analysis that employed the entire lower lip movement trajectory for a six-syllable phrase (Smith et al., 1995). After linearly amplitude- and time-normalizing each multicomponent movement trajectory, an average trajectory for the set of trials within one condition was computed. Standard deviations of the set were computed as a function of normalized time. The average trajectory reveals aspects of the underlying *pattern* of movement, whereas the cumulative sum of the standard deviations (the spatiotemporal index, STI) indicates the degree to which the set of trajectories converges on a single underlying template, or the *stability* of the movement sequences.

Since publication of that initial work, we have used these analytic techniques to examine a number of issues in speech motor control, including changes in patterning and stability related to (a) alteration of a single phoneme (Goffman & Smith, 1999), (b) maturation over the childhood years (Smith & Goffman, 1998; Goffman & Smith, 1999) and aging (Wohlert & Smith, 1998), (c) increased linguistic processing demands (Maner, Smith, & Grayson, in press), and (d) stuttering (Kleinow & Smith, in press). We have found the technique of linear normalization followed by computation of a composite index of spatiotemporal stability to be useful in capturing aspects of speech movement control that were not accessible with analytic techniques employed in earlier studies of speech motor control processes. The STI is proposed not as a replacement for traditional measures but as an additional analysis that provides, in a single value, information about the performer's composite output. The index is composite in that it reflects variability attributable to spatial and temporal aspects of control; it is also composite in the sense that variability over the entire movement trajectory is integrated into a single value.

Northwestern Syntax Screening Test (NSST) on several grounds, one of which was that the test may have limited applicability because of the nature of the sample used for standardization, namely middle- to upper middle-class children from one geographical area. In addition, the norms do not extend beyond age six to eleven (Lee, 1977). Both the researcher *and* the clinician must recognize the limitations of the test and use the test accordingly. To reiterate, the point is simply that the critical reader of a research article must determine whether the instruments used are appropriate to the sample investigated.

### Experimenter Bias in Research Measurement.

Another measurement consideration is the problem of experimenter bias, or the Rosenthal Effect, in the making of research measurements (Rosenthal, 1966; Rosenthal & Rosnow, 1969). As discussed in Part I, the Rosenthal Effect can be of two types: (1) experimenter attributes that can interact with an independent variable to influence participants' behavior or (2) experimenter expectancies that bias an observer's measurement of the behavior of participants. The first type actually changes participants' behavior, whereas the second type does not change the participants' behavior but changes the way it is measured. It is important to note that expectancy effects have been identified in a wide variety of areas, including learning studies, reaction-time studies, psychophysical studies, and animal research (Christensen, 2004).[1]

There are several different methods that an experimenter can use to reduce or control experimenter bias. The critical reader of research should be alert to these methods and attempt to identify them *somewhere* in the Method section. One way of controlling experimenter expectancy is to use a blind technique whereby the experimenter knows the hypothesis but does not know in which treatment condition the participant is. Barber (1976) makes a distinction between an investigator (designs, supervises, analyzes, and reports the study) and an experimenter (tests participants and collects data) and urges, as another way of controlling experimenter bias, that the investigator and experimenter *not* be the same person. Still another method is to automate procedures and, where possible, to record and analyze responses by mechanical or electrical devices. Experimenter bias can also be reduced, according to Barber (1976), by the use of strict experimental protocols and by frequent checks to determine if the protocol, designed by the investigator, is being followed by the experimenter. To control for experimenter attributes, different experimenters, with different attributes, can be used in a given study. Or a study can be replicated using a different experimenter, especially if experimenter attributes are believed to have confounded the data of the first study.

Surprisingly little attention has been paid to the problem of experimenter bias in communicative disorders research. One study (Hipskind & Rintelmann, 1969) did investigate the effect of experimenter bias on pure-tone and speech audiometry and found no influence of attempts to bias experienced or inexperienced testers with true or false information about prior audiometric results. No systematic research has been published to identify areas of speech and hearing research that are more or less susceptible to experimenter bias, however. A few studies may be found in the communicative disorders literature that have introduced some control procedures to attempt to reduce or eliminate problems of experimenter bias.

---

[1]There is some controversy over the existence and magnitude of experimenter-expectancy effects. For a detailed discussion of this issue, the reader is urged to see Barber and Silver (1968) and Barber (1976).

The examples shown in the next three excerpts may help readers to identify how researchers have tried to reduce experimenter bias threats to internal validity. Excerpt 8.21 shows two portions of the Method section taken from a multidiscipline study of functional hearing loss, an area where tester or investigator bias has long intruded. The last sentence of the first part of the excerpt is the key one and indicates that of the several investigators involved in the evaluation of participants (including a psychologist and a psychiatrist), only the audiologists knew what participants were in the control (nonfunctional) group or in the experimental (functional) group. The other experimenters did "blind" evaluations. How did the audiologists control for their bias? Because they knew which participants were in which group, experimenter expectancy could not be totally controlled. However, expectancies with regard to certain aspects of the data were controlled, in part, as shown in Excerpt 8.21. Test-retest measurements constituted an important part of the audiologic evaluation and the RVA controlled, to some extent, experimenter bias from influencing the test-retest measurements. In addition, a rigid test protocol was followed by the entire research staff.

The next example, shown in Excerpt 8.22, is from a study of stuttering in monozygotic and dizygotic twins. Note that two diagnoses had to be made: one for zygosity and one for stuttering. In both instances "blind" judges were used who had no knowledge of the other diagnosis while making the diagnosis for which they were responsible. Also note the use of

---

**EXCERPT  8.21**

Methodological and procedural inadequacies of subject selection in previous studies have been fully discussed (Chaiklin & Ventry, 1963). In this study an effort was made to develop precise sampling procedures, objective general and medical eligibility criteria, and specific audiometric criteria.

A monthly schedule of appointments (covering a 25-mo period) was established specifying the random order in which subjects for the two major groups would be hospitalized for evaluation. The appointment designations referred not to individual subjects but only to the order in which subjects for the two groups would be evaluated. Twice as many functional as nonfunctional subjects were included in the schedule. The order in which subjects were scheduled was known only to the project audiologists. Thus all research evaluations, except the audiological evaluation, were performed without examiners knowing to which group a subject was assigned.

. . . . . . . . . . .

All inpatient examinations for both groups were conducted in the suite containing the I. A. C. 1201 booth. In addition, this suite contained a Grason-Stadler Békésy audiometer Model E 800, and an accessory Random Variable Attenuator (RVA) that allowed six different values of attenuation (0 to 25 dB in 5-dB steps) to be introduced into the earphone line before each repeat measurement.

The face of the RVA is blank but there is provision for quick read-out of the amount of attenuation introduced into the line. The six attenuation values are arranged randomly on the RVA's selector switch. Before a repeat measurement the experimenter rotated the dial to introduce one of the attenuation values. After the repeat measurement the RVA value was determined and then subtracted from the hearing level dial reading to produce the correct measurement figure. The use of the RVA made test–retest measurements relatively free from tester bias. The RVA was designed and constructed by Mr. L. G. Pew, Electro-Acoustic Co., San Carlos, California.

From "Introduction and Research Plan," by J. B. Chaiklin and I. M. Ventry, 1965, *Journal of Auditory Research, 5,* pp. 181–182 & 188. Reprinted by permission of the authors.

EXCERPT 8.22

**Diagnosis of Zygosity**

Twin pairs were classified as either monozygotic (MZ) or dizygotic (DZ), based on the following four criteria: (a) blood grouping for nine systems: ABO, Rhesus, MNSs, P, Lutheran, Kell, Lewis, Duffy, Kidd (Race & Sanger, 1968). Permission for blood tests was granted by 22 pairs, six of whose HLA tissue typing was also available; (b) total ridge counts and maximal palmar ATD angle (Holt, 1968); (c) cephalic index (Weiner & Lourie, 1969); and (d) height.

In seven pairs, DZ classification was certain because of the presence of at least one blood type difference. For each remaining pair, the probability of dizygosity was calculated, given the observed intrapair differences and similarities on the four criteria (Maynard-Smith & Penrose, 1955; Race & Sanger, 1968). The calculated probability of dizygosity was less than .05 in all but three of the pairs classified as MZ and greater than .95 in all but four of the pairs classified as DZ. Final classification was based on the probabilities examined in conjunction with intrapair differences in iris color, hair color and form, earlobe attachment, and finger ridge patterns. Zygosity was assessed by two judges, one of whom had direct contact with the twins, while the other made the diagnosis on the basis of profile and full-face photographs and all the relevant data. Thus, the second judge had no information about stuttering concordance. The zygosity classifications of the two judges agreed in every case.

**Speech Samples and Diagnosis of Stuttering**

For each subject, two 500-word speech samples were recorded: a monologue with standard instructions ("Tell the story of a book or film"); and a conversation with the experimenter on standardized topics. The recordings of the 60 subjects were arranged on audiotape in random order, and stuttering was diagnosed by a speech pathologist who had never met the twins and had no knowledge of twin pair membership or zygosity, thus ensuring independence of stuttering diagnosis and zygosity classification.

From "Concordance for Stuttering in Monozygotic and Dizygotic Twin Pairs," by P. M. Howie, 1981, *Journal of Speech and Hearing Research, 24,* p. 318. Copyright 1981 by the American Speech-Language-Hearing Association. Reprinted with permission.

---

two judges for zygosity, one of whom had contact with the twins and one of whom did not, in order to have no information available to that judge about stuttering concordance.

The third example illustrates the importance of eliminating experimenter bias during acoustic measurement procedures. Excerpt 8.23 is from a study that examined the effect of familiarity on word durations in children's speech over a four-week period. Novel words were introduced to the children in the "early" sessions of the experiment, and the durations of their productions were compared to the durations of the same words that were produced during the "late" sessions of the experiment. An acoustic analysis was used to obtain the word durations. In an effort to eliminate potential experimenter bias, the person conducting the acoustic measurements did not know whether the words came from the early or late experimental sessions.

The problem of experimenter bias is basically a problem in determining the *validity* of the measures made by an experimenter. The more free of bias an experimenter is, the more valid are the measurements made by that experimenter. An issue that is closely related to experimenter bias, then, is the *reliability* of the experimenter in making these measurements.

### EXCERPT 8.23

Word and vowel duration were measured using a Kay 5500 sonograph with a wideband setting (300 Hz). Measurements were made from a master tape constructed by dubbing from a mixed order of session tapes. The primary judge was not aware of the designation of tokens as early or late. Both the amplitude and the spectrographic display were used in determining the beginning and endpoints of measurement. Word onsets were measured from the first visible increase of amplitude from zero and the corresponding onset of voicing or the burst on the spectrographic display or from the onset of visible noise in the case of fricatives. Word offsets were measured at the end of closure or the release of final stops.

From "Effect of Familiarity on Word Duration in Children's Speech: A Preliminary Investigation," by R. G. Schwartz, 1995, *Journal of Speech and Hearing Research, 38,* p. 79. Copyright 1995 by the American Speech-Language-Hearing Association. Reprinted with permission.

Researchers can check an experimenter's reliability in one of two ways. *Inter-experimenter* reliability is the consistency among two or more experimenters in making a measurement. *Intra-experimenter* reliability is the consistency of one experimenter in remaking a particular measurement. Excerpt 8.24 describes two procedures designed to assess the inter-listener and intra-listener reliability of 20 untrained judges' rating of selected aspects of dysphonic voices. Notice that Chronbach's alpha coefficients were used to assess inter-listener reliability and Pearson correlation coefficients were used to assess intra-listener reliability.

### EXCERPT 8.24

**Reliability**

A conservative measure of the internal consistency of a group of items, Cronbach's alpha coefficient (Cronbach, 1970), was used to assess interlistener reliability. This measure involves measuring the correlation between each individual listener's rating for each stimulus with the group mean of all the other listeners. The value may vary between 0 and 1. For the present study, Cronbach's alpha was 0.95 for breathiness ratings, 0.96 for roughness ratings, and 0.98 for abnormality ratings, indicating adequate interlistener reliability for each of the three listening tasks.

Intralistener agreement was evaluated by computing Pearson correlation coefficients between ratings on first and second presentations of each randomized sample for each listener. Individual coefficients ranged between 0.26 and 0.95, with a mean coefficient of 0.69 for the breathiness ratings, 0.74 for the roughness ratings, and 0.81 for the abnormality ratings. These values were comparable to those obtained in other studies and undoubtedly reflect not only listener ability but the contextual effect of different random orders on first and second presentations. For example, Kreiman et al. (1992) obtained a range of .47–.71 for test-retest reliability.

From "Perception of Dysphonic Voice Quality by Naive Listeners," by V. I. Wolfe, D. P. Martin, and C. I. Palmer, 2000, *Journal of Speech, Language, and Hearing Research, 43,* p. 700. Copyright 2000 by the American Speech-Language-Hearing Association. Reprinted with permission.

One final example should suffice. Caruso and his colleagues investigated the effects of three different levels of cognitive stress on the articulatory coordination abilities of persons who stutter and fluent speakers. Articulation coordination abilities were assessed using a variety of acoustic measurements. Excerpt 8.25 shows that both intrajudge and interjudge acoustic measurement reliabilities are assessed. Reliability coefficients are not reported. Rather, the actual measurement-remeasurement differences are reported. As such, the consumer of research knows the exact magnitude of both the intrajudge and interjudge measurement differences and can, thus, interpret directly the measurement reliability. Conversely, intrajudge and interjudge reliability of the identification of disfluencies is reported using a well-established agreement index.

***Test Environment.***   The environment within which research measurements are made may be an important aspect of measurement in many studies. Test environment may affect both internal and external validity. With regard to internal validity, test environment should be specified if measurements can vary from one environment to another. Also, the constancy of environments across all measures should be ascertained if measurements need to be made in different environments. If environmental variables need to be controlled, sufficient detail should be provided to allow the environment to be replicated in future research. Excerpt 8.26 describes the recording environment used in a study to examine children's phoneme identification in naturally produced nonsense syllables under reverberation and noise conditions. The clear and complete details of the room would allow the recording environment to be replicated in future research.

---

**EXCERPT  8.25**

## Reliability

A random subset of approximately 10% of the speech samples from stutterers and nonstutterers under all three conditions were re-analyzed by the examiner and also analyzed by a second judge to assess reliability. The mean intrajudge measurement difference and range (shown in parentheses) for each acoustic measure were as follows: word duration—1.41 msec (0–29 msec); vowel duration—4.59 msec (0–26 msec); consonant-vowel transition extent—15.00 Hz (0–62 Hz); consonant-vowel transition duration—4.00 msec (0–22 msec); first formant center frequency—12.26 Hz (0–62 Hz); second formant center frequency—14.83 Hz (0–93 Hz). The mean interjudge measurement dif-

ference for each acoustic measure was as follows: word duration—1.88 msec (0–33 msec); vowel duration—3.11 msec (0–39 msec); consonant-vowel transition extent—13.74 Hz (0–93 Hz); consonant-vowel transition duration—4.67 msec (0–30 msec); first formant center frequency—4.63 Hz (0–62 Hz); second formant center frequency—18.59 Hz (0–93 Hz). Measures of agreement (Sander, 1961) were computed for the identification of dysfluencies (agreement/disagreement + agreement). Intrajudge agreement was 90% and interjudge agreement was 92% for judgments of dysfluency.

## EXCERPT 8.26

**Environment for Recording of Speech Stimuli**
The reverberant recordings were made in a 448 m³ (14 m × 10 m × 3.2 m) lecture hall. The lecture hall had a linoleum floor, cinder-block walls, and acoustic tiling on the ceiling. During the recording of the speech stimuli, the lecture hall was empty except for the experimenters, equipment, and desks in the room. The ambient noise levels were consistent (i.e., within 2 dB) throughout the lecture hall, which was verified by making sound-level measurements at the front, middle, and back of the lecture hall, using a precision modular sound level meter (Bruel & Kiaer, Model No. 2231S), its octave-band filter (Bruel & Kjaer, Model No. 1625), and sound measurement module (Bruel & Kjaer, Model No. BZ7109). The ambient noise level was 40 dB SPL with the following levels obtained through the octave-band filters: 37 dB with a 125-Hz center frequency (cf), 33 dB with 250-Hz cf, 24 dB with a 500-Hz cf, 9 dB with a 1000-Hz cf, 9 dB with a 2000-Hz cf, 10 dB with a 4000-Hz cf, and 11 dB with an 8000-Hz cf.

The precision modular sound level meter, octave-band filter, and reverberation module (Bruel & Kjaer, Model No. BZ7108) were used to determine the average reverberation time of the lecture hall. The sound level meter with reverberation module, positioned in one corner of the room, created frequency-specific pulses. These pulses were sent to an amplifier, and transduced through a loudspeaker into the lecture hall (Optimus, Model No. 650). The 0.25-inch condenser microphone of the sound level meter transduced the frequency-specific pulses as they reverberated throughout the lecture hall. The sound level meter and the reverberation module calculated the frequency-specific pulses' rate of decay. The estimated reverberation time of the lecture hall through the following octave band filters were 1.29 s with a 250-Hz cf, 1.24 s with a 500-Hz cf, 1.40 s with a 1000-Hz cf, 1.34 s with a 2000-Hz cf, 1.28 s with a 4000-Hz cf, and 1.04 s with an 8000-Hz cf. The average reverberation time of the lecture hall was calculated to be 1.3 s by averaging the individual reverberation times obtained through the 500-, 1000-, and 2000-Hz octave-filter bands. The nonreverberant recordings (one in quiet and one in noise) were made in an anechoic chamber. The instrumentation used for these recordings was identical to those used for the reverberant recordings described below.

From "Children's Phoneme Identification in Reverberation and Noise," by C. E. Johnson, 2000, *Journal of Speech, Language, and Hearing Research, 43,* p. 147. Copyright 2000 by the American Speech-Language-Hearing Association. Reprinted with permission.

Research studies in communicative disorders report the kind of test room used and the background noise levels because of the importance of maintaining an adequately low background noise level to eliminate masking in audiology studies and to yield noise-free recordings for speech analysis. Studies of lipreading often report the illumination characteristics of the room because of the importance of lighting for lipreading. Any time environmental variables can affect measurements taken in a given research study, they should be specified.

With respect to external validity, the environment may serve as a "reactive arrangement" so that generalizations may be limited to individuals functioning only in that particular environment. The question facing the critical reader is whether the test environment is so different from environments to which the reader wishes to generalize as to preclude such generalization. An adequate description of the environment in which testing or treatment takes place can help the reader judge the possible reactivity of the environment. It would be even better for the researcher to discuss the possible threat to external validity of reactive arrangements or to test the generality of results to other environments with a systematic replication.

Excerpt 8.27 is from a study that examines treatment selected outcomes of prolonged-speech therapy for stuttering. The first paragraph of Excerpt 8.27 was taken from the Introduction section of the article and the second paragraph was taken from the Discussion section. In the first paragraph, the authors discuss the importance of different times and settings regarding external validity issues to stuttering treatment research, and in the second paragraph they discuss certain external validity concerns regarding their results and the results of other treatment outcomes research.

In summary, the test environment is an important part of the Materials section of an article for two reasons. First, the environment may be important in determining the internal validity of the study by assessing the degree to which the environment affects the measurements

## EXCERPT 8.27

There was a resurgence of interest in legato speech in the 1960s with the influence of the behavioral paradigm on stuttering treatment. Goldiamond (1965) demonstrated in single case studies that stuttering could be eliminated at a very slow speech rate using DAF, and that the resulting stutter-free speech could be shaped toward more natural-sounding speech. Goldiamond called this legato speech pattern prolonged speech (PS). Since then, stuttering treatment centers in North America, Europe, and Australia have developed individual behavioral treatment programs using variants of Goldiamond's PS to control stuttering (see Ingham, 1984). Like the commercial stuttering schools, these programs are typically intensive in nature. Participants control their stuttering at a slow speech rate that is then systematically shaped toward more normal-sounding speech. This stutter-free speech is then used outside the clinic. Despite the similarity of some aspects of these programs to the stuttering schools, most treatment programs now incorporate procedures designed to assist clients to generalize and maintain the benefits of the clinic-based stage of treatment. And, as stated by Ingham (1993), behavioral stuttering treatments should include "the quantification of treatment targets, plus the systematic evaluation of relevant behaviors across clinically important settings and over clinically meaningful periods of time" (p. 135).

. . . . . . . . . . .

A final issue raised by the present results concerns external validity. It is likely that clinicians who specialize in the treatment of stuttering will achieve better results than generalist clinicians who attempt the same treatments (Onslow & Packman, in press). This is a particular concern with the present report because work has only just begun to search for the distinguishing features of the PS pattern used in this treatment (Onslow, van Doorn, & Newman, 1992; Packman, Onslow, & van Doorn, 1994). This lack of objective description of the PS pattern will not facilitate any efforts that generalist clinicians make to conduct the treatment reported here (Onslow & Ingham, 1989). This concern is bolstered by the results of attempts to conduct PS programs in settings other than the specialist facilities in which they were developed (Franck, 1980; Mallard & Kelley, 1982). Treatment outcomes in these reports give good reason to question the extent to which published outcome data pertain to other clinics (Onslow, 1996). It is necessary to explore this matter directly in an empirical fashion and if nonspecialist clinicians generally fail to achieve results equivalent to those achieved by specialist clinicians, then it is necessary to determine the training required to bridge that gap.

made. Second, the nature of the research environment is important in determining the external validity of the results with regard to generalizing to other settings.

*Instructions.*     The final consideration in this section has to do with instructions. Instructions to participants can be thought of as part of instrumentation because instructions are the tools by which the researcher attempts to elicit the desired response or behavior and to maintain a consistent response set across participants. Inadequate, inappropriate, poorly worded instructions thus pose an instrumentation threat to internal validity. In many circumstances, instructions are rather straightforward and, in fact, are specified in the administration of standardized test instruments. In other instances, the researcher may have to develop a set of instructions. The intent of the instructions, the thrust of the instructions, if not the instructions themselves, need to be specified by the researcher. The critical evaluator needs to ask two questions: (1) Are the instructions appropriate to the task at hand? and (2) Is sufficient detail provided to allow for replication or for clinical application?

Excerpt 8.28 is a fairly lengthy section that details the instructions given to two different groups of raters in a study that investigates the construct validity of interval rating procedures for judging speech naturalness from audiovisual recordings. The equal-appearing interval (EAI) rating procedure that is used replicated an earlier study by Martin and Haroldson (1992). As such, the instructions given to the EAI raters were taken verbatim from Martin and Haroldson's study. The instructions given to the raters using the direct magnitude estimation (DME) procedures were similar to those used in a study by Metz, Schiavetti, and Sacco (1990) that evaluated the construct validity of interval scaling procedures for judging speech naturalness from audio recordings.

The example shown in Excerpt 8.29 is from a study of the effects of time-interval judgment training on stuttering measurement. The authors describe their instructions in detail and provide the text of written instructions that were provided to the participants making judgments of stuttering. The instructions are presented in sufficient detail for another investigator to replicate the procedure.

In conclusion, the major emphasis of this section on materials has been to identify instrumentation threats to internal validity. Inadequate instrumentation and inadequate materials can vitiate the value of an elegant design, but, to reiterate, a poor problem cannot be salvaged with even the most sophisticated instrumental array. Thus, the need for the enlightened consumer of research to put the Materials section of the research article into proper perspective. The Materials section is important but constitutes only one portion of the research article.

# Procedures

The Procedure section of the research article usually concludes the Method section. It is here that the researcher describes what is done to the participants with the materials. It must be recognized that for convenience and simplicity, we have divided the present chapter into the three *typical* parts of a Method section. Reading just a few issues of selected journals will

**EXCERPT 8.28**

### Equal-Appearing Interval (EAI) Rating

Twenty raters were assigned randomly to use the EAI rating procedure. No more than five raters participated in a given session. In general, the rating procedures and instructions were the same as those employed in the Martin et al. (1984) and the Martin and Haroldson (1992) studies. Raters were seated in front of a video monitor and given a packet of 20 numbered 9-point naturalness scales on which 1 was labeled "highly natural" and 9 was labeled "highly unnatural." Raters were asked to read the following instructions:

> We are studying what makes speech sound natural or unnatural. You will see and hear a number of short speech samples. The samples will be separated by a few seconds of silence. Each sample will be introduced by the sample number. Your task is to rate the naturalness of each speech sample.
>
> If the speech sample sounds highly natural to you, circle the 1 on the scale. If the speech sample sounds highly unnatural, circle the 9 on the scale. If the sample sounds somewhere between highly natural and highly unnatural, circle the appropriate number on the scale. Do not hesitate to use the ends of the scale (1 or 9) when appropriate.
>
> "Naturalness" will not be defined for you. Make your ratings based on how natural or unnatural the speech sounds to you.

### Direct Magnitude Estimation (DME)

The other 20 raters participated in the DME rating procedure. Again, no more than five raters participated in a session. The DME rating procedures and instructions were similar to those used with DME raters in the Metz et al. (1990) experiment. Raters were seated in front of a video monitor and given a protocol sheet on which were listed samples 1 through 20 with a blank space beside each number. Raters were asked to read the following instructions:

> We are studying what makes speech sound natural or unnatural. You will see and hear a number of short speech samples.

> The samples will be separated by a few seconds of silence. Each sample will be introduced by the sample number. Your task is to rate the naturalness of each speech sample.
>
> When you have seen and heard the first sample, give its naturalness a number—any number you think is appropriate. You will then be presented the second sample to rate. If the second sample sounds more natural than the first sample, give it a lower number. If the second sample sounds more unnatural than the first sample, give it a higher number. Try to make the ratio between the two numbers correspond to the ratio of the naturalness between the two samples. The higher the number, the more unnatural the second sample sounds relative to the first sample; the lower the number, the more natural the second sample sounds relative to the first sample. If you assigned the first sample the number "10," and the second sample sounds twice as natural, give the second sample a rating of "5." If the third sample sounds twice as unnatural as the first sample, give the third sample a rating of "20."
>
> "Naturalness" will not be defined for you. Make your ratings based on how natural or unnatural the speech sounds to you.

We followed the suggestions of Engen (1971) for the use of DME with no standard/modulus so that raters were free to rate the first speaker with any number they chose and to scale the speech naturalness of all subsequent speakers with numbers proportional to the perceived naturalness or unnaturalness of each speaker. Further details on the use of direct magnitude estimation with and without standard/modulus can be found in Engen (1971); Lane, Catania, and Stevens (1961); and Schiavetti, Sacco, Metz, and Sitler (1983). In a manner similar to that described by Metz et al. (1990), both the DME and EAI raters practiced their respective rating procedures by scaling the relative lengths of a number of horizontal lines.

## EXCERPT  8.29

At the beginning of each session, the judge was seated in a quiet room, before a table, facing an 18-inch color television video monitor. On the table were printed instructions, the remote control for the volume of the video monitor, and a computer mouse. The mouse was connected to a Pentium series computer which controlled the playback from the laser videodisk player and recorded the subject's button-press judgments about the speech samples.

At the beginning of each assessment session, judges were instructed that they would watch and listen repeatedly to nine 2-min speech samples, one from each of 9 different persons who stutter. They were instructed to press either button on the computer mouse to mark the location and duration of individual stuttering events:

> If, in your judgment, the speaker has a stuttering, then press the mouse button as soon as that stutter begins and hold it down throughout the duration of that stutter. You should try to hold the button down throughout each stuttering and then release it as soon as the stutter ends. Of course, sometimes an occasion of stuttering might be so brief that you will

only have time to press the button down and release it almost immediately, which is fine.

Stuttering was not defined for the judges, but they were instructed that not all disruptions or interruptions in speech are stutterings and that normal or acceptable disruptions were not to be counted as stuttering.

After the experimenter was satisfied that the judge understood these instructions, the judge was given the opportunity to practice the task up to four times with one randomly selected speaker. When the judge reported feeling comfortable with the task, the assessment task itself was begun, and the judge then watched and judged all nine 2-min speech samples.

During each assessment session the judge completed the entire assessment task (i.e., identifying the location and duration of stuttering in nine 2-min samples) three times, with a 5-min break between repetitions. The three assessment sessions combined, therefore, included nine repetitions of the entire assessment task, referred to below as the nine trials of this study. Sample order was randomized by the SMAAT software for each judge, for each trial.

From "Effects of Time-Interval Judgment Training on Real-Time Measurement of Stuttering," by A. K. Cordes and R. J. Ingham, 1999, *Journal of Speech, Language, and Hearing Research, 42,* p. 866. Copyright 1999 by the American Speech-Language-Hearing Association. Reprinted with permission.

---

quickly reveal that there may be considerable overlap among parts; some procedures may be described in the Materials section, subject-selection procedures might be handled in the Procedures section, and so on. Despite the variety of formats used, the critical reader's responsibility is to identify how the researcher has dealt with the threats to internal and external validity detailed in Part I. Because the preceding sections of this chapter have dealt primarily with the threats to validity posed by subject-selection procedures and instrumentation (materials), this section will deal with the remaining threats to validity.

It should be apparent by now that principal ways to reduce threats to validity are through the use of an appropriate experimental design or through the use of special precautions when employing a descriptive design. For example, the one-group pretest–posttest design is far weaker than the randomized pretest–posttest control-group design. A between-subjects design with faulty subject-selection criteria is far less adequate than a within-subjects design where appropriate attention has been given to counterbalancing or randomizing test conditions. However, a within-subjects design can be faulted if, for example, randomization or counterbalancing has not been used. The point, then is for the critical evaluator to identify the type of design employed by the researcher and to assess the adequacy of the design, keeping in mind the advantages and disadvantages of the various designs described in Part I. To help develop this critical skill, the remainder of the chapter includes some rather lengthy excerpts from the research literature. Our accompanying narrative shows how the reader can identify the type of research design used and how the researcher has dealt with threats to validity.

## Within-Subjects Experimental Design

Excerpt 8.30 is taken from the Method section of a study by Conture on the effects of loudness and frequency spectrum (two independent variables) on stuttering frequency, reading rate, and vocal level (three dependent variables). The design is within-subjects because all the participants were exposed to all levels of the independent variables and there was only

### EXCERPT 8.30

#### Subjects
The subjects were nine adult male stutterers who were receiving speech therapy at the Wendell Johnson Speech and Hearing Center at the University of Iowa. All nine subjects had hearing threshold levels of better than 15 dB (re ANSI, 1969) at 500, 1000, and 2000 Hz.

#### Stimulus Material
The stimulus material consisted of five prose readings taken from the same level of the *Reader's Digest Reading Skill Builder* series (ninth-grade level, Part 3). A random sample of 100 words was taken from each of the five readings and rated according to Brown's (1945) "word weights." The similarity of the average word weight among the five readings indicated that the five passages were suitably equated with regard to Brown's four linguistic factors (Conture, 1972).

#### Experimental Conditions
Each subject read during four sessions separated by at least 24 hours. There were two conditions in three sessions and one condition in the fourth. At the beginning of the first session, and at the start of every subsequent session, each subject performed a fixed frequency

(4000 Hz) Bekesy tracing for two minutes in each ear. The middle one-minute segment from each ear was used to determine whether a subject's exposure to noise from the previous session might have produced a temporary threshold shift (TTS). If a shift of 5 dB or greater was noted on this task at the beginning of any session, then the subject was asked to leave and to come back another day.

After the TTS check, the subject began to read aloud continuously from the prepared readings while two conditions were presented. The sequence of presentation of the six experimental conditions and one control condition was as follows: the subject read for five minutes (adjustment period), then for another five minutes (preexposure period), followed by a 10-minute rest period. The same sequence was presented after the rest period, except that a different condition was presented during the exposure period. Sessions 2, 3, and 4 were identical to Session 1 except for the type of experimental or control conditions presented during the exposure period. The sequence of conditions and the particular passage that was read during a condition were all determined by chance through the use of a table of random numbers.

one group of participants. Each individual participated in all four sessions in this experiment, and several important design strategies were used to reduce threats to internal validity. Note, first, that a measure of TTS was used each day to ensure that no threshold shifts would contaminate the data with a carry-over effect from the previous day's noise exposure. Also note that rest periods were used to reduce short-term maturation (fatigue), and an adjustment period was used before the preexposure period to stabilize participants' speaking behavior. The sequences of conditions and passages read during each condition were both randomized to control for sequencing effects. This within-subjects experimental design, then, shows several concerted attempts to minimize threats to internal validity.

## Between-Subjects Experimental Design

Excerpt 8.31 was taken from a study of the efficacy of group treatment in adults with chronic aphasia. Twenty-eight participants with aphasia were randomly assigned to one of two treatment groups: (a) immediate treatment (IT) or (b) deferred treatment (DT). Participants in the IT group received immediate assessment and treatment, whereas participants in the DT group received immediate assessment but deferred treatment. The DT group received treatment following completion of the IT group's four-month treatment program. The reader should recognize this design as a randomized pretest–posttest control group design, where the DT group serves as the control group. At first glance, this design can be diagramed as follows, maintaining the notation system described in Part I:

$$R \; O_1 \; X_{IT} \; O_2$$

$$R \; O_3 \; X_{DT} \; O_4$$

Here $X_{IT}$ represents immediate treatment and $X_{DT}$ represents delayed treatment, or the control group. The overall design of the study, however, avoids the ethical concerns of denying treatment to a group of people by administering treatment at a later date during the conduct of the investigation.

Factors that can jeopardize internal validity are well controlled in the design discussed in Excerpt 8.31 because of the random assignment of participants to the two treatment conditions. The general equality of the two groups of participants is shown in Tables 1 and 2.

The example of a between-subjects design shown in Excerpt 8.31 is from an experimental investigation of the effects of treatment that involved a rather long-term study of the participants. Most short-term experiments, like the one by Conture of the effects of noise on stuttering shown in Excerpt 8.30, use within-subjects designs because allowing participants to act as their own controls by participating in all experimental conditions eliminates problems of differential subject-selection. The example shown in Excerpt 8.32 illustrates a short-term experiment on the effects of practice and instructions on lingual vibrotactile thresholds using a between-subjects design. A between-subjects design was used because of the probability that a permanent carry-over effect could not be eliminated with counterbalancing or randomization of the conditions presented to the participants. Note the authors' rationale for using the between-subjects design instead of counterbalancing conditions because participants could not become naive again after having been exposed to the instructions. Thus, a within-subjects design would be exposed to the danger of carryover of the effect of one instruction set onto another subsequent instruction set in later conditions.

E X C E R P T  **8.31**

## Method

### Participants

All of the aphasic clients who participated in the study were chronically aphasic (more than 6 months post-onset) and had completed individual speech-language treatment that was available to them through their insurance coverage. All aphasic individuals had sustained a single, left-hemisphere cerebrovascular accident that was documented in the medical record; were 80 years of age or younger; had no major medical complications or history of alcoholism; were within and/or inclusive of the 10th and 90th overall percentile on the SPICA at entry; were premorbidly literate in English; and agreed to participate in the study.

Ninety individuals responded to our call for research participants and were screened on the telephone for the basic selection criteria. From this telephone screening, 45 people were asked to complete testing on our dependent measures. Following receipt of complete medical records, individuals with multiple brain lesions or diagnosed alcoholism were excluded. The remaining 28 participants meeting subject selection criteria were enrolled in the treatment study.

### Design

Participants were randomly assigned to one of two conditions. Immediate treatment (IT) participants received immediate assessment and immediate communication treatment. Deferred treatment (DT) participants received immediate assessment but deferred communication treatment. The DT group began their treatment following the completion of the IT groups' 4-month treatment trial. In order to control for the effect of social contact and to ensure that none of the participants was isolated at home during the DT interval, DT participants attended 3 or more hours weekly of social group activities of their choice, such as movement classes, creative/performance arts groups, church activities, and support groups. DT participants were reassessed on all measures following this "socialization" period, just before their deferred treatment.

Once randomly assigned to IT or DT groups, participants were assigned to either mild-moderate or moderate-severe aphasia groups based on their initial aphasia severity as measured by the SPICA overall percentile. Participants with moderate aphasia (defined as a SPICA overall percentile between 50 and 65) could be assigned to either the mild-moderate or moderate-severe groups. Therefore, an attempt was made to balance the participant groups for age, education level, and time post-onset. The result was four groups of 7 individuals each (two groups immediate and two groups deferred). Individuals with mild or moderate aphasia formed both an IT and DT group, and individuals with moderate or severe aphasia made up the remaining two groups. Five individuals dropped out of the study before they completed their treatment: 1 in the IT mild-moderate group because of transportation difficulties; 1 in the DT mild-moderate group with medical complications; and 3 because of time constraints (1 in the IT mild-moderate group, 1 in the DT mild-moderate group, and 1 in the DT moderate-severe group). In addition, 1 participant in the DT group enrolled following initial testing but before DT began. A total of 24 participants successfully completed the 4-month treatment trial. Participants in the IT and DT groups did not differ significantly in age, education, months post-onset, or SPICA overall percentile [all $p > .20$, all $t(11) \leq 1.27$]. See Table 1 and Table 2 for individual participant information and descriptive data on the IT and DT groups.

*(continued)*

**TABLE 1**   Participant characteristics including age, sex, months post-onset (MPO), WAB aphasia classification, SPICA overall percentile, education level (in years), WAB AQ, and CADL scores at intake in the mild-moderate and moderate-severe immediate- and deferred-treatment groups

| Sex | Classification | Age | MPO | SPICA% | Education | WAB AQ | CADL |
|---|---|---|---|---|---|---|---|
| | | | *Immediate (n = 12)* | | | | |
| Mild-Moderate | | | | | | | |
| M | Broca's | 46 | 7 | 57 | 16 | 61.5 | 120 |
| M | Anomic | 67 | 103 | 80 | 20 | 88 | 125 |
| M | Unclassified | 58 | 77 | 78 | 15 | 85.9 | 134 |
| F | Anomic | 38 | 17 | 76 | 14 | 80.8 | 131 |
| F | Anomic | 72 | 13 | 90 | 16 | 92.9 | 136 |
| *M (SD)* | | 56.2 (14.2) | 43.4 (43.7) | 76.2 (12.0) | 16.2 (2.3) | 81.8 (12.2) | 129.2 (6.6) |
| Moderate-Severe | | | | | | | |
| F | Trans. Motor | 79 | 36 | 35 | 16 | 61.4 | 96 |
| F | Broca's | 58 | 33 | 35 | 15 | 13.1 | 57 |
| M | Trans. Motor | 60 | 21 | 58 | 14 | 72.8 | 116 |
| M | Broca's | 49 | 29 | 30 | 12 | 18.9 | 106 |
| F | Broca's | 51 | 12 | 30 | 16 | 24.2 | 64 |
| M | Broca's | 63 | 16 | 61 | 12 | 45.9 | 124 |
| M | Conduction | 58 | 26 | 47 | 14 | 55.9 | 98 |
| *M (SD)* | | 59.7 (9.8) | 24.7 (8.8) | 42.3 (13.1) | 14.1 (1.7) | 41.7 (23.2) | 94.4 (25.2) |
| | | | *Deferred (n = 12)* | | | | |
| Mild-Moderate | | | | | | | |
| M | Anomic | 52 | 336 | 60 | 16 | 80.2 | 113 |
| F | Anomic | 80 | 36 | 64 | 11 | 75.1 | 102 |
| F | Unclassified | 70 | 43 | 78 | 16 | 94.3 | 129 |
| F | Anomic | 58 | 23 | 67 | 12 | 87.7 | 130 |
| F | Anomic | 71 | 14 | 88 | 16 | 92.8 | 131 |
| M* | Anomic | 52 | 134 | 76 | 20 | 76.4 | 129 |
| *M (SD)* | | 63.8 (11.5) | 97.7 (124.5) | 72.2 (10.4) | 15.2 (3.3) | 84.4 (8.3) | 122.3 (12.0) |
| Moderate-Severe | | | | | | | |
| M | Broca's | 47 | 10 | 42 | 18 | 57.4 | 121 |
| M | Conduction | 48 | 19 | 54 | 14 | 67.3 | 107 |
| F | Broca's | 65 | 59 | 23 | 18 | 20.7 | 70 |
| F | Broca's | 71 | 137 | 50 | 18 | 63.5 | 104 |
| M | Conduction | 59 | 42 | 46 | 16 | 65.3 | 114 |
| M | Conduction | 55 | 7 | 54 | 16 | 54.4 | 123 |
| *M (SD)* | | 57.5 (9.5) | 45.7 (49.0) | 44.8 (11.7) | 16.7 (1.6) | 54.8 (17.4) | 106.5 (19.4) |

*Subject enrolled late into study; information is from pretreatment testing session.

**TABLE 2  Descriptive data for participants at intake in the immediate- and deferred-treatment groups**

| | Immediate treatment (n = 12) | | | Deferred treatment (n = 12) | | |
|---|---|---|---|---|---|---|
| | *M* | *SD* | *Range* | *M* | *SD* | *Range* |
| Age (years) | 58.3 | 11.4 | 38–79 | 60.7 | 10.6 | 47–80 |
| Education (years) | 15 | 2.1 | 12–20 | 15.9 | 2.6 | 11–20 |
| Months post-onset | 32.5 | 28.7 | 7–103 | 71.7 | 94.2 | 7–336 |
| SPICA % | 56.4 | 21.2 | 30–90 | 58.5 | 17.7 | 23–88 |

From "The Efficacy of Group Communication Treatment in Adults with Chronic Aphasia," by R. J. Elman and E. Bernstein-Ellis, 1999, *Journal of Speech, Language, and Hearing Research, 42,* pp. 413–414. Copyright 1999 by the American Speech-Language-Hearing Association. Reprinted with permission.

EXCERPT  8.32

## Procedure

The 30 subjects were divided randomly into three groups of 10 each. Each group was assigned to a condition involving a different instructional set for obtaining their lingual vibrotactile thresholds. A counterbalancing design, although desirable, could not be employed since naiveté was a prerequisite for each subject to be used in the study. Once a subject received an instructional set, that subject would no longer be naive; therefore, it would be difficult to determine whether the instructions previously given interacted with a new instructional set. The instructional sets were as follows:

*Condition 1—Strict instructions.* Subjects were given simple but relatively strict instructions to raise their hands as soon as they felt the stimulus on their tongue.

*Condition 2—Comprehensive instructions.* Subjects were given more comprehensive instructions in which the idea of threshold was stressed. This set of instructions told the subjects to raise their hands as soon as they felt the stimulus, no matter how faint it appeared to be. They were encouraged to respond even if they only thought the stimulus was present.

*Condition 3—Comprehensive instructions with examiner reinforcement.* Subjects were given the same instructions as in the second condition, but appropriate examiner feedback was supplied regarding the accu-

racy of their responses. If their responses did not conform to what we have experienced as fitting within the range of previously generated normative threshold data, appropriate feedback was provided. The following subject responses and examiner feedback occurred during this experimental condition:

*Subject Responses*

1. False alarm.
2. Should be responding earlier.
3. Appropriate response.

*Examiner Feedback*

1. Make sure you are feeling the tickling before you raise your hand.
2. You probably feel the stimulus before you raise your hand.
3. You are responding right about where I would expect you to.

Examiner feedback used in Condition 3 was based on normative lingual vibrotactile threshold data obtained from 110 normal young adults (Telage, Fucci, & Arnst, 1972).

From "Effects of Practice and Instructional Set on the Measurement of Lingual Vibrotactile Thresholds," by D. Fucci, L. H. Small, and L. Petrosino, 1983, *Journal of Speech and Hearing Research, 26,* p. 290. Copyright 1983 by the American Speech-Language-Hearing Association. Reprinted with permission.

Note also that the authors dealt with the problem of differential subject-selection by randomly assigning participants to one of the three conditions.

## Mixed (Between-Subjects and Within-Subjects) Design

The example shown in Excerpt 8.33 illustrates a mixed design in which one independent variable is studied with a between-subjects design and another independent variable is studied with a within-subjects design. This investigation examines differences and relationships among phonological awareness, morphological awareness, and reading abilities in children with and without language disorders. Both the between-subjects and within-subjects components of the study are clearly seen in the Results section of the article. In the between-subjects component, children with language delays (LD) are compared with gender matched children of the same language age (LA) and chronological age (CA). In the within-subjects component, all participants' scores on a variety of measures (PPVT, TOLD, and so on) were used as variables to predict reading scores.

### EXCERPT 8.33

### Results

*Base Production Task*

**Foil Performance**

All but one child demonstrated a clear understanding of the task requirements. This CA child and her LA and LD matches were excluded from analyses. There was essentially no difference in accuracy between Set A and Set B, and results for the two stimulus sets were combined. Although the CA group was reasonably accurate in their foil performance ($M = 88.2\%$), the LA group and especially the LD group showed fairly low accuracy in correctly stating that the foils did not contain a smaller, related word ($M = 76.9\%$ and $58.9\%$, respectively). For instance, many children incorrectly identified *pan* as a smaller, related word in *pansy*. All CA children and 19 of the 22 LA children showed above 50% accuracy with both pseudo-base and no-base foils. Only 13 children with LD showed above 50% accuracy with the foils. Thus, although children with LD could identify smaller words in derivatives, many had minimal morphological knowledge of the semantic relation linking bases and derivatives.

**Differences Among Groups and Derivatives**

Each group's accuracy was substantially affected by phonological opacity (Figure 1). A two-way ANOVA (group × opacity) was used to compare total number of accurate responses. The ANOVA indicated a signifi-

cant group effect [$F(2, 63) = 9.80$, $p < .0001$], a significant opacity effect [$F(1, 63) = 395.24$, $p < .0001$], and a significant group × opacity interaction effect [$F(2, 63) = 18.55$, $p < .0001$]. A Tukey test indicated that the interaction effect was due to the CA group's outperforming the LD group for opaque derivatives ($MSE = 10.04$, 63 *df*, $p < .0001$). The difference among groups for transparent derivatives was not significant.

*Suffix Identification Task*

**Foil Performance**

All children showed a clear understanding of the task and stated that they knew what a suffix was. There was no difference in accuracy between Set A and Set B, and results for the two stimulus sets were combined. As for the Base Production task, foil accuracy was higher for the CA group ($M = 69.8\%$) than for the LA ($M = 52.7\%$) and LD groups ($M = 34.8\%$). Fifteen CA children, 10 LA children, and only 5 children with LD showed above 50% foil accuracy.

**Differences Among Groups and Derivatives**

As was true for the Base Production task, phonological opacity markedly affected children's ability to identify suffixes correctly (Figure 2). The CA group performed a little below the level adults obtained for transparent derivatives in the pilot testing, achieving 86% accuracy for these stimuli. Because there were three possible responses in the Suffix Identification task, children could

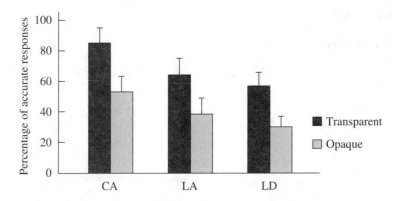

**FIGURE 1** **Percentage accuracy for the Base Production task. Error bars indicate 1 *SD* above the mean.**

achieve 33% accuracy by guessing alone. Thus, both the LA and LD groups' accuracy with opaque derivatives (39% and 31%, respectively) approximated the level of accuracy due to chance.

A two-way ANOVA showed a significant group effect [$F(2, 66) = 14.73, p < .0001$], a significant opacity effect [$F(1, 66) = 134.30, p < .0001$], and a nonsignificant group × opacity interaction effect [$F(2, 66) = 1.16, p = .32$]. A Tukey Test ($MSE = 13.66, 66\ df, p = 0.3$) indicated that the group effect was due to the CA group's outperforming the LA and LD groups.

**Contributions to Variance in Reading Scores**

Stepwise regression analyses (from Systat, version 6.0) were used to determine the relation between perfor-

mance on the Base Production and Suffix Identification tasks and reading scores. One regression predicted scores on the Word Identification (WI) subtest of the WRMT; another regression predicted scores on the Passage Comprehension (PC) subtest. As is conventional age (in months) and receptive vocabulary (PPVT score) were entered as control variables into the regressions. To reduce the number of predictor variables and ensure a reliable prediction equation (Stevens, 1996), scores from the Base Production and Suffix Identification tasks were added to create one transparent and one opaque predictor variable. All scores were standardized as $z$ scores before entering them into the regressions.

Importantly, one criterion for inclusion in the LD group was the presence of a spoken language

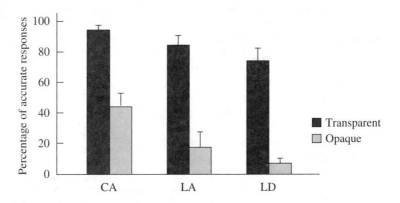

**FIGURE 2** **Percentage accuracy for the Suffix Identification task. Error bars indicate 1 *SD* above the mean.**

*(continued)*

**EXCERPT  8.33  Continued**

**TABLE 1  Correlations between variables**

|         | Age | PPVT  | TOLD  | Transp. | Opaque | WI     | PC     |
|---------|-----|-------|-------|---------|--------|--------|--------|
| Age     | —   | −.270 | −.384 | .095    | .251   | −.409  | −.352  |
| PPVT    |     | —     | .784* | .471*   | .536*  | .603*  | .723*  |
| TOLD    |     |       | —     | .441*   | .541*  | .792*  | .872*  |
| Transp. |     |       |       | —       | .564*  | .449*  | .428*  |
| Opaque  |     |       |       |         | —      | .594*  | .639*  |
| WI      |     |       |       |         |        | —      | .847*  |
| PC      |     |       |       |         |        |        | —      |
| **Partial correlations, controlling for age, PPVT, and TOLD** | | | | | | | |
| Transp. |     |       |       | —       | .281   | .273   | .089   |
| Opaque  |     |       |       |         | —      | .567*  | .519*  |
| WI      |     |       |       |         |        | —      | .537*  |
| PC      |     |       |       |         |        |        | —      |

*Note.* PPVT = Peabody Picture Vocabulary Test. TOLD = Test of Language Development. Transp. = Transparent score. Opaque = Opaque score. WI = World Identification subtest of the Woodcock Reading Mastery Tests. PC = Passage Comprehension subtest of the Woodcock Reading Mastery Tests. In the WI subtest, children see a written word in isolation and then say the word. In the PC subtest, children silently read a short passage and then identify the key word that is missing from the passage.

*$p < .01$

impairment as well as a reading impairment. Conversely, children in the CA and LA groups had neither a spoken language nor reading impairment. Thus, it was anticipated that expressive/receptive language skill (TOLD Spoken Language Quotient) would be a substantial predictor of reading achievement. To examine the predictive value of the morphological tasks beyond that of TOLD score, TOLD score was entered as the third step after age and PPVT scores in separate regression analyses predicting WI and PC scores.

Table 1 shows the Pearson correlations between each of the five predictor variables and two dependent variables. Scores on the transparent and opaque derivatives were significantly correlated with each other and with PPVT, TOLD, WI, and PC scores. Neither derivative score was significantly correlated with age. Partial correlations showed that the correlations between performance on the opaque derivatives and the two reading scores were still significant when age, PPVT score, and TOLD score were controlled. Results of the stepwise regressions for the WI and PC

scores are shown in Tables 2 and 3.[1] In each table, the $R^2$ value refers to the proportion of variance contributed by each predictor at the point at which it was entered in the regression. (For example, PPVT score accounted for 26.2% of the variance in WI score once the variance contributed by age had been accounted for. Cumulatively, age and PPVT accounted for 42.9% of the total variance.) Each table shows the results of two separate regressions. In the first regression, TOLD

[1]To confirm the value of combining scores from the two tasks, regression analyses also were run with scores for the Base Production and Suffix Identification tasks entered as separate predictors. Scores for transparent stimuli in the Base Production task and Suffix Identification task did not add any significant contribution to the total variance in WI or PC score after age and PPVT score had been entered. Scores for opaque stimuli in the Suffix Identification task added a significant but very minor contribution to the variance beyond that contributed by the opaque stimuli in the Base Production task (2.3% for the WI score, 4.2%, for the PC score).

TABLE 2 **Results of two stepwise regressions predicting Word Identification (WI) scores**

| Step | $R^2$ | Cumulative $R^2$ | p level |
|---|---|---|---|
| *Regression 1* | | | |
| Age | .167 | .167 | <.001 |
| PPVT score | .262 | .429 | <.001 |
| Transparent score | .069 | .498 | .005 |
| Opaque score | .199 | .697 | <.001 |
| *Regression 2* | | | |
| Age | .167 | .167 | <.001 |
| PPVT score | .262 | .429 | <.001 |
| TOLD score | .211 | .640 | <.001 |
| Transparent score | .037 | .667 | .029 |
| Opaque score | .094 | .761 | <.001 |

*Note.* PPVT = Peabody Picture Vocabulary Test. TOLD = Test of Language Development. The *p* levels refer to the significance levels for predictor variables at the point at which they were entered into the regression.

TABLE 3 **Results of two stepwise regressions predicting Passage Comprehension (PC) scores**

| Step | $R^2$ | Cumulative $R^2$ | p level |
|---|---|---|---|
| *Regression 1* | | | |
| Age | .124 | .124 | .004 |
| PPVT score | .425 | .549 | <.001 |
| Transparent score | .022 | .571 | .081 |
| Opaque score | .165 | .736 | <.001 |
| *Regression 2* | | | |
| Age | .124 | .124 | .004 |
| PPVT score | .425 | .549 | <.001 |
| TOLD score | .216 | .765 | <.001 |
| Transparent score | .002 | .767 | .486 |
| Opaque score | .062 | .829 | <.001 |

*Note.* PPVT = Peabody Picture Vocabulary Test. TOLD = Test of Language Development. The *p* levels refer to the significance levels for predictor variables at the point at which they were entered into the regression.

score was excluded, and the transparent and opaque scores were entered as the third and fourth steps. In the second regression, TOLD score was entered as the third step, and the transparent and opaque scores were entered as the fourth and fifth steps.

From "The Role of Phonological Opacity in Reading Achievement," by J. Windsor, 2000, *Journal of Speech, Language, and Hearing Research, 43,* pp. 55–57. Copyright 2000 by the American Speech-Language-Hearing Association. Reprinted with permission.

## Within-Subjects Time-Series Experiment

The next example is taken from a study that investigates potential reductions in caregiver-identified problem behaviors in persons with Alzheimer's disease (AD) and hearing loss pre- and post-hearing-aid fitting. Excerpt 8.34 describes an AB multiple-baseline design to evaluate the effects of hearing-aid use on selected problem behaviors of individuals with AD and hearing loss. As explained in Excerpt 8.34, this is a pre-/posttreatment design with varying lengths of baseline (A) and treatment phases (B). The A segment consists of caregiver frequency counts of problem behaviors (e.g., making negative statements, repeating questions, and so on) over a period of many days prior to hearing-aid fitting. The B segment consists of caregiver frequency counts of the same problem behaviors following hearing-aid fitting. Eight participants with AD and hearing loss were evaluated individually in this

E X C E R P T   8.34

### Design

A multiple-baseline design across individuals with multiple dependent variables was used to evaluate the effects of hearing-aid intervention on the problem behaviors of individuals with AD and hearing loss. This is a pre/post-treatment design with differential lengths of baseline and treatment phases (McReynolds & Kearns, 1983). Differential phase length allows the demonstration that the behavior does not change with the passage of time, but only changes at the point of in-

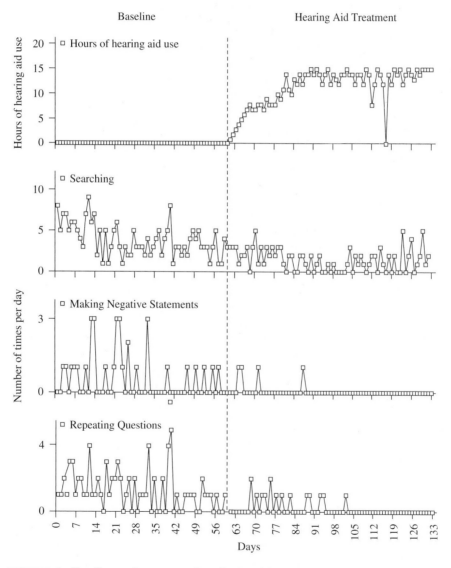

**FIGURE 2    Baseline and treatment data for Participant 1.**

tervention. During baseline, caregivers counted the frequency of one to four "hearing-related" problem behaviors on a daily basis. Baseline data (pre-hearing-aid treatment) were collected for 1.5 to 2.5 months in order to accumulate a representative sample of the participants' behaviors. After this time period, the hearing-aid intervention began (hearing-aid treatment phase). Caregivers continued to collect daily data on the problem behaviors for approximately 2 months post-treatment. Introduction of the hearing-aid inter-

vention was staggered across individuals according to the multiple baseline design.

A single-subject design methodology was chosen to evaluate treatment effects, allowing individuals to be their own controls, and thereby making a control group unnecessary. Considering the varied data regarding the auditory systems of patients with Alzheimer's disease and the varied stages of the disease, it is unlikely that an appropriate control group could be defined.

From "Reduction in Caregiver-Identified Problem Behaviors in Patients with Alzheimer's Disease Post-Hearing-Aid Fitting," by C. V. Palmer, S. W. Adams, M. Bourgeois, J. Durrant, and M. Rossi, 1999, *Journal of Speech, Language, and Hearing Research, 42,* pp. 314 & 319. Copyright 1999 by the American Speech-Language-Hearing Association. Reprinted with permission.

study. Excerpt 8.34 describes the design of the study and shows the results from one of the participants.

Excerpt 8.35 is taken from a study designed to evaluate the effect of improved classroom signal-to-noise ratios (SNR) on appropriate and inappropriate behaviors of young school-aged children. Classroom signal-to-noise ratios were controlled in this experiment using soundfield amplification. The design used in this study extends the simple AB format by including another A segment following the B segment, or ABA. The second A segment provides the opportunity to observe behavior maintenance following removal of the treatment condition, in this case, classroom soundfield amplification.

The ABA format described in Excerpt 8.35 permitted observation of appropriate (task management) and inappropriate (competing/inappropriate responses) behaviors prior to classroom soundfield amplification (first A segment), observation of these same behaviors during classroom soundfield amplification (B segment), and finally, observation of the behaviors following removal of classroom soundfield amplification (second A segment). The figure shown in Excerpt 8.35 illustrates that appropriate and inappropriate behaviors increased and decreased, respectively, during the B segment. Following removal of the classroom soundfield amplification, the students maintained improved task management, but showed an increase in inappropriate behaviors.

The next examples is the Procedures section taken from a within-subjects time-series study by Williams on the relationship between productive phonological knowledge and generalization of learning patterns in nine phonologically disordered children. Excerpt 8.36 describes a multiple-baseline design to evaluate the effects of consonant cluster training on the production of that cluster, as well as potential production generalization to a different consonant cluster. A basic AB design is used. During the baseline segment (A), both consonant clusters were measured to provide an index of each participant's pretreatment production performance. During the treatment segment (B), test probes were administered

**Experimental Design and Analysis**

An A (baseline), B (soundfield treatment), A (maintenance) withdrawal design was used in this experiment. Single-subject designs were designed specifically for evaluating questions of treatment efficacy, of which this experimental question is an example (Kazdin, 1982).

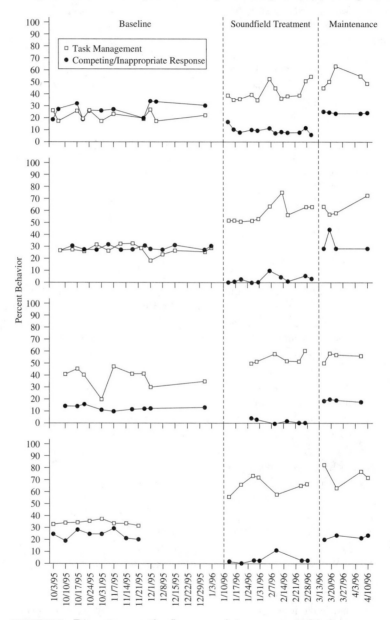

FIGURE 2 **Percent competing/inappropriate response and task management for four first-grade students. Each graph contains the complete data for one student.**

## E X C E R P T  8.35  Continued

Although the soundfield system was placed at the beginning of the school year (September), observation was not started until mid-October or November. This one-to-two month period allowed the students time to adjust to a new school environment before baseline data were collected. Treatment commenced after data points over at least three consecutive baseline observations remained within 5% of each other for each student in each observation category. Whenever a classroom was in the treatment condition, the teacher used the soundfield system throughout the entire school day. Actual observation started within one week of the system's being turned on. Treatment was withdrawn when observation results for each student had once again remained within 5% for three consecutive observation intervals. Students were then observed post-treatment (maintenance) for 4 to 5 more weeks. Post-treatment observation started within 1 week of the system's being turned off. The soundfield equipment including the teacher microphone was in place during baseline, treatment, and withdrawal. The system was turned on only during treatment.

for both consonant clusters at the end of every third training session. Training was initiated on one of the consonant clusters at the start of the B segment and continued until the child achieved 70 percent production accuracy or had completed twenty-one training sessions. When the child had completed training on the first cluster, training on the second cluster began. Excerpt 8.36 also shows the test probe results for three of the nine participants in the Williams study. Observe the relatively stable baselines during the A segment and the influence of training a particular consonant cluster in the B segment.

Time-series designs can also be used to evaluate simultaneously the effectiveness of multiple treatment methods. Excerpt 8.37 describes how the time-series design was used to evaluate the relative effectiveness of speech training using speech spectrographic display instruction versus noninstrumental instruction.

Finally, Excerpt 8.38 shows portions of the Method and Results sections of an article by Costello and Hurst that used a time-series design in an experiment with three participants over a longer period of time. The participant for whom the data are shown participated in twenty-seven sessions over a period of about nine weeks. This particular example illustrates several other points about time-series designs. First, the speakers participated over a longer term for more extended analysis of their behavior. The Experimental Design section explains how the ABABAC time-series design was executed. Second, the design used two reversals of baseline (A) and experimental segment (B), with several sessions included in each segment. Note the first paragraph of the Experimental Design section where the authors discuss the reasons for using this repeated reversals design. Third, the authors studied the effects of the experimental manipulations on different dependent variables (two stuttering behaviors for Participant 1 and three behaviors each for Participants 2 and 3). This allowed them to check the effect of manipulations on "target" behavior, as well as generalization to other behaviors. After the second baseline, the manipulation was changed to the nontarget behavior to evaluate the effect on both behaviors.

## Experimental Design

A multiple-baseline design across behaviors was used with a counterbalanced training order. The two cluster classes, [st] and [tr], were the two behaviors forming the dependent variable. The independent variable treatment was applied to the first behavior while the second behavior continued to be measured in baseline. Training was shifted to the second behavior when training was completed for the first behavior.

In this design, both behaviors were measured initially during a baseline period, then treatment was applied to the first behavior while the second behavior remained in baseline. When treatment on the first behavior was completed, the second behavior was treated. Thus, there were two points of evidence in the multiple baseline across behaviors design that demonstrated experimental control: (a) the point that occurred at the end of baseline and the beginning of treatment for the first behavior and (b) the point that occurred at the end of baseline for the second behavior and the beginning of treatment for that behavior (McReynolds & Kearns, 1983).

## Procedures

Prior to training, each child's phonological knowledge was assessed using the procedures of standard generative phonology as described in Dinnsen (1984), Elbert and Gierut (1986), and Kenstowicz and Kisseberth (1979). The analyses were based on data from a 20-min conversational sample and a 306-item analysis probe (adapted from Gierut, 1985). The items were elicited by utilizing a cueing hierarchy that began by requesting spontaneous production of the target item. If needed, additional cues (i.e., sentence completion, delayed imitation, direct imitation) were systematically provided to elicit the form. The analysis probe sampled each English phoneme a minimum of five times in all permissible word positions, included potential minimal or near-minimal pairs and morphophonetic alternations, and included word-initial and word-final consonant clusters. Each child's phonological system was described in terms of phonetic and phonemic inventories, phonological rules, phonotactic constraints, and underlying representations.

Following the description of each child's unique phonological system, a hierarchy of knowledge was constructed that compared the child's system to the target phonological system. From this analysis, it was determined that all subjects exhibited nonambient knowledge, or incorrect underlying representations, of the sounds [s] and [r]. According to the classification system discussed by Dinnsen et al. (1987), Elbert and Gierut (1986), and Gierut et al. (1987), these sounds were characterized by inventory constraints. Hierarchies constructed for each child prior to treatment are presented in Table 3 and discussed in the Results section.

A generalization probe was constructed to measure each subject's baseline and generalization performance on /s/ and /r/ clusters. The probe consisted of 40 items each of /s/ and /r/ word-initial clusters. Included were the five /st/ and five /tr/ training words plus five untrained /st/ and /tr/ word-initial clusters. Five additional /s/ and /r/ clusters of the following were included: /sl/, /sp/, /sk/, /sm/, /sn/, /sw/, /pr/, /dr/, /gr/, /kr/, /θr/, and /fr/. The generalization probe is shown in the Appendix.

The generalization probe was administered on three separate occasions prior to treatment, which constituted the baseline period. After the initiation of training, the probe was administered at the end of every third training session. A delayed imitation elicitation procedure was utilized. For example, "Do you climb a tree or a banana?"

The training items consisted of five initial /st/ words and five initial /tr/ words, as shown in the Appendix. Training continued for each cluster until the child achieved 70% accuracy for the target cluster on the generalization probe or until a total of 21 sessions were completed.

Training consisted of three phases. In Phase 1, children imitatively produced the pictorially represented training items following the clinician's model. A continuous reinforcement schedule was utilized. Phase 2 was identical to Phase 1 except the reinforcement schedule was shifted to a variable reinforcement schedule in which approximately every third correct response was reinforced. During Phase 3, the children spontaneously produced the training items when the experimenter presented the pictures without a verbal model. The variable schedule of reinforcement was continued in this phase. Criterion to move from each phase was 90% accuracy of production across three training sets. A training set consisted of 20 responses, and each training session involved five training sets, or 100 trials.

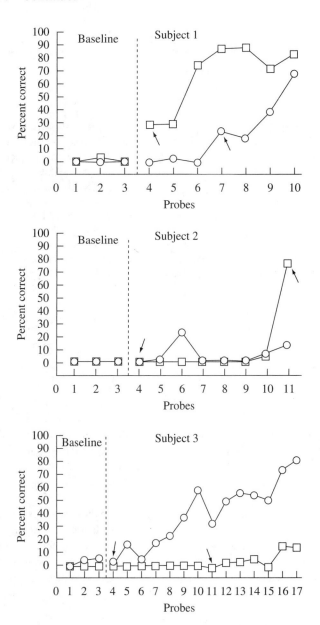

**FIGURE 1  Generalization learning curves for all subjects for target /s/ and /r/ clusters. Squares represent target /s/ clusters and circles represent target /r/ clusters. The arrows indicate initiation of treatment.**

E X C E R P T   8.37

## Methods

### Experimental Design

A modified alternating-treatment design (Barlow & Hersen, 1984; McReynolds & Kearns, 1983) with replication across subjects and speech targets, was employed to address the main research questions of this study. In this design, each speech training method (NI and SD) was assigned to one speech target (/m/ or /t/), for each of 4 subjects. Each treatment condition (i.e., method and target combination) was replicated across two subjects. The effectiveness of each training method was determined by examining changes in trend, slope, level, and variability across baseline and treatment phases within each subject. Within-subject comparisons of pre- and post-training generalization scores were also made, and maintenance of improvement was assessed for each subject at 2- and 6-week intervals after the completion of training. The relative effectiveness of each treatment was examined across the subjects by determining how often NI and SD instruction resulted in improved target acceptability, generalization to untrained words, and maintenance of acceptable productions. A final probe at 10 weeks post-training examined the effects of 10 minutes of independent speech practice with spectrographic feedback on the production of targets previously trained with SDs.

From "A Comparison of Speech Training Methods with Deaf Adolescents: Spectrographic versus Noninstrumental Instruction," by D. J. Ertmer and J. E. Maki, 2000, *Journal of Speech, Language, and Hearing Research, 43,* p. 1511. Copyright 2000 by the American Speech-Language-Hearing Association. Reprinted with permission.

Figure 1 in Excerpt 8.38 illustrates the data for the first participant. The two dependent variables (stuttering behaviors) are indicated by the two lines with open and filled circles. Note reasonable stability of both behaviors in the first A segment, a decrease in both behaviors in the first B segment, an increase back toward the first baseline levels in the second A segment, and another decrease in both behaviors in the second B segment. Both behaviors increased again in the third A segment and decreased in the C segment, although tremor disfluencies (which became the nontarget behavior in the C segment) began to increase again when they were no longer punished. Excerpt 8.38 illustrates the many possibilities for variation with multiple treatments, and multiple dependent variables with time-series designs. One caution that must be entertained in discussing these variations is that multiple-treatment interference is a threat to external validity that can best be dealt with through multiple replications to ferret out individual treatment effects and interactions among treatments.

## Between-Subjects Comparative Research

The basic structure of a descriptive study using a comparative design has already been illustrated in the subject-selection section of this chapter (see Excerpts 8.5 and 8.6). Because of the frequency with which this type of design has been employed, another brief example is appropriate with respect to procedural considerations.

Excerpt 8.39 is from a comparative study that examines the effect of emotional content on verbal pragmatic aspects of discourse production in right-brain-damaged, left-

Experimental sessions were approximately 40 minutes in length. Subjects 1 and 3 attended sessions three days per week, while Subject 2 came for sessions four days per week. Subject 1 participated in 27 sessions, Subject 2 in 51, and Subject 3 attended 39 sessions.

*Experimental Design.* The stuttering behavior of each subject was studied through a within-subject repeated reversals experimental design. For each subject, two or three selected types of stuttering behavior were separately and concurrently measured and one of them was directly manipulated by a punishment procedure. Experimental and baseline/reversal conditions were systematically alternated over several sessions yielding a repeated reversals design, often referred to as an ABAB design (Hersen & Barlow, 1976, p. 185). This design allows repeated observations of the effects of the independent variable on the form of stuttering behavior being manipulated (the target disfluency), as well as on the unmanipulated disfluency types being measured concurrently.

*Baseline condition.* During baseline (Condition A) the clinician instructed the subject to speak in monologue or to read for the entire 40 minutes. Noncontingent (never following a moment of stuttering) social reinforcers in the form of smiles and nods from the clinician were provided on the average of every 60 seconds while the subject was speaking. Further, the clinician maintained continuous attention to the subject's speaking throughout each session by maintaining eye contact. During the baseline sessions the experimenter differentially counted the frequency of occurrence of each selected stuttering topography. Baseline sessions were continued until stuttering was stable or was not systematically decreasing. Stability was said to have been achieved when the within-session average disfluency rate of each disfluency type showed variation no greater than plus or minus one disfluency per minute in three consecutive sessions. When the baseline data indicated stability, the experimental condition was introduced. All changes in conditions were introduced within sessions.

*Experimental condition.* As in the baseline sessions, subjects continued speaking in monologue or reading during experimental (Condition B) sessions, and the clinician provided continuous social reinforcement in

the form of attention as long as the subject was speaking fluently. However, during experimental sessions every occurrence of the target disfluency was consequated by one of two punishment procedures. In one, referred to as time-out from positive reinforcement (Costello, 1975), each occurrence of the target disfluency was immediately followed by the clinician saying, "Stop," and looking away from the subject for ten seconds. The subject was required to stop speaking immediately. After the time interval had elapsed the clinician looked up, smiled, and said, "Begin." In the other punishment procedure each occurrence of the target disfluency was followed by the immediate presentation of a one-second burst of a 50-dB, 4000-Hz tone through headphones, a procedure similar to that described by Flanagan, Goldiamond, and Azrin (1958).

During the experimental condition the experimenter continued counting the frequency of occurrence of all of the selected stuttering behaviors for each subject. The experimental condition was continued until the data were stable or until the direction and nature of change were clear. At this time Condition A was reintroduced in order to assess whether changes produced by the introduction of the independent variable could be reversed by its withdrawal. Following this the experimental condition was reintroduced in order to demonstrate further the control of the independent variable over the dependent variables by replication of the original effect.

*Subsequent manipulations.* Following the last reversal session (Condition A) for Subject 1, the target disfluency was changed to the previously nonmanipulated disfluency form. This was continued for three sessions. For Subject 2, during the final experimental condition, all disfluencies regardless of topography became the targets for punishment by time-out. This condition continued until the end of the study.

. . . . . . . . . . .

*Experimental Findings.* The data from each of the three subjects indicate that stuttering behaviors tended to covary directly with one another. When a punishing stimulus was applied to one topography of disfluency, other topographies were seen to decrease in frequency of occurrence, even though they were never directly manipulated.

*(continued)*

*Subject 1.* Figure 1 shows the session-by-session data collected for Subject 1 across all experimental conditions. The speaking modality for this subject was reading and the two topographies of disfluency selected for measurement were: (1) jaw tremors; and (2) unitary repetitions of phonemes, syllables, and monosyllabic words. Jaw tremors were chosen as the target disfluency for the application of punishment contingencies during experimental conditions.

Condition A (baseline) was conducted for five complete sessions. Jaw tremors averaged 18.20/min while repetitions averaged 4.45/min. After the first ten

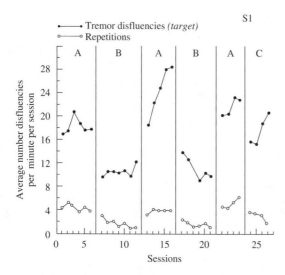

FIGURE 1 **Disfluency data for Subject 1. The ordinate indicates the number of disfluencies per minute averaged across each session; the abscissa represents individual sessions, except where changes in condition occurred. The last data point in each condition is from the same session as the first data point in the subsequent session. Experimental conditions are indicated at the top of the graph and are separated by dark vertical lines. The selected stuttering topographies measured for Subject 1 are defined in the legend at the top of the graph, and the one which served as the target disfluency is also indicated.**

minutes of Condition A in session 6, Condition B was initiated. A time-out interval of ten seconds was presented contingent upon every instance of tremors. The experimental condition was in effect for seven sessions wherein a decrease in the frequency of occurrence of tremors was noted, as well as a progressive decrease in the frequency of occurrence of untreated repetitions. Condition A was reinstated for five sessions after the first ten minutes of session 12. An immediate increase in the frequency of tremors and of repetitions demonstrated the functionality of the punishing stimulus and the reliability of the direct covariation phenomenon. During session 16 the experimental condition was reinstated for six sessions. Time-out contingencies applied to all tremors once again produced a decrease in the frequency of occurrence of these behaviors and direct covariation of untreated repetitions, thus replicating the effects of the first experimental condition and further verifying the response class relationship between tremor and repetition disfluencies for this subject. During the third session of this condition (session 18), the time-out interval was decreased from ten to five seconds, with no apparent influence on the data. Reversal Condition A was once again instated during session 21 for four sessions, resulting in an immediate increase in the frequency of occurrence of tremors and repetitions to their original baseline levels. It is unlikely that changes in speaking rate (word output) systematically varying across conditions would have accounted for these ABABA results because speaking rate has been shown to remain independent of disfluency rates in studies using procedures similar to those of this study (e.g., Costello, 1975; Martin, 1968).

In Condition C, introduced during session 24 for four sessions, time-out was no longer presented contingent upon tremors, but rather contingent upon repetitions, heretofore untreated. The frequency of occurrence of repetitions was observed to decrease. A corresponding initial decrease in the rate of now untreated tremors was noted, but this was followed by a gradual increase toward the baseline level. Thus the direct covariation observed to occur reliably across behaviors when tremors were treated was not replicated clearly when the treatment target was changed.

**EXCERPT 8.39**

In this study, we attempted to clarify whether there is a breakdown in the verbal pragmatic aspects of narrative discourse in right-brain-damaged patients and in left-brain-damaged aphasics. Further, we attempted to determine the extent to which emotional versus nonemotional (i.e., visuospatial and procedural) content contributes to pragmatic discourse deficits when they occur.

To characterize the pragmatic rules used to produce discourse, seven verbal pragmatic features were evaluated: topic maintenance, conciseness, specificity, lexical selection, revision strategy, quantity, and relevancy. The pragmatic features used in this analysis have been described by Grice (1975), who proposed that people adapt to certain cooperative principles when they communicate. Accordingly, raters in this analysis evaluated a speaker's adherence to the rules that enable an efficient exchange of information between communication partners. A variation of this pragmatic analysis has been used previously by Prutting and Kirchner (1987) for describing populations with communication disorders.

In the current study, a picture-story task (Bloom et al., 1992) was used to elicit narratives from all subjects in emotional and nonemotional conditions. The nonemotional conditions included a visuospatial one and a procedural/neutral one for baseline comparison.

**Method**

*Subjects.* Brain-damaged subjects were 21 right-handed adults, 9 with unilateral right hemisphere pathology (RBDs) and 12 with unilateral left hemisphere pathology (LBDs). Twelve neurologically healthy adults served as normal controls (NCs). All subjects were recruited from hospitals and rehabilitation agencies within the greater New York City area.

In order to be included in the study, patients had to meet the following criteria: (a) unilateral left or right hemisphere damage resulting from a single thrombotic or embolic cerebrovascular accident (CVA) confirmed by CT scan; (b) at least 6 months post CVA onset; (c) righthanded by self-report and confirmed by a score of +80 or higher on the Modified Edinburgh Handedness Inventory (Oldfield, 1971); (d) monolingual English speaker; (e) at least 11 years of education; (f) no history of psychiatric or prior neurological

disorder, dementia, or substance abuse; and (g) no uncorrected peripheral visual or auditory impairment. Nominal controls also met the above criteria with the exception of (a) and (b).

The LBDs were referred by speech-language pathologists on the basis that the patients demonstrated a mild to moderate aphasia as measured by standard aphasia batteries (i.e., Goodglass & Kaplan, 1983; Schuell, 1965). Global or severe aphasic patients were not included because subjects needed to produce sufficient discourse for analysis. The RBDs were recruited through medical chart review and were referred through speech-language pathologists. None of the RBDs demonstrated any clinical signs of aphasia or specific deficits on the four subtests of the auditory comprehension section of the Boston Diagnostic Aphasia Examination (Goodglass & Kaplan, 1983).

In order to be included in the study, subjects were tested to ensure that they had adequate cognitive, perceptual, temporal-sequencing, and auditory comprehension abilities. For cognitive screening, subtests of the Wechsler Adult Intelligence Scale—Revised (WAIS-R) (Wechsler, 1981) were selected to tap into the presumably intact functions of the nonlesioned hemisphere—a WAIS-R Verbal subtest for the RBDs and a WAIS-R Performance subtest for the LBDs. The Information subtest was administered to the RBDs, the Block Design was administered to LBDs, and both subtests were administered to the NCs. These two particular subtests were selected because of their high correlation with the overall WAIS-R IQ scores. An age-corrected scaled score of 8 or better on each subtest was required to participate in the study. For visual perceptual screening, the Visual Form Discrimination Test (Benton, Hamsher, Varney, & Spreen, 1983) was administered. In order to participate, a score of 26 or better (of 32 possible points) was required. Screening data are displayed in Table 1.

A picture sequence task was designed as a screening device to ensure that a subject could adequately process temporal information. The content of the picture sequences was equivalent in length and complexity to the pictures used in the study to elicit discourse. Three sets of three-picture sequences were presented. In order to participate in the study, a subject was required to demonstrate appropriate left-to-right placement of the cards for at least two of the three sets.

**E X C E R P T   8.39   Continued**

**TABLE 1   Screening, demographic, and lesion site variables for each subject group**

| | | | Subject Group | | | | | |
|---|---|---|---|---|---|---|---|---|
| | | | *RBDs* | | *LBDs* | | *NCs* | |
| *Category* | *Variable* | *Measure* | *M* | *SD* | *M* | *SD* | *M* | *SD* |
| Screening | Intelligence | WAIS-R age-corrected scaled score (≥8)[a] | 10.3 | 1.9 | 10.3 | 1.6 | 11.8 | 1.4 |
| | Visual perception | BVFDT (≥26) | 28.1 | 2.9 | 29.5 | 1.8 | 29.4 | 1.8 |
| | Handedness | MEHI (≥80) | 97.2 | 6.7 | 97.5 | 4.5 | 94.6 | 8.4 |
| | Auditory comprehension | BDAE (≥60 for LBDs, ≥80 for RBDs) | 90.2 | 6.6 | 79.9 | 10.8 | | |
| Demographic | Gender | males/females | 6/3 | | 9/3 | | 8/4 | |
| | Age | years | 64.2 | 7.5 | 63.3 | 10.4 | 62.8 | 8.0 |
| | Education | years | 12.8 | 1.6 | 12.8 | 2.2 | 13.2 | 2.0 |
| | Occupation | 9-point scale[b] | 5.1 | 1.5 | 4.7 | 1.6 | 5.1 | 2.2 |
| Lesion site | Frontal | number of subjects | 2 | | 3 | | — | |
| | Parietal | | 3 | | 3 | | — | |
| | Temporal | | 1 | | 2 | | — | |
| | Parietal/frontal | | 2 | | 1 | | — | |
| | Parietal/temporal | | 1 | | 3 | | — | |

*Note.* [a]WAIS-R Information subtest for RBDs, Block Design subtest for LBDs, and Information and Block Design subtests for NCs. [b]Hollingshead Scale (1977), where 1 = unskilled worker, 5 = clerical or sales worker, and 9 = major professional. WAIS-R = Wechsler Adult Intelligence Scale–Revised. BVFDT = Benton Visual Form Discrimination Test. MEHI = Modified Edinburgh Handedness Inventory. BDAE = The mean percentile score for the four subtests from the auditory comprehension section of the Boston Diagnostic Aphasia Examination.

Additional language screening was conducted on the LBDs (aphasics) to control for complicating linguistic factors. On the Auditory Comprehension Subtests of the Boston Diagnostic Aphasia Examination (Goodglass & Kaplan, 1983), a mean percentile score of 60 or better was required to be included in the study (see Table 1). To ensure that the LBDs had sufficient quantity of verbal output, the Picture Description Subtest of the Minnesota Test for the Differential Diagnosis of Aphasia (Schuell, 1965) was administered. A minimum score of 2 ("uses phrases and sentences and names at least 10 objects correctly") was required on this measure.

The three subject groups were matched for gender, age, education, and occupational status (see Table 1). No significant group differences were found when one-way analyses of variance (ANOVAs) or chi square tests were conducted on the four demographic variables. RBDs ($M = 39.2 \pm 31.9$) and LBDs ($M = 44.7 \pm 51.9$) did not differ significantly on months post CVA onset at the time of testing. The number of patients with lesions in a particular site is specified in Table 1. Sites include the frontal lobe, parietal lobe, temporal lobe, parietal and frontal lobes, and parietal and temporal lobes. Site of lesion information was taken directly from the neuroradiological report of the CT scan results in the medical chart of each person. Fisher exact tests revealed that the distributions of patients with and without lesions in each of these sites were not significantly different from each other.

## Procedures

*Picture story test.* Discourse was elicited in response to three sets of sequential pictures presented with the examiner seated directly across from the subject. Each stimulus set contained three 5 × 5-inch line drawings mounted horizontally on cardboard (Bloom et al., 1992). The stimulus sets were designed to elicit emotional content (a story about a girl whose dog is hit by a car), visuospatial content (about moving a box by climbing on books piled on a chair), or procedural/neutral content (about how to fry an egg). Each stimulus set was designed to contain seven predictable content elements. The stimulus sets were piloted on three naive normal subjects to ensure that the seven content elements, and not others, were reliably produced.

To orient the subjects to the storytelling task, the examiner first displayed a practice set of pictures and modeled a narrative (Bloom et al., 1992). Using the procedures described above, the practice stimulus set and modeled narrative were designed to contain approximately equal amounts of emotional, visuospatial, and procedural content elements. After the examiner modeled the sample narrative, subjects were then instructed to tell a story about each of the three stimulus sets. Stimulus set presentation order was randomized within subject and across groups. The development and rationale of the picture story test are further described in Bloom et al. (1992).

The stories were audiotaped and transcribed verbatim for analysis. The audiotapes were reviewed independently by two trained professionals. Percentages of agreement were calculated for each transcript (Sackett, 1978) and revealed a 96.7% mean level of interrater reliability. Written transcripts were used to eliminate the effects of prosody.

brain-damaged, and normal adults. The research question describes the groups of adults to be studied and the dependent variables to be compared. The Subjects part of the Method section describes the three groups of adults, indicates how they were selected, and displays data regarding relevant participant characteristics in Table 1. Additionally, the brain-damaged adults were screened extensively before being included in the study to ensure that they could adequately participate in the study. The results of the screening tests and group matching procedures (demographic information) are also presented in Table 1. The Procedures section of the Method section details the manner in which discourse was elicited and how emotional content was varied.

## Developmental Research

The characteristics of developmental research were discussed in Part I. Three basic designs for developmental research were discussed: cross-sectional (between-subjects design), longitudinal (within-subjects design), and semilongitudinal (mixed design). In this section, we will present excerpts from each of these three different types of developmental studies to illustrate the way participants were selected and procedures were outlined for studying the development of their behavior.

Excerpt 8.40 is taken from a study that examines the development of communicative functions of young children with and without hearing loss, who were learning spoken English.

## EXCERPT 8.40

The purpose of the present study was to evaluate whether the use of communicative functions observed in children with hearing losses who are learning spoken language reflect the same usage as that by normally developing children at younger ages or whether the children with hearing losses are putting their emerging linguistic skills—improvements in rate, vocabulary, syntax—to different uses in social situations. Specifically, age differences were examined in the emergence and use of informative/heuristic functions from 12 to 54 months of age. In addition, a relatively large number of normally hearing children were observed in order to document typical development with the same measurement techniques.

It was also of interest to examine the relationship between the use of informative/heuristic functions and the acquisition of vocabulary and syntax. It was predicted that when compared with normally hearing children, those with hearing losses would be delayed in achieving language milestones including rate of communication, breadth of vocabulary, and frequency of combining words. It was further predicted that, when children with hearing losses reach the same level in these language milestones as normally hearing children, they would be using those communicative behaviors for different social purposes.

. . . . . . . . . . .

**Characteristics of the Children with Hearing Loss**
The average age of diagnosis of hearing loss was 11.2 months (range 0–23 months). Causes of deafness in this sample were as follows: meningitis (4), likely genetic (6), cytomegalovirus (4), ototoxicity (1), head injury (1) and unknown (27). None of the children were known to have normal hearing beyond 15 months of age. All children were enrolled in a parent-infant program or nursery classroom with an auditory-oral instructional approach. Three of the children wore vibrotactile aids along with hearing aids. Five children had cochlear implants; of these, all had received their implant within the previous 8 months, with a mean length of use of 3.8 months at the time of the observation. All of the other children wore binaural hearing aids. All children were consistent in the use of their sensory

aids. All of the children in this group had profound hearing losses with the mean better ear PTA at 103.93 (SD = 8.65; ANSI, 1969), except for 2 children with losses in the severe-profound category (with 86 and 88 dB better ear thresholds). One of these children scored above average on most of the measures to be reported and the other scored below average. The average aided sound field threshold was 49.67 (SD = 9.30), though it should be noted that this number is not considered particularly reliable for the youngest age groups.

Forty-one of the 43 children in the hearing-impaired sample were administered the Communication Scale of the Vineland Adaptive Behavior Scale (Sparrow, Balla & Cicchetti, 1984), with their mother or classroom teacher serving as informant. Almost all of these children exhibited substantial communication delays on this measure compared to their normally hearing age mates (average standard score = 68.63, SD = 12.82, range 49–99). Individual data on children in this group is presented in Table 1.

**Characteristics of the Normally Hearing Children**
The normally hearing children were recruited through local birth records. All of these children were administered a hearing screening at 500, 1000, and 2000 Hz and were found to have hearing within normal limits. Two language screening instruments were administered to each normally hearing child. All children were administered the Communication Scale of the Vineland Adaptive Behavior Scale; all children in the 12–30-month groups were administered the Receptive-Expressive Emergent Language Test (Bzoch & League, 1991) and the Peabody Picture Vocabulary Test (Dunn & Dunn, 1981) was administered to all children in the 36–54-month age groups. A child was excluded if his/her score on both measures was more than 20 standard score points above or below the mean. This group tended to score higher on the vocabulary measure than on the communication measure although still within the average range. For purposes of comparison with the hearing loss group (described above), the mean score on the Vineland's Communication Scale was 102.34 (SD = 9.96, range 80–120).

**TABLE 1    Characteristics of participants with hearing loss**

| Age in months | Participant number | Sensory aid | Aided PTA | Aided SFT[a] | Cause of deafness | Diagnosis age in months |
|---|---|---|---|---|---|---|
| 12 | 1 | BHA | 105 | 45 | unknown | 6 |
| 12 | 2 | BHA | 94 | 48 | genetic | 1 |
| 12 | 3 | BHA | 110 | 60 | unknown | 6 |
| 12 | 4 | BHA | 97 | 48 | genetic | 8 |
| 12 | 5 | BHA | 100 | 50 | meningitis | 9 |
| 18 | 6 | BHA | 110 | 60 | unknown | 14 |
| 18 | 7 | BHA | 95 | 55 | unknown | 5 |
| 18 | 8 | BHA | 86 | 62[a] | meningitis | 11 |
| 18 | 9 | BHA | 105 | 45 | unknown | 10 |
| 18 | 10 | BHA | 100 | 63[a] | cytomegalovirus | 2 |
| 18 | 11 | BHA | 108 | 52[a] | unknown | 9 |
| 24 | 12 | BHA | 102 | 38[a] | unknown | 14 |
| 24 | 13 | BHA | 107 | 55 | unknown | 11 |
| 24 | 14 | BHA | 95 | 45 | cytomegalovirus | 0 |
| 24 | 15 | BHA/TA | 100 | 45 | unknown | 17 |
| 24 | 16 | BHA | 110 | 55 | unknown | 13 |
| 24 | 17 | BHA | 93 | 40 | unknown | 11 |
| 30 | 18 | BHA | 108 | 53[a] | unknown | 17 |
| 30 | 19 | BHA | 105 | 50 | genetic | 22 |
| 30 | 20 | BHA | 117 | 60 | unknown | 9 |
| 30 | 21 | BHA | 120 | 60 | unknown | 0 |
| 30 | 22 | BHA | 108 | 75 | meningitis | 11 |
| 36 | 23 | BHA | 90 | 35 | ototoxic | 8 |
| 36 | 24 | BHA | 101 | 45 | unknown | 16 |
| 36 | 25 | BHA | 97 | 35 | unknown | 6 |
| 36 | 26 | BHA | 110 | 45 | unknown | 10 |
| 36 | 27 | BHA | 105 | 40 | unknown | 23 |
| 42 | 28 | BHA | 107 | 60 | unknown | 18 |
| 42 | 29 | BHA | 115 | Unav. | cytomegalovirus | 13 |
| 42 | 30 | CI/HA | 117 | 44[a] | unknown | 13 |
| 42 | 31 | CI | 113 | 40 | unknown | 9 |
| 42 | 32 | BHA | 95 | 45 | genetic | 19 |
| 48 | 33 | BHA | 97 | 45 | unknown | 16 |
| 48 | 34 | BHA/TA | 113 | 60 | genetic | 16 |
| 48 | 35 | CI/HA | 118 | 44[a] | unknown | 17 |
| 48 | 36 | CI | 115 | 48[a] | unknown | 5 |
| 48 | 37 | BHA | 93 | 45 | unknown | 11 |

*(continued)*

EXCERPT   **8.40**   **Continued**

TABLE 1   **Continued**

| Age in months | Participant number | Sensory aid | Aided PTA | Aided SFT[a] | Cause of deafness | Diagnosis age in months |
|---|---|---|---|---|---|---|
| 48 | 38 | BHA | 102 | 40 | unknown | 18 |
| 54 | 39 | BHA/TA | 100 | 45 | cytomegalovirus | 0 |
| 54 | 40 | CI | 108 | 35 | meningitis | 13 |
| 54 | 41 | BHA | 88 | 40 | head injury | 15 |
| 54 | 42 | BHA | 97 | 43 | unknown | 8 |
| 54 | 43 | BHA | 113 | 65 | genetic | 22 |

*Note.* PTA = pure tone average; SFT = sound field threshold; BHA = binaural hearing aids; CI = cochlear implant; TA = tactile aid. Unav. = unavailable.
[a] aided SFT was unavailable; aided PTA was provided instead.

From "Age Differences in the Use of Informative/Heuristic Communicative Functions in Young Children with and without Hearing Loss Who Are Learning Spoken Language," by J. Nicholas, 2000, *Journal of Speech, Language, and Hearing Research, 43,* pp. 381–382 & 383. Copyright 2000 by the American Speech-Language-Hearing Association. Reprinted with permission.

The study was cross-sectional, in that it used a between-subjects design to compare the development of certain language behaviors of two different groups of children who ranged in age from 12 to 54 months. The purpose of the study was to evaluate potential similarities or dissimilarities in the emergence of certain communicative functions in these two groups of children. The excerpted material shows a brief statement of the specific purpose of the study followed by a portion of the Method section that describes the participants. Specific characteristics of each child with hearing impairment are provided in Table 1.

Portions of a longitudinal developmental study are shown in Excerpt 8.41. This study examines the concept of agent in the emerging language of three children as they developed from about age eleven months to age two years. The first part of the excerpt shows the research questions posed. This is followed by a description of the three participants who were studied and the method of observing them. Note that the children were observed ten times over a twelve-month period of development. The observation sessions and the children's ages at each session are detailed in Table 2 shown in Excerpt 8.41. Whereas the cross-sectional study shown in Excerpt 8.40 used a between-subjects design, this longitudinal study used a within-subjects design to observe the children repeatedly over the developmental span and to watch their behavior change directly. Note that a larger number of participants was employed in the cross-sectional study ($N = 30$) and a smaller number of participants was used in the longitudinal study ($N = 3$), as is usually the case.

The final example of a developmental study (Excerpt 8.42) is taken from a study by Wilder and Baken of respiratory patterns in infants and illustrates the use of a semilongitudinal design. The first paragraph of the excerpt provides a description of the ten participants

## EXCERPT 8.41

The research that follows examines the emergence of the cognitive concept of agent as hypothesized in Table 1. This was done by observing those overt, nonverbal behaviors (i.e., gestures) assumed to be indicative of the cognitive notion of agent, and subsequently describing the evolution of these behaviors over time in three children. Specifically the following questions were addressed: What gestural behavioral sequences indicate the child's nonverbal concept of agent? To what extent does actual development of the cognitive notion of agent match the hypothesized 5-level developmental sequence proposed in Table 1?

### Method

To discover behavioral changes which emerge over the course of a child's early development, a descriptive, longitudinal study was conducted. The methodology used a modification of the traditional observation approach (Bloom, 1970, 1973; Bloom, Lightbown, & Hood, 1975; Bowerman, 1973; Brown, 1973; Carter, 1974; Greenfield & Smith, 1976). Rather than using only diary-like observations of free unstructured sessions in which no specific activities are scheduled for administration and observation, this study included several activities having a high probability of eliciting the behaviors hypothesized in Table 1, depending on the child's current concept of agent (Edwards, 1974; Ingram, 1971; Lock, 1976; Piaget, 1952, 1954; Snyder, 1975; Sugarman, 1973).

### Subjects

The three subjects were selected on the basis of a normal prenatal and perinatal history, meeting developmental milestones as determined by the *Bayley Scales of Infant Development* (Bayley, 1969) and the Uzgiris and Hunt scales (Uzgiris & Hunt 1975), and by a normal medical history. At the beginning of the study, all three children were 11 months old, and according to the author's interpretation of the Uzgiris and Hunt scales their performance was most characteristic of Piaget's sensorimotor Stage IV (see Appendix A). The subjects, two boys and one girl, were from upper-middle-class families; the mothers of all three children either worked or attended school, resulting in the children spending at least part of the day with babysitters. One boy had an older sibling,

whereas the other two subjects had none. At the beginning of the study, all three subjects were producing prelinguistic vocalizations (i.e., consonant-vowel combinations, fussing, whining); according to the parents, none of the children had used any consistent phonetic forms to label people, objects, events, or activities. All three children were using crawling as their predominant means of locomotion during the first observation session, and walking during the second.

### Procedures

The children were videotaped in their respective homes 10 times over 12 months at approximately 1-month intervals; each session lasted 1 hour. Table 2 indicates the age of the children at each videotaping session. The observations for two children extended from the prelinguistic vocalization period (11 months) to their beginning use of 2-word utterances, particularly agent + action, agent + object, action + object constructions. The observations for one of the children extended from his use of vocalization (11 months) to his use of successive single-word utterances. During each session the mother-child pair and the investigator were present.

The children were observed during each hour-long videotaping session under two conditions: a free-play situation and an elicitation situation. The tasks in the elicitation situation were designed to supplement the data obtained in the free-play situation by providing specific opportunities for agentive behaviors to occur. They are described in detail in Appendix B. The basic structure of these agentive elicitation tasks remained the same over the 12-month period whereas specific objects within a task frequently changed from session to session. This provided some degree of structure and continuity across taping sessions and across subjects; it also allowed for more reliable observations of changes in agentive behavior (Greenfield & Smith, 1976; Schlesinger, 1974). During each session a minimum of 10 agentive elicitation tasks were presented—2 tasks for each of the 5 levels of behavior described below. These agentive elicitation tasks were interspersed throughout the free-play session. This format allowed for both free-play by the children, as well as their elicited responses to particular tasks.

*(continued)*

**EXCERPT  8.41  Continued**

**TABLE 2  Videotaped sessions per child; given are typical age (months) versus actual age (months:days)**

| Session | Typical Age | Actual Age | | |
|---|---|---|---|---|
| | | Denise | Michael | Christopher |
| 1 | 11 | 10:24 | 10:23 | 11:6 |
| 2 | 12 | 11:26 | 11:23 | 11:30 |
| 3 | 13 | 12:29 | 12:28 | 13:3 |
| 4 | 14 | 13:28 | 13:27 | 14:1 |
| 5 | 15 | 14:24 | 14:22 | 15:12 |
| 6 | 16 | 15:30 | 15:28 | 16:11 |
| 7 | 17 | 17:10 | 16:24 | 17:20 |
| 8 | 18 | 18:22 | 17:27 | 18:20 |
| 9 | 20 | 20:16 | 19:17 | 20:8 |
| 10 | 22 | 22:4 | 22:1 | 22:20 |

From "The Ontogenesis of Agent: Cognitive Notion," by L. B. Olswang and R. L. Carpenter, 1982, *Journal of Speech and Hearing Research, 25,* pp. 298–300. Copyright 1982 by the American Speech-Language-Hearing Association. Reprinted with permission.

**EXCERPT  8.42**

## Method: Subjects

The population for this study was composed of 4 male and 6 female infants who presented unremarkable pre-, peri-, and postnatal histories, and who had 5-minute Apgar scores of 8 or higher. Each child's development was monitored during the course of the study using selected items from Gesell's developmental scales (Gesell & Amatruda, 1947); the gross motor maturation of all subjects remained within normal limits. Hearing acuity was not formally assessed, but all infants responded appropriately to auditory stimuli.

The study used a semilongitudinal approach. The age of subjects at the time of entry into the population ranged from 2 to 161 days; each infant was observed over a period of approximately four months at intervals averaging 28 days. From the 62 individual observation sessions a statistical consultant selected four consecutive observations of each of the ten infants, providing a statistically useful sample of respiratory behavior over the age range in question (2–255 days). For data analysis these observations were grouped into eight 32-day age intervals, roughly representing age in months. Observation of each of the infants used in the analysis of data are summarized in Figure A.

EXCERPT 8.42 Continued

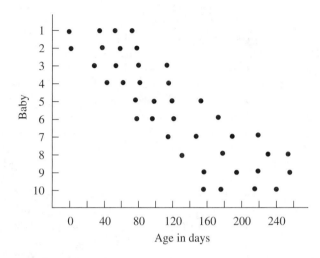

FIGURE A   Distribution of the forty sample observations among the study population.

From "Respiratory Patterns in Infant Cry," by C. N. Wilder and R. J. Baken, Winter 1974–75, *Human Communication, No. 3,* pp. 21 & 31. Reprinted with permission of the authors.

and serves to emphasize the point that the infants were developmentally normal and had normal hearing sensitivity. The second paragraph and Figure A in Excerpt 8.42 capture the essence of the semilongitudinal design. For instance, the measurement of Participant 1 began at two days of age and continued at various intervals until the child was about eighty days old. Participant 9, on the other hand, entered the study at 161 days of age and measurements ended when the child was 255 days old. Each participant was followed for about the same length of time (the longitudinal, within-subjects aspect), but participants had different ages at the time of participation in the study (the cross-sectional, between-subjects aspect). Thus, the semilongitudinal design is a compromise between the cross-sectional and longitudinal designs that incorporates aspects of each one. Note, for example, that the number of participants studied is neither as high as the cross-sectional example in Excerpt 8.40 nor as low as the longitudinal example shown in Excerpt 8.41. The semilongitudinal design tries to maximize the advantages of both the cross-sectional design and the longitudinal design while minimizing their disadvantages.

## Correlational Research

Correlational research plays an important role in communicative disorders. Correlational studies are found in research on test reliability and validity, in factor analyses of large groups of variables, in studies aimed at predicting behavior from knowledge of certain variables, and in studies of the interrelations of many clinical variables. There is a broad spectrum of correlational research to be found in the field and no single example can typify correlational research. Nevertheless, a specific example would be helpful to illustrate briefly the manner in which a researcher might go about assembling important variables for correlational analysis.

Excerpt 8.43 is taken from a study of the relationship between speech and language impairments and reading disabilities. The basic goal of the research was to determine whether there was a relationship between specific language and articulation impairments and reading disabilities as assessed by word-identification and word-attack skills tests. The Subjects section of the Method section describes the participants and their performance on several tests of speech and language (Table 1). The Reading Achievement section describes the reading skills tests that were used. Minimization of threats to internal and external validity is difficult in such a correlational study because the researcher does not have the ability to manipulate the independent (predictor) variables. That is to say, these predictor variables are attribute variables, the values of which depend on participant selection and careful measurement procedures. The author has described the participant selection and measurements carefully and the use of standardized tests helps reduce internal validity threats in the measurements of the predictor variables.

## Retrospective Research

In Part I, we cited some of the problems associated with retrospective research studies. Excerpt 8.44 presents the Method section from a retrospective study of clinical data that examined three groups of individuals with different types of hearing loss to determine whether peaked audiograms found in persons with Meniere's disease are pathognomonic of the disease. The Method section is important because it details participant selection criteria that are significant for both internal and external validity. Although the specific nature of audiometric testing is not provided, the medical diagnoses of persons with Meniere's disease and acoustic tumors and the settings where the testing was conducted provides credible evidence of a representative participant population. Nonetheless, the reader of retrospective research must be painstaking, indeed, when reading the Method section, for such research may stand or fall on this section alone.

## Survey Research

We come next to the evaluation of survey research. Although there is an extensive body of literature on survey research methodology, questionnaire development, interview techniques, and the like (e.g., see Babbie, 2000; Davis, 1971; and Slonim, 1960), such research does not appear with much frequency in the literature. Thus, we will focus here on only a

## Method

*Subjects.* Fifty-six children with speech-language impairments (S-LI) and 30 children with normal speech-language abilities participated in this investigation. In the S-LI group, there were 40 males and 16 females. At the beginning of the study, subjects in the S-LI group were in kindergarten and were an average age of 6 years, 2 months old. Each of the subjects in this group had been referred for a speech-language evaluation in one of two Midwest public school districts. In addition to the evaluation the children in this group received in the schools, a battery of standardized speech-language tests was administered for this investigation. This battery included three measures of receptive language abilities: Peabody Picture Vocabulary Test—Revised (Dunn & Dunn, 1981), Token Test for Children (DiSimoni, 1978), Grammatical Understanding subtest of the Test of Language Development—2 (Newcomer & Hammill, 1988), and three measures of expressive language abilities: Expressive One-Word Picture Vocabulary Test (Gardner, 1979), Structured Photographic Expressive Language Test—II (Werner & Kresheck, 1983), combined performance on the Sentence Imitation and Grammatical Closure subtests of the Test of Language Development—2, and a measure of articulation: Goldman-Fristoe Test of Articulation (Goldman & Fristoe, 1986). In addition, the Block Design and Picture Completion subtests of the Wechsler Preschool and Primary Scale of Intelligence (Wechsler, 1967) were administered.[1]

Children in the S-LI group had a variety of speech and language difficulties. The standardized test battery indicated that the majority of the subjects ($n = 41$) demonstrated a language impairment. A language impairment was operationally defined as performance of at least one *SD* below the mean on at least two of three receptive language measures and/or two of three expressive language measures. Nineteen subjects displayed impairments on both receptive and expressive language tests, 12 subjects showed language difficulties

primarily on receptive measures, and 10 subjects displayed impairments primarily on expressive language tests. In some analyses for the present study, the above children with language impairments are referred to as the LI subgroup. The remaining 15 subjects in the S-LI group did not meet the criteria for a language impairment but demonstrated articulation problems and/or were enrolled in articulation therapy during the kindergarten school year (referred to as the AI subgroup). Twelve of these subjects performed below average on the Goldman-Fristoe Test of Articulation (mean percentile = 16.9 %, range < 1–33%). The other three subjects had been enrolled in articulation therapy throughout the kindergarten year and had resolved their articulation difficulties by the time of our assessment. Nevertheless, enrollment in articulation therapy was considered sufficient criterion for inclusion in this investigation. Some of the subjects in the LI subgroup (37%) also had articulation impairments. However, these subjects were included with the other subjects demonstrating language impairments (i.e., LI subgroup) when examining differences between subgroups. All subjects in the S-LI group demonstrated nonverbal abilities within the normal range. School records also indicated that children in this group had hearing and corrected vision within normal limits and no history of emotional disorders.

Thirty children without a history of speech-language impairments or a referral for such impairments also participated in this study. These children served as a comparison group to evaluate the performance of the S-LI group on measures of reading achievement. The normally developing subjects were enrolled in the same classrooms or schools as subjects in the S-LI group and were approximately the same age (6 years, 1 month at the beginning of the study). There were 18 males and 12 females in this group. Each of these children performed within normal limits on the battery of speech-language tests and measures of nonverbal ability.

The means and standard deviations for the normal and S-LI groups on the speech-language and nonverbal tests are presented in Table 1. Also shown in Table 1 are the means and standard deviations for the LI and AI subgroups within the S-LI group.

. . . . . . . . . . . .

## Reading achievement

Reading achievement was assessed in the first and second grades. The Word Identification (Word Id) and

---

[1]For children older than 6-½ years, the Block Design and Picture Completion subtests from the Wechsler Intelligence Scale for Children—Revised (Wechsler, 1974) were administered. Testing was limited to the Block Design and Picture Completion subtests because of the time constraints and testing concerns imposed by the school systems. Previous researchers have also relied on the use of these subtests as a measure of nonverbal abilities (Bishop & Adams, 1990).

*(continued)*

Word Attack subtests from the Woodcock Reading Mastery Tests—Revised (Woodcock, 1987) were administered to subjects in the spring of first and second grade. These subtests required subjects to read a list of words or pseudo-words presented in isolation, and as such, served as measures of written word recognition. In second grade, subjects were also given the Gray Oral Reading Test—Revised (GORT-R) (Wiederholt & Bryant, 1986). In addition to an oral reading quotient, this test provided a measure of speed and accuracy of word recognition in context and a measure of reading comprehension. The GORT-R was not administered in the first grade because the majority of the subjects with S-LI had limited reading abilities at that time.

All subjects in the S-LI and normal groups completed the reading tests during first grade. Six subjects in the S-LI group and 1 subject in the normal group moved away and were unavailable for testing in the second grade. In addition, some of the subjects with S-LI re-

peated their kindergarten year ($n = 5$), whereas others were placed in developmental first grade classes prior to going to first grade ($n = 18$). Developmental first (D-1) classes have been instituted in some school districts to allow young or slowly developing children (often vaguely defined) an extra year of maturation before beginning first grade and formal reading instruction. Children in D-1 programs in our school districts repeated kindergarten classes during half of the school day and received primarily the nonacademic curriculum (e.g., art, music) of first grade during the other half of the day. In the case of the subjects repeating kindergarten or placed in D-1 classes, standardized speech-language tests and measures of phonological awareness and rapid naming were administered during the second year of kindergarten (or D-1 classes). The results of this testing served as these subjects' kindergarten data and were subsequently used for data analysis.

**TABLE 1  Mean standard scores (and standard deviations) on standardized tests in kindergarten for the normal and speech-language impaired (S-LI) groups and the language-impaired (LI) and articulation-impaired (AI) subgroups within the S-LI group**

|  | Normal | S-LI | LI | AI |
|---|---|---|---|---|
|  | N = 30 | N = 56 | n = 41 | n = 15 |
| PPVT | 108.3 | 90.8 | 85.0 | 106.9 |
|  | (7.5) | (14.6) | (10.8) | (11.2) |
| Token | 499.0 | 494.0 | 493.3 | 498.7 |
|  | (3.8) | (4.0) | (2.8) | (2.9) |
| TOLD-2 | 104.3 | 87.5 | 81.7 | 103.1 |
|  | (10.9) | (14.2) | (10.5) | (10.9) |
| EOWPVT | 113.4 | 97.7 | 92.3 | 112.7 |
|  | (11.50) | (13.8) | (9.0) | (13.9) |
| SPELT-II | 108.5 | 84.9 | 78.2 | 103.1 |
|  | (13.1) | (17.8) | (11.7) | (19.4) |
| Picture completion | 12.9 | 11.5 | 10.8 | 13.3 |
|  | (1.8) | (2.4) | (2.2) | (2.2) |
| Block design | 12.4 | 10.2 | 9.4 | 12.3 |
|  | (1.6) | (2.4) | (2.0) | (2.3) |

*Note.* PPVT = Peabody Picture Vocabulary Test—Revised; Token = Token Test for Children; TOLD-2 = Test of Language Development—2, Syntax Quotient; EOWPVT = Expressive One-Word Picture Vocabulary Test; SPELT-II = Structured Photographic Expressive Language Test—II.

From "The Relationship between Speech-Language Impairments and Reading Disabilities," by W. H. Catts, 1993, *Journal of Speech and Hearing Research, 36,* pp. 949–950 & 951. Copyright 1993 by the American Speech-Language-Hearing Association. Reprinted with permission.

EXCERPT 8.44

## Method

A retrospective review of charts from the Minnesota Ear, Head, and Neck Clinic and the Fairview-University of Minnesota Hospital was undertaken to gather the audiometric data utilized by this study. The participants were assigned to one of three groups based upon their clinical diagnosis as follows: (Group 1) participants with Meniere's disease, charts were obtained from both the Minnesota Ear, Head, and Neck Clinic and the Fairview-University of Minnesota Hospital; (Group 2) participants with confirmed acoustic tumors, charts were obtained from the Fairview-University of Minnesota Hospital; (Group 3) participants from a general clinical population, charts were obtained from the Fairview-University of Minnesota Hospital. All participants were adults whose ages ranged from 20 to 96 years; they were selected as per the group criteria given below. The average ages of the participants with Meniere's disease, those from the general clinical population, and those with tumors were 50.3, 51.1, and 45.3 years, respectively. The audiometric data for each participant were entered into a spreadsheet program (Microsoft Excel 97) for subsequent analysis. The participants' pure-tone threshold configurations were analyzed via Boolean logic formulas and then assigned to one of five categories: falling, flat, peaked, rising, and other. Further analysis was performed on data from all three groups to evaluate (a) the effects of bilateral high-frequency hearing loss on the Meniere's disease audiometric configuration, (b) the performance of the clinical diagnostic criterion for Meniere's disease proposed by the AAO (Committee on Hearing and Equilibrium, 1995) versus those employed by this study, and (c) the usefulness of audiometric configurations for diagnosing Meniere's disease.

Patients at both the Fairview-University of Minnesota Hospital and the Minnesota Ear, Head, and Neck Clinic are carefully tested for acoustic tumors when audiometric results or patient symptomology are suggestive of a tumor's existence. Criteria for referral include unilateral tinnitus, asymmetrical sensorineural hearing loss, dizziness, or unusually poor word-recognition performance with respect to the patient's pure-tone thresholds. At the Minnesota Ear, Head, and Neck Clinic, patients meeting one or more of the aforementioned criteria will undergo either ECochG/ Auditory Brainstem Response (ABR) or Magnetic Resonance Imaging (MRI) testing to rule out the existence of an acoustic tumor. Similarly, patients at the Fairview-University of Minnesota Hospital will undergo MRI testing if any of the above criteria are met. Because of the careful screening procedures implemented at these two clinics and the low prevalence of acoustic tumors in the general population, we are confident that the results obtained in this study from the Meniere's disease and general clinical population groups have little, if any, chance of being confounded by the existence of an acoustic tumor.

The charts of 321 patients diagnosed with clinical Meniere's disease were reviewed to find 80 adults (age $\geq$ 20 years) with unilateral Meniere's disease as per the criteria listed below. The remaining 241 unselected participants did not meet our criteria.

The diagnosis of these patients by a physician was based on history and symptoms. The 80 participants selected were considered to have unilateral Meniere's disease based on the following criteria: (a) an asymmetric sensorineural hearing loss, that is, the thresholds differed by 15 dB or more between ears at a minimum of two frequencies; (b) thresholds in the better ear less than or equal to 20 dB HL at 0.25 and 0.5 kHz; (c) a reported symptom of rotational vertigo; and (d) a reported symptom of aural fullness only in the poorer-hearing ear. Although we do not know precisely how long all of the participants have had Meniere's disease, all indicators point to the conclusion that our study's Meniere's disease participants harbor an early form of this disease. We arrived at this conclusion via three means. First, persons with Meniere's disease exhibit rising or peaked audiograms early in the course of the disease, but flat audiograms are most prevalent over time (Anderson, Huffman, & McCabe, 1969; Eliachar, Keels, & Wolfson, 1973; Enander & Stable, 1967; Paparella et al., 1982; Pfaltz & Matefi, 1981). None of the participants with Meniere's disease in this study have flat audiograms. Second, 30 to 50% of persons with Meniere's disease in one ear will develop this disease in the other ear within 3 to 5 years (Paparella & Grieble, 1984; Schwaber, 1997). We selected only unilateral cases, and given the above

**EXCERPT  8.44  Continued**

information, it is reasonable to expect that many of the participants selected have early Meniere's disease.

Third, clearly abnormal ECochG findings generally occur only early in the evolution of the disease (Margolis et al., 1995). The 19 participants with Meniere's disease from the Fairview-University of Minnesota Hospital all had positive ECochG results. When the pure-tone thresholds of the Minnesota Ear, Head, and Neck Clinic's Meniere's disease participants are compared to those from the Fairview-University of Minnesota Hospital, we see little difference in these groups' average thresholds and their standard deviations. Because all three of these factors have been met, we concluded that our participants with Meniere's disease are representative of persons with an early form of the disease.

A second group included 89 adults (age ≥ 20 years) seen consecutively at the Fairview-University of Minnesota Hospital. This general clinical population included those with normal hearing as well as those with hearing losses of various etiologies; however, participants with Meniere's disease, an acoustic tumor, or a conductive loss were not included in this group. A conductive loss was defined as an air-bone gap of 20 dB or more at a single frequency, 15 dB or more at two or more frequencies, or 10 dB or more at three or more frequencies. No other exclusion criteria were implemented for this group. The ears for this group's participants were assigned as better- or poorer-hearing ears based upon each ear's pure-tone threshold average for the octave frequencies from 0.25 kHz to 8.0 kHz. This was done so that asymmetrical hearing losses occurring in the general clinical population could be compared to hearing losses related to Meniere's disease or acoustic tumors.

A third group included 56 adults (age ≥ 20 years) diagnosed with unilateral acoustic tumors who were seen at the Fairview-University of Minnesota Hospital between the years of 1987 and 1996. The existence of a tumor was confirmed by surgery. All audiometric data used from this group were obtained from pre-surgical audiometric tests. The data for this group were originally gathered for a study of acoustic reflex thresholds (ARTs), and as such, this group contains only those acoustic tumor patients for whom ART measures were attempted. This group includes tumor patients both with and without measurable ARTS.

From "The Peaked Audiometric Configuration in Meniere's Disease: Disease Related?" by D. T. Ries, M. Rickert, and R. S. Schlauch, 1999, *Journal of Speech, Language, and Hearing Research, 42,* pp. 831–832. Copyright 1999 by the American Speech-Language-Hearing Association. Reprinted with permission.

few selected issues that need to be identified by the critical evaluator of survey research and hope that the interested reader who wishes to delve more deeply into the area will consult the sources just noted.

The choice of a survey research design should be consistent with, and appropriate to, the purpose of the study. The first question the critical reader must raise, then, is whether the research reported was best conducted by means of a survey design or whether there were alternate, and perhaps better, research designs that could have been used to answer the research questions. Assuming that the survey design was appropriate, the next question deals with the adequacy of the sample surveyed. As we pointed out in Part I, it is difficult, if not impossible, to survey the entire population of interest (e.g., all speech pathologists in the United States, all speech and hearing facilities in the country). As a result, survey researchers often draw a sample of participants that presumably is representative of the total population. On the surface, this may appear to be a relatively simple task; in reality, the task can be quite complex. Fortunately, there are a variety of sampling techniques that can be employed. These include random sampling, stratified sampling, cluster sampling, systematic sampling, and the like. We cannot address here the technical aspects of sampling or the advantages and disadvantages of various sampling techniques. Suffice it to say that the critical reader must address the issue of the adequacy of the sample used in survey research. It may not be readily apparent but the sampling issue in survey research is analogous to the differential-selection-of-subjects threat to internal validity, as well as the subject-selection threat to external validity.

The mortality threat to internal validity is a common problem in survey research. Mortality in this context is represented by the number of people surveyed who failed to respond to the survey instrument. Babbie (2000) pointed out that a response rate of at least 50 percent can be considered adequate for analysis and reporting purposes, that a response rate of 60 percent is good, and that a response of 70 percent or greater is very good. If the nonresponse rate is high, the researcher may have a biased sample, a sample that may not be representative of the population of interest, and a sample of responders who are quite different, on important dimensions, from individuals who failed to respond. It is for these reasons that survey researchers spend considerable time, effort, and money on attempts to enlist the cooperation of individuals who failed to respond to the initial request to participate in the survey. The careful reader of survey research must identify the mortality rate and determine whether the number of nonresponders poses a threat to both internal and external validity.

The instrumentation threat to internal validity is directly related to the adequacy of the survey instrument, be it a questionnaire or an interview. Good questionnaire development is a difficult and complex task, one not readily undertaken by the novice. Are the questions clear and unambiguous? Do the questions address the issues under study? Are the questions objective and nonthreatening? Do the questions lead to nonbiased responses? In an attempt to ensure the adequacy of a questionnaire, researchers often pretest the instrument. That is, a small sample of representative individuals is given a trial questionnaire for their reactions, their suggestions, and their comments. The pretest is an extremely important part of questionnaire development and the critical reader should be alert to the researcher's reference to the use of a pretest. It should be noted that the questionnaire itself is usually not available for the reader's inspection but should be made available to an interested reader if requested from the researcher. In longer articles or in books reporting the results of survey research, the questionnaire is usually included for the reader's inspection. Remember, a questionnaire survey is only as good as the questions asked.

The survey research interview has several advantages over the questionnaire format. Interviewing permits probing to obtain more or different data, allows for greater depth, and enables the interviewer to assess rapport and communication between interviewer and respondent and to determine whether these factors affect the data-collection process. On the other hand, interviews are costly and time-consuming, the interviewer needs to be trained, and the interaction between interviewer and respondent can have a strong influence on the data collected. In this context, of course, the interviewer and the interview format (e.g., structured versus unstructured interviews) can pose an instrumentation threat to internal validity.

Excerpt 8.45 is from an article that reports the results of a survey conducted to determine the frequency and adverse effects of voice disorders on job performance and attendance in teachers and the general population. The authors' motivation for conducting the study was predicated on the fact that extant literature on the topic was limited by small sample sizes, absence of comparison groups, and/or nonrandomly selected participants. The Method section of the article, presented here, clearly shows how the authors intend to redress the problems in the extant literature.

E X C E R P T   8.45

## Method

### Sampling Procedures

Teachers and nonteachers in Utah and Iowa were selected for study. The State Office of Education for the State of Iowa provided a list of currently employed elementary and secondary school teachers (grades K to 12), ages 20–66 years. A similar list of teachers was provided by specific school districts in Utah. The lists included information about current school assignment, address and telephone number, teacher age, gender, race and education, number of years taught, current subjects taught, type of school (public, private, parochial), and employment status (i.e., full- or part-time). All of the individuals contacted completed a half-hour telephone interview conducted by Iowa State Statistical Laboratory interviewers. The initial contact was made through a mailing to the teacher's home, describing the study and human subject requirements. About 5 days later, contact was made with the potential interviewee by telephone. At this time, the study was briefly described again, questions were answered, and a convenient time was scheduled to conduct the telephone interview.

The general (nonteacher) population was randomly sampled and surveyed so that population-based prevalence estimates of voice disorders, and their effects, could be generated. This sample consisted of both working and nonworking individuals in each state who met the age criterion (i.e., 20–66 years) and had never taught at any educational level or type (e.g., college, aerobic instructor). The Iowa State Statistical

Laboratory also conducted the telephone interviews of this nonteacher referent group using the identical questionnaire. Details of this procedure and the sampling method used (i.e., the random digit dialing procedure) are described elsewhere (Roy et al., 2004). Response rates for both the teacher and nonteacher groups were very high in both states. Response rates of completed interviews in Iowa were 95% for teachers and 92% for nonteachers. Corresponding response rates in Utah were 98% for teachers and 87% for nonteachers. In both states, the nonresponses were due to lack of an identifiable home telephone number for the telephone interview and to lack of interest or time because of other burdens.

### Description of the Interview/ Questionnaire

To determine the prevalence and effects of voice disorders in teachers and the general population, a standardized questionnaire was administered. For the purpose of this study, we defined a voice disorder for the participants as the experience of the voice not working, performing, or sounding as it normally should, so that it interfered with communication.[2] The interview instrument was designed to be similar to those used in the periodic United States Public Health Service National Health and Nutrition Examination Survey prevalence surveys of health status in random samples of the U.S. population, which are also conducted by telephone, and which serve as the standard for many epidemiological studies. Validation information and a complete description of the questionnaire are reported in Roy et al. (2004). To assess the functional impact of voice disorders in teachers and the general population, specific questions were included in the interview to elicit the participant's opinion of the effects of the voice symptoms/disorder on their employment and career. These questions were asked to determine: (a) the frequency of selected voice symptoms and signs, and (b) how frequently participants had experienced adverse work-related effects due to a voice disorder. Specific questions elicited information regarding (a) the presence and frequency of 10 specific current or past voice symptoms/signs typically associated with voice disorders (e.g., hoarseness, vocal fatigue, trouble speaking or singing softly, difficulty projecting the voice, loss of singing range, discomfort while using the voice, monotone voice, increased effort associated with speaking, chronic throat dryness, and chronic throat soreness) and 4 other laryngopharyngeal symptoms/signs (frequent throat clearing, bitter or acid taste, swallowing difficulties, a wobbly or shaky voice); (b) whether the partici-

pant attributed the aforementioned symptoms/signs to their occupation; (c) whether the participant's voice affects, limits, or restricts his or her ability to perform various tasks or work-related activities; and (d) whether the participant reports past and/or anticipated occupation/career changes due to a voice disorder.

Demographic variables considered in this study were age and gender. Because the association between the percentage of participants with voice disorders and age was not linear, we categorized this variable as 20–29, 30–39, 40–49, 50–59, and 60 years and older. Race/ethnicity was not considered in the study because of the very high percentage of participants who were White, non-Hispanic (i.e., 97.9% of teachers and 94.4% of nonteachers)

[2]The precise definition of a voice disorder, as provided by the interviewer to the respondents was, "For the purpose of this study, we consider a voice problem to be any time your voice does not work, perform or sound as you feel it normally should, so that it interferes with communication."

From "Voice Disorders in Teachers and the General Population: Effects on Work Performance, Attendance, and Future Career Choices," by N. Roy, R. M. Merrill, S. Thibeault, S. D. Gray, and E. M. Smith, 2004, *Journal of Speech, Language, and Hearing Research, 47,* pp. 543–544. Copyright 2004 by the American Speech-Language-Hearing Association. Reprinted with permission.

## EVALUATION CHECKLIST

**Instructions:** The four-category scale at the end of each part of the *Method* section checklist may be used to rate these parts of an article. The *Evaluation Items* help identify those topics that should be considered in arriving at the ratings. Comments on these topics, entered as *Evaluation Notes,* should serve as the basis for the ratings. An additional scale is provided to allow for an overall rating of the *Method* section.

*Evaluation Items (Participants)*                        *Evaluation Notes*

1. Sample size was adequate.

2. Selection and exclusion criteria were adequate and clearly defined.

3. Participants were randomly selected and randomly assigned.

*Evaluation Items (Participants)*                          *Evaluation Notes*

4. Overall or pair matching was employed.

5. Differential subject-selection posed no threat
   to internal validity.

6. Regression effect controlled for participants
   selected on basis of extreme scores.

7. Interaction of subject-selection and treatment
   posed no threat to external validity.

8. General comments.

*Overall Rating (Participants):*

|  |  |  |  |
|---|---|---|---|
| Poor | Fair | Good | Excellent |

*Evaluation Items (Materials)*                          *Evaluation Notes*

1. Instrumentation (hardware and behavioral)
   was appropriate.

2. Calibration procedures were described and
   were adequate.

3. Evidence presented on reliability and validity
   of hardware and behavioral instrumentation.

4. Experimenter and human observer bias was
   controlled.

5. Test environment was described and was
   adequate.

6. Instructions were described and were adequate.

7. There were adequate selection and measurement
   of independent (classification, predictor)
   variables.

8. There were adequate selection and measurement
   of dependent (criterion, predicted) variables.

9. General comments.

*Overall Rating (Materials):*

|  |  |  |  |
|---|---|---|---|
| Poor | Fair | Good | Excellent |

*Evaluation Items (Procedures)*                           *Evaluation Notes*

**1.** Research design was appropriate to purpose
of study.

**2.** Procedures reduced threats to internal validity
arising from:
**(a)** history
**(b)** maturation
**(c)** reactive pretest
**(d)** mortality
**(e)** interaction of above

**3.** Procedures reduced threats to external validity
arising from:
**(a)** reactive arrangements
**(b)** interactive pretest
**(c)** subject-selection
**(d)** multiple treatments

**4.** General comments.

*Overall Rating (Procedures):*

| —— | —— | —— | —— |
|------|------|------|-----------|
| Poor | Fair | Good | Excellent |

*Overall Rating (Method):*

| —— | —— | —— | —— |
|------|------|------|-----------|
| Poor | Fair | Good | Excellent |

# REFERENCES

Arndt, W. B. (1977). A psychometric evaluation of the Northwestern Syntax Screening Test. *Journal of Speech and Hearing Disorders, 42,* 316–319.

Babbie, E. R. (2000). *Survey research methods.* Belmont, CA: Wadsworth.

Barber, T. X. (1976). *Pitfalls in human research.* New York: Pergamon.

Barber, T. X., & Silver, M. J. (1968). Fact, fiction, and the experimenter bias effect. *Psychological Bulletin Monograph Supplement, 70*(6, Pt. 2).

Christensen, L. B. (2004). *Experimental methodology* (9th ed.). Boston: Allyn & Bacon.

Davis, J. A. (1971). *Elementary survey analysis.* Upper Saddle River, NJ: Prentice Hall.

Hipskind, N. M., & Rintelmann, W. F. (1969). Effects of experimenter bias upon pure-tone and speech audiometry. *Journal of Auditory Research, 9,* 298–305.

Lee, L. L. (1977). Reply to Arndt and Byrne. *Journal of Speech and Hearing Disorders, 42,* 323–327.

Levitt, H. (1983). Issue X: Advancing technology. *Proceedings of the 1983 National Conference on Undergraduate, Graduate, and Continuing Education. ASHA Reports, 13,* 87–89.

Martin, R. R., & Haroldson, S. K. (1992). Stuttering and speech naturalness: Audio and audiovisual judgments. *Journal of Speech and Hearing Research, 35,* 521–528.

McCauley, R. J., & Swisher, L. (1984). Psychometric review of language and articulation tests for preschool children. *Journal of Speech and Hearing Disorders, 49,* 34–42.

Metz, D. E., Schiavetti, N., & Sacco, P. R. (1990). Acoustic and psychophysical dimensions of the perceived speech naturalness of nonstutterers and posttreatment stutterers. *Journal of Speech and Hearing Disorders, 55,* 516–525.

Pedhazur, E. J., & Schmelkin, L. P. (1991). *Measurement, design, and analysis: An integrated approach.* Mahwah, NJ: Lawrence Erlbaum Associates.

Plutchik, R. (1983). *Foundations of experimental research* (3rd ed.). New York: Harper & Row.

Rosenthal, R. (1966). *Experimenter effects in behavioral research.* New York: Appleton-Century-Crofts.

Rosenthal, R., & Rosnow, R. L. (Eds.). (1969). *Artifact in behavioral research.* New York: Academic Press.

Rosenthal, R., & Rosnow, R. L. (1975). *The volunteer subject.* New York: John Wiley & Sons.

Slonim, M. J. (1960). *Sampling.* New York: Simon & Schuster.

# CHAPTER 9

# The Results Section

Basic terms, concepts, and procedures used in organizing and analyzing data derived from research in communicative disorders were described in Chapter 6. This chapter will consider the evaluation of the Results section of a research article through the use of examples that illustrate many of those basic terms, concepts, and procedures.

An important consideration in the evaluation of the Results section is the manner in which the results are related to the research problem. It is imperative that the Results section be organized in a clear fashion with regard to the general research problem and the various subproblems delineated under it. Without clear articulation of the results and problem, even relatively simple data may be confusing and frustrating to the reader, whereas tight organization of the results around the research problem may make complex data comprehensible to most readers. Just as the writer has a responsibility to maintain the problem as the focus of the Results section, the reader must constantly bear the problem in mind while reading and evaluating the Results section.

## Organization of Results

Upon completion of data collection, the researcher's first task is to organize the raw data to present a coherent picture of the results to readers. This section will present examples from the communicative disorders literature that illustrate some of the ways in which raw data have been organized for presentation. In reality, an author may have gone through several steps of organizing and reorganizing raw data on paper before arriving at a solution that enables the results to be presented in as clear, complete, and efficient a manner as possible within the confines of a short journal article. What the reader eventually sees in print is usually a processed version of the raw data that gives a clear indication of the general behavior or characteristics of participants in the various conditions of the research design. The results may be organized for the reader by tabular or graphic presentation of the frequency distribution of the data or through the use of summary statistics that describe the distribution.

### Frequency Distributions:
### Tabular and Graphic Presentations

It was stated in Chapter 6 that whenever variables are measured in a research study, the obtained values of the measurements form a distribution. The distribution may be in the form of category frequencies (for nominal data), ranks (for ordinal data), or score values (for

315

interval or ratio data). Both tabular and graphic presentation of the frequency distribution may be effective means of data organization for comparing results within-subjects or between-subjects. Although any frequency distribution may be presented in either tabular or graphic form, there are some advantages unique to each type of illustration. In general, frequency distributions presented in graphic form (i.e., frequency histograms or polygons) give a more immediate overall picture of the distribution and have a more dramatic effect on the reader in showing the characteristics of the distribution. On the other hand, frequency distributions presented in a table are generally more convenient for inspection of specific values of the data or for making exact within-subjects and between-subjects comparisons. In some articles, authors have taken advantage of both types of presentations and included both a tabular and a graphic presentation of a frequency distribution.

Excerpt 9.1 is from a study of prelinguistic vocalization and later expressive vocabulary in young children with developmental delay in which children's language was mea-

## EXCERPT 9.1

The children vocalized an average of 3.95 times per minute ($SD$ = 2.95). The rate of vocalizations per minute that included a consonant was 1.14 ($SD$ = 1.22). The rate of communication acts with vocalizations per minute was 1.11 ($SD$ = .99). The child's rate of expressive vocabulary was measured 12 months later. The means include children who did not produce words in the testing sessions. During the structured interactions at the end of the study, all but 7 children used words. The rate of expressive vocabulary was .66 words per minute ($SD$ = .8). The average number of words used was 13 ($SD$ = 15.35). The range was 0–79. In the unstructured play session, 12 children didn't talk. The average number of words used during the 15-minute session was 11.31 ($SD$ = 15.54). The range was 0–87. (See Table 1 for a breakdown of word use in each session.)

TABLE 1    **Number of words used in each setting by number of children**

| | Number of children in each setting | |
| --- | --- | --- |
| *Number of words* | *Structured interaction* | *Unstructured play* |
| 0 words | 7 | 12 |
| 1–9 words | 28 | 25 |
| 10–19 words | 12 | 9 |
| 20–29 words | 5 | 4 |
| 30–39 words | 3 | 5 |
| 40–49 words | 0 | 1 |
| 50 and above | 3 | 2 |

sured in two settings: structured interaction versus unstructured play. The excerpt includes a tabular frequency distribution of the number of words used in each setting, a brief textual description of the data distribution, and summary statistics for central tendency and variability. The table shows number of words used in the left column, divided into intervals of 10 words each (except that the lowest level is 0 words and the highest level is 50 words and above) and two columns, one for each setting, that include the number of children whose data fell into each 10-word interval. Examination of the frequency distribution shows that about twice as many children were nonverbal in the unstructured play than in the structured interaction but that the mode, or most frequently occurring value (the 1–9 word interval), was the same in both distributions (i.e., twenty-eight children in the structured interaction and twenty-five children in the unstructured play used between 1 and 9 words). Because most children were clustered between 0 and the 20–29 word intervals and a few children were spread out across the range from 30–39 to 50 and above, the frequency distributions for the two settings are both positively skewed. A good exercise for students would be to take these data and draw a frequency histogram and a frequency polygon on graph paper to see the skewness in the tabular data displayed graphically.

The next excerpt (9.2) shows a frequency distribution presented in the form of a histogram. This illustration shows the SICD Expressive Age posttreatment improvement (measured as proportional change relative to pretreatment development) of twenty children in

EXCERPT 9.2

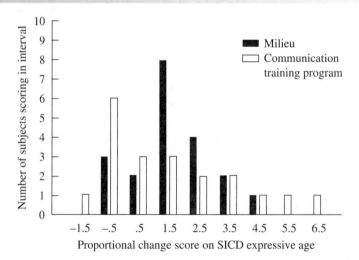

FIGURE 1 Histogram of proportional change score for the SICD-E by treatment group.

From "An Exploratory Study of the Interaction between Language Teaching Methods and Child Characteristics," by P. J. Yoder, A. P. Kaiser, and C. L. Alpert, 1991, *Journal of Speech and Hearing Research, 34,* p. 162. Copyright 1991 by the American Speech-Language-Hearing Association. Reprinted with permission.

a milieu language training program and twenty children in a communication training program. The bar heights in the histogram indicate the number of participants in each group who achieved each of the SICD proportional change scores shown on the abscissa. The dark bars indicate the number of children in the milieu group who achieved each score change, and the light bars indicate the number of children in the communication training program who achieved each score change. Inspection of the histogram reveals (1) the distribution of milieu participants' scores is close to a normal distribution in shape; (2) the distribution of communication training program participants' scores is positively skewed; (3) the central tendencies are similar in the two groups (the means were 1.61 for milieu and 1.78 for communication training program); and (4) variability among participants is smaller in the milieu group ($SD$ = 1.22) and larger in the communication training program group ($SD$ = 2.14).

The histogram in Excerpt 9.2 gives a more immediate and dramatic picture of the overall results than does the table shown in Excerpt 9.1. On the other hand, closer inspection of the exact frequency of participants obtaining each specific score is easier when inspecting the frequency table.

Excerpts 9.1 and 9.2 illustrate how tabular or graphic frequency distributions would appear in a journal article when the dependent variable data are scores at the interval or ratio level of measurement. The next two excerpts (9.3 and 9.4) show frequency distributions for data at the nominal and ordinal levels of measurements. In other words, they show the distribution of frequencies of categories (nominal level) or frequencies of rankings (ordinal level).

Excerpt 9.3 is from a study of conflict resolution abilities of children with normal language versus children with specific language impairment. The excerpt illustrates the use of a frequency distribution table for displaying the number of older and younger participants in each language group who used each one of a number of conflict resolution strategies during a role-playing exercise. The role-playing strategies are represented as the categories of a nominal dependent variable and are listed on the left side of the table. Younger and older children in each language group ($NL$ = normal language; $SLI$ = specific language impairment) constitute the four columns identified at the top of the table. The number in each cell indicates the number of children in the indicated group column who used the role-playing strategy indicated in the corresponding row. For example, seven young normal language children used the "physical" strategy (column 1, row 1) and fifteen older specific language impaired children used the "insistence" strategy (column 4, row 2). The Chi-square test in the footnote indicates that only the categories of "requests for explanation" and "reasons/moral persuasion" were used more by children with normal language than by children with specific language impairment. The Chi-square test will be illustrated with more in-depth discussion later in the chapter when we discuss examples of data analysis.

Excerpt 9.4 illustrates the use of frequency histograms to show the distribution of data for a dependent variable at the ordinal level of measurement. The example is from a study of quality judgments of speech transduced through hearing aids. The histograms show the frequency of listeners' response rankings from best to worst (1 to 5 on the abscissa) of each of five different hearing aids (labeled $A$ through $E$). The height of each bar represents the number of times each hearing aid was ranked at each position from best to worst by the listeners. Inspection of Figure 2 in Excerpt 9.4 reveals that hearing aid $E$ was most often ranked as the best aid and hearing aid $D$ was most frequently ranked as the

EXCERPT 9.3

**TABLE 10 Number of children with normal language (NL) and children with specific language impairment (SLI) who used conflict resolution strategies with role-enactment tasks**

| | NL | | SLI | |
|---|---|---|---|---|
| *Role Play Strategies* | *Young* | *Old* | *Young* | *Old* |
| Physical | 7 | 3 | 8 | 7 |
| Insistence | 15 | 15 | 14 | 15 |
| Threats/insults | 7 | 4 | 8 | 5 |
| Commands/demands | 12 | 14 | 11 | 14 |
| Assertions | 15 | 15 | 15 | 15 |
| Compliance | 9 | 6 | 5 | 11 |
| Counter | 6 | 6 | 3 | 3 |
| Mitigation/aggravation | 7 | 5 | 4 | 7 |
| Conditional | 1 | 0 | 1 | 0 |
| Compromise | 1 | 4 | 3 | 2 |
| Requests for explanation* | 10 | 15 | 7 | 8 |
| Reasons/moral persuasion** | 9 | 13 | 8 | 6 |
| Other | 9 | 12 | 13 | 12 |

$*\chi^2 = 7.50, p < 0.01; **\chi^2 = 4.44, p < 0.05.$

From "Conflict Resolution Abilities of Children with Specific Language Impairment and Children with Normal Language," by L. J. Stevens and L. S. Bliss, 1995, *Journal of Speech and Hearing Research, 38,* p. 607. Copyright 1995 by the American Speech-Language-Hearing Association. Reprinted with permission.

worst aid. Hearing aids *C, B,* and *A* received more frequent rankings in the intermediate stages between best and worst.

The frequency histograms shown in Excerpts 9.2 and 9.4 and the frequency tables shown in Excerpts 9.1 and 9.3 all show the absolute frequencies at each score, ranking, or category. Readers may also expect to encounter frequency distributions that present all data as relative frequencies, expressed as a percentage or proportion of total cases in the distribution, as shown in Excerpts 9.5, 9.6, and 9.7.

Excerpt 9.5 is from a national survey of clinicians' use of methods for assessment of children's phonemic awareness (PA) skills. Data on the absolute and relative frequency (%) of use of different methods of assessment are shown in Table 6. The absolute and relative frequency (%) of use of different formal tests by those clinicians who responded that they used formal tests (41.8 percent of survey respondents) are shown in Table 7. The different methods of assessment tabulated and the formal tests that were used are categories of two different nominal level dependent variables, and frequencies are reported for each

**EXCERPT 9.4**

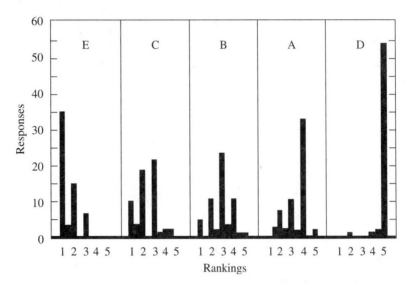

**FIGURE 2   Histograms representing frequency distributions of listener's response rankings of the aids, A through E. Each bar on the graph shows the number of times an aid was ranked in a given position, based upon the ratings across all listeners. Thirty subjects judged the aids on two different listening sessions, making 60 the total number of possible responses per aid. This figure is the responses for the female voice.**

From "Quality Judgments of Hearing Aid Transduced Speech," by H. L. Witter and D. P. Goldstein, 1971, *Journal of Speech and Hearing Research, 14,* p. 315. Copyright 1971 by the American Speech-Language-Hearing Association. Reprinted with permission.

category of use. Readers will notice that both the methods of assessment and the formal tests are listed in these tables in rank order of their frequency of use from most to least from top to bottom of the tables.

Excerpt 9.6 shows the use of a relative frequency histogram to display voice onset time (VOT) data for the voiced plosive /b/ for three groups of participants of different ages. The ordinates for the three histograms are labeled as Relative Frequency (%), and the abscissa of each histogram indicates VOT in milliseconds from –10 on the left to +30 on the right. The height of each bar in the histogram, then, does not represent the number of participants at each VOT value, but rather the percentage of participants in each group at each VOT value.

Excerpt 9.7 is from a study of otitis media with effusion and illustrates the use of a frequency polygon for displaying the percent of children at each pure tone average hearing level in each of the first three years of life. The three lines on the graph each represent the

## PA Assessment Procedures

Respondents were asked to indicate which PA assessment methods were used most frequently at their work setting (see Table 6). As can be seen, PA skills were most often assessed using a formal, standardized test (41.8%). Approximately 27% of the respondents indicated that children's PA skills were assessed using informal procedures that were developed within the work setting, but without any normative information. Approximately 20% of the respondents indicated that they used either a published criterion-referenced test or a published test without standardization information to assess children's PA skills. Only 8% of the respondents indicated the use of PA assessment procedures developed at their work setting that included locally derived normative information.

**TABLE 6  Frequency (and percentage) of respondents' report of the use of various methods of phonemic awareness (PA) assessment at their work setting.**

| Method of assessment | Frequency (%) | |
|---|---|---|
| Formal standardized test | 114 | (41.8) |
| Informal procedures without local norms | 74 | (27.1) |
| Criterion-referenced published test | 35 | (12.8) |
| Published test without standardization information | 23 | (8.4) |
| Informal procedures developed with local norms | 22 | (8.1) |
| Not assessed in my setting | 4 | (1.5) |

To obtain additional information on assessment practices, respondents were presented with a list of published tests that are currently available to assess PA and were asked to indicate all those used at their work setting. Those tests and the percentage of respondents indicating each option are presented in Table 7. The most frequently reported formal PA assessment measures included the Phonological Awareness Test (Robertson & Salter, 1995), the Lindamood Auditory Conceptualization Test (Lindamood & Lindamood, 1979), and the Test of Phonological Awareness (Torgesen & Bryant, 1994).

**TABLE 7  Frequency (and percentage) of participants reporting the use of various formal measures of phonemic awareness (PA) skills at their work setting.[a]**

| Assessment instrument | Frequency (percentage of use) | |
|---|---|---|
| Phonological Awareness Test (Robertson & Salter, 1995) | 101 | (37.0%) |
| Lindamood Auditory Conceptualization Test (Lindamood & Lindamood, 1979) | 89 | (32.6%) |
| Test of Phonological Awareness (Torgesen & Bryant, 1994) | 83 | (30.4%) |
| Comprehensive Test of Phonological Processes in Reading (Wagner & Torgesen, 1997) | 26 | (9.5%) |
| Rosner Test of Auditory Analysis (Rosner, 1975) | 25 | (9.2%) |
| Yopp-Singer Test of Phoneme Segmentation (Yopp, 1988) | 17 | (6.2%) |
| Not assessed in my setting | 3 | (1.1%) |

[a]Respondents were asked to choose all that apply.

EXCERPT  9.6

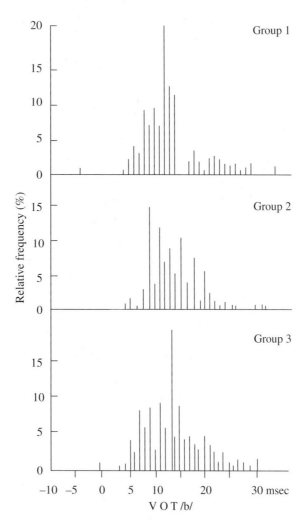

**FIGURE 1     Relative frequency distribution for all productions of /b/ for three experimental groups. Group 1, aged 25 through 39; Group 2, aged 65 through 74; Group 3, over 75.**

EXCERPT **9.7**

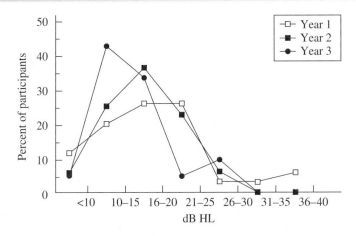

**FIGURE 1** Distribution of average hearing levels for children with OME in Years 1, 2, and 3. Data are presented according to hearing level (HL) categories in decibels (dB). Four-frequency (500, 1000, 2000, and 4000 Hz) average values displayed were derived by categorizing each participant's mean hearing levels across each study year.

From "Effects of Otitis Media with Effusion on Hearing in the First 3 Years of Life," by J. S. Gravel and I. F. Wallace, 2000, *Journal of Speech, Language, and Hearing Research, 43,* p. 638. Copyright 2000 by the American Speech-Language-Hearing Association. Reprinted with permission.

data for the children in the first, second, and third year of life and the lines plot the percent of participants who fell at each 5 dB interval of pure tone average hearing level. Because most participants clustered between <10 and 21–25 dB HL and only a few children were spread out across the range from 26–30 to 36–40 dB HL, all three distributions are positively skewed. Readers will also notice that as age increases from 1 to 3, the distributions shift further to the left indicating improved hearing in later years because the leftward shift means more of the older children had pure tone averages at the lower hearing levels.

These relative frequency distributions give a very clear picture of the distribution (central tendency and variability) of the data, but readers should be careful to note whether they are reading absolute number of participants or relative number of participants (e.g., percentage) at each score value.

Excerpt 9.8 shows the use of a table that includes both a frequency distribution and a cumulative frequency distribution of the scores of persons who stutter and normally fluent speakers on a scale of communication attitudes. Attitude scores are shown in the left-hand column, with the lower scores at the top of the table and the higher scores at the

EXCERPT 9.8

**TABLE 1    Frequency ($f$) and cumulative relative frequency ($crf$) distributions of S-scale scores in the nonstuttering and stuttering groups**

| Score | Nonstutterers ($n = 144$) | | Stutterers ($n = 120$) | |
|---|---|---|---|---|
| | $f$ | $crf$ | $f$ | $crf$ |
| 1 | 0 | 0.00 | | |
| 2 | 7 | 0.05 | | |
| 3 | 5 | 0.08 | | |
| 4 | 11 | 0.16 | | |
| 5 | 9 | 0.22 | 0 | 0.00 |
| 6 | 6 | 0.26 | 1 | 0.01 |
| 7 | 5 | 0.30 | 0 | 0.01 |
| 8 | 9 | 0.36 | 1 | 0.02 |
| 9 | 6 | 0.40 | 1 | 0.02 |
| 10 | 7 | 0.45 | 1 | 0.03 |
| 11 | 7 | 0.50 | 2 | 0.05 |
| 12 | 4 | 0.53 | 0 | 0.05 |
| 13 | 5 | 0.56 | 1 | 0.06 |
| 14 | 6 | 0.60 | 4 | 0.09 |
| 15 | 3 | 0.62 | 2 | 0.11 |
| 16 | 6 | 0.67 | 2 | 0.12 |
| 17 | 6 | 0.71 | 4 | 0.16 |
| 18 | 5 | 0.74 | 4 | 0.19 |
| 19 | 2 | 0.76 | 5 | 0.23 |
| 20 | 4 | 0.78 | 3 | 0.26 |
| 21 | 5 | 0.82 | 4 | 0.29 |
| 22 | 3 | 0.84 | 2 | 0.31 |
| 23 | 2 | 0.85 | 2 | 0.32 |
| 24 | 3 | 0.88 | 6 | 0.38 |
| 25 | 5 | 0.91 | 8 | 0.44 |
| 26 | 1 | 0.92 | 6 | 0.49 |
| 27 | 3 | 0.94 | 4 | 0.52 |
| 28 | 0 | 0.94 | 6 | 0.58 |
| 29 | 3 | 0.96 | 3 | 0.60 |
| 30 | 1 | 0.97 | 12 | 0.70 |
| 31 | 2 | 0.98 | 8 | 0.77 |
| 32 | 2 | 0.99 | 3 | 0.79 |
| 33 | 1 | 1.00 | 7 | 0.85 |
| 34 | — | — | 11 | 0.94 |
| 35 | — | — | 3 | 0.97 |
| 36 | — | — | 2 | 0.98 |
| 37 | — | — | 2 | 1.00 |
| *Mean* | 13.24 | | 26.65 | |
| SD | 8.20 | | 7.24 | |

From "Assessing Communication Attitudes among Stutterers," by R. L. Erickson, 1969, *Journal of Speech and Hearing Research, 12,* p. 719. Copyright 1969 by the American Speech-Language-Hearing Association. Reprinted with permission.

bottom of the table. The next column to the right ($f$) shows the number of normally fluent speakers who obtained each score. The next column ($crf$) shows the cumulative relative frequency (expressed as a decimal fraction of the number of participants) of the normally fluent speakers obtaining each score on the attitude scale. The next two columns on the right-hand side show the data for the persons who stutter displayed in the same format. In addition, summary statistics (means and standard deviations) are shown at the bottom of the table for both groups of participants. Inspection of the table reveals both the degree of separation and overlapping of the two groups in their scores on this communication attitude scale.

As seen in the foregoing examples, frequency distributions can be a valuable addition to the Results section, because they provide a description of the overall distribution of the data. We noted in Chapter 6 that the selection of a format for organizing the data may depend partly on the author's style and partly on the requirements of the data. Nevertheless, the format chosen should (1) present the data accurately, (2) be clearly labeled for easy reading and interpretation, and (3) relate well to the textual description of the data.

One other point should also be mentioned: the problem of accounting for missing data. Occasionally some data may be lost or not available for analysis, perhaps owing to equipment failure or failure of some participants to complete all tasks (i.e., mortality). Authors should make a point of explaining to readers what happened in the particular study to account for any missing data. They should also comment on the implications (if any) of missing data for the validity of the study. Whenever the number of data entries in tables or figures varies from the number stated in the text or varies from condition to condition, the author should explain the reason for the discrepancy in the text or, perhaps, in a footnote. Some authors may offer an explanation of missing data or fluctuations in number of scores in the Method section, whereas other authors may wait and explain discrepancies as they arise in the Results section. Again, this is usually a matter of individual style, but all authors have a responsibility to their readers to explain number discrepancies or missing data somewhere in the article.

## Summary Statistics: Central Tendency and Variability

A second way of organizing data in addition to, or instead of, the use of frequency distributions is the use of summary statistics. Summary statistics are parsimonious because they describe the overall distribution of a body of data in a simple numerical form that uses less space than does the presentation of the entire frequency distribution. Also, the summary statistics help to provide the foundation on which most analysis techniques are based, and, therefore, the selection of appropriate summary statistics is critical to appropriate analysis of the data. Most articles encountered in the communicative disorders literature present data that are organized through the use of summary statistics.

Summary statistics are used to describe the central tendency and variability of a distribution of data with a few numbers. The central tendency statistics describe what is "typical" or "average" in a distribution, and the variability statistics describe how the data spread out from the "typical" or "average" case in the distribution. In many articles, different conditions or groups of participants are compared so that summary statistics are used to organize the data for each condition or group. Later, analysis of relationships or differences will refer to the summary statistics of each condition or group for the purpose of making comparisons.

Various summary statistics are available for describing distributions, and the selection of appropriate statistics depends on such factors as the level of measurement of the data, the number of observations, and normality or skewness of the distribution. Normal or nearly normal distributions of a fairly large number of interval or ratio measurements are usually summarized by reporting the mean and standard deviations of the measurements. Lack of one or more of these data characteristics (i.e., small *N*, skewed distribution, or nominal or ordinal level of measurement) usually means that data should be summarized with the median or the mode as a measure of central tendency and some form of the range (e.g., total range or interquartile range) as a measure of variability.

In some instances, summary statistics may be included only in the textual narrative, especially if only a few numbers are presented. The more usual case, however, involves presentation of summary statistics in tabular or graphic form, or, sometimes, in both forms. Graphic presentation of summary statistics has the advantage of providing an easily viewed overall summary of results for different conditions or groups of participants. Differences between groups, changes in dependent variables as a function of changes in independent variables, or differences in performances on different measures can often be immediately impressed on the reader by a well-formulated graphic presentation of summary statistics. On the other hand, graphic figures may suffer from a disadvantage: the difficulty in locating exact values of the summary statistics for each condition or group, especially when the ordinate or the abscissa is labeled with gross intervals. Some figures are labeled only at every tenth- or fifth-score interval and interpolation of exact scores between such gross intervals may be difficult. Tabular presentation of summary statistics may be less dramatic or immediately impressive to the reader, but it does have the advantage of allowing easier retrieval of exact values of summary statistics for any group or condition.

The process of tabular and graphic presentation of summary statistics is illustrated in Excerpts 9.9 and 9.10, which show a table and a figure presenting summary statistics on the effects of listening conditions on speech recognition from two different studies.

The table in Excerpt 9.9 shows consonant identification (in percent correct) for four different age groups listening at four different sensation levels (SLs) in four different listening conditions. Each of the 64 (4 ages by 4 levels by 4 conditions) cell entries has the mean across listeners followed by the standard deviation across listeners in parentheses. In addition, at the bottom of each SL data group, the mean (and standard deviation) across the four age groups for each listening condition is tabulated. Despite the complexity of the data, the clarity and organization of this table make the data quite comprehensible.

The figure in Excerpt 9.10 shows nonsense syllable recognition scores (in percent correct) obtained in quiet and noise conditions for three groups of elderly listeners: a normal hearing group (EN), a group with hearing impairment and good word recognition (EHIG), and a group with hearing impairment and poor word recognition (EHIP). The height of each of the six bars indicates the mean performance of each group in each of the two listening conditions. The rank order of syllable recognition performance in both conditions is the same: EN followed by EHIG followed by EHIP, but the performance is clearly better in the quiet than in the noise condition for all listeners. In addition, an important feature of this bar graph is the inclusion of the standard deviations of each measure for

TABLE 1   Listeners' mean consonant identification scores and standard deviations (in parentheses) as a function of listening condition, SL, and age group

| | Listening Condition | | | | | | | |
| | Control | | Reverberation | | Noise | | Rever. + Noise | |
|---|---|---|---|---|---|---|---|---|
| **30 dB SL** | | | | | | | | |
| **Group** | | | | | | | | |
| Adults | 63.4 | (13.4) | 55.4 | (9.7) | 58.2 | (12.4) | 55.4 | (11.2) |
| 14–15 years | 58.9 | (14.3) | 47.5 | (10.3) | 51.4 | (11.4) | 46.1 | (7.5) |
| 10–11 years | 57.8 | (12.2) | 47.2 | (9.9) | 50.6 | (10.0) | 43.1 | (10.5) |
| 6–7 years | 47.5 | (13.5) | 39.2 | (13.7) | 40.7 | (12.2) | 35.9 | (9.4) |
| Mean | 56.9 | (14.7) | 47.3 | (12.5) | 50.2 | (13.2) | 45.1 | (11.0) |
| **40 dB SL** | | | | | | | | |
| **Group** | | | | | | | | |
| Adults | 74.7 | (10.4) | 62.4 | (8.2) | 62.0 | (10.3) | 53.3 | (9.7) |
| 14–15 years | 69.6 | (11.2) | 58.2 | (9.6) | 57.0 | (9.7) | 48.6 | (8.5) |
| 10–11 years | 67.1 | (11.1) | 52.2 | (9.0) | 53.9 | (10.2) | 46.2 | (11.3) |
| 6–7 years | 58.1 | (11.7) | 46.8 | (8.7) | 43.7 | (10.2) | 39.9 | (8.0) |
| Mean | 67.4 | (12.7) | 54.9 | (10.7) | 54.1 | (12.2) | 47.0 | (10.7) |
| **50 dB SL** | | | | | | | | |
| **Group** | | | | | | | | |
| Adults | 80.5 | (6.9) | 62.2 | (9.3) | 66.0 | (8.9) | 58.1 | (8.0) |
| 14–15 years | 75.4 | (10.7) | 61.0 | (9.3) | 59.6 | (8.7) | 48.6 | (7.6) |
| 10–11 years | 70.3 | (11.1) | 55.7 | (9.1) | 56.8 | (10.9) | 46.3 | (8.9) |
| 6–7 years | 61.3 | (10.3) | 50.3 | (9.9) | 46.9 | (9.5) | 42.9 | (11.2) |
| Mean | 71.9 | (12.3) | 57.3 | (10.6) | 57.3 | (11.8) | 49.0 | (10.7) |
| **60 dB SL** | | | | | | | | |
| **Group** | | | | | | | | |
| Adults | 80.1 | (7.9) | 65.3 | (8.7) | 65.7 | (8.2) | 58.3 | (7.7) |
| 14–15 years | 77.9 | (7.5) | 60.3 | (9.9) | 59.9 | (9.1) | 52.3 | (7.8) |
| 10–11 years | 72.5 | (11.4) | 57.4 | (10.4) | 55.3 | (9.4) | 45.0 | (9.0) |
| 6–7 years | 64.5 | (10.8) | 52.2 | (10.5) | 46.8 | (10.2) | 40.4 | (10.4) |
| Mean | 73.7 | (11.4) | 58.8 | (11.0) | 56.9 | (11.6) | 49.0 | (11.2) |

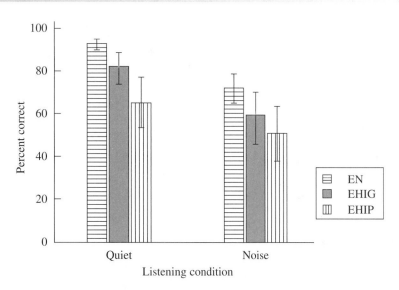

FIGURE 1    **Mean NST scores and standard deviations of the three listener groups, in quiet and noise (EN = elderly normal, EHIG = elderly listeners with hearing impairment and good word-recognition scores, EHIP = elderly listeners with hearing impairment and poor word-recognition scores).**

From "Frequency and Temporal Resolution in Elderly Listeners with Good and Poor Speech Recognition," by S. L. Phillips, S. Gordon-Salant, P. J. Fitzgibbons, and G. Yeni-Komshian, 2000, *Journal of Speech, Language, and Hearing Research, 43,* p. 223. Copyright 2000 by the American Speech-Language-Hearing Association. Reprinted with permission.

each of the three groups in each condition. The standard deviation markers are the thin lines with horizontal caps (often called *error bars*) at the top of each bar in the graph. Standard deviations are smallest for the normal hearing group and larger for the hearing impaired groups, especially for those listeners with poor speech recognition, and are somewhat smaller for the quiet than the noise conditions.

Figure 1 in Excerpt 9.11 is an illustration taken from a study of audiometry with infants that uses a line graph to present both central tendency and variability data together in one graph. The independent variable on the abscissa is signal level in dB regarding the infant's clinical threshold (*CT*) with a control condition (no sound presented) indicated on the left. The dependent variable shown on the ordinate is the mean response latency in seconds of the infant's unidirectional head turn toward a loudspeaker and adjacent reinforcer during a visual reinforcement audiometry (VRA) task. The two lines indicate the mean performance of 20 eight-month-old infants (dotted line) and 20 twelve-month-old infants (solid line)

**EXCERPT 9.11**

**Response Latency**

Figure 1 shows the average response latency at each signal level for the two age groups. The graph illustrates three important features of the data. First, latency decreased systematically with increases in near-threshold SPL. Brackets on the graph represent one standard deviation (SD) above and below mean thresholds. In general, the SDs show that intersubject variability also decreased with increasing signal level.

Second, latency means and SDs in –10 trials were equivalent to the same measures in control (C) trails. Average latency in C trials, approximately 4 sec, was predictable based on random response over a period of 8 sec. Third, latencies were equivalent between age groups. In fact, the latencies were remarkably similar considering the variability often associated with infant behavior.

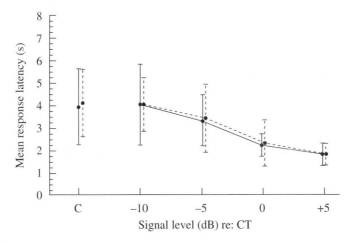

FIGURE 1    **Mean response latency values for 8-month-old (dotted line) and 12-month-old (solid line) infants under control and signal conditions. Brackets represent one standard deviation above and below mean latencies.**

From "Operant Response in Infants as a Function of Time Interval Following Signal Onset," by M. A. Primus, 1992, *Journal of Speech and Hearing Research, 35,* p. 1423. Copyright 1992 by the American Speech-Language-Hearing Association. Reprinted with permission.

under the control (no sound) and the signal (four intensity levels) conditions. The vertical bars connected to each line represent plus-or-minus one standard deviation above and below the mean for each age group at each value of the independent variable. The dotted vertical lines show the standard deviations for the eight-month-old infants, and the solid vertical lines show the standard deviations for the twelve-month-old infants. The accompanying text in the excerpt describes the pattern of data illustrated in the figure. Readers can compare the mean performance of the groups at each intensity level and also determine whether the groups differ in variability and central tendency. For example, not only does mean response latency decrease with intensity, but variability among infants does so as well.

As mentioned earlier, not all articles will contain data that will be organized with only means and standard deviations as the summary statistics. The summary statistics may be presented in the form of medians and ranges, either accompanying or replacing the means and standard deviations, because of reasons such as small sample sizes, skewed distributions, or unequal variances among participant groups or experimental conditions. Excerpt 9.12 presents a table from the Results section of a study of the durations of prolongations and repetitions of children who stutter. Nine dependent variables listed under the left-hand column are based on data gathered from recordings of fourteen children who stutter. The three data columns to the right show the mean, standard deviation (in parentheses), median, and range for each of the nine dependent variables. The medians were close to the means for some of the dependent variables, as is the case with normal distributions, but were somewhat below the means for other dependent variables, indicating some positive skewness. As mentioned earlier, summary statistics help to provide a foundation for later use of data analysis techniques for examining differences and relationships. Means and standard deviations are usually used to summarize data that will be analyzed with parametric statistics, and alternate summary statistics such as the median and range are usually employed to summarize data that will be analyzed with nonparametric statistics. The accompanying text in the excerpt describes the author's rationale for choosing the nonparametric approach; this example will be referred to again in this chapter in the section on data analysis.

Excerpt 9.13 is from a study of the Preschool Language Scale—3 (PLS-3) performance of African American children. Table 1 shows summary statistics for all four moments of the distributions—central tendency, variability, skewness, and kurtosis—for comprehension and expressive scores as well as total PLS-3 scores for both African American children and European American children. Figure 1 shows the frequency distribution displayed as a histogram for the total scores with a smoothed normal distribution polygon overlaid for comparison purposes. In addition, the summary statistics are displayed in the background field of the figure. Readers will notice that the data description in the text explains why skewness and kurtosis were computed in order to examine the normality of the distributions.

## Some Characteristics of Clear Data Organization

Results that are included in the text, table, and figures of an article should be organized in a manner that allows the reader to understand immediately the author's empirical statement regarding the problem posed in the introduction to the article. Readers should expect some of the following characteristics of clear data organization when reading the Results section of an article.

First, table and figure captions should be brief but informative, and they should quickly convey the organization of the particular illustration. After reading the caption, the reader should know immediately where to find data entries for each participant group, experimental condition, or dependent variable that is included in the illustration. The caption should act as a clear road map to direct the reader through the illustration in the most efficient manner possible. Occasionally, a complex illustration may require a longer

**EXCERPT 9.12**

**Data Analysis**

Means (with standard deviations), medians and ranges were obtained for all eight measures of speech (dis)fluency. Further, Kendall rank-order correlation coefficients (T) were calculated to allow examination of possible relationships between and among these measures, along with age and interval from reported onset. Nonparametric analyses were chosen for several reasons, most notably to avoid violating assumptions of normalcy of distribution and homogeneity of variance. Further, differences in the absolute number of sound prolongations and sound/syllable repetitions contributed by each child for analysis suggested the appropriateness of nonparametric procedures. It should be noted that prior to statistical analysis, the two measures expressed in percentage of frequencies of occurrence (i.e., frequency of disfluency and SPI) were submitted to arc-sine transformations.

**Results**

Table 1 shows the data obtained for each of the 14 children for all measures. Table 2 provides a summary of the group means (and standard deviations), medians and ranges for all measures of speech (dis)fluency.

**TABLE 2  Means (with standard deviations), medians, and ranges of measures of speech (dis)fluency obtained from 14 stuttering children**

| Measure | Mean (S.D.) | Median | Range |
| --- | --- | --- | --- |
| Duration of sound prolongation (in msec) | 706 (296) | 623 | 442–1063 |
| Duration of sound/syllable repetitions | 724 (145) | 720 | 403–1003 |
| Number of repeated units per instance of sound/syllable repetition | 2.45 (.53) | 2.25 | 2.0–3.8 |
| Rate of repetition per instance of sound/syllable repetition (in repetitions per sec) | 3.48 (.923) | 3.30 | 2.2–5.7 |
| Frequency of speech disfluency per 100 words | 19.9% (10.17) | 16.0% | 10–49% |
| SPI | 46% (.20) | 45% | 3–79% |
| Overall speech rate (in words per minute) | 107 (22.8) | 107 | 51–142 |
| Articulatory rate (in words per minute) | 141.12 (22.7) | 140.32 | 107–184.5 |
| Articulatory rate (in syllables per second) | 2.73 (.419) | 2.72 | 2.09–3.4 |

caption. There is nothing wrong with a lengthy caption *per se* as long as it is clearly written and the length is justifiable in helping the reader to understand the illustration. The Information for Authors page of every issue of *JSLHR* emphasizes the importance of captions by stating:

> Table titles and figure captions should be concise but explanatory. The reader should not have to refer to the text to decipher the information.

EXCERPT   9.13

## Results

TABLE 1   Distribution properties of the PLS-3 for African American and European American children.

|  | African American children (n = 701) | | | European American children (n = 50) | | |
|---|---|---|---|---|---|---|
|  | PLS-3 Auditory Comprehension standard score | PLS-3 Expressive Communication standard score | PLS-3 Total score | PLS-3 Auditory Comprehension standard score | PLS-3 Expressive Communication standard score | PLS-3 Total score |
| M | 86.17 | 88.61 | 86.09 | 88.62 | 89.96 | 88.20 |
| SD | 12.67 | 12.58 | 12.79 | 11.41 | 14.30 | 13.24 |
| Median | 86 | 87 | 85 | 90 | 87 | 85 |
| Range | 54–139 | 56–134 | 52–141 | 67–124 | 65–132 | 66–131 |
| Skewness | .56 | .62 | .46 | .44 | .84 | .81 |
| Kurtosis | 1.08 | .39 | .49 | .69 | .46 | .94 |

*Note.* PLS-3 = Preschool Language Scale—3.

### Distribution Properties

Distribution properties for the PLS-3 Total, Auditory Comprehension, and Expressive Communication scores by ethnicity are presented in Table 1. In addition, Figure 1 shows the distribution of PLS-3 Total scores for the 701 African American children. The mean for the African American sample was 86.09, with a standard deviation of 12.79. The mean for the African American sample was approximately 1 $SD$ below the standardized sample ($M = 100$, $SD = 15$). The median score was 85. This 14-point difference from the normative mean is statistically significant, $t(700) = -28.92$, $p < .001$. Eighty-seven percent of the African American children in this sample scored below the normative sample mean of 100. Fifty-two percent of African American children scored more than 1 $SD$ below this mean. Based on a conservative cutoff of 2 $SD$ below the normative mean as an indicator of language delay (i.e., standard score = 70), 10% of the children in the African American sample showed signs of a significant language delay. An independent $t$ test indicated that the PLS-3 Total scores of the African American children were not significantly different from those of the European American children from similar SES backgrounds, $t(749) = -1.76$, $p = .77$.

In order to test whether the distribution of PLS-3 scores within this sample deviated from normality, particularly because of a floor effect, we examined skewness and kurtosis values. As shown in Table 1, the skewness value of .46 and kurtosis value of .49 for the PLS-3 Total scores of the African American sample were both quite close to zero, indicating a relatively normal distribution of scores. Only the kurtosis value for the PLS-3 Auditory Comprehension scores exceeded 1.0 (kurtosis = 1.08). Skewness and kurtosis values for the normative sample are not provided in the technical manual of the PLS-3. We therefore compared skewness and kurtosis values in the African American sample to those obtained in the smaller European American sample. Our findings showed that the skewness and kurtosis values were generally similar across the two groups.

**FIGURE 1    Frequency distribution of PLS-3 Total scores**

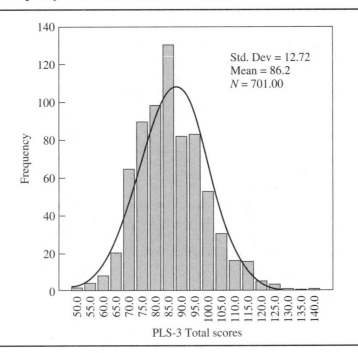

From "The Performance of Low-Income African American Children on the Preschool Language Scale—3," by C. H. Qi, A. P. Kaiser, S. E. Milan, Z. Yzquierdo, and T. B. Hancock, 2003, *Journal of Speech, Language, and Hearing Research, 46,* pp. 580–581. Copyright 2003 by the American Speech-Language-Hearing Association. Reprinted with permission.

Readers should expect the table titles and figure captions that they read to be prepared according to this statement. There should also be a key either in the caption or in the field of a figure that identifies the meaning of the symbols used in the figure. For example, the figure in Excerpt 9.11 includes solid and dotted lines, and the figure's caption indicates which line refers to which age group. In Excerpt 9.10, a key is set in the field of the graph that identifies which bar refers to which participant group. Readers should expect to find such keys in either the caption or the field of a figure to provide ready understanding of the organization of the figure.

Second, each table or figure should be capable of standing alone as an illustration of the results. That is, the table should be sufficiently clear and complete so that the reader can spend some time studying it without having to refer constantly to the text to understand it. The text may summarize and analyze the results in the illustration, but the illustration should be well constructed so that it can act as an independent display of the results. If the reader has great difficulty understanding an illustration without constantly referring back to the text to make sense of the illustration, there is probably something wrong with its construction.

Third, a good illustration should dovetail with the description of the data in the text. The textual narrative should contain references to the illustrations, usually in consecutive order of presentation. This narrative will often summarize overall patterns of results and may mention specific values of data in the illustration. The text and illustrations should be parallel in the results presentation so that the reader does not have to jump back and forth in the Results section to understand the organization of the results in relation to the research problem. A clear Results section contains a narrative with tables and figures integrated into the text so that the flow of the narrative is not interrupted awkwardly by the references to illustrations.

A fourth point is that figures should be accurately proportioned so that the visual impression created for the reader actually reflects the data. Fortunately, the editorial boards of professional journals usually scrutinize figures to ensure accurate representation of results. Nonetheless, readers should be sure that values represented in tables or text are carefully presented in figures so that the overall effect is not a distortion of actual data values.

Finally, tables and figures should be as consistent and complete as possible. All available data or summary statistics should be displayed in similar manner for all groups or conditions to facilitate within-subjects and between-subjects comparisons. Consistency of tabular entries or graphic configurations are important for meaningful comparisons between such elements as experimental and control groups. Once a particular organization has been set up, readers should be able to follow it through different illustrations in an efficient manner. If it is necessary for an author to change the organization in presenting a large number of illustrations, the new organization should be clearly described so that readers are not confused by the change.

Many research articles present only descriptive statistics to organize the data with no further analysis included in the Results section. There may be a variety of reasons for an author's decision to exclude the analysis techniques. For example, the descriptive statistics used to organize the data may show such striking differences or lack of differences that further data analysis might only belabor the obvious. Or the research questions might have been phrased in such a way that descriptive measures of central tendency and variability would suffice for answering them. In any case, consumers of research should be aware that they may encounter articles that present only a descriptive organization of the data and that this may be entirely appropriate in many cases.

## Analysis of Data

Once the data of a study have been organized so that readers may peruse them to grasp the pattern of results in relation to the original research problem, certain statistical procedures may be employed to analyze the results. These statistical procedures may be generally classified as the analysis of relationships and the analysis of differences, although these two kinds of analysis may overlap somewhat, as pointed out in Chapter 6. This section will begin with examples of data analysis using correlational statistics to examine relationships among variables and then proceed to examples of data analysis using inferential statistics (also called significance tests) to examine differences between groups or conditions.

## Correlational Analysis

Researchers often wish to examine (1) the strength and direction of relationships among two or more variables and (2) the manner in which performance on one variable may be predicted from performance on another variable. The first examination is accomplished through the calculation of correlation coefficients and the plotting of scattergrams (also called scatterplots), and the second examination is accomplished through the use of regression analysis. Correlation and regression are intimately related statistical procedures that are often completed together as one analysis package to examine relationships among variables. Some researchers, however, complete only one of the two analyses because they may be more interested in the strength and direction of the relationship than in predicting performance on one variable from another (or vice versa).

Correlation and regression analysis may be done in the relatively simple case of the relationship between two variables or it may be attempted for the more complicated case of the relationships among several variables. We will begin with examples of bivariate correlation and regression analysis to show how the results can be presented in a journal article and then progress to more complicated multivariate examples.

As mentioned in Chapter 6, the scattergram graphically depicts the relationship between two variables by showing the intersection point of the two measurements for each participant. If the two variables are positively correlated, participants would tend to have high scores on both measures, medium scores on both measures, or low scores on both measures so that the pattern of dots on the scattergram slopes upward to the right of the graph. If the two variables are negatively related, participants who score high on one variable tend to have low scores on the other variable so that the pattern of dots on the scattergram slopes downward to the right of the graph. Uncorrelated variables result in a scattergram that has dots spread around the graph in no particular order.

The strength of the relationship between the two variables can be roughly observed in the scattergram. A tight clustering of the dots around the center of an upward sloping pattern indicates a strong positive correlation, whereas a more diffuse pattern of dots spread around the center of an upward sloping pattern indicates a weaker positive correlation. By the same token, the clustering or dispersion of the dots around the center of a downward sloping pattern indicates the strength or weakness of a negative correlation.

Excerpt 9.14 includes two scattergrams that depict the relationship between objective and subjective speech intelligibility scores indexed with the rationalized arc-sine unit (RAU) transform, a procedure often used to transform proportional or percentage scores into a format that is more suitable for statistical data analysis. Listeners' ability to understand speech was measured with an objective transcription procedure and a subjective scaling procedure, and each listener contributed multiple listening trials to the data pool with different listening passages.

The first scattergram in the excerpt (Figure 2) shows data from a group of twenty-eight persons with normal hearing who listened to speech at several different signal-to-babble

## EXCERPT 9.14

The data comprised two objective intelligibility scores and two corresponding subjective intelligibility estimates for 28 subjects. To homogenize the variances of these percentage data, all values were transformed into rationalized arcsine units (raus) before analysis as Studebaker (1985) described. The scale for rationalized arcsine units extends from –23 to 123. Values in the range from 20 to 80 are within about one unit of the corresponding percentage score.

Figure 2 illustrates the relationship between the objective and subjective intelligibility data for normal hearers. Each symbol depicts one pair of scores. There are two pairs of scores per subject. Despite some individual variation, and one aberrant subject shown by the open squares, these data are well described by the diagonal line, suggesting that objective and subjective intelligibility scores were essentially equal for these listeners. The linear correlation coefficient between subjective and objective scores was .82 (this correlation was .87 if the aberrant subject was excluded from the analysis).

. . . . . . . . . . . .

The speech intelligibility data consisted of 4–6 pairs of objective and subjective scores per subject. Figure 10 illustrates the relationship between subjective and objective scores. Each symbol depicts one pair of scores. The correlation between the two types of scores was .85; the regression line is shown.

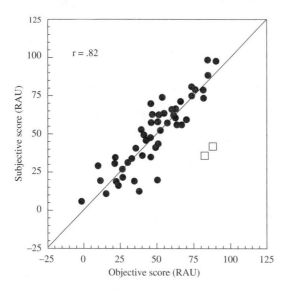

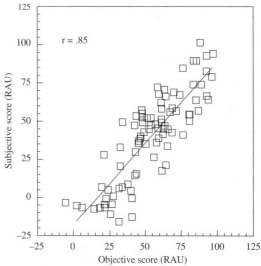

**FIGURE 2**   **Objective and subjective intelligibility data for 28 normal-hearing listeners. Each symbol depicts one pair of scores. There are two pairs of scores per subject.**

**FIGURE 10**   **Objective and subjective intelligibility data for 15 hearing-impaired listeners, 13 of them from the group depicted in Figure 4. Each symbol depicts one pair of scores.**

ratios in order to provide a range of speech intelligibility scores. Each filled circle represents a pair of intelligibility scores (one objective and one subjective). The diagonal line indicates where all circles would have fallen if the correlation were perfect (i.e., an $r$ of +1.00) and if the regression equation had a slope of 1.00 and a $y$-intercept of 0, indicating the same score on both the objective and subjective intelligibility measures. This diagonal line is not the regression line of the actual data but is used for comparative purposes to show how close the score pairs are to being identical for each subject. The correlation is indicated in the field as $r = 0.82$, a strong positive correlation. Also note the authors' comments that all the data were clustered fairly close to the diagonal, except for one participant whose performance appeared to be aberrant (open squares in the scattergram); if that participant's scores were eliminated, the $r$ would have been slightly higher (+0.87). The second figure in the excerpt shows the scattergram for a group of hearing-impaired listeners and includes the correlation coefficient (+0.85) and the actual regression line drawn in the scattergram for these data. The two scattergrams and correlations reveal that the strength and direction of the relationship between objective and subjective intelligibility scores were similar for the hearing-impaired and normal-hearing listeners.

Excerpt 9.15 shows the results of a detailed correlation and regression analysis of the relationships among auditory and phonatory variables. The abstract explains the methods of measuring and comparing the auditory and phonatory variables, and textual excerpt and figure show the detailed results of the regression analysis. Each panel in the figure is a scattergram demonstrating the relationship between a different auditory measure on each abscissa and the two laryngeal reaction time measures (LRT) on the ordinate. The data points for BLRT and an auditory measure are indicated in each scattergram by filled squares, and the data points for MLRT and an auditory measure are indicated in each scattergram by open squares. Each scattergram has two regression lines drawn through it, one for BLRT and one for MLRT prediction from each auditory measure. The dark lines are for regression equations associated with correlations significantly above zero and the light line for a regression equation associated with a correlation not found to be significantly above zero. The keys on the right of each panel show the regression equations for each prediction, the $R$-square (percentage of shared variance), and the probability that the correlation is above zero. Note the detailed description presented in the figure caption, which is necessary because of the sheer volume of information presented in the figure.

Not all relationships are fit best with a linear regression equation. Sometimes the relationship between two variables is curvilinear and the regression equation that best fits the data and predicts the dependent variable from the independent variable is a formula for generating a curve such as a quadratic, logarithmic, or exponential function. Excerpt 9.16 shows data from a study of developmental phonological disorders, plotting percentage of consonants produced correctly by normally developing children (open circles) and children with delays (filled circles) against a normalized relative age measure. The ages of development for early-, middle-, and late-developing sounds for both groups were indexed relative to age of early developing sounds for normal-developing children to derive a new independent variable called *relative age*. The figure shows the curvilinear regression equation for predicting percentage correct consonant production (dependent variable) from the relative age measure (independent variable) and also indicates the $r^2$ derived from the

## EXCERPT 9.15

Interaction between auditory and phonatory systems was explored in normal speakers by comparing laryngeal reaction time (LRT) with interpeak intervals from the auditory brainstem response (ABR) obtained using high and low stimulus presentation rates. Thirty-four subjects with no history of neurological or speech-language disorders and normal hearing sensitivity participated. Interpeak intervals were derived from ABR's recorded for each ear at rates of 21.1 and 91.1 clicks/s. LRT responses were obtained by instructing subjects to sustain an /s/ and then phonate an /a/ as fast as possible following visual cues. Two measures of reaction time performance were derived, Mean Laryngeal Reaction Time (MLRT) and Best Laryngeal Reaction Time (BLRT). Linear regression analyses were completed between each measure of reaction time performance

and each ABR interpeak interval. Using either LRT measure, two significant ($p < .05$) positive linear relationships were found. One involved the interpeak interval between Waves III and V and the other involved the interpeak interval between Waves I and V. Both were recorded at high stimulus presentation rates. These results support the small body of literature from normal speakers, stutterers, and spasmodic dysphonics suggesting interaction between the auditory and phonatory systems at the brainstem level.

. . . . . . . . . . . .

Figure 1 displays the following: (a) the individual data points ($n = 25$) for the dependent variables BLRT and MLRT and the independent variable IPI III–V L90, and the lines of best fit; (b) the individual

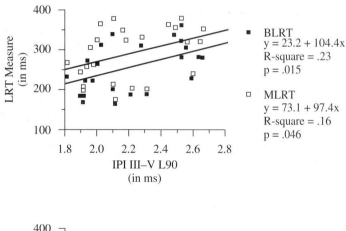

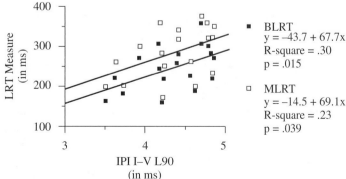

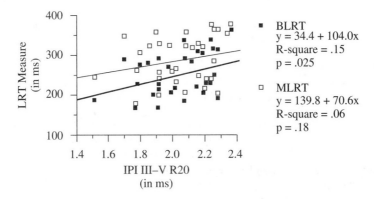

**FIGURE 1** The upper graph illustrates the lines of best fit for the individual data points (*n* = 25) of the dependent variables of BLRT (dark squares) and MLRT (open squares) in ms versus the independent variable of ABR interpeak interval IPI III–V L90 in ms. The middle graph illustrates the lines of best fit for the individual data points (*n* = 19) of the dependent variables of BLRT (dark squares) and MLRT (open squares) in ms versus the independent variable of ABR interpeak interval IPI I–V L90 in ms. The lower graph illustrates the lines of best fit for the individual data points (*n* = 33) of the dependent variables of BLRT (dark squares) and MLRT (open squares) in ms versus the independent variable of ABR interpeak interval IPI III–V R20 in ms. The linear relationship between MLRT and the ABR measure did not reach statistical significance, so the line is lighter than for the relationship between BLRT and the ABR measure. The regression equation, the *R*-square value, and the level of significance between the two variables are written underneath the dependent variable name, to the right of each graph.

data points (*n* = 19) for the dependent variables BLRT and MLRT and the independent variable IPI I–V L90, and the lines of best fit; and (c) the individual data points (*n* = 33) for the dependent variables BLRT and MLRT and the independent variable IPI III–V R20, and the lines of best fit.

As can be seen from Figure 1, the slopes of the linear relationships were positive, meaning that longer ABR interpeak intervals predicted poorer LRT performance (i.e., longer BLRTs or MLRTs) and shorter ABR interpeak intervals predicted better LRT performance (i.e., shorter BLRTs or MLRTs).

## EXCERPT  9.16

Figure 7 is a plot of the resulting fit for the regression equation along with unconnected plots for the age-shifted percentage of consonants correct data from Figure 6. The resulting equation accounts for a decisively high 93.3% of the variance, with a standard error of 6.83%. By traditional statistical criteria, it appears to be appropriate to claim that this equation and its corresponding fit provide a valid characterization of speech-sound normalization in both normal and speech-delayed children. The trend in Figure 7 is consistent with the position that there is a single course of normalization for both groups of children, differing only in temporal markers among the three speech-sound classes and between group assignment. This finding is markedly consistent with the first of the three hypotheses about speech-sound development proposed by Bishop and Edmundson (1987) and the findings of Curtiss, Katz, and Tallal (1992) for syntax.

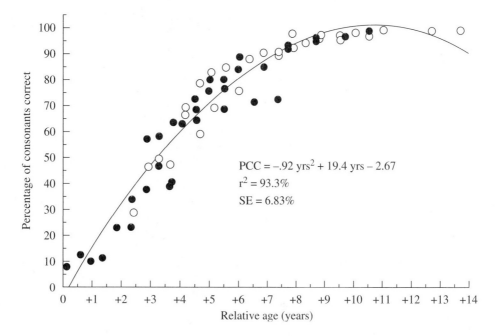

**FIGURE 7    Regression analysis of the age-shifted percentage of consonants correct data in Figure 6.**

correlation between $X$ and $Y$ (i.e., the percentage of shared variance between $X$ and $Y$) and the standard error of the prediction from the regression equation.

Excerpt 9.17 contains a table and three scattergrams that illustrate the use of the Spearman correlation with rank-order data in a study of vocal characteristics and male–female quality of the voice. Rank-order data were used in the analysis of the relationships among three variables: rating of male–female voice quality, fundamental frequency of the voice, and vocal tract resonance. Spearman rank-order correlations (rhos) are entered in the table for each of the three pairings of the variables: male–female voice quality with fundamental frequency, male–female voice quality with vocal tract resonance, and fundamental frequency with vocal tract resonance. These three relationships are indicated under the table heading "Comparison." The three columns of Spearman rhos include the correlations calculated for male speakers only, female speakers only, and male and female speakers combined. These same relationships are also depicted in the corresponding scattergrams. Male data are indicated by filled circles and female data are indicated by the open circles. The correlations for male and female data combined correspond to the entire scattergram for each variable pair.

The correlations of male–female voice quality with fundamental frequency are the highest ones, and the scattergram in Figure 2 depicts these correlations and shows the tightest clustering of the pattern of dots. In fact, the dot pattern clusters more tightly for the females than for the males, and the correlation for the female speakers only is higher than the correlation for male speakers only. The correlation for male and female data combined is highest of all because this correlation is based on a larger number of observations with a greater range of scores on both variables. The correlations of male–female voice quality with vocal tract resonance and of vocal tract resonance with fundamental frequency are much lower, and a more widely dispersed pattern of dots can be seen in Figures 3 and 4 in Excerpt 9.17, which are the corresponding scattergrams for these correlations. Significance of all the correlations is indicated by the asterisks in Table 1 that identify those correlations that were significantly different from zero at the 0.01 level. Readers should find it a relatively simple matter to compare the correlations and scattergrams for each pair of variables for each group because of the effective manner in which the correlational analysis has been displayed.

The Pearson correlations shown earlier were computed from interval or ratio level data, and the Spearman correlations (Excerpt 9.17) were computed from ordinal level data. It was mentioned in Chapter 6, that correlational analysis may be performed with nominal level data through the use of the $\chi^2$ statistic to evaluate the significance of the association between nominal level variables. Excerpt 9.18 illustrates this use of $\chi^2$. In this example, the authors investigate the relationship between adolescents' knowledge of the nouns in unfamiliar proverbs and comprehension of the proverbs. The excerpt shows tabulated data for performance of three age groups on a proverb comprehension test (PCT) and a word knowledge test (WKT). The text in the excerpt explains the scoring of the WKT and PCT and how these were arranged as nominal variables in the contingency tables for each age group. Chi-square results are then reported indicating significant relationships between word knowledge and proverb comprehension for each age group.

TABLE 1    Spearman rank-order correlation coefficients (RHOs) between degree of male-female voice quality (M-F voice quality), fundamental frequency ($F_0$), and vocal tract resonances (VTR)

| | Rhos | | |
|---|---|---|---|
| Comparison | Males and Females | Males Only | Females Only |
| M-F voice quality with $F_0$ | 0.94* | 0.65* | 0.88* |
| M-F voice quality with VTR | 0.59* | 0.00 | 0.27 |
| VTR with $F_0$ | 0.56* | 0.14 | 0.17 |

*$p < 0.01$.

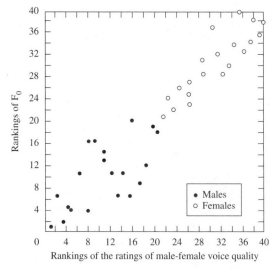

FIGURE 2    Rankings of listener ratings of degree of male-female voice quality compared with rankings of fundamental frequency.

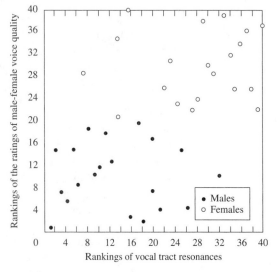

FIGURE 3    Rankings of individual vocal tract resonances compared with rankings of listener ratings of degree of male-female voice quality.

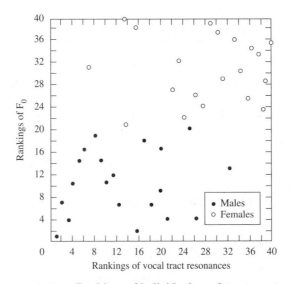

**FIGURE 4   Rankings of individual vocal tract resonances compared with rankings of fundamental frequency.**

Many studies examine the relationships among several variables simultaneously rather than just two at a time; that is, they are multiple correlation studies rather than bivariate. In this case, correlation coefficients are calculated for all possible combinations of two variables and are displayed in a correlation matrix that lists all variables down the vertical axis and across the horizontal axis of the table. The correlation coefficient for each pair is entered in the cell of the table that represents the intersection of the two variables, one from the vertical and one from the horizontal list. Discussion of the results may then center on the relative strength of the relationships among various pairs of variables. In addition, regression analysis may be done using various combinations of independent variables in a single regression equation to predict a given dependent variable listed in the matrix. A multiple correlation matrix and accompanying multiple regression analysis is exemplified by the study of the relationships among several acoustic measures and speech intelligibility that is shown in Excerpt 9.19. The excerpt displays text describing the correlational analysis, a table of regression data, and the intercorrelation matrix for a set of independent variables that are acoustic characteristics used to predict the dependent variable of speech intelligibility. The text describes how the regression analysis selected the four best independent variables for predicting the speech intelligibility variable, and Table 5 shows which variables were selected, the slope and intercept coefficients to be entered in

Given the statistically significant correlation coefficients obtained between abstract proverbs and abstract nouns, it was of interest to examine the relationship between students' comprehension of specific proverbs and their knowledge of the key words contained in those same expressions. Accordingly, students' comprehension of each of the 10 abstract proverbs was examined in relation to their knowledge of the corresponding nouns. Recall that on the PCT, a student could earn a score of 0 or 1 for each proverb, and that on the WKT, a student could earn 0, 1, or 2 points on the nouns in that proverb. For example, for the expression, "Envy is destroyed by true friendship," a score of 0 or 1 could be earned for the proverb, and scores of 0 or 1 could be earned for each word (*envy, friendship*), yielding up to 2 points for the key vocabulary. Using the frequencies with which each of those scores occurred, a $2 \times 3$ (proverb $\times$ word) contingency table was constructed for each group (see Figure 1), and a chi-square test was performed to examine the association between comprehension of abstract proverbs and knowledge of key words in them. The results were statistically significant for all three groups [Age 12: chi-square (2) = 15.39, $p < .001$; Age 15: chi-square (2) = 13.45, $p < .001$; Age 18: chi-square (2) = 22.87, $p < .001$].

| Age 12 | | Words | | | |
|---|---|---|---|---|---|
| **Proverb** | | **0** | **1** | **2** | **Total** |
| **0** | | 35 | 106 | 101 | 242 |
| **1** | | 20 | 87 | 151 | 258 |
| **Total** | | 55 | 193 | 252 | 500 |

| Age 15 | | Words | | | |
|---|---|---|---|---|---|
| **Proverb** | | **0** | **1** | **2** | **Total** |
| **0** | | 11 | 47 | 109 | 167 |
| **1** | | 9 | 58 | 266 | 333 |
| **Total** | | 20 | 105 | 375 | 500 |

| Age 18 | | Words | | | |
|---|---|---|---|---|---|
| **Proverb** | | **0** | **1** | **2** | **Total** |
| **0** | | 4 | 24 | 70 | 98 |
| **1** | | 4 | 37 | 361 | 402 |
| **Total** | | 8 | 61 | 431 | 500 |

**FIGURE 1   Contingency tables reporting the frequency with which abstract proverbs were interpreted correctly or incorrectly in relation to the number of words understood.**

From "How Adolescents Comprehend Unfamiliar Proverbs: The Role of Top-Down and Bottom-Up Processes," by M. A. Nippold, M. M. Allen, and D. I. Kirsch, 2000, *Journal of Speech, Language, and Hearing Research, 43,* p. 627. Copyright 2000 by the American Speech-Language-Hearing Association. Reprinted with permission.

### Analysis

All acoustic measures were incorporated into a multiple regression framework to determine which acoustic measures or combination of measures accounted significantly for the variance in the perceptual intelligibility measures. The potential predictor (independent) variables in the multivariate analysis were the seven acoustic measures (e.g., voice onset time, vowel duration). The criterion or predicted (dependent) variables were the intelligibility percentages. The intelligibility percentage scores were converted to arcsine values prior to the analysis. An all possible subsets regression analysis program was employed (Dixon, 1981). This regression analysis examines subsets of varying size (subset size is the number of independent variables included in the equation), so that the "best" subset of predictor variables can be determined. In addition, this procedure allows the investigator to specify the identity and the ordering of predictor variables entered into the equation.

### Results

By regression analysis, it was determined that 62.6% of the variance in the phonemic intelligibility scores was accounted for by four variables: fricative-affricative contrast, front-back vowel contrast, high-low vowel contrast, and tense-lax vowel contrast. Table 5 presents these subset data. Included are $R^2$, the square of the correlation between the dependent variable $y$ and the predicted value of $y$, and adjusted $R^2$.

The inter-correlation matrix is given in Table 6. The four variables that comprised this "best" subset yielded a multiple correlation of 0.79 with the measured intelligibility scores.

The all-possible-subsets approach allowed a critical comparison of the data provided for subsets with combinations of one through seven variables. The addition of variables beyond four did not result in an appreciable increase in predictive efficiency. The subset containing all given acoustic variables (equivalent to the full equation multiple regression analysis with all dependent variables entered) accounted for 62.9% of the variance. Practical clinical and theoretical concerns did not warrant the addition of three contrast variables for an increase of only 0.3% of the variance.

The large multiple correlation between speech intelligibility and four acoustic aspects of speech, the fricative-affricate contrast and the three vowel contrasts, indicated that these four factors strongly influence intelligibility. A general conclusion of this research relating acoustic factors to word intelligibility is that the vowel parameters of duration and F1 and F2 formant locations, and the fricative-affricate durational parameters, are major predictors of the scored intelligibility of speech.

**TABLE 5**  **Multiple regression analysis: Squared multiple correlation ($R^2$), adjusted $R^2$, Mallows' Cp, coefficient of each variable, and $t$ statistic for the best subset of predictor variables**

| $R^2$ | Adjusted $R^2$ | CP |
|---|---|---|
| 0.626155 | 0.490211 | 2.08 |

| Variable | Coefficient | $T$ statistic |
|---|---|---|
| fric.-affr. | 0.520324 | 2.29 |
| front-back | −0.172504 | −2.80 |
| high-low | 0.0874958 | 1.38 |
| tense-lax | −0.283510 | −2.68 |
| intercept | 169.448 | |

*(continued)*

E X C E R P T   **9.19**   **Continued**

**TABLE 6**   **Correlations between acoustic value for each contrast (voice-voiceless initial, voice-voiceless final, stop-nasal, fricative-affricate, front-back vowel, high-low vowel, tense-lax vowel, and intelligibility)**

|  |  | vvic | vvfc | snc | fac | fbv | hlv | tlv | int |
|---|---|---|---|---|---|---|---|---|---|
|  |  | *1* | *2* | *3* | *4* | *5* | *6* | *7* | *8* |
| vvic | 1 | 1.000 |  |  |  |  |  |  |  |
| vvfc | 2 | − 0.223 | 1.000 |  |  |  |  |  |  |
| snc | 3 | − 0.530 | 0.703 | 1.000 |  |  |  |  |  |
| fac | 4 | 0.214 | − 0.080 | − 0.322 | 1.000 |  |  |  |  |
| fbv | 5 | 0.449 | − 0.456 | − 0.307 | 0.377 | 1.000 |  |  |  |
| hlv | 6 | − 0.337 | 0.461 | 0.228 | − 0.309 | − 0.589 | 1.000 |  |  |
| tlv | 7 | − 0.087 | 0.745 | 0.472 | 0.344 | − 0.153 | 0.263 |  |  |
| int | 8 | − 0.238 | − 0.010 | − 0.187 | − 0.031 | − 0.574 | 0.408 | − 0.214 | 1.000 |

From "Acoustic-Phonetic Contrasts and Intelligibility in the Dysarthria Associated with Mixed Cerebral Palsy," by B. M. Ansel and R. D. Kent, 1992, *Journal of Speech and Hearing Research, 35,* pp. 303–304. Copyright 1992 by the American Speech-Language-Hearing Association. Reprinted with permission.

the regression equation for each independent variable, and the resultant $R^2$ statistics. Table 6 shows the intercorrelation matrix, which presents the Pearson correlations for all the possible pairings of the variables.

Excerpt 9.20 shows a similar intercorrelation matrix, but the correlations entered in Table 3 of the excerpt are not Pearson correlations. Each correlation coefficient is a Kendall's rank-order Tau, a nonparametric correlation calculated from ordinal data that is very similar to the Spearman Rho illustrated in Excerpt 9.17. The textual excerpt describes why a nonparametric approach was used and indicates that the discussion of the results will emphasize the relative strengths of the relationships among the disfluency measures and the age and onset interval data. The emphasis in this excerpt is on the strength and direction of the various relationships rather than on prediction of one variable from a combination of other variables.

In some cases, the emphasis in presenting the results of the correlational analysis is placed more squarely on the prediction equation, especially when an important practical implication of the research concerns the prediction of one variable from another. Excerpt 9.21 displays a table taken from a study of the relationships among thresholds at various pure-tone frequencies and speech reception thresholds (SRT). This table shows the correlations between predicted SRT and actual SRT (i.e., the multiple correlations) for each combination of predictor variables. The table also displays the regression equations for predicting SRT from each combination of pure-tone thresholds. A separate listing of these correlations and regression equations is made for each of the different audiometric configurations. Three sets of equations are included: zero-order, first-order, and second-order.

## EXCERPT 9.20

### Data Analysis

Means (with standard deviations), medians and ranges were obtained for all eight measures of speech (dis)fluency. Further, Kendall rank-order correlation coefficients (T) were calculated to allow examination of possible relationships between and among these measures, along with age and interval from reported onset. Nonparametric analyses were chosen for several reasons, most notably to avoid violating assumptions of normalcy of distribution and homogeneity of variance. Further, differences in the absolute number of sound prolongations and sound/syllable repetitions contributed by each child for analysis suggested the appropriateness of nonparametric procedures. It should be noted that prior to statistical analysis, the two measures expressed in percentage of frequencies of occurrence (i.e., frequency of disfluency and SPI) were submitted to arc-sine transformations.

. . . . . . . . . . . .

### Correlational Analysis

Table 3 presents Kendall rank-order correlation coefficients between mean age, interval between reported onset of stuttering and data collection, and eight measures of speech (dis)fluency for the stuttering children (N = 14) who participated in this study.

Eleven correlations were statistically significant at the .05 level or better. The main purpose of using correlational analyses with these data was to observe and describe relationships between and among specific (non)speech behaviors as a way of uncovering salient behaviors for future research. Therefore, because of the descriptive nature of this study, adjusted alphas were not used. The remainder of this section will be devoted to a discussion of the 11 correlations which reached significance.

**TABLE 3    Kendall Rank-Order Correlation Coefficients (T) between age, interval from onset, and measures of (dis)fluent speech**

|          | Age | Interval | SP  | SSR  | Units | Rate  | FREQ | SPI  | OVER   | ARTIC |
|----------|-----|----------|-----|------|-------|-------|------|------|--------|-------|
| Age      | —   | .49*     | .36 | −.14 | .23   | .11   | .24  | .26  | −.12   | .17   |
| Interval | —   | —        | .12 | −.05 | .26   | .07   | .25  | .22  | −.23   | .01   |
| SP       | —   | —        | —   | .05  | .09   | .01   | .31  | .45* | −.54** | −.42* |
| SSR      | —   | —        | —   | —    | .18   | −.42* | .02  | .01  | −.16   | −.02  |
| UNITS    | —   | —        | —   | —    | —     | .41*  | −.15 | −.15 | .04    | .20   |
| RATE     | —   | —        | —   | —    | —     | —     | −.23 | −.07 | .28    | .12   |
| FREQ     | —   | —        | —   | —    | —     | —     | —    | .47* | −.45*  | −.24  |
| SPI      | —   | —        | —   | —    | —     | —     | —    | —    | −.49** | −.43* |
| OVER     | —   | —        | —   | —    | —     | —     | —    | —    | —      | .71** |
| ARTIC    | —   | —        | —   | —    | —     | —     | —    | —    | —      | —     |

*Note.* SP = Mean duration of sound prolongations; SSR = Mean duration of sound/syllable repetitions; Units = Mean number of repeated units per instance of sound/syllable repetition; Rate = Mean rate of repetition per instance of sound/syllable repetition; Freq = Mean frequency of speech disfluency in 100 words; SPI = Sound Prolongation Index; Over = Overall speech rate in wpm; Artic = Articulatory rate in sps.

$*p < 0.05$

$**p < 0.01$

From "Duration of Sound Prolongation and Sound/Syllable Repetition in Children Who Stutter: Preliminary Observations," by P. M. Zebrowski, 1994, *Journal of Speech and Hearing Research, 37,* pp. 257 & 259. Copyright 1994 by the American Speech-Language-Hearing Association. Reprinted with permission.

EXCERPT   9.21

TABLE 7    Coefficients of correlation and regression equations for prediction of speech reception threshold (SRT) from pure-tone thresholds (T's) for six groups classified according to audiometric pattern*

| Classification | Coefficient | SRT = Regression Equation |
|---|---|---|
| *Zero-Order* | $r$ | |
| Flat | 0.975 | $0.4 \text{ dB} + 0.94 \, T_{1000}$ |
| Gradual | 0.931 | $3.4 \text{ dB} + 0.84 \, T_{1000}$ |
| Marked | 0.873 | $12.0 \text{ dB} + 0.87 \, T_{500}$ |
| Rising | 0.929 | $0.0 \text{ dB} + 0.92 \, T_{1000}$ |
| Trough | 0.951 | $-10.6 \text{ dB} + 1.03 \, T_{1000}$ |
| Atypical | 0.882 | $4.8 \text{ dB} + 0.76 \, T_{1000}$ |
| *First-Order* | $R$ | |
| Flat | 0.978 | $-0.3 \text{ dB} + 0.77 \, T_{1000} + 0.19 \, T_{2000}$ |
| Gradual | 0.952 | $2.6 \text{ dB} + 0.39 \, T_{500} + 0.53 \, T_{1000}$ |
| Marked | 0.891 | $7.3 \text{ dB} + 0.63 \, T_{500} + 0.26 \, T_{1000}$ |
| Rising | 0.955 | $1.6 \text{ dB} + 0.60 \, T_{1000} + 0.43 \, T_{4000}$ |
| Trough | 0.962 | $-12.5 \text{ dB} + 0.68 \, T_{1000} + 0.41 \, T_{2000}$ |
| Atypical | 0.927 | $2.0 \text{ dB} + 0.37 \, T_{500} + 0.51 \, T_{1000}$ |
| *Second-Order* | $R$ | |
| Flat | 0.979 | $-1.1 \text{ dB} + 0.18 \, T_{500} + 0.62 \, T_{1000} + 0.18 \, T_{2000}$ |
| Gradual | 0.956 | $-0.1 \text{ dB} + 0.38 \, T_{500} + 0.41 \, T_{1000} + 0.16 \, T_{2000}$ |
| Marked | 0.894 | $3.0 \text{ dB} + 0.62 \, T_{500} + 0.21 \, T_{1000} + 0.11 \, T_{2000}$ |
| Rising | 0.958 | $1.7 \text{ dB} + 0.48 \, T_{1000} + 0.21 \, T_{2000} + 0.38 \, T_{4000}$ |
| Trough | 0.966 | $-10.9 \text{ dB} + 0.21 \, T_{500} + 0.44 \, T_{1000} + 0.45 \, T_{2000}$ |
| Atypical | 0.937 | $-0.5 \text{ dB} + 0.40 \, T_{500} + 0.41 \, T_{1000} + 0.11 \, T_{2000}$ |

*The threshold for each frequency is designated by the appropriate subscript (for example $T_{1000}$ = threshold for 1000 Hz). The right-hand section of each equation consists of a correction constant (first term) followed by one or more terms consisting of a beta coefficient multiplied by a threshold value.

From "Audiometric Configuration and Prediction of Threshold for Spondees," by R. Carhart and L. S. Porter, 1971, *Journal of Speech and Hearing Research, 14,* p. 491. Copyright 1971 by the American Speech-Language-Hearing Association. Reprinted with permission.

The zero-order equations are used to predict SRT from the one pure-tone threshold that is most highly correlated with SRT. The first-order equations are used to predict SRT from the two pure-tone thresholds that are most highly correlated with SRT, and the second-order equations are used to predict SRT from the three pure-tone thresholds that are most highly correlated with SRT. The prediction may become more accurate as more predictor variables are added to the regression equation, so several orders of equations are often run through in this fashion to find the most accurate prediction equation. Once the most accurate equation is found, it can be used to predict SRT from the pure-tone data of new patients who fall into the various categories of audiometric configuration. In the text of this article, the authors have suggested the best equations for making these predictions with patients having different types of audiometric configurations when various pure-tone data are available.

The focus in this last example is more on prediction of one variable from the others than on the analysis of strength and direction of the relationship among the variables. Both of these concepts are important and intimately related aspects of correlational analysis, but different authors may emphasize one of them over the other, depending on the purposes of a particular study. Traditionally, the analysis of the strength and direction of the relationship through presentation of correlation coefficients and scattergrams has been more prevalent in the research literature, but there has been more interest developing in the regression aspect of correlational analysis in recent years.

## Analysis of Differences

Now that we have illustrated some of the typical formats in which correlational analysis may be presented in the Results section of a research article, we will present some examples of the use of inferential statistics to examine between-subjects differences or to examine within-subjects differences between conditions. We will begin with cases of simple two-sample comparisons and progress to cases with more complicated comparisons of several samples.

The format for the presentation of inferential statistics to test the significance of differences may vary somewhat from article to article. Some authors prefer to include inferential statistics in a table that combines frequency distributions and summary statistics. The table may include values of central tendency and variability for the different groups or conditions that were compared and the values of the inferential statistics that were used to test the significance of the differences. The significance levels of the inferential statistics may be included in the table or may be placed in a footnote to the table. In other articles, the inferential analysis may be described in the narrative of the Results section, perhaps with the values of the inferential statistics and significance levels presented in parentheses. Such a narrative analysis may often make references to the summary statistics presented in a table of data organization. Some authors simply mention in the text that inferential tests were used and that differences were significant without specifically stating the values of the statistics or the significance levels that were reached. This latter alternative certainly provides less information than would be desirable for a complete evaluation of the article, but it has apparently come into vogue as a space-saving device because journal space is at such a premium.

The examples that follow will illustrate some of the diverse manners in which authors present inferential analysis in research articles in communicative disorders. Although these examples do not provide an exhaustive treatment of the possible formats that readers may encounter in the literature, they should enable consumers of research to appreciate the general manner in which statistical inference may be presented in journal articles and enable them to locate and examine inferential analysis in the articles they will read in the future.

As mentioned in Chapter 6, bivalent or two sample differences may often be evaluated statistically. These might involve between-subjects comparison of two different groups or within-subjects comparison of the same group under two different conditions. The two samples, then, represent two different levels of an *independent* or *classification* variable. These two samples may be compared to each other on one or, in some cases, on more than one *dependent* variable. When the data used in such comparisons meet the requirements of the parametric statistical tests, the *t*-test (sometimes called the "Student's test" after the pseudonym of its inventor, W. S. Gosset) is used to make the bivalent comparison. When the data do not meet the requirements of the parametric model, nonparametric tests for the bivalent comparisons are used instead.

Whenever two *different* groups are compared, the particular *t*-test used is called an independent *t*-test or a *t*-test for unrelated measures or uncorrelated groups. In addition to this independent *t*-test, there is another *t*-test called the dependent *t*-test or the *t*-test for related measures or correlated groups. This dependent *t*-test is used for making within-subjects comparisons on the *same* group, such as comparison of scores on a test before and after treatment. As mentioned in Chapter 6, larger values of the resultant *t*-statistic indicate a more significant difference between groups or conditions (i.e., a larger value of *t* would have a lower probability of occurrence if the two samples were indeed the same under the null hypothesis). Conversely, small values of *t*-scores indicate less-significant differences.

Excerpt 9.22 shows an example of the use of the *t*-test to compare the means of two *different* groups (i.e., the independent *t*-test), and Excerpt 9.23 shows an example of the use of the *t*-test to compare the means of one group performing under two *different* conditions (i.e., the dependent *t*-test). In Excerpt 9.22 a group of children with specific language impairment (SLI group) was compared to a group of children without language impairment who were matched to the SLI group in mean length of utterance (the MLU group). The dependent variable analyzed was number of unique noun stems. The independent *t*-test was used because the groups contained entirely different participants; thus, their scores were

---

**E X C E R P T   9.22**

**Lexical productivity**

One way that youngsters can achieve a spuriously high percent of correct use is to rely heavily on only a few frequently used words that may be memorized forms. One way to evaluate this possibility is to count the number of different words that appear with the plural affix. Thus, the number of unique noun stems that appeared with regular plural inflection was tabulated for each child, and group means and standard deviations were calculated. Fixed forms, such as groceries, were excluded. The mean for the SLI group was 4.4, with an *SD* of 3.2; for the MLU group the mean was 5.1, and the *SD* was 2.4. The means for the

two groups did not differ significantly ($t = -1.21$, $p = .231$). In these samples, the SLI group of children produced plural markings with a total of 100 different words; the MLU-matched children, 105. It is important to emphasize that these are unique noun stems, obtained in spontaneous utterances. Thus both groups of children generated a large number of unique and varied noun types that were marked for plurality, and the groups were not differentiated by the total number of different words. It does not appear, then, that the SLI group is differentiated from their MLU-matched controls on the basis of lexical productivity.

From "Morphological Deficits of Children with SLI: Evaluation of Number Marking and Agreement," by M. L. Rice and J. B. Oetting, 1993, *Journal of Speech and Hearing Research, 36,* p. 1253. Copyright 1993 by the American Speech-Language-Hearing Association. Reprinted with permission.

E X C E R P T   **9.23**

**Results**

Approximately 3,650 child utterances were transcribed and scored. The structural and conversational characteristics of these utterances were examined for systematic variations between the freeplay and interview contexts. Pairwise *t* tests were performed when appropriate to facilitate statistically the interpretation of the data obtained. The results were as follows.

**Structural Characteristics**

*Syntax.* The children produced more utterances within the interview context (*M* = 226 utterances) than the freeplay context (*M* = 139 utterances), as shown in Table 2. A pairwise *t* test indicated that the context differences were significant statistically [$t(9) = 8.75; p < .01$].

From "Language Sample Collection and Analysis: Interview Compared to Freeplay Assessment Contexts," by J. L. Evans and H. K. Craig, 1992, *Journal of Speech and Hearing Research, 35,* p. 347. Copyright 1992 by the American Speech-Language-Hearing Association. Reprinted with permission.

independent of each other, or uncorrelated. In Excerpt 9.23 one group of children was tested in two different conditions: an interview context and a free play context. The dependent variable analyzed was number of utterances. The dependent *t*-test was used because there was only one group containing the same children tested twice; thus, their scores in one condition were not independent of their scores in the other, or were correlated in the two conditions. Both excerpts present the analysis in a clear and straightforward comparison of the two means (and the two standard deviations in Excerpt 9.22) with the *t*-statistics and associated probabilities blended right into the text of the Results sections.

The *t*-test is most appropriate for comparing two means, but sometimes multiple *t*-tests are used either to compare two groups on a number of different dependent variables or to compare more than two groups. Caution should be exerted in making such comparisons, however, because the level of significance needs to be adjusted for the additional probability of making a Type I error associated with making multiple comparisons. A commonly used correction factor for multiple comparisons is the Bonferroni procedure, which takes the number of multiple comparisons into account in setting the correct alpha level. Excerpt 9.24 shows how the Bonferroni correction was applied to multiple *t*-tests to compare two groups of speakers on a number of different dependent variables. Means, standard deviations, and ranges are shown in the table for six dependent variables measured for the two independent groups of speakers. The textual excerpt shows the *t*-test analysis for the three dependent variables displayed in the right three columns of the table (jitter, shimmer, and H/N ratio). Excerpt 9.25 shows how the Bonferroni correction was applied to *t*-tests and correlations in a study comparing different pairs of speakers on a number of dependent variables. In addition, the study used an arc-sine transformation of the percentage scores, a commonly employed distribution normalization procedure used with proportion or percentage scores to make them more suitable for parametric statistical analysis. The table shows the means and standard deviations for the six dependent variables for the four different groups of speakers, and the excerpt shows the cautions used in approaching the multiple comparisons with the Bonferroni and arc-sine procedures.

## EXCERPT 9.24

Based on pilot data commensurate with Steinsapir et al.'s (1986) study that indicated greater levels of perturbation in the voices of black speakers, independent (unpaired) one-tailed t-tests were used on each acoustic measure of vocal noise to test this hypothesis. Because the three measures (frequency perturbation, amplitude perturbation, and H/N ratio) are not independent, a Bonferroni adjustment to the .05 alpha level was made to control for error (Miller, 1981).

Mean relative jitter (RAP, in percent) for the black subjects averaged 0.40%, with a fairly large standard deviation (0.36%). The white subjects' RAP averaged 0.28%, with much smaller intersubject variability ($SD = 0.12\%$). Although the standard deviation for the black subjects was almost as high as the mean and three times greater than that for the white subjects, the mean RAP of both subject groups was lower than the 0.57% reported by Takahashi and Koike (1975) for normal Japanese males. The standard deviation they report (0.13%), however, is similar to that of the white subjects in the present study. Despite greater frequency perturbation in the black voice samples, the difference between the two subject groups was not statistically significant.

The average shimmer measured in the black and in the white samples was 0.33 dB and 0.28 dB, respectively. The difference in mean shimmer was statistically significant ($t = 2.15$, $df = 98$, $p = .016$). Both means fall well within the ranges reported in the literature for healthy young adult men (e.g., Horiguchi, Haji, Baer, & Gould, 1987; Horii, 1980, 1982; Kitajima & Gould, 1976; Orlikoff, 1990a).

The mean harmonics-to-noise (H/N) ratio for the black voice samples was 14.77 dB, which was significantly lower than the mean H/N ratio of 16.32 dB for the white samples ($t = -2.58$, $df = 98$, $p = .005$).

TABLE 2   Means, standard deviations, and ranges for the mean vocal fundamental frequency ($F_0$, in Hz), first (F1) and second (F2) formant frequencies (in Hz), jitter (RAP, in percent), shimmer (in dB), and harmonics-to-noise (H/N) ratio (in dB) for the black and white vowel samples used in this study

|  | $F_0$ | F1 | F2 | Jitter | Shimmer* | H/N* Ratio |
|---|---|---|---|---|---|---|
| *Black Samples* | | | | | | |
| M | 108.85 | 660 | 1181 | 0.40 | 0.331 | 14.77 |
| SD | 14.48 | 60 | 90 | 0.36 | 0.150 | 3.38 |
| Range | 84.91–141.04 | 560–797 | 1052–1501 | 0.14–2.33 | 0.110–0.662 | 6.68–20.96 |
| *White Samples* | | | | | | |
| M | 107.55 | 662 | 1181 | 0.28 | 0.275 | 16.32 |
| SD | 15.11 | 72 | 88 | 0.12 | 0.111 | 2.56 |
| Range | 82.75–148.46 | 515–898 | 1030–1411 | 0.17–0.89 | 0.095–0.704 | 10.49–21.45 |

*Level of significance = .02.

From "Speaker Race Identification from Acoustic Cues in the Vocal Signal," by J. H. Walton and R. F. Orlikoff, 1994, *Journal of Speech and Hearing Research, 37,* pp. 740–741. Copyright 1994 by the American Speech-Language-Hearing Association. Reprinted with permission.

**EXCERPT 9.25**

A commercial software package (SYSTAT, Wilkinson, 1989) was used to perform a series of *t* tests to compare characteristics of the language samples obtained, frequencies of disfluencies, speaking rates, interrupting behaviors, and response time latencies of the four speaker groups (stuttering children [C-St], nonstuttering children [C-Nst], mothers of stutterers [M-St], and mothers of nonstutterers [M-NSt]). Sets of six *t* test comparisons (four independent and two correlated) at an alpha level of 0.01 for each individual comparison and 0.06 for all six comparisons in each set as a family (i.e., Bonferroni adjusted for multiple comparisons) were performed for each of these variables. The four independent sample *t* tests in each set included comparisons of C-St and C-Nst, M-St and M-Nst, C-St and M-St, and C-Nst and M-St. The two correlated sample *t* tests in each set compared C-St and M-St, and C-Nst and M-NSt. For percentages of within-word and between-word disfluencies as well as the frequency of all disfluencies combined, arcsine transformations were performed to make differences in percent more suitable for subsequent parametric statistical analysis (Studebaker, 1985). Post hoc nonparametric

Spearman rank-correlational coefficients with Bonferroni adjustments for multiple comparisons were determined to assess relations between speaking rate, interruptions, and RTL and between these three paralinguistic variables and children's disfluencies.

. . . . . . . . . . .

**Results**

*Characteristics of the Language Samples.* Table 2 illustrates means and standard deviations for numbers of conversational turns, utterances, words, syllables, morphemes, and mean lengths of utterances (MLU) produced by stuttering children, nonstuttering children, mothers of stuttering children, and mothers of nonstuttering children. No significant differences were found in any of the *t* test comparisons for numbers of conversational turns, utterances, words, syllables or morphemes. Mothers of nonstuttering children were found to produce significantly longer MLUs ($M = 4.338$; $SD = 0.50$) than their own children ($M = 3.405$; $SD = 0.65$; $t = 3.454$; $p < 0.01$), and than the stuttering children ($M = 3.311$; $SD = 0.80$; $t = 3.816$; $p < 0.01$).

**TABLE 2    Means and standard deviations for numbers of conversational turns, utterances, words, syllables and morphemes and mean lengths of utterances (MLU) for stuttering (C-St) and nonstuttering (C-NSt) children and their mothers (M-St and M-NSt)**

| | Speaker group | | | | | | | |
|---|---|---|---|---|---|---|---|---|
| | *C-St* | | *C-NSt* | | *M-St* | | *M-NSt* | |
| Measures | *M* | *SD* | *M* | *SD* | *M* | *SD* | *M* | *SD* |
| Conversational turns | 57.2 | 17.6 | 61.9 | 17.9 | 55.1 | 16.8 | 62.0 | 18.6 |
| Utterances | 99.0 | 21.2 | 100.6 | 19.7 | 96.7 | 37.2 | 100.7 | 39.5 |
| Words | 301.3 | 13.5 | 302.6 | 2.8 | 338.4 | 145.4 | 410.4 | 196.5 |
| Syllables | 358.1 | 16.1 | 360.1 | 12.6 | 407.0 | 171.4 | 483.7 | 221.2 |
| Morphemes | 312.5 | 20.0 | 327.7 | 9.0 | 375.2 | 161.0 | 447.5 | 203.6 |
| MLU | 3.31 | 0.8 | 3.41 | 0.6 | 3.85 | 0.5 | 4.34 | 0.5 |

From "Speaking Rates, Response Time Latencies, and Interrupting Behaviors of Young Stutterers, Nonstutterers, and Their Mothers," by E. M. Kelly and E. G. Conture, 1992, *Journal of Speech and Hearing Research, 35,* pp. 1260–1261. Copyright 1992 by the American Speech-Language-Hearing Association. Reprinted with permission.

## EXCERPT 9.26

### Data Analysis

As will be discussed, the stuttering and nonstuttering children in this study contributed unequal and/or small numbers of speech disfluencies of all types, including the disfluency types of primary interest, namely sound/syllable repetitions, sound prolongations, and whole-word repetitions. These unequal or small samples can be attributed to either low production of disfluent speech in general (as in the case of the nonstuttering children), or to speech disfluencies that were acoustically unmeasurable. In order to account for discrepancies in sample sizes and make appropriate between-group comparisons, the non-parametric Mann-Whitney U test (Siegel, 1956) was used to compare the stuttering and nonstuttering children in (a) duration of sound/syllable repetitions, (b) duration of sound prolongations, (c) number of repeated units per instance of sound/syllable repetition, (d) number of repeated units per instance of whole-word repetition, and (e) proportions of different speech disfluency types. In contrast, between-group comparisons of mean frequency of speech disfluency (that is, the average frequency of disfluency in three contiguous 100-word samples) were obtained through an independent-groups $t$ test with adjusted degrees of freedom.

### Results

*Duration of Sound/Syllable Repetitions.* The 10 stuttering children produced a total of 89 sound/syllable repetitions. Of these 89 sound/syllable repetitions, 5 were acoustically unmeasurable either because of faint or indistinct acoustic energy as displayed on the video-sound spectrograph or because of the investigator's inability to clearly observe either the beginning or end points associated with a particular speech disfluency (Zebrowski et al., 1985). As Figure 1 shows, the mean duration of the young

stutterers' measurable ($N = 84$) sound/syllable repetitions was 556 ms ($SD = 370$ ms; range = 155–1878 ms).

Nine of the 10 nonstuttering children produced a total of 21 sound/syllable repetitions, 3 of which were unmeasurable. The mean duration of the nonstuttering children's measurable ($N = 18$) sound/syllable repetitions was 520 ms ($SD = 245$ ms; range = 187–967 ms). Results of Mann Whitney U analysis indicated no significant between-group differences (Mann Whitney $U = 38$, $C = 12$; $p > .01$) in the duration of sound/syllable repetitions.

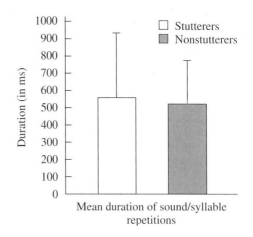

**FIGURE 1   Mean duration (in ms) of acoustically measured sound/syllable repetitions produced by stuttering ($N = 10$) and nonstuttering ($N = 9$) children in one 300-word sample of conversational speech obtained from each child. Lines indicate one standard deviation above the mean.**

The illustration in Excerpt 9.26 shows the use of the Mann–Whitney $U$ test, a non-parametric test, to make a between-subjects comparison. The Mann–Whitney $U$ test, as mentioned in Chapter 6, is often referred to as a nonparametric alternative to the independent $t$-test because it is used to make a two-sample comparison between groups when the requirements for the *t*-test cannot be met by the data. In the example shown in Excerpt 9.26, two different groups are compared: a group of children who were beginning stutterers and an age- and gender-matched group of children who did not stutter. The Data Analysis section explains why the Mann–Whitney *U* was used in place of the *t*-test for five of the six dependent variables, and the Results section displays the text and figure for the analysis of one of these five variables, namely duration of sound/syllable repetitions. Note that the means of the two groups were fairly similar, that there was wide variability in both groups (more so for the children who stutter), and that the Mann–Whitney *U* statistic indicated no significant difference between the groups.

As mentioned previously, the Mann–Whitney *U* test is often referred to as a nonparametric alternative to the independent *t*-test because it is used to make a bivalent between-subjects comparison. It should be noted, however, that the Mann–Whitney *U* statistic is calculated in a manner different from the manner in which the *t*-statistic is calculated. Smaller values of the Mann–Whitney *U* statistic indicate a more significant difference between groups and, conversely, larger values of Mann–Whitney *U* are nonsignificant.

When a nonparametric alternative to the *t*-test is used, the author may decide to include a central tendency measure other than the mean or a variability measure other than the standard deviation in the summary statistics table. This is because the mean and standard deviation are usually associated with parametric statistics. In the example in Excerpt 9.26 the author includes the mean as the measure of central tendency but uses the range in addition to the standard deviation as a measure of variability.

The Mann–Whitney *U* test operates on the ranks of the participants in the two groups rather than on their actual test scores. Thus, the level of measurement used for the dependent variable is ordinal. The Mann–Whitney *U* test would be an appropriate alternative to the *t*-test when the original dependent variable data are at the ordinal level of measurement or when interval- or ratio-level original data are transformed to the ordinal level of measurement for use with a nonparametric test because one of the other assumptions of a parametric test (e.g., normal distribution) cannot be met. The Wilcoxon Matched-Pairs Signed-Ranks Test (to be illustrated in the next excerpt) also makes use of ranks rather than actual scores, so that it is also appropriate for analyzing data at the ordinal level of measurement.

Excerpt 9.27 contains an illustration of the use of the Wilcoxon Matched-Pairs Signed-Ranks Test to make a bivalent within-subjects comparison. The Wilcoxon Matched-Pairs Signed-Ranks Test is often referred to as a nonparametric alternative to the dependent *t*-test because it is used to make a comparison of the performance of one group of participants in two different conditions when the data are not appropriate for the use of parametric statistics. In the study shown in Excerpt 9.27, two treatment procedures for stuttering were investigated: (a) speech motor training (SMT) and (b) extended length of utterance (ELU). Six children who stuttered were compared in stuttering frequency using the "percent-syllables-stuttered" (%SS) measure before and after speech motor training. In addition, six other children who stuttered were compared in stuttering frequency before and after a treatment employing extended length of utterance. Two Wilcoxon Matched-Pairs, Signed-Ranks Tests were used to make the pretest–posttest comparisons in stuttering frequency—one Wilcoxon test for the speech motor training group and one Wilcoxon test for the extended length of utterance treatment group. Both Wilcoxon Matched-Pairs, Signed-Ranks Tests showed significant differences from before to after treatment for both types of treatment.

## EXCERPT   9.27

### Changes in Stuttering

Group data indicating changes in stuttering frequency following 24 sessions of SMT are shown in Table 5. The median decrease in %SS from 7.8 to 4.61 was 3.19 (41%). Using Wilcoxin matched-pair analysis, this reduction was significant at $p <.05$. The median rather than the mean was used to reduce the influence of one child (E6) whose %SS increased. Table 6 shows the pre- and posttreatment frequency of stuttering for each individual participant and the percent change for each participant. This procedure gives more weight to the milder stutterers for whom a given amount of absolute reduction in stuttering results in a greater percentage change. Using these individual percent changes, the median reduction was 36.5%

Group data indicating changes in stuttering frequency after 24 sessions of ELU treatment are included in Table 5. The median decrease from 4.25 %SS to 1.89 was 2.36 (56%). Wilcoxin matched-pair analysis indicated that this reduction was significant at $p = .04$. ELU reduced stuttering 63.5% (see Table 6, last column).

**TABLE 5   Median stuttering frequency pre– and post–24 treatment sessions of Speech Motor Training (SMT) or Extended Length of Utterance (ELU) treatment.**

|  | Pre- | Post- | Diff. | Wilcoxon, $N = 6$ |
|---|---|---|---|---|
| | **Speech motor training** | | | |
| Frequency (%SS) | 7.8 | 4.61 | 3.19 | $(z, -2.0; p, .04)$ |
| | **Extended length of utterance** | | | |
| Frequency (%SS) | 4.25 | 1.89 | 2.36 | $(z, -2.1; p, .04)$ |

**TABLE 6   Percent reduction for individual children in stuttering frequency (%SS) following Speech Motor Training (SMT) or Extended Length of Utterance (ELU) treatment.**

| Participant number | Speech motor training | | | Extended length of utterance | | |
|---|---|---|---|---|---|---|
| | *Pre-* | *Post-* | *%diff.* | *Pre-* | *Post-* | *%diff.* |
| Reduction in %SS | | | | | | |
| 1 | 7.85 | 4.97 | −37 | 11.34 | 3.24 | −71 |
| 2 | 7.74 | 4.24 | −45 | 5.36 | 1.68 | −69 |
| 3 | 3.74 | 1.37 | −63 | 10.14 | 4.28 | −58 |
| 4 | 13.49 | 11.20 | −17 | 2.60 | 1.20 | −54 |
| 5 | 4.84 | 3.10 | −36 | 3.14 | 2.10 | −33 |
| 6 | 13.58 | 14.71 | +8 | 2.74 | .48 | −83 |
| Median | 7.8 | 4.61 | −36.5 | 4.25 | 1.89 | −63.5 |
| Inter-quartile | 4.84 to 13.49 | 3.1 to 11.2 | −17 to −45 | 2.74 to 10.14 | 1.2 to 3.24 | −54 to −71 |

From "Acoustic Duration Changes Associated with Two Types of Treatment for Children Who Stutter," by G. D. Riley and J. C. Ingham, 2000, *Journal of Speech, Language, and Hearing Research, 43,* pp. 971–972. Copyright 2000 by the American Speech-Language-Hearing Association. Reprinted with permission.

Notice that the authors used the conversion of the Wilcoxon $T$ to a $z$-score to make the comparisons, even though the sample sizes were smaller than twenty-five. Table 5 shows the median %SS before and after treatment and the pre–post difference for both treatments and the Wilcoxon $z$-scores with associated alpha probabilities. The negative z-scores in Table 5 indicate that stuttering frequency decreased from pretest to posttest for both types of stuttering treatment. Table 6 shows the raw data for individual children as well as medians and interquartile ranges as the appropriate summary statistics for central tendency and variability when nonparametric analysis will be used.

As mentioned in Chapter 6, the $\chi^2$ statistic has a variety of uses. We have already seen it used as a measure of association in the example in Excerpt 9.18 in the correlational analysis section of this chapter. The example in Excerpt 9.28 shows the use of the $\chi^2$ statistic as an inferential test of the significance of the difference between two groups on nominal level dependent variables that are dichotomized into two categories. The $\chi^2$ statistic may also be encountered when more than two groups are compared or when groups are compared on a nominal variable that can be categorized in more than two ways. These comparisons can sometimes become somewhat cumbersome or difficult to interpret if there are too many categories but can be useful with a few categories. The $\chi^2$ statistic is similar to the $t$-test in the determination of its significance; that is, higher values of the $\chi^2$ statistic are needed to indicate statistical significance, and lower values indicate the lack of significant differences between the groups.

In the example from the prevalence survey of voice disorders shown in Excerpt 9.28, comparison is made between teachers and nonteachers on several variables that describe participant background characteristics. In addition, comparisons are made between the teachers and nonteachers in frequency and duration of voice disorders. Because these particular dependent variables were all measured at the nominal level, $\chi^2$ tests were used to test the significance of the differences between the teachers and nonteachers on each variable. Table 1 in the excerpt lists the variables in the left column and then shows the number and percent of teachers and nonteachers who fell into each nominal category of each variable (e.g., Gender: Male vs. Female; Family history: Yes vs. No; etc.). The three columns to the right indicate the $\chi^2$ value for each comparison as well as the degrees of freedom ($df$) and alpha level probability ($p$) for each variable. Because only two groups of participants (teachers vs. nonteachers) were compared on each variable, note that the degrees of freedom for each comparison corresponds to the number of levels of each variable minus one. For example, there are two gender groups and $df = 1$ for that comparison; there are three ethnicity categories and $df = 2$ for that comparison. The text in the excerpt explains which variables differed between teachers and nonteachers and which variables showed no differences between the two groups. For example, fewer teachers reported using tobacco products and the $\chi^2$ was large (149.5) and significant ($p < .001$), whereas the reported history of asthma was about the same for both teachers and nonteachers, and the $\chi^2$ was small (1.30) and nonsignificant ($p = .250$). The text in the excerpt also describes very clearly many of the differences found between teachers and nonteachers in frequency and duration of voice disorders and uses the $\chi^2$ test to make specific comparisons between teachers and nonteachers in the various age groupings.

The bivalent statistical inference tests previously discussed were used for making comparisons between two different groups in a between-subjects research design or for

EXCERPT 9.28

## Results

### Participant Background Characteristics

The results reported are based on analysis of 2,531 participants who completed the voice disorder interview in Iowa and Utah during 1998 to 2000. Of this number, 49.1% were teachers ($n$ = 1,243), 50.9% were nonteachers ($n$ = 1,288), 35.5% were men ($n$ = 899), 64.5% were women ($n$ = 1,632), and 82.9% were from Iowa and 17.1% were from Utah. Participants ranged in age from 20 to 66 years ($M$ = 44.2, $SD$ = 10.7).

Teachers, compared with nonteachers, were more likely to be women, to be in the age range of 40–59 years, to be White, to have 16 or more years of education, and to have a higher income (see Table 1). The percentage of teachers identified in Iowa was similar to that in Utah. Teachers compared with nonteachers were also more likely to experience respiratory allergies, one or more colds annually, and one or more episodes of laryngitis annually; were less likely to have used tobacco products for a year or longer; and were less likely to have ever drunk an average of one or more alcoholic beverages a week for one year or longer. There was no statistical difference in the prevalence of asthma, sinus infections, postnasal drip, or family history of voice disorders between teachers and nonteachers.

### Frequency and Duration of Voice Disorders

Of the 1,088 individuals (i.e., 43% of the total sample) who reported experiencing a voice disorder during their lifetime, 18.6% had chronic (4 weeks or more) voice disorders and 81.4% had acute (less than 4 weeks) voice disorders. The prevalence of voice disorders increased with age, peaked in the age group of 50–59 years, and then decreased (see Figure 1). The prevalence of reporting a voice disorder during their lifetime was significantly greater in teachers compared with nonteachers (57.7% for teachers vs. 28.8% for nonteachers), $\chi^2(1)$ = 215.2, $p$ < .001 (see Table 2), as was the prevalence of reporting a current voice problem (11.0% for teachers vs. 6.2% for nonteachers), $\chi^2$ = 18.2, $p$ < .001. This higher lifetime prevalence persisted across the age span (see Figure 2). Furthermore, teachers, compared with nonteachers, were more likely to report current voice problems across the age continuum. Percentages for teachers and nonteachers were 7.2% versus 4.2% for ages 20–29,) $\chi^2$ = 1.06, $p$ = .303; 8.2% versus 4.3% for ages 30–39, $\chi^2$ = 3.7, $p$ = .053; 10.3% versus 6.9% for ages 40–49, $\chi^2$ = 3.1, $p$ = .078; 14.4% versus 8.2% for ages 50–59, $\chi^2$ = 5.5, $p$ = .019; and 11.1% versus 7.3% for ages 60 and older, $\chi^2$ = 0.9, $p$ = .351. There was no statistical difference between Iowa and Utah in the prevalence of voice problems among teachers.

Of those participants who indicated they had previously experienced a voice disorder, teachers were less likely to report chronic voice disorders but more likely to report multiple voice disorder episodes, even after adjusting for the potential confounding effect of age (see Table 2). Among all study participants, a significantly higher percentage of teachers (14.3%, $n$ = 178) versus nonteachers (5.5%, $n$ = 71) had visited a physician or speech-language pathologist about any type of voice disorder,) $\chi^2$ = 55.3, $p$ < .001.

**TABLE 1    Frequency distributions of teachers compared with nonteachers according to selected characteristics**

| Variable | Teachers | | Nonteachers | | $\chi^2$ | $df$ | $p$ |
|---|---|---|---|---|---|---|---|
| | No. | % | No. | % | | | |
| Gender | | | | | 21.3 | 1 | <.001 |
| Male | 386 | 31.0 | 513 | 39.8 | | | |
| Female | 857 | 69.0 | 775 | 60.2 | | | |

*(continued)*

**E X C E R P T  9.28  Continued**

TABLE 1  (Continued

| Variable | Teachers | | Nonteachers | | $\chi^2$ | df | p |
|---|---|---|---|---|---|---|---|
| | No. | % | No. | % | | | |
| Age | | | | | 91.2 | 4 | <.001 |
| 20–29 | 83 | 6.7 | 189 | 14.7 | | | |
| 30–39 | 255 | 20.5 | 302 | 23.4 | | | |
| 40–49 | 455 | 36.6 | 404 | 31.4 | | | |
| 50–59 | 378 | 30.4 | 256 | 19.9 | | | |
| 60+ | 137 | 5.8 | 137 | 10.6 | | | |
| Race/ethnicity | | | | | 20.8 | 2 | <.001 |
| White, non-Hispanic | 1217 | 97.9 | 1216 | 94.4 | | | |
| Hispanic | 13 | 1.05 | 37 | 2.9 | | | |
| Other | 13 | 1.05 | 35 | 2.7 | | | |
| School grade | | | | | 1624 | 4 | <.001 |
| <16 | 0 | 0.0 | 977 | 78.9 | | | |
| 16 | 368 | 29.6 | 204 | 15.8 | | | |
| >16 | 875 | 70.4 | 107 | 8.3 | | | |
| Gross annual income ($) | | | | | 274.2 | 3 | <.001 |
| <20K | 7 | 0.6 | 169 | 13.5 | | | |
| 20K to <40K | 222 | 18.2 | 419 | 33.5 | | | |
| 40K to <60K | 460 | 37.8 | 321 | 25.7 | | | |
| >60k | 528 | 43.4 | 341 | 27.3 | | | |
| State | | | | | 0.3 | 1 | .586 |
| Iowa | 1036 | 83.4 | 1063 | 82.5 | | | |
| Utah | 207 | 16.6 | 225 | 17.5 | | | |
| Respiratory allergies | | | | | 8.3 | 1 | .004 |
| No | 962 | 77.4 | 1056 | 82.0 | | | |
| Yes | 281 | 22.6 | 232 | 18.0 | | | |
| Asthma | | | | | 1.3 | 1 | .250 |
| No | 1126 | 90.6 | 1149 | 89.2 | | | |
| Yes | 117 | 9.4 | 139 | 10.8 | | | |
| Colds[a] | | | | | 12.6 | 2 | .002 |
| Never | 15 | 1.2 | 20 | 1.6 | | | |
| <1 | 109 | 8.8 | 168 | 13.0 | | | |
| 1+ | 1119 | 90.0 | 1100 | 85.4 | | | |
| Sinus infection[a] | | | | | 1.3 | 2 | .530 |
| Never | 429 | 34.5 | 470 | 36.5 | | | |
| <1 | 229 | 18.4 | 239 | 18.6 | | | |
| 1+ | 584 | 47.0 | 579 | 44.9 | | | |

**E X C E R P T   9.28   Continued**

**TABLE 1   Continued**

| Variable | Teachers | | Nonteachers | | $\chi^2$ | df | p |
| --- | --- | --- | --- | --- | --- | --- | --- |
| | No. | % | No. | % | | | |
| Laryngitis[a] | | | | | 205.3 | 2 | <.001 |
| Never | 521 | 41.9 | 866 | 67.3 | | | |
| <1 | 287 | 23.1 | 254 | 19.7 | | | |
| 1+ | 435 | 35.0 | 168 | 13.0 | | | |
| Postnasal drip | | | | | 7.2 | 3 | .066 |
| Not at all | 210 | 16.9 | 262 | 20.3 | | | |
| Occasionally | 721 | 58.0 | 744 | 57.8 | | | |
| Seasonally | 188 | 15.1 | 177 | 13.7 | | | |
| Chronically | 124 | 10.0 | 105 | 8.2 | | | |
| Tobacco[b] | | | | | 149.5 | 1 | <.001 |
| No | 940 | 75.6 | 673 | 52.3 | | | |
| Yes | 303 | 24.4 | 615 | 47.7 | | | |
| Alcohol drinking[c] | | | | | 12.5 | 1 | <.001 |
| No | 819 | 65.9 | 761 | 59.1 | | | |
| Yes | 424 | 34.1 | 527 | 40.9 | | | |
| Family history | | | | | 3.3 | 1 | .070 |
| No | 1186 | 95.9 | 1248 | 97.2 | | | |
| Yes | 51 | 4.1 | 36 | 2.8 | | | |

[a]On average, per year.

[b]Based on the question, "Have you ever used any tobacco products for a year or longer?"

[c]Based on the question, "Have you ever drunk an average of one or more alcoholic beverages a week for one year or longer?"

From "Prevalence of Voice Disorders in Teachers and the General Population," by N. Roy, R. M. Merrill, S. Thibeault, R. A. Parsa, S. D. Gray, and E. M. Smith, 2004, *Journal of Speech, Language, and Hearing Research, 47,* pp. 284–286. Copyright 2004 by the American Speech-Language-Hearing Association. Reprinted with permission.

comparing the same participants' performances in two different conditions in a within-subjects research design. However, when more than two samples are compared simultaneously (as in multivalent or parametric research studies), these two-sample comparison statistics are usually replaced by a statistical procedure for making simultaneous comparisons of more than two samples of data. The analysis of variance (ANOVA) was described in Chapter 6 as an appropriate statistical test for analyzing differences among three or more groups or among three or more conditions. For example, a multivalent between-subjects experiment might have three different groups representing three levels of the independent variable; a multivalent within-subjects experiment might have one group measured under three different conditions that reflect three levels of the independent variable. A parametric experiment might have two groups (representing two levels of a between-subjects independent variable) performing under two different conditions (representing two levels of a within-subjects independent variable).

The ANOVA allows the researcher to test the main effect of each independent variable and the interaction effects among the independent variables. The number of independent variables tested in an ANOVA is usually referred to as the number of *ways* of the ANOVA (e.g., a one-way ANOVA tests only one independent variable, a two-way ANOVA tests two independent variables simultaneously, a three-way ANOVA tests three independent variables simultaneously). As indicated in Chapter 6, ANOVAs are available for making between-subjects comparisons, within-subjects comparisons (sometimes called *repeated measures* comparisons because the measurement with each participant is repeated in each condition), and a combination of a between-subjects comparison on one independent variable and a within-subjects comparison on another independent variable (called a *mixed model* ANOVA).

Excerpt 9.29 illustrates the use of a one-way ANOVA making a between-subjects comparison in a study of age differences in auditory/articulatory correspondences. Forty-five children were measured, fifteen each in the age groups five, six, and seven years old, on metaphonological tasks designed to study their knowledge of auditory and articulatory correspondences. Table 1 in the excerpt shows the means, standard deviations, and ranges of the performances of the three age groups on a nonverbal matching task in which children had to match an auditory and a visual stimulus without using a verbal response. As can be seen from the table, the mean performances increased from the younger to the older

---

**EXCERPT 9.29**

### Results

*Nonverbal Matching*

The mean number of correct responses on the nonverbal matching task was computed for each age group (see Table 1 for descriptive statistics). The results of a one-way analysis of variance (ANOVA) revealed significant differences among group means ($F(2, 42) = 34.22$, $p < .001$). A Scheffe post-hoc comparison (Weinberg & Goldberg, 1979) revealed significant differences between ages 5 and 7 ($F = 32.66$, $p < .001$) and between ages 6 and 7 ($F = 16.00$, $p < .001$).

**TABLE 1  Number of correct responses on nonverbal matching task by three age groups**

| Age group | *M* | *SD* | Range |
|---|---|---|---|
| 5 ($N = 15$) | 10.93 | 1.751 | 8–14 |
| 6 ($N = 15$) | 12.67 | 2.664 | 8–17 |
| 7 ($N = 15$) | 16.73 | 1.223 | 14–18 |

children. The results of the one-way, between-subjects ANOVA are described in the textual excerpt. The overall $F$ indicates significant differences across the age variable, and specific Sheffe contrast tests indicated that the two younger groups were different from the older group but not from each other (i.e., groups aged five and six differed from children aged seven). A one-way between-subjects ANOVA is the simplest, most straightforward version of this statistical procedure and more complex designs build on this concept of simultaneous statistical inference with one test.

Excerpt 9.30 includes a bar graph that was used to display summary statistics (means) and a textual description of the results of a two-way (2 × 2) repeated measures ANOVA in a study of the influence of metrical patterns of words on phoneme production accuracy. The two independent variables that are manipulated in this within-subjects design are stress pattern and word position. Mean proportion of production errors is indicated on the ordinate and two different syllable stress patterns and phoneme positions are indicated on the abscissa. The bar heights indicate the mean proportion of consonant errors made by 20 children for words with stressed versus unstressed initial and final syllables. The presentation of results in the bar graph format provides readers with a clear overall picture of the influence of stress and syllable position on consonant errors. In addition, one unique feature of this bar graph is the inclusion of the actual mean above each bar (e.g., 0.55 for Stressed-Initial syllable type, and so on), which allows readers to see the exact values of the means as would be conveyed by a tabular format. The textual description of the results of the ANOVA very clearly explains the significant main effects of position and stress, the two-way interaction between them, and the follow-up tests that were done to compare specific pairs of means.

The next example in Excerpt 9.31 shows a two-way ANOVA design with a between-subjects comparison made on each independent variable. The first independent variable is fluency, with two levels represented by two different groups: children who stutter versus children who do not stutter. The second independent variable is age, with five levels represented by the five different groups: seven, eight, nine, ten, and eleven-plus years of age. The dependent variable is a thirty-five-item Dutch version of the Communication Attitude Test (CAT-D), in which a higher score indicates a more negative attitude toward speech and a lower score indicates a more positive attitude toward speech. Table 1 displays the means and standard deviations of the two groups (further subdivided by gender, which is not analyzed in the ANOVA because of the small number of females who stutter—see textual excerpt for an explanation of this), and Table 2 displays the means and standard deviations of different age groups. Table 3 is the ANOVA summary table and indicates a significant $F$-ratio for group and group by age interaction, but an insignificant $F$-ratio for age as an independent variable main effect. Figure 1 shows the obvious difference in means between the two fluency groups at each age level; notice also that standard deviations show some overlap at the younger ages but almost no overlap at the older ages. The figure also shows how the groups diverged as age increased: CAT-D scores of children who stutter increased with older ages and normally fluent children's CAT-D scores decreased with age. Table 4 displays the contrast tests comparing fluency groups at each age and the mean squares and $F$-ratios all show greater group differences at the older ages. This divergent age pattern for the two groups resulted in an averaging of CAT-D scores for ages across groups that made age a nonsignificant factor: in other words, CAT-D scores averaged across groups did not vary significantly as age increased. The text explains the ANOVA results quite clearly and thoroughly and makes careful reference to the tables and figure in presenting each difference.

## EXCERPT 9.30

**Overall error rates**

The second set of analyses focused on the accuracy of the consonants produced. A repeated measures ANOVA with stress (stressed vs. unstressed) and serial position in the word (first vs. second position) as within-subject variables was applied to the proportions of incorrect consonants (including omissions) calculated for each condition. The proportions were normalized by arcsine transformation for the statistical analyses. Means are presented as untransformed proportions. These data are illustrated in Figure 3. Significant main effects were found for both stress [$F(1, 19) = 6.46, p < .025$] and for serial position [$F(1, 19) = 7.00, p < .025$]. In general, consonants in unstressed syllables ($M = .64$)

were more frequently incorrect than those in stressed syllables ($M = .50$), and consonants in first position ($M = .63$) were more often inaccurate than those in the second position ($M = .49$). Importantly, though, there was significant interaction between these two factors [$F(1, 19) = 5.81, p < .05$]. Post hoc Newman Keuls' tests ($p < .05$) revealed that consonants in unstressed first position syllables ($M = .74$) were significantly less accurate than consonants in stressed first position syllables ($M = .55$), consonants in stressed second position syllables ($M = .46$), and those in unstressed second position syllables ($M = .51$). No other significant differences were found.

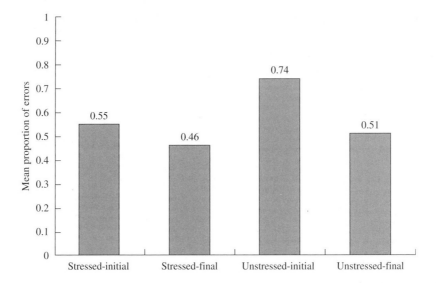

**FIGURE 3    Mean proportion of consonant errors according to syllable type.**

From "Metrical Patterns of Words and Production Accuracy," by R. G. Schwartz and L. Goffman, 1995, *Journal of Speech and Hearing Research, 38,* pp. 882 & 883. Copyright 1995 by the American Speech-Language-Hearing Association. Reprinted with permission.

Excerpt 9.32 illustrates the use of an analysis of variance for the comparison of two groups of participants (children with normal articulation versus children with impaired articulation) performing under three different conditions (responding to digits, random words, and words in sentences). A mixed model ANOVA was used to compare the performances of the two groups of children (between-subjects comparison) as the first main effect. The

One of the purposes of the present study was to compare the speech attitudes of stuttering and nonstuttering children at different age groups. Toward this end, both subject groups were subdivided into five age levels (7, 8, 9, 10, and 11-plus years). The sample size in each of these five age groups for the stutterers was 24, 13, 10, 9, and 14, respectively, and for the nonstuttering controls, 62, 40, 42, 41, and 86, respectively. A two-way analysis of variance was used to evaluate whether the CAT-D scores of the stuttering and the nonstuttering children differed statistically across the five age levels and whether there was a significant group × age interaction.

### Results

The mean CAT-D scores, and their standard deviations, for the stutterers and the nonstuttering children are presented in Table 1. The stuttering children obtained notably higher mean test scores than did their controls; indeed, the overall CAT-D score for the stutterers was almost twice that of the nonstuttering children.

Also shown in Table 1 are the mean scores for the male and the female subjects. The descriptive difference between the groups was present also for the sexes. Both the boys and the girls who stuttered scored higher on the CAT-D than did their nonstuttering peers.

Interestingly, within the group of stutterers, the females obtained a notably higher CAT-D score than did the males. This sex difference was not apparent among the nonstuttering children (see also Brutten & Dunham, 1989). This finding may suggest the presence of gender differences in speech attitudes among stutterers. However, because the number of female stutterers studied in the present investigation was so small, a separate analysis of their scores was not justified.

Another purpose of the present study was to analyze whether the differences in CAT-D scores of the two subject groups were influenced by the age level of the children. In this respect, the data summarized in Table 2 show that the average CAT-D score of the stuttering children was descriptively higher than that of their nonstuttering peers at each of the five age levels studied.

A two-way analysis of variance (BMDP4V) was used to test whether the observed difference between the CAT-D scores of the two subject groups across all age levels was statistically significant, and whether a significant group × age level interaction existed (Table 3).

**TABLE 1   Descriptive statistics of the CAT-D scores for the stuttering and the nonstuttering children as a group and subdivided by sex**

| Group | N | M | SD |
|---|---|---|---|
| *Stutterers* | | | |
| Male | 63 | 15.95 | 7.28 |
| Female | 7 | 23.29 | 2.69 |
| Total | 70 | 16.69 | 7.29 |
| *Nonstutterers* | | | |
| Male | 134 | 8.57 | 5.22 |
| Female | 137 | 8.85 | 5.84 |
| Total | 271 | 8.71 | 5.53 |

**TABLE 2   Descriptive statistics of the CAT-D scores for the stuttering and the nonstuttering children at each of five age levels**

| Group | N | M | SD |
|---|---|---|---|
| *Stutterers* | | | |
| 7 years | 24 | 14.79 | 6.62 |
| 8 years | 13 | 17.23 | 9.86 |
| 9 years | 10 | 17.60 | 6.35 |
| 10 years | 9 | 18.56 | 6.80 |
| 11 years + | 14 | 17.57 | 6.93 |
| *Nonstutterers* | | | |
| 7 years | 62 | 9.98 | 5.57 |
| 8 years | 40 | 10.35 | 4.49 |
| 9 years | 42 | 10.62 | 5.92 |
| 10 years | 41 | 8.20 | 5.17 |
| 11 years + | 86 | 6.34 | 5.12 |

TABLE 3   Two-way analysis of variance of the CAT-D scores of the
stuttering and the nonstuttering children at five different age levels

| Source | SS | df | MS | F | p |
|--------|-----|-----|-----|-----|-----|
| Group | 3228.93 | 1 | 3228.93 | 97.66 | .00 |
| Age | 146.05 | 4 | 36.51 | 1.10 | .35 |
| Group × age | 358.06 | 4 | 89.52 | 2.71 | .03 |
| Error | 10943.97 | 331 | 33.06 | | |

A significant main effect was found between the CAT-D scores of the stuttering and the nonstuttering children, $F(1, 331) = 97.66$; $p < 0.05$. In other words, the stuttering children, as a group, obtained significantly higher scores on the CAT-D than did the control subjects. The ANOVA also revealed a significant group × age level interaction, $F(4, 331) = 2.71$; $p < .05$. Thus, the difference in the CAT-D scores of the two subject groups was dependent upon the age level of the children. A simple effects analysis (BMDP4V), the results of which are summarized in Table 4, was used to examine this interaction effect in more detail.

The between-group difference in CAT-D scores was found to be statistically significant at each of the five age levels. That is to say, the stuttering children at each level scored significantly higher on the CAT-D than did their nonstuttering peers. However, as the significant group × age level interaction indicated (Table 3), the magnitude of the between-group difference at the various age levels was not equal. This finding is consistent with the descriptive data, summarized in Table 2, that show that the between-group difference in the mean CAT-D scores was larger at the older age levels than at the younger ones. Closer inspection of the scores in Table 2 suggested that this growing discrepancy between the two groups was due to a differential trend in CAT-D scores among the subjects at the different age levels. The stuttering children tended to show somewhat higher CAT-D scores with increasing age, a trend which was most apparent at the younger age groups. An opposite trend could be observed among the nonstutterers. The mean CAT-D scores of the nonstuttering children decreased after age 9. Figure 1 makes this trend difference in the performance of the two subject groups apparent.

TABLE 4   Simple effects analysis of the CAT-D scores of the stuttering and the
nonstuttering children at five different age levels

| Source | SS | df | MS | F | p |
|--------|-----|-----|-----|-----|-----|
| Group—7 yrs | 399.94 | 1 | 399.94 | 12.10 | .00 |
| Group—8 yrs | 464.52 | 1 | 464.52 | 14.05 | .00 |
| Group—9 yrs | 393.62 | 1 | 393.62 | 11.90 | .00 |
| Group—10 yrs | 792.16 | 1 | 792.16 | 23.96 | .00 |
| Group—11 yrs+ | 1519.54 | 1 | 1519.54 | 45.96 | .00 |
| Error | 109343.97 | 331 | 33.06 | | |

*(continued)*

**E X C E R P T   9.31   Continued**

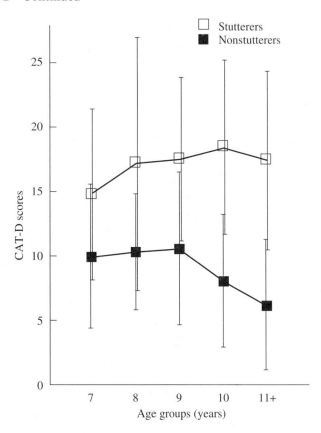

**FIGURE 1    Line graph of the mean CAT-D scores (squares)
and their standard deviations (extensions) for the stuttering
and the nonstuttering children at five different age levels.**

From "Speech-Associated Attitudes of Stuttering and Nonstuttering Children," by L. F. De Nil and G. J. Brutten,
1991, *Journal of Speech and Hearing Research, 34,* pp. 62–63. Copyright 1991 by the American Speech-Language-
Hearing Association. Reprinted with permission.

second main effect examined was the difference between the three stimulus presentation
conditions (within-subjects comparison). Finally, the interaction effect between subject
groups and stimulus conditions was evaluated. The results of these three parts of the analysis of variance are shown in the figure, table, and text included in the excerpt.

Figure 1 in Excerpt 9.32 is a bar graph depicting the mean number of stimuli correctly recalled by the two groups of children in each of the stimulus conditions. The table
is a complete ANOVA summary table similar to the one described in Chapter 6. The
between-subjects and within-subjects main effects and the interaction effect are listed in
the left column and the degrees of freedom, mean squares, *F*-ratios, and significance levels

**EXCERPT 9.32**

## Results

*Number of Items Recalled.* Figure 1 is a graph of the mean number of items recalled correctly by the two groups of children for the three types of stimulus material. A groups-by-stimulus-material-type analysis of variance (ANOVA), with repeated measures on material type (Winer, 1962), was performed on the number of items recalled to determine which of the recall performance differences were statistically significant. Results of the ANOVA (summarized in Table 1) were that the groups-by-stimulus-material interaction was significant ($p < 0.01$), as were each of the main effects. Because of the significant interaction, group means for

each of the stimulus-material-type conditions were analyzed. The group with good articulation recalled significantly more items than did the group with poor articulation when the word items were cast as sentences ($F = 29.61$; $df$ 1, 108; $p < 0.01$). The two groups did not perform differently on the digit or random-word tasks. Both groups were found to recall significantly ($p < 0.01$) more items on the sentence task than on the digit or random-word tasks. (See Figure 1.)

**TABLE 1   Summary of ANOVA to test for differences in mean number of items recalled for 28 children with poor articulation and 28 children with good articulation for three stimulus material types**

| Source | df | MS | F | p |
|---|---|---|---|---|
| *Between Subjects* | 55 | 2.22 | — | — |
| Groups (B) | 1 | 36.21 | 22.77 | <0.01 |
| Error (S within B) | 54 | 1.59 | — | — |
| *Within Subjects* | 112 | 10.11 | — | — |
| Stimulus material (A) | 2 | 338.04 | 206.11 | <0.01 |
| Stimulus material × groups (A × B) | 2 | 9.13 | 5.57 | <0.01 |
| Error (A × S within B) | 108 | 1.64 | — | — |

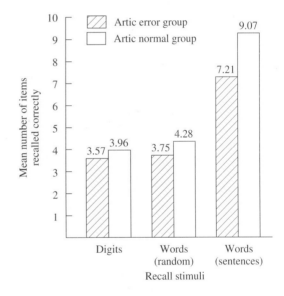

**FIGURE 1   The mean number of items (string length) recalled correctly by the articulation-error ($N = 28$) and articulation-normal ($N = 28$) groups for each of the three types of stimulus material.**

are listed in the other columns for each main effect and interaction. In such an ANOVA, significant differences are indicated by large *F*-ratios and nonsignificant differences are indicated by smaller *F*-ratios, although the absolute value of a significant *F* depends on the number of degrees of freedom associated with each comparison.

The *F* was significant for the main effect of the between-subjects comparison, indicating that the groups performed differently on the recall task. The within-subjects *F* for the comparison of the effects of the different stimulus materials was significant, indicating that recall performance was not the same for the different stimuli. The stimulus material by groups interaction was also significant, indicating that the two groups of children performed differently on the different types of material. This interaction effect is further explored in the text with references to the figure. The authors indicate in the text that follow-up comparisons with contrast tests of specific pairs of means (e.g., normal versus articulation-impaired children on recall of words in sentences) reveal that the two groups of children did not perform differently on recall of digits or random words but that they did perform differently on recall of words in sentences. This finding is the essence of the interaction effect and the most important result of this analysis of variance.

Inspection of Figure 1 in Excerpt 9.32 confirms the notion that the two groups of children were different in their recall of words in sentences but not in their recall of either digits or random words. A greater separation of the means of the two groups can be seen for the words in sentences than for the digits or random words when the figure is inspected closely. In this example, a rather thorough recounting of the analysis of variance is provided that includes the ANOVA summary table, the figure, and a narrative description of the comparisons.

Excerpt 9.33 shows the results of a three-way analysis of variance and includes the ANOVA summary table, a three-dimensional bar graph of the means, a table showing summary statistics (means and standard deviations) for all levels of three independent variables, and a textual description of the results of the three-way ($3 \times 3 \times 2$) between-subjects (i.e., *non*-repeated measures) ANOVA in a study of the influence of age, education, and living environment (independent variables) on naming ability (dependent variable). The text clearly explains the three main effects and the three-way interaction between the independent variables. The interaction can clearly be seen in the bar graph where the bar-height patterns for institutionalized, low-education participants and for noninstitutionalized, high-education participants differ from all the other bar-height patterns.

Excerpt 9.34 shows text and table regarding the results of a series of four parametric one-way analyses of variance and a Kruskal Wallis nonparametric analysis of variance in a between-subjects study of narrative development in late talkers. The independent variable is the talker group, which has three levels: children with normal language development (NL), children with a history of expressive language delay (HELD), and children with expressive language delay (ELD). There are five dependent variables, four of which (information score, MLU, lexical diversity, and cohesive adequacy), the authors determined, met the assumptions of parametric statistics. The authors explain that the narrative stage dependent variable was an ordinal level measure, however, so the nonparametric ANOVA was substituted for the parametric and the Mann–Whitney *U* test was used in place of the parametric Tukey test for follow-up contrasts. The text clearly explains the significant F statistics for the parametric ANOVAs and the significant *H* statistic for narrative stage. *H* is a statistic calculated from ordinal ranks rather than from interval or ratio scores that substitutes for the *F* statistic in the Kruskal Wallis ANOVA. The footnote in the table clearly explains how superscripts were used to indicate which differences between groups were significant and which were not and these patterns are also described in the text.

Excerpt 9.34 showed the Kruskal Wallis nonparametric ANOVA, which is used in place of a between-subjects, nonrepeated measures ANOVA when the data do not meet the

## EXCERPT 9.33

In order to further define the effects of living environment, age, and education on BNT scores, a 3 × 3 × 2 factorial analysis of variance was conducted. The variable Age was recoded into 3 groups: Age Group 1 (*n* = 100) included ages 65–74; Age Group 2 (*n* = 119) included ages 75–84; and Age Group 3 (*n* = 104) included ages 85–97. The three Education Groups included Group 1: 6–9 years (*n* = 100); Group 2: 10–12 years (*n* = 119); and Group 3: 13–21 years (*n* = 104). The third factor was living environment, and subjects were classified as institutionalized and noninstitutionalized.

Table 1 shows the significant main effects for Age, Education, and Living Environment. There were no significant two-way interactions. There was a significant three-way interaction. Table 2 displays the means and standard deviations of the Living Environment × Age × Education subgroups. The standard deviations indicate an overlap in BNT scores among the subgroups. The mean BNT scores of the subgroups are also displayed in bar graphs in Figure 1. Noninstitutionalized subgroups appear on the left side of Figure 1, and the institutionalized subgroups on the right side. The subgroups are also classified according to age: "Young" (65–74 years), "Middle" (75–84 years), and "Old" (85–97 years). Notice that education is lowest (6 to 9 years) in the front and highest (12+ years) in the back of Figure 1.

### Subjects with 6 to 9 Years of Education

The front row of Figure 1 shows that subjects with a low level of education obtained relatively low mean scores on the BNT. For noninstitutionalized subjects with a low level of education, BNT scores declined further with increasing age. In contrast, the institutionalized subjects with a low level of education showed little difference in mean BNT scores according to age. The youngest institutionalized subjects with a limited education did not appear to benefit from their relative youth as much as other relatively young institutionalized subjects with more education.

### Subjects with 10 to 12 Years of Education

The second row of Figure 1 shows that age had a similar impact on both noninstitutionalized and institutionalized subjects with a middle level of education. The youngest subjects obtained the highest mean BNT scores, and the oldest subjects obtained the lowest mean BNT scores. However, there were differences in mean BNT performance according to living environment; these were more pronounced for the old and middle subgroups than for the young subgroups. The institutionalized subjects performed more poorly than the noninstitutionalized subjects.

### Subjects with Education beyond the High School Level

The back row of Figure 1 shows that there was little difference in BNT performance in terms of age or living environment for the well educated. (The only exception was the oldest institutionalized subjects, who performed poorly regardless of level of education.)

**TABLE 1  Summary of analysis of variance for BNT scores**

| Source | df | MS | F |
|---|---|---|---|
| Living Environment (A) | 1 | 3208.76 | 43.16* |
| Age Groups (B) | 2 | 1169.01 | 15.72* |
| Education (C) | 2 | 2362.03 | 31.77* |
| A × B | 2 | 19.66 | .26 |
| A × C | 2 | 87.92 | 1.18 |
| B × C | 4 | 24.64 | .33 |
| A × B × C | 4 | 236.66 | 3.18* |

*$p < .05$

(continued)

**E X C E R P T   9.33    Continued**

**TABLE 2    BNT norms according to living environment, education, and age**

| Age | Education Level | | | |
| --- | --- | --- | --- | --- |
| | 6–9 | 10–12 | 12+ | All education levels |
| Noninstitutionalized[1] | | | | |
| 65–74 | 47.58 (SD = 6.14, n = 12) | 53.00 (SD = 6.63, n = 22) | 53.10 (SD = 6.55, n = 20) | 51.83 (SD = 6.77, n = 54) |
| 75–84 | 42.79 (SD = 10.99, n = 19) | 50.73 (SD = 5.72, n = 22) | 48.55 (SD = 7.96, n = 20) | 47.54 (SD = 8.99, n = 61) |
| 85–97 | 36.00 (SD = 12.46, n = 17) | 45.53 (SD = 10.70, n = 19) | 49.88 (SD = 7.19, n = 16) | 43.75 (SD = 8.89, n = 52) |
| Total | 41.58 (SD = 11.36, n = 48) | 49.95 (SD = 8.29, n = 63) | 50.55 (SD = 7.40, n = 56) | |
| Institutionalized[2] | | | | |
| 65–74 | 35.14 (SD = 6.77, n = 14) | 46.95 (SD = 8.78, n = 19) | 49.54 (SD = 6.42, n = 13) | 44.09 (SD = 9.59, n = 46) |
| 75–84 | 36.90 (SD = 11.84, n = 19) | 39.95 (SD = 10.05, n = 19) | 48.30 (SD = 6.62, n = 20) | 41.82 (SD = 10.71, n = 58) |
| 85–97 | 34.53 (SD = 9.78, n = 19 ) | 38.11 (SD = 7.48, n = 18) | 40.20 (SD = 7.62, n = 15) | 37.40 (SD = 8.60, n = 52) |
| Total | 35.56 (SD = 9.80, n = 52) | 41.73 (SD = 9.51, n = 56) | 46.10 (SD = 7.87, n = 48) | |

[1]n = 167   [2]n = 156

EXCERPT 9.33 Continued

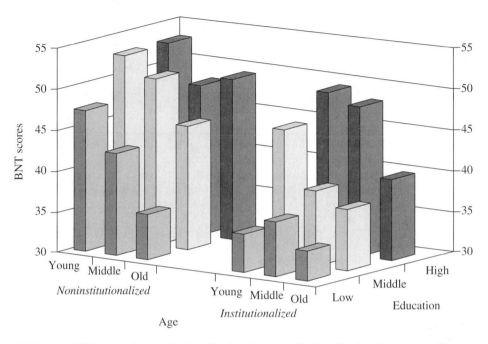

FIGURE 1 BNT scores for institutionalized and noninstitutionalized subjects according to age and education.

From "Effects of Age, Education, and Living Environment on Boston Naming Test Performance," by J. Neils, J. M. Baris, C. Carter, A. L. Dell'aira, S. J. Nordloh, E. Weiler, and B. Weisiger, 1995, *Journal of Speech and Hearing Research, 38,* pp. 1145–1147. Copyright 1995 by the American Speech-Language-Hearing Association. Reprinted with permission.

assumptions for a parametric inferential analysis. When a within-subjects, repeated measures ANOVA is needed, but the data do not meet the assumptions for a parametric inferential analysis, the nonparametric alternative is the Friedman Analysis of Variance. The example shown in Excerpt 9.35 examines whether two levels of context (contextualized vs. decontextualized) and two types of discourse tasks (cooking vs. narrative) would affect the behavior of children who stutter on three different dependent variables. The two crossed bivalent independent variables of context and discourse make four conditions for a 2 × 2 ANOVA: CC = contextualized cooking, DC = decontextualized cooking, CN = contextualized narrative, and DN = decontextualized narrative. Three separate Two-Way Friedman Analyses of Variance by Ranks were run, one for each of three different dependent variables (stuttering type, linguistic nonfluencies, and mazing). Table 7 in Excerpt 9.35 shows the results of the ANOVA: the dependent variables stuttering type and mazing showed significant differences overall, but the linguistic nonfluencies dependent variable failed to reach significance across the two independent variables. Table 8 in the excerpt shows the follow-up with multiple comparisons of each condition to determine which specific pairs were significantly different from each other. Notice that the Wilcoxon Signed-Ranks Test (with the $z$-score conversions of the $T$ statistics) was used for these repeated measures contrasts much as the Mann–Whitney $U$ test

## EXCERPT 9.34

### Results

For each of the three follow-up assessments, the results on four of the variables studied (Information score, MLU per T-unit, Lexical Diversity, and Cohesive Adequacy) were subjected to a one-way ANOVA. Pair-wise differences were examined with Tukey tests. Because of the ordinal nature of the Narrative Stage score, a Kruskal Wallis nonparametric ANOVA was used to examine group differences on this measure. The Mann-Whitney U-test was used as a nonparametric analog of the Tukey tests.

### Kindergarten

Table 4 presents results of the narrative analyses for the year the subjects were in kindergarten. Approximately two thirds of the children originally identified as SELD had moved within the normal range (above the 10th

percentile on DSS) of expressive language by kindergarten (the HELD group). There were significant differences among the three groups ($p < .05$) on Lexical Diversity, $F(1, 52) = 5.70$; Cohesive Adequacy, $F(1, 52) = 3.68$; and Narrative Stage, $H = 6.70$, at the kindergarten assessment. The NL group scored significantly higher than both the HELD and ELD groups on Lexical Diversity. The HELD and ELD groups were not significantly different on this measure. Children with NL scored significantly higher than those with ELD on Cohesive Adequacy, but the children with HELD were not significantly different from either of the other two groups. The children with NL scored significantly higher than both those with HELD and with ELD on the narrative stage measure, but the children with HELD and ELD were not significantly different. As indicated in Table 4, there were no other significant differences.

**TABLE 4   Mean (and standard deviation) narrative scores and comparison for three groups: Kindergarten**

| Variable | NL [n = 25] | HELD [n = 17; 63%[1]] | ELD [n = 10; 37%[1]] |
|---|---|---|---|
| Information score | 11.9 (3.2) | 11.4 (3.1) | 9.1 (4.7) |
| MLU per T-unit | 7.2 (1.0) | 6.9 (1.3) | 6.6 (1.2) |
| Lexical diversity[2] | 15.5[a] (6.1) | 11.0[b] (3.5) | 10.3 (4.6)[b] |
| Cohesive adequacy[2] (% complete ties) | 84.7[a] (16.6) | 76.7[a,b] (23.4) | 62.1[b] (31.7) |
| Narrative stage[2] | 4.1[a] (0.8) | 3.8[b] (0.7) | 3.1[b] (1.2) |

*Note.* NL = Normal Language, HELD = History of Expressive Language Delay, ELD = Chronic Expressive Language Delay.

[1]percentage of original SELD subjects who were placed in this subgroup.

[2]groups are significantly different at $p < .05$. Groups with differing superscripts were significantly different on post-hoc pair-wise comparisons. Those with the same superscripts were not.

From "Narrative Development in Late Talkers: Early School Age," by R. Paul, R. Hernandez, L. Taylor, and K. Johnson, 1996, *Journal of Speech and Hearing Research, 39,* pp. 1299–1300. Copyright 1996 by the American Speech-Language-Hearing Association. Reprinted with permission.

## Effects of Context on Disfluency Type in Children Who Stutter

The third question asked whether CWS would exhibit differences in the types of disfluencies used across the two levels of contextualization and two types of discourse tasks. Friedman's Two Way Analysis of Variance by Ranks ($F_r$) was used to answer this question because of the small number of scores in each condition ($n = 12$) and because the sample did not contain a matched control group (see Table 7). Separate analyses were completed for each type of disfluency because the question of interest was examining each type of disfluency by itself, rather than whether the three types were affected together by varying conditions.

**TABLE 7   Results of the Friedman's ($F_r$) Two-Way Analysis of Variance by Ranks Test for proportion of occurrence of three types of disfluency between four conditions: Contextualized Cooking (CC), Decontextualized Cooking (DC), Contextualized Narrative (CN), and Decontextualized Narrative (DN).**

| Disfluency type | df | Number of samples | $F_r$ | p |
|---|---|---|---|---|
| Stuttering type | 3 | 12 | 8.385 | .0387* (corrected for ties) |
| Linguistic nonfluencies | 3 | 12 | 5.118 | .1634 (corrected for ties) |
| Mazing | 3 | 12 | 7.983 | .0464* (corrected for ties) |

*Statistically significant difference at the .05 level of significance.

Stuttering-type disfluency was significantly different across the four conditions [$F_r(3) = 8.385$, $p = .0387$], corrected for ties. This result may be influenced by 3 of the 12 participants, who had considerably higher proportions of stuttering (ranges between 11% and 18% stuttering) than did the rest of the group (ranges between 0% and 9% stuttering). A nonsignificant difference was found for proportion of linguistic nonfluencies between the four conditions [$F_r(3) = 5.118$, $p = .1634$]. Finally, a significant difference was noted for proportion of maze behavior between the four conditions [$F_r(3) = 7.983$, $p = .0464$]. This value also represents a correction for ties, as there were two tied groups in the sample.

To determine which conditions were significantly different from one another, the Wilcoxon Signed Ranks Test was used to make multiple comparisons of proportion of occurrence for stuttering-type disfluency and mazing between the four conditions. Results are presented in Table 8. Stuttering was significantly different in conditions between the contextualized cooking condition and both narrative conditions. For mazing, conditions CC and DC were significantly different from one another, as were CC and DN and DC and CN. The rest of the paired comparisons were nonsignificant.

**TABLE 8   Results of the Wilcoxon Signed Ranks Test for multiple comparisons of stuttering-type disfluency and mazing among the four conditions: Contextualized Cooking (CC), Decontextualized Cooking (DC), Contextualized Narrative (CN), and Decontextualized Narrative (DN).**

| Comparison of contexts | z | p |
|---|---|---|
| Stuttering-type disfluency | | |
| CC vs. DC | −1.07 | .2845 |
| CC vs. CN (corrected for ties) | −2.394 | .0167* |
| CC vs. DN (corrected for ties) | −2.434 | .0149* |
| DC vs. CN (corrected for ties) | −.314 | .7536 |
| DC vs. DN (corrected for ties) | −1.727 | .0841 |
| CN vs. DN (corrected for ties) | −.535 | .593 |
| Mazing | | |
| CC vs. DC | −2.401 | .0164* |
| CC vs. CN | −.314 | .7537 |
| CC vs. DN | −2.04 | .0414* |
| DC vs. CN | −2.04 | .0414* |
| DC vs. DN | −.706 | .4802 |
| CN vs. DN | −1.6 | .1095 |

*Statistically significant difference between the two conditions at the .05 level of significance.

was used in Excerpt 9.34 for the follow-up contrast tests with the nonrepeated measures Kruskal Wallis ANOVA.

As mentioned in Chapter 6, when multiple dependent variables are used in a parametric analysis, it may be advisable in some circumstances to use a multivariate analysis of variance (MANOVA) rather than the univariate model (i.e., one dependent variable at a time) to determine the simultaneous effects of the independent variables on the dependent variables,

---

**E X C E R P T   9.36**

### Results

#### Group Differences

A two-way multivariate analysis of variance (MANOVA) was conducted to determine whether the four Age × Language groups differed on the three measures: reticence as measured by the TBRS, language skills as measured by the CASL composite score, and emotion regulation skills as measured by the Emotion Regulation subscale of the ERC. Age (younger and older) and language group (typical and SLI) served as independent variables, and the three test measures as dependent variables. A significant main effect for language group was found, approximate $F(3, 81) = 45.98$, $p < .001$, $\eta^2 = .629$.[2] No other significant effects were found. We conducted follow-up univariate tests for each dependent variable to further evaluate the language group effect. For each of these follow-up tests, the Bonferroni procedure was used to adjust alpha levels.

Means and standard deviations for the language, emotion regulation, and reticence measures of the follow-up analyses are presented in Table 1. Significant language group main effects were found for each of the following three measures: reticence, $F(1, 83) = 26.12$, $p < .001$, $\eta^2 = .235$; CASL composite, $F(1, 83) = 136.05$, $p < .001$, $\eta^2 = .615$; and emotion regulation, $F(1, 83) = 26.70$, $p < .001$, $\eta^2 = .243$. From Table 1, it may be seen that, for all three measures, the group with SLI performed more poorly than did the typical group. These findings replicated the results of previous research (Fujiki et al., 1999; Fujiki et al., 2002).

**TABLE 1    Means and standard deviations for language, emotion regulation, and reticence scores.**

| Participant group | CASL composite | Emotion regulation | Reticence[a] |
|---|---|---|---|
| Younger, typical | | | |
| M | 111.38 | 28.05 | 1.19 |
| SD | 14.72 | 2.50 | 1.44 |
| Older, typical | | | |
| M | 111.09 | 27.57 | 1.26 |
| SD | 11.69 | 4.24 | 1.71 |
| Younger, SLI | | | |
| M | 83.67 | 23.19 | 3.33 |
| MSD | 11.58 | 4.75 | 2.94 |
| Older, SLI | | | |
| M | 79.18 | 23.45 | 4.26 |
| SD | 9.14 | 4.28 | 2.91 |

*Note.* CASL = Comprehensive Assessment of Spoken Language (Carrow-Woolfolk, 1999).

[a]Higher reticence scores indicate greater withdrawal.

---

[2]As the reader is likely more familiar with the $F$ statistic, we report the $F$ approximation derived from the Wilks's lambda statistic associated with the MANOVAs reported herein (see Tabachnick & Fidell, 2001, for a discussion).

especially when the dependent variables are correlated with each other. Excerpt 9.36 shows results from a study of the relationship between language, reticence, and emotional regulation in children with specific language impairment (SLI). Children in two age groups with and without SLI were compared simultaneously on three dependent variables: the Comprehensive Assessment of Spoken Language (CASL), the Emotion Regulation Checklist (ERC), and the Teacher Behavior Rating Scale (TBRS). Table 1 in the excerpt shows the means and standard deviations of the three dependent variables for each of the four groups of children (younger typical, older typical, younger SLI, and older SLI). The text describes the use of the MANOVA for the analysis of the overall effect and follow-up $F$-tests for the specific comparisons of the different groups on the different dependent variables. Note the use of the approximated $F$-statistic derived from the MANOVA Wilks's Lambda based on the rationale that readers are more familiar with the $F$-statistic. This is probably because MANOVA has not been used as commonly as ANOVA in communicative disorders research until recent years. In fact, Tabachnick and Fidell (2001), the authors of the book cited in the footnote in Excerpt 9.36, stated that MANOVA is now becoming increasingly popular for analyzing complicated data sets and more widely used in many areas of behavioral research as more sophisticated computer programs become available.

Note also that the authors reported the effect size (Eta squared = $\eta^2$) for the overall MANOVA for the three dependent variables ($\eta^2 = .629$), which was in the medium to large range, as discussed in Chapter 6. They also reported the individual effect sizes for the analysis of each dependent variable, which were fairly small for reticence ($\eta^2 = .235$) and emotional regulation ($\eta^2 = .243$) but larger for the language variable ($\eta^2 = .615$). As mentioned in Chapter 6, it was not common until recent years to find effect sizes reported in the communicative disorders literature, but more journal articles are reporting this statistic in consonance with the effect size statement in the *APA Publication Manual* cited in Chapter 6 (American Psychological Association, 2001, pp. 25–26). Effect size statistics are not limited to MANOVA, but can be calculated for a number of other inferential statistical tests as well, including, for example, univariate ANOVA and the $t$-test.

This leads us to our final example in Excerpt 9.37, which illustrates the reporting of effect sizes using Cohen's $d$ statistic to accompany a series of Bonferroni $t$-tests. The study shown in this excerpt compared the performance of children and adults in their mental images for transparent and opaque idiomatic expressions. Table 5 in the excerpt shows the percent of each type of image (irrelevant, literal, or figurative) evoked by transparent or opaque idioms for both the children and the adults. The Bonferroni $t$-tests indicated significant differences between children and adults on irrelevant images (more for children than adults) and on figurative images (more for adults than children), but no significant difference between them on literal images. Effect sizes (Cohen's $d$) for the two significant differences are reported as large for irrelevant images and moderate for figurative images.

## Some Characteristics of Clear Data Analysis

The analysis of data in a Results section should present a clear picture of the strength and direction of relationships or of the significant differences that were found. Readers should expect some of the following characteristics of clear analysis of data.

**E X C E R P T   9.37**

To further explore the relationship between comprehension and imagery, the types of images (irrelevant, literal, or figurative) evoked by the transparent and opaque expressions were tabulated for all idioms that each participant had answered correctly on the Idiom Comprehension Task. The resulting raw numbers were converted to percentages to adjust for differences in performance on the comprehension task. These data are shown in Table 5. A series of independent $t$ tests, with Bonferroni corrections for multiple $t$ tests and an adjusted alpha of .008, were performed to compare the groups. The results indicated that, for both types of idioms, the children, despite comprehending the expressions, produced a significantly greater percentage of irrelevant images than the adults [transparent, $t(78) = 4.12, p < .0001$; opaque, $t(78) = -3.87, p = .0002$], and the adults produced a significantly greater percentage of figurative images than the children [transparent, $t(78) = -3.43, p = .0010$; opaque, $t(78) = -3.04, p = .0032$]. However, the groups did not differ significantly in the percentage of literal images for either type of idiom [transparent, $t(78) = 1.03, p > .05$; opaque, $t(78) = 0.83, p > .05$]. The effect sizes were large (Cohen, 1988) for irrelevant images ($d = .93$ for transparent; $d = .88$ for opaque) and moderate for figurative images ($d = .77$ for transparent; $d = .68$ for opaque).

**TABLE 5   Images of each type (in %) produced on the Mental Imagery Task for all idioms that were answered correctly on the Idiom Comprehension Task ($n = 40$ per group).**

| Image type | Children | Adults |
|---|---|---|
| *Irrelevant (score = 0)* | | |
| Transparent | 24.54 | 10.24 |
| Opaque | 28.64 | 14.41 |
| *Literal (score = 1)* | | |
| Transparent | 47.92 | 40.99 |
| Opaque | 44.79 | 38.98 |
| *Figurative (score = 2)* | | |
| Transparent | 27.54 | 48.77 |
| Opaque | 26.58 | 46.89 |

From "Mental Imagery and Idiom Comprehension: A Comparison of School-Age Children and Adults," by M. A. Nippold and J. K. Duthie, 2003, *Journal of Speech, Language, and Hearing Research, 46,* pp. 794–795. Copyright 2003 by the American Speech-Language-Hearing Association. Reprinted with permission.

Illustrations that are used in the analysis of relationships or differences should conform to the same standards that were discussed earlier in the section on organization of data. Table and figure captions should be brief but informative. Tables and figures should be capable of standing alone in presenting the analysis, and the narrative should dovetail easily with the illustrations in the discussion of the data analysis.

The analysis of relationships should employ statistical techniques that are appropriate to such factors as the level of measurement of the data and the number of observations. Readers should be aware of the general appropriateness of indices such as the Pearson and Spearman correlation coefficients, the $\chi^2$, and the contingency coefficient that are used in the analysis of relationships. The significance levels of the correlations that are reported should be included when necessary, and consumers may also expect authors to comment on the practical meaning of correlations, as well as their statistical significance. This may often be accompanied by reference to the index of determination ($r^2$) in discussing the overlap of variance among variables.

The evaluation of intercorrelation matrices or of multiple regression analyses may be particularly difficult for novice consumers. Authors may aid consumers in this task through careful presentation and discussion of these analyses, especially in the integration of the narrative with the illustrations. Despite this, evaluation of multiple correlation and regression analyses will usually require more time and effort from consumers. Frequent exposure to multiple correlation studies should serve to sharpen the reader's evaluative skills in this area.

The analysis of differences should employ statistical techniques that are appropriate to the level of measurement used, the number of observations, the number of comparisons, and so forth. Readers should be aware of the appropriateness of parametric and nonparametric inference tests. Readers should also be cognizant of the appropriate uses of two-sample comparison statistics and of the need for analysis of variance techniques for simultaneous comparisons. These analyses should present a clear and consistent summary of significant and nonsignificant differences and of main and interaction effects when necessary. Such analyses often include reference to both a table and a figure to clarify the narrative explanation of the differences found. Multiple comparisons with complex interactions may present some difficulty to novice consumers; once again, authors may aid these readers through careful integration of tables, figures, and text.

# EVALUATION CHECKLIST

**Instructions:**  The four-category scale at the end of this checklist may be used to rate the *Results* section of an article. The *Evaluation Items* help identify those topics that should be considered in arriving at the rating. Comments on these topics, entered as *Evaluation Notes,* should serve as the basis for the overall rating.

*Evaluation Items*                                          *Evaluation Notes*

1. Results were clearly related to research problem.

2. Tables and figures were integrated with text.

3. Summary statistics were used appropriately.

4. Organization of data was clear.

5. Statistical analysis was appropriate to:
   (a) level of measurement
   (b) number of observations
   (c) type of sample
   (d) shape of distribution

6. There was appropriate use of correlational and inferential analysis.

*Evaluation Items*                                                                 *Evaluation Notes*

  **7.** There was clear presentation of significant and
     nonsignificant correlations.

  **8.** There was clear presentation of significant and
     nonsignificant differences and effect sizes.

  **9.** General comments.

*Overall Rating (Results):*

| _____ | _____ | _____ | _____ |
| Poor | Fair | Good | Excellent |

# REFERENCES

American Psychological Association. (2001). *Publication manual of the American Psychological Association* (5th ed.). Washington, DC: American Psychological Association.

Tabachnick, B. G., & Fidell, L. S. (2001). *Using multivariate statistics* (4th ed.). Boston: Allyn & Bacon.

# The Discussion and Conclusions Section

The last section of an article, usually titled *Discussion* or *Conclusions* or both, is written with somewhat more license than are the other sections, and readers may often notice more variation among authors in the organization of this section. In fact, consumers of research may encounter shorter articles that combine the results and conclusions into one section. Nevertheless, there are some general topics that are usually addressed at the end of an article, and consumers of research should be aware of the importance of these in the culmination of a research article. Five general topics will be included in our evaluation checklist for the Discussion and Conclusions section:

> Relationship of Conclusions to Preceding Parts of the Article
> Relationship of Results to Previous Research
> Theoretical Implications of the Research
> Practical Implications of the Research
> Implications for Future Research

Each of these general topics will be discussed separately in the next five sections.

## Relationship of Conclusions to Preceding Parts of the Article

The Discussion section should contain some material that relates the conclusions directly to the *Problem, Method,* and *Results* of the investigation and that unites the preceding sections into a coherent whole.

### The Research Problem

The conclusions of a research article should be directed clearly toward the *research problem* that was presented in the first section of the article. Complete restatement of the problem and rationale would be cumbersome at this point in an article, but in many of the better articles in the literature, the discussion commences with a brief reminder of the problem and a general statement of the conclusion of the investigation regarding the problem or research questions.

Excerpts 10.1 and 10.2 present introductory paragraphs from two Discussion sections that neatly remind readers of the research problem and quickly summarize the results

**Discussion**

It has been argued that personality, emotions, and psychological problems contribute to or are primary causes of voice disorders and that voice disorders in turn create psychological problems and personality effects. This investigation compared a non-voice-disordered otolaryngology control and four voice-disordered groups on self-report measures of personality and emotional adjustment. At the superfactor trait level, the FD and VN groups differed in significant ways from one another, from the other voice-disordered groups, and from the non-voice-disordered control group. Results largely support the contention that individuals with certain personality traits may be susceptible to developing FD or VN. In contrast, less support was found for the disability (scar) hypothesis, which argues that voice disorders lead to general personality changes. This raises the question as to how the results can be interpreted within the general theoretical framework presented in the companion article (Roy & Bless, 2000b).

From "Personality and Voice Disorders: A Superfactor Trait Analysis," by N. Roy, D. M. Bless, and D. Heisey, 2000, *Journal of Speech, Language, and Hearing Research, 43,* p. 760. Copyright 2000 by the American Speech-Language-Hearing Association. Reprinted with permission.

in relation to the problem. The conclusions of both studies reflect clearly and directly on the research problems and set the stage for further discussion of the limitations and implications of the research. Excerpt 10.1 is from a study of various voice disorders, including functional dysphonia (FD) and vocal nodules (VN) and Excerpt 10.2 is from a study comparing the effects of sentence-structure priming on children who stutter (CWS) and children who do not stutter (CWNS).

## The Method of Investigation

The Discussion section should also present some remarks concerning the *method* of the investigation and how it relates to the conclusion of the study. Any limitations of the research imposed by the particular method should be considered. Qualifying remarks may be found concerning the participants, materials, or procedures employed and how they may limit the conclusions that may be drawn from the data.

Of particular concern is the manner in which the author discusses the potential threats to internal and external validity in the investigation and how these threats may have been reduced in the design of the study. As readers will have surmised, every empirical investigation may be subject to some threats to internal and external validity, and the better studies are those that minimize these threats. Minimization implies, however, that there is usually some residue of jeopardy to internal and external validity. This residue should be addressed in the Discussion section in order to qualify the conclusions and, perhaps, to suggest future research possibilities to improve or extend the findings of the investigation. The better studies in the literature, then, are those that not only reduce the threats to internal and external validity but also discuss the residue of jeopardy with some candor in qualifying the results. Of course, if an inordinately large number of research design limitations are discussed, readers may question the wisdom of the journal editor for publishing the

EXCERPT 10.2

## Discussion

The primary purpose of this investigation was to examine experimentally the time course of syntactic production processes in young CWS and CWNS. This study was prompted, in part, by speculation that stuttering may be related to slowness, inefficiencies, or dyssynchronies within linguistic formulation components (Perkins, Kent, & Curlee, 1991; Postma & Kolk, 1993), as well as various empirical studies indicating that stuttering events appear to be related, at least in part, to the linguistic features of an utterance (e.g., Melnick & Conture, 2000; Yaruss, 1999; Zackheim & Conture, 2003). A modified version of the sentence-structure priming paradigm (Bock, 1990; Bock et al., 1992) was used to examine experimentally the time course of syntactic processes in CWS and CWNS, the findings of which are considered below.

### Main Findings: An Overview
The present study resulted in four main findings: (a) temporal processing of sentences for 3- to 5-year-

old children appears to be influenced by experimental manipulation (i.e., syntactic priming) of sentence retrieval, integration, and/or production; (b) CWS demonstrated a greater syntactic-priming effect (approximately 212 ms) than CWNS (approximately 51 ms); (c) CWS produced fewer accurate responses than CWNS during the sentence-structure priming task; and (d) CWS who produced more stuttering-like disfluencies during conversational speech exhibited slower SRTs (during accurate picture descriptions) in the absence of a syntactic prime, but there was no apparent relationship between the frequency of conversational stuttering and a syntactic-priming effect. The general implications of each of these four findings will be discussed immediately below.

study in the first place. In other words, as the limitations become more extensive and significant, the value of the research is reduced accordingly.

Excerpts 10.3 and 10.4 illustrate the ways in which authors have considered various limitations of the method of investigation and discussed appropriate qualifications of their conclusions based on these limitations. Excerpt 10.3, from a study of problem behaviors of children with language disorders, addresses limitations concerning cause–effect inferences drawn from descriptive versus experimental research and restrictions of generalization to other settings, measures, and persons. Excerpt 10.4 is from a study of listeners' attitudes toward speakers with voice and resonance disorders and discusses several limitations concerning internal and external validity.

## The Results of the Investigation

The conclusions in the Discussion section should be drawn directly and fairly from the results. Although the Discussion section should not be merely a rehashing of the results,

EXCERPT   10.3

**Limitations of the Study**

There are several limitations of the present study. First, the results are descriptive and correlational; no cause-and-effect relationships between language delays and behavior patterns could be established. For example, the significant $r = -.32$ between externalizing behavior and auditory comprehension suggests that language delays are related to an externalizing behavioral problem. It may be, however, that another child characteristic (e.g., lack of social skills) causes the child to exhibit certain externalizing behavior. In this case, lack of social skills, rather than low auditory comprehension ability, would be the cause of the child's high level of externalizing problem behaviors. Both language delays and problem behaviors may be the concomitant outcomes of the multiple risk factors associated with poverty or of underlying cognitive deficits.

A second limitation is that there were no direct measures of language use with peers by target children, which could have provided more specific information linking behavior to language performance in the classroom context. For example, it seems important to examine what the target children are saying and how explicit or well formed these utterances are during peer interactions. In future studies, simultaneous language sampling during observations should also be used to provide a clearer picture of children's language use during problem behavior episodes.

Third, there was limited observation assessment of children's internalizing behaviors. Internalizing behaviors may be relatively subtle and difficult to measure accurately without considerable knowledge of individual children and their family backgrounds. The low frequency of internalizing behaviors and their context-specific characteristics makes them difficult to observe reliably. The coding scheme used in our study, like those used in most preschool observational studies, included very few internalizing behaviors. Thus, it was not possible to test adequately the relationship between teacher reports of internalizing behaviors and observed internalizing behaviors or to explore fully the relationship between language and internalizing behavior.

Finally, sample characteristics qualify the findings of this study. The Head Start sample was predominantly low-income African American, with a very small percentage of low-income European American and Hispanic children represented. The findings cannot be generalized to other populations. Further research with samples from other ethnic groups or middle- or upper-income families is needed to determine the applicability of the present findings to such groups. In addition, as regional differences might mitigate the findings from this study, the results could not be generalized to all African American children in Head Start programs. The study could be replicated in the future, examining children from rural or northern areas.

authors often refer to the data to support their conclusions. Occasionally, authors may even include a table or figure in the Discussion section to summarize their own results and, perhaps, the results of other studies to aid in the presentation of the conclusions. The important point is that the conclusions should be tied directly and fairly to empirical results, and comments that are not empirically based should be labeled as speculations, not as conclusions. Speculations are often important in the generation of new research and contribute to the cre-

## EXCERPT 10.4

**Limits to Validity**

There are several limits to the internal validity of this study that should be considered when interpreting the results. The speakers with voice and resonance disorders were not matched in age, as this was not possible with the available clinical population. Instead each one of the three control speakers was selected to fit within the young, middle-aged, and old categories represented among the disordered speakers. This is a concern because Deal and Oyer (1991) found that the voices of older speakers (with no disorder) tended to be rated as less pleasant than those of younger speakers. Other threats to internal validity include the fact that some speakers may have had differences in intonation that the listeners responded to. Finally, although the listeners were asked multiple-choice questions for the purposes of ensuring they read the information materials, their responses do not ensure that they truly processed that knowledge and applied it during the semantic differential task.

Some features that limit the external validity of this study also should be noted. The results cannot be generalized to listeners' attitudes about all speakers with voice and resonance disorders. Rather, they should be applied only to the disorders and severities of conditions used in this study and are relevant only when these disorders occur in female voices. Deal and Oyer (1991) compared listeners' perceptions of male

and female voices (with no disorder) and found that listeners tend to perceive men's voices more positively than women's voices.

Another limitation to external validity is that the results may not reflect the attitudes of individuals exposed to other types of information about voice and resonance disorders or to people exposed to information disseminated via other mediums. The results of this study also may not generalize to situations where a greater amount of intervention is provided than was offered in this study. The listeners also must be considered when evaluating external validity. Although a large number of listeners were used, they did not represent a randomly selected group of people. Thus, the results may be biased toward responses more typical of young, middle-class, female university student participants.

Finally, the experimental task performed in this study was not an actual interaction between a listener and speaker. This restricts the extent to which the results can be generalized to attitudes based on actual face-to-face interactions in which a listener would form an impression of a speaker based on the speaker's voice, message content, physical appearance, affect, and mannerisms. In this context, voice quality becomes only one of many factors that influence a listener's perceptions of a speaker.

---

ativity that is important in designing new research, but authors and readers alike must be aware of the difference between solid conclusions drawn directly from empirical data and intuitive speculations about the nature of phenomena.

In Excerpt 10.5 the author reviews the results for each of the three research questions that were stated in her introduction and excerpted in Chapter 7. The consonant identification performance data referred to are the same results shown clearly in the table of means and standard deviations for all conditions in Excerpt 9.9 in Chapter 9.

In Excerpt 10.6 the authors clearly review the results of their experiment on the effects of utterance length and syntactic complexity on speech motor stability of the fluent

## EXCERPT 10.5

**Discussion**

This study investigated children and young adults' consonant and vowel identification abilities in reverberation, noise, and combined listening conditions. Three experimental questions were posed regarding the SL for maximum performance and differences in consonant, vowel, and feature recognition between children's vs. young adults' age groups in the various listening conditions. Results showed that all age groups achieved maximum consonant identification performance at 50 dB SL. Vowel identification scores were unaffected by SL. Statistical analyses revealed that children's ability to identify consonants varied according to listening condition. For example, children's consonant identification abilities reached adult-like levels of performance at about age 14 years in the reverberation-only and noise-only listening conditions. However, in the reverberation-plus-noise listening condition, children's consonant identification abilities may not mature until the late teenage years. The ability to identify vowels, on the other hand, develops much earlier. A feature analysis showed that for all three consonant features (voicing, manner, and place), identification scores were highest in the control condition, similar for the reverberation-only and noise-only conditions, and lowest in the reverberation-plus-noise condition. Voicing was easier for listeners to identify than manner or place of articulation features in reverberation and noise. The ability to identify speech in reverberation and noise reaches adult-like levels of performance at different ages for different components of the speech signal.

From "Children's Phoneme Identification in Reverberation and Noise," by C. E. Johnson, 2000, *Journal of Speech, Language, and Hearing Research, 43,* p. 152. Copyright 2000 by the American Speech-Language-Hearing Association. Reprinted with permission.

speech of persons who stutter. In addition, the excerpt includes a paragraph titled Conclusions that they add at the end of their article, which functions somewhat like an abstract at the beginning of an article to give a brief overview of the article at the end. This excellent summarizing device is used more often in research journals, especially for longer and more complex articles.

Results are not always clear-cut, however. Occasionally the researcher may run into puzzling results that are difficult to interpret. In that case, the researcher is faced with the dilemma of trying to explain a difficult result and may need to speculate on the problem of interpretation of results and suggest future research for solving the dilemma. Excerpt 10.7, from a study of auditory speech perception, shows how the authors tried to grapple with a puzzling result. Note how they have offered several possible explanations for the result and suggest future research to clear up the issue.

## Relationship of Results to Previous Research

The Discussion section should relate the results of the investigation to the findings of previous research. Scientific research is a cumulative endeavor that relies on the results of many studies for a broad understanding and explanation of phenomena. One research study cannot cover sufficient territory to answer completely all of the relevant questions re-

## EXCERPT 10.6

### Discussion

The primary goal of this experiment was to examine the possible interaction between the variables of utterance length and linguistic complexity and the motor performance of adults who do and do not stutter. The stability of lower lip movements across multiple repetitions of the phrase "buy Bobby a puppy," measured by the spatiotemporal index (STI), as well as measures of phrase duration were recorded across conditions of increased length and syntactic complexity. Results indicate that adults who stutter demonstrated significantly higher STI values across conditions than their nonstuttering peers. In addition, syntactic complexity influenced the lower lip motor stability during fluent speech of people who stutter differently than the speech stability of nonstuttering adults. For the stuttering group, increases in syntactic complexity negatively influenced the stability of speech movements across repeated task performance. Longer utterances employing a nonsentence surround, however, did not significantly affect the speech kinematics of either speaker group. These observations provide evidence that certain linguistic processes may affect the speech motor execution of some subgroups of speakers. The speech systems of people who stutter may be more likely to be susceptible to these effects.

Though the speech motor output of the normally fluent speakers was generally unaffected by increasing linguistic loads, the speech motor systems of many adults who stutter may be especially susceptible to such linguistic processing demands. It is possible that the complexity of the stimulus sentences was not great enough to significantly affect the speech motor output of adults who do not stutter, and that sentences of greater complexity could negatively impact the stability

of normally fluent adults. Adults who stutter, however, may have a lower threshold for speech motor breakdowns, and smaller changes in variables that affect speech motor execution may have relatively large effects on spatiotemporal stability. This observation can explain individual differences in the effects of syntactic complexity on the speech motor stability of people who stutter, as illustrated below, and lends support to multifactorial models of stuttering.

. . . . . . . . . . .

### Conclusion

The present investigation focused on the influences of increasing length and syntactic complexity on the speech motor stability of normally fluent adults and adults who stutter. The results indicated that, unlike the control participants, the speech motor stability of people who stutter decreased when the length and syntactic complexity of stimulus utterances increased. Because linguistic processes appeared to affect the speech kinematics of adults who stutter, the results of this study have significant implications when applied to multifactorial models of speech production as well as to theories concerning the development and maintenance of stuttering. Stuttering is a heterogenous, multifactorial disorder. Many disparate variables may interact to affect the speech motor systems of people who stutter. These factors include autonomic responses, speech motor planning factors, and, as seen in this study, linguistic variables such as length and complexity. To fully understand the nature of stuttering and to aid in proper diagnosis and treatment, continued research investigating how such variables can affect the speech motor systems of people who stutter is necessary.

garding a given topic. Therefore, it is important for a researcher to inform consumers of research about the relationship of their findings to other research findings in the literature.

The Discussion section should provide both completeness and accuracy of references to previous research. Completeness demands that the author be aware of the literature in the area of his or her investigation and that he or she relate the findings to as many relevant studies as possible within the space limitations of the journal article format. In some cases, reference to certain previous research may have to be omitted if the manuscript is too long, and only the most directly related articles can be covered. References to previous research findings should also be accurate. Occasionally, an author may seriously misinterpret the findings of a previous study and go awry in discussing the relationship of his or her findings to that study. If such errors go undetected, the development of knowledge on a given topic may become confusing and misleading to consumers of research.

It is also important for authors to provide an objective and balanced account of both the agreements and disagreements of their results with those of previous research. Sometimes the findings of a particular article dovetail nicely with previous results in the research literature. For example, the results of a study with children may show evidence of an orderly developmental trend in some behavior or characteristic when compared with the results of studies with children of other ages. On the other hand, an article may present results that are at odds with previous research. For example, a replication study may find a pattern of results different from those that have been previously reported. Or a study employing a new procedure to study a well-researched phenomenon may reveal that previous data can be obtained only with a certain procedure and that procedural changes may yield conflicting answers to the same question.

Those points on which there is agreement may provide material for the discussion of theoretical and practical implications of the research, as we will see in the next section of this chapter. When there is disagreement, however, authors have a special responsibility to the readers to try to explain *why* there were disagreements between their results and those of previous research. For example, there might have been methodological or statistical differences between two investigations that could explain the discrepant results and such differences should be explored in the Discussion section. Often, authors may suggest avenues for future research that may help to explain why two studies show discrepant results.

Occasionally, the discussion of the relationship of results to previous research must cover some difficult territory. Subtle differences between studies must be analyzed to determine if the differences found are really meaningful or if they represent small fluctuations in human performance due to sampling or measurement errors. Also, obvious differences between studies may involve controversial topics that are subject to theoretical bias. The important point is for consumers to look for an objective attitude on the part of an author who is discussing discrepancies between the results of various studies. The writer of a research article has a responsibility to readers to present a balanced and objective analysis of the discrepancies and agreements between his or her findings and the body of research in existence on a particular topic. The writer should also be certain to identify the theoretical bias in the field on *both* sides of the issue at hand to indicate the merits of *each* side in the interpretation of a cumulative body of research data.

How can the reader determine if previous research has been completely and accurately described and if the discussion of agreements and disagreements has been fairly and objectively treated? First, consumers need to be aware of the important research that already exists on the topic covered in an article they are reading. Students and clinicians new to the field will develop this awareness over time as they read and assimilate more and more research. Second, for consumers who have questions about previous research, the best course of action is to find the references cited in the article's bibliography or reference list (that is one reason for appending a bibliography to an article) and read the original ref-

**EXCERPT  10.7**

The present results do not seem to support the finding of ter Keurs et al. (1993), in which normally hearing and hearing-impaired listeners (with flat losses) performed similarly for speech processed to have poor spectral resolution. However, that study used speech in a relatively high level of background noise, and it is difficult to separate the possible effects of noise masking from those of reduced spectral resolution upon the perception of the speech cues themselves. Whereas the present experiment's results might seem unusual, a parallel phenomenon has been observed in research with cochlear implants. In a study by Fishman, Shannon, & Slattery (1997), normally hearing and listeners with cochlear implants were compared in a recognition task using one-, two-, three-, and four-channel speech. For the implant users, the number and combinations of active electrodes were varied in order to produce varying degrees of spectral resolution. The best implant users produced recognition scores that were nearly the same as those of the normally hearing group for all conditions. However, the more poorly performing implant users produced results strikingly similar to the hearing-impaired listeners of the present study. That is, the performance was equal to that of the normally hearing listeners for the one-channel speech, but when even minimal spectral resolution was added, such as two-channel speech, the performance was poorer than that of listeners with normal hearing. These results, along with those of the present study, make clear that many listeners with cochlear implants, as well as many listeners with sensorineural hearing loss, are unable to take full advantage of even minimal spectral resolution in speech.

These results are somewhat puzzling; one would expect that most listeners with sensorineural hearing loss (or multichannel cochlear implants), if they have some hearing response across the entire frequency range, would have at least two channels of spectral resolution, based upon previous psychoacoustic work in this population. One strong possibility is that psychoacoustic measures of frequency selectivity, electrode interactions, or both, as performed in listeners with sensorineural hearing loss or in cochlear implant patients, are misleading researchers into believing that their spectral resolution is considerably better than it actually is for signals such as speech. In

ter Keurs et al. (1993), no relation was found between psychophysically measured frequency resolution and the degree of smearing required to degrade recognition of speech in noise, which could be taken as support for the irrelevance of psychoacoustic measures of frequency resolution to the prediction of speech recognition. The results of Experiment 2 in the present study, in which band-reject filtered two-channel speech was used in an attempt to reduce spread of information from one band to another, did not yield any improvement in scores for the hearing-impaired listeners. This does suggest that a simple explanation based upon reduced frequency resolution in the hearing-impaired listener may be inadequate.

If an explanation of the present results based upon reduced frequency selectivity is not adequate, why did the listeners with hearing impairment perform more poorly than the normally hearing listeners for all conditions with more than one channel of spectral resolution? We can only offer some reasonable speculations on the underlying causes at this point. It is possible that the sensitivity thresholds at certain frequencies in hearing-impaired listeners do not represent responses from a cochlear place corresponding to the test frequency. Cochlear damage has been shown to shift the characteristic frequency of auditory nerves (Liberman & Dodds, 1984), and numerous cases of auditory thresholds in hearing-impaired subjects have been linked to responses from the "wrong" place on the basilar membrane (Santi, Ruggero, Nelson, & Turner, 1982; Thornton & Abbas, 1980; Turner, Burns, & Nelson, 1983). Thus, hearing-impaired listeners might not be receiving an accurate representation of the place of the various speech channels. It is possible, therefore, that although some listeners with hearing impairment have only moderately impaired frequency selectivity, this frequency information might be inaccurate and therefore not particularly helpful in speech recognition.

Another possibility is that the central auditory system is somehow deficient in listeners with sensorineural hearing loss. This is suggested by the finding that the listeners with hearing impairment in the present study had difficulty combining the temporal-envelope information across multiple channels. The fact that the listeners with hearing impairment in the

*(continued)*

## E X C E R P T   10.7   Continued

present study were generally older than those with normal hearing might be a contributing factor in such a central deficit for the listeners in this study. However, if this explanation were proposed for younger listeners with hearing loss, it would represent a very different theoretical approach to sensorineural hearing loss than is generally accepted today. Further research is certainly needed to clarify these important issues.

erences (and the articles listed in those bibliographies) to check an author's interpretation of previous research.

The next two excerpts, taken from Discussion sections, illustrate balanced and objective approaches to the consideration of agreements and disagreements of the results with previous research. Excerpt 10.8 from a study of prevalence of voice disorders in teachers and nonteachers shows general agreement with previous findings except for a small difference in prevalence among teachers. The authors attempt to account for this prevalence variation on the basis of sample size and geographical differences between the studies. Excerpt 10.9 is taken from a study of spatiotemporal index (STI) variability measures in normal speakers and those with dysarthria. The author points out how the results differed

## E X C E R P T   10.8

Comparison of our results to prevalence estimates reported in previous studies for teachers and the general population is complicated, because of differences in how a voice disorder was defined and methods of data collection. In most studies, a clear operational definition of a voice disorder was not reported, and use of comparison groups in studies with teachers has been infrequent. In some studies, the teacher had to consult a physician or speech-language pathologist to qualify as having a voice disorder. These limitations aside, our prevalence estimate for current voice disorders in teachers (11%) is somewhat lower than that of Smith et al. (1997), who found that 14.6% of teachers, compared with 5.6% of nonteachers, reported a current voice disorder, and lower than that of Russell, Oates, and Mattiske (1998), who reported that 15.9% of teachers surveyed complained of a current voice disorder. The difference between our prevalence estimates and those of Smith and colleagues (1997) may be partly explained by their substantially smaller sample size that was limited to Utah teachers, rather than the two states combined as in the present study. However, Smith, Lemke, et al. (1998) later reported a lower rate of current voice disorders (i.e., 9%) in a larger group of teachers (*n* = 554). Our prevalence estimate of current voice disorders in the general population (6.2%) is consistent with that of Smith and colleagues (1997, 1998)—the only other investigators who used a nonteacher comparison group.

EXCERPT 10.9

This study was designed to assess the effect of rate manipulation on the variability of speech movement sequences in dysarthria. The results for individuals with mild and moderate-to-severe dysarthria were compared with normal controls. Regardless of rate condition, the normal controls consistently demonstrated the lowest STI values. Both groups with dysarthria were the least variable in the stretched condition and the most variable in the fast condition. There were no significant differences in STI values between the group with mild dysarthria and the normal controls; however, the group with moderate-to-severe dysarthria demonstrated significantly higher STI values than either of the other groups.

The STI values obtained in the present investigation for the normal controls in the habitual condition are somewhat higher than those of normal controls in previous research (Smith & Goffman, 1998; Wohlert & Smith, 1998), although normative data for this measure remain limited. As in Wohlert and Smith's study, the normal controls produced the lowest STI values in the habitual condition. In contrast to previous investigations (Kleinow et al., 2001; Wohlert & Smith, 1998), where the normal controls demonstrated the highest STI values in the slow condition, in the present study they showed the highest STI values in the fast condition. It is possible that methodological differences contributed to this discrepancy. In previous work, the investigators instructed their participants to say the phrase "Buy Bobby a puppy" at

"half your normal rate" in the slow condition. In the present study, very specific strategies and modeling procedures were used to elicit a reduced speaking rate, to ensure comparability to common treatment strategies. For the breaks condition, the experimenter modeled "Buy Bobby a puppy" with brief pauses between each word. For the stretched condition, the experimenter modeled prolonged vowels with no breaks between words. It is likely that the specific elicitation procedure used for all participants, including the normal controls, contributed to the reduced variability in this condition.

The STI values for individuals with mild and moderate-to-severe dysarthria are greater than those reported for individuals with IPD (Kleinow et al., 2001) in the habitual, fast, and slow conditions. This is not surprising, because the authors reported that the majority of individuals with IPD demonstrated mild symptoms based on the Hoehn and Yahr (1967) scale. They were not classified according to dysarthria severity.

The STI values for individuals with mild and moderate-to-severe dysarthria are also greater than those reported for healthy older adults (Wohlert & Smith, 1998) in habitual, fast, and slow conditions. The authors concluded that the greater variability seen in older adults reflected an age-related decline in motor ability. The higher values obtained in the present work across conditions most likely reflect the decline in motor ability due to dysarthria.

From "The Effect of Pacing Strategies on the Variability of Speech Movement Sequences in Dysarthria," by M. A. McHenry, 2003, *Journal of Speech, Language, and Hearing Research, 46,* p. 708. Copyright 2003 by the American Speech-Language-Hearing Association. Reprinted with permission.

from some previous data gathered from normal speakers and persons with idiopathic Parkinson disease (IPD). Differences in methods of instruction to participants may account for the differences in normal speakers and differences in severity of dysarthria, and the decline in motor ability due to aging versus dysarthria may account for differences in the clinical and aging participants.

Sometimes results may not be in agreement with an author's previous research and this presents a challenge to explain why results differ across the same author's studies. Excerpt 10.10 is from a study of speech recognition in older listeners with hearing impairment (OHI) and shows how the author met this challenge by discussing two variables that

**E X C E R P T    10.10**

Finally, for a complete understanding of aging and speech recognition, we should consider why this study showed poorer performance with increased age whereas others (e.g., Souza & Turner, 1994) have not. This difference in results cannot be attributable wholly to the confounding influence of hearing threshold. A possible explanation lies in the age of the test group (Pichora-Fuller & Schneider, 1998). For example, the OHI group in the current study had an average age of 79 years, whereas the OHI group tested in the Souza and Turner study averaged 69 years old. In a recent study, Humes and Christopherson (1991) noted poorer performance for 76–86-year-old listeners than for a 65–75-year-old group. Additionally, Gordon-Salant

(1987a) has suggested that age effects depend on both task demands and the complexity of the acoustic stimulus, which may vary across studies.

Another potential explanation for the poorer speech recognition of the older listeners with hearing loss concerns the auditory history of these subjects. The majority of the younger listeners with hearing loss reported congenital or early-onset hearing loss, whereas the older listeners acquired their loss relatively late in life. It is possible that the younger listeners with hearing loss developed better compensatory listening strategies because of their lifelong experience with hearing loss.

From "Older Listeners Use of Temporal Cues Altered by Compression Amplification," by P. E. Souza, 2000, *Journal of Speech, Language, and Hearing Research, 43,* p. 671. Copyright 2000 by the American Speech-Language-Hearing Association. Reprinted with permission.

differed between two of her studies, the participants' ages and hearing loss histories, that could explain discrepancies in the results of the studies.

## Theoretical Implications of the Research

It is important for the author of a research article to state clearly the theoretical implications of findings with regard to past and current thinking in the field. In the last section, we discussed the relationship of the results to previous research. The theoretical implications of the results are closely tied to this relationship because the results of a single article are often juxtaposed with those of previous research to form the nomothetic network developed for any particular topic.

Implications may be drawn regarding the validity of a previously stated theory. Research results of a particular article may be supportive of an existing theory and further support may be gleaned from the agreement of that research article with previous research. Through the accumulation of more data in agreement with the predictions made by a particular theory, the theory gradually develops more plausibility as a valid explanation of the phenomenon under study. On the other hand, results of a particular study (and, possibly, other previous research) may be in disagreement with a particular theory. In such a case, the theory may need revision to account for discrepancies between the predictions made by the theory and the empirical evidence. In fact, so many data in disagreement with the theory may accumulate over the years that a theory may eventually be discarded because of its failure to find empirical support.

Theoretical implications are not limited to the discussion of previous theories in light of the data of a research article. The author may take the public opportunity to generate a new theory or to modify an old one so radically that it would no longer be recognizable in its revised form as a relative of the old theory. The data of a new article may be so provocative as to require new and original thinking for the explanation of the phenomenon under study. Readers will recall that two types of theory were mentioned in Chapter 1: those that are advanced before research is executed and await empirical confirmation and those that synthesize the existent empirical data. Both types of theory may be entertained in the Discussion and Conclusions section when the theoretical implications of the research are discussed.

Where can the reader expect to find the discussion of the theoretical implications in the research article? This depends on the style of the particular author. Some authors prefer to combine the discussion of the relationship of results to previous research with the discussion of theoretical implications at the beginning of the Conclusions section. This especially makes sense if the results of a particular investigation are to be combined with those of previous research in commenting on a theory. Others prefer to separate the discussion of theoretical implications from the discussion of relationship of results to previous research. Some authors even give considerable attention to theoretical issues in the introduction, literature review, or rationale before reporting data and refer back to this material in the theoretical implications portion of the conclusion. The important point is that the author needs to lend theoretical perspective to the empirical data and to articulate the theoretical implications of his or her findings so that readers understand where the research fits in the nomothetic network regarding the particular topic.

Excerpt 10.11 is from a study of the effects of contextualization on the fluency of children who stutter, children with language impairment, and typically developing children. The results, as summarized in the first two paragraphs of the excerpt, had both theoretical and clinical implications, which are discussed in the next two paragraphs. These findings provide support for an existing theory, the Demands and Capacities model, that has been discussed for a number of years in the stuttering literature. This model has generated significant research literature and much of the research to test this theory is summarized in the introduction of this article as the development of the rationale for the study. The theoretical conclusions concerning the model in the Discussion section tie in clearly with the original rationale presented in the introduction.

Excerpt 10.12 is the entire Discussion section from a videofluoroscopic study of oropharyngeal swallowing in younger and older women. The results are discussed directly with regard to the original independent variables of this study (age and volume) and a comparison is made to data from a previous study of men to examine sex as a descriptive independent variable. Conclusions regarding the effects of the three independent variables are stated immediately. The data on the women in this study and from the men in the previous study by the same authors are compared in Figure 2, which could logically be included as part of the Discussion section of the article, rather than part of the Results section, because this figure makes comparisons across the extensive data of the two different studies. This extended effort to present and compare the results of the two studies leads to substantial conclusions with theoretical implications for the interaction of age and sex in compensatory adjustments. Interesting suggestions are made regarding the possibility that reduced muscular reserve in men relative to women may make them more vulnerable to dysphagia with the onset of illness or injury because they may not be able to compensate for aging

EXCERPT 10.11

Stuttering behaviors for this population followed similar patterns. Only small mean differences were obtained for the four task conditions, with significance found only between the easiest task condition (i.e., contextualized cooking) and the two story-retelling tasks. The mean proportion of stuttering behaviors produced within the decontextualized cooking task was not significantly different from either the contextualized cooking task or from either narrative condition. This suggests that narrative discourse may place more demands on the speaker than does procedural, or scripted, discourse. It is possible that discourse form may represent another form of linguistic demand that influences stuttering, not unlike syntactic complexity.

Across all tasks, children with language impairment and children with normally developing fluency skills exhibited greater amounts of linguistic nonfluencies and mazing than stuttering behavior, with mazing the most predominant form of disfluency across all three groups of participants. It is expected that children with language impairment and children with normally developing fluency skills would not exhibit stuttering-type disfluencies. However, it was unexpected that mazing would be the predominant form of disfluency for all three groups—even the children who stutter. The means illustrate higher proportions of mazing in the decontextualized conditions, suggesting that decontextualization of the topic poses greater demand for language formulation than does contextualized information.

These patterns have relevance for clinical work with children who stutter; in general, the contextualized tasks elicited the fewest instances of mazing and stuttering, with trends in linguistic nonfluencies following the same patterns but not with differences that reached a level of significance. For children who stutter, results yielded evidence of greater language formulation difficulties occurring with greater decontextualization and less familiarity of the topic. If clinicians are attempting to carefully control therapy tasks so that linguistic demands are minimized, consideration of discourse type and amount of contextualization available may be in order.

The relationship between language and fluency is complex. Findings from the current study would support the Demands and Capacities model (Starkweather, 1987) as well as Karnoil's hypothesis that stuttering arises from a need for more time to plan or revise utterances in response to increasing linguistic demands. In this study, all three groups of children exhibited mazing behavior as the most frequent form of disfluency, with the most mazing noted in decontextualized conditions. Children who stutter exhibited a significantly higher proportion of stuttering in the two narrative conditions than in the contextualized cooking condition. According to Demands/Capacities, the increased demands placed by narrative discourse and decontextualization would explain these results. When fitting these findings to Karnoil's model, the changes in linguistic complexity as a result of changes in contextualization and discourse genre do indeed influence time needed to plan and revise utterances, as symbolized by the high proportions of mazing and changes in stuttering behaviors.

changes as well as women. In addition, the authors pointed to future research directions to resolve some unknown issues about swallowing in older men and women, including studies of viscosity, texture, and taste; the potential for differential swallowing effects of disease; and the need to control for age and sex in future swallowing research. The authors of this comprehensive Discussion section have done an excellent job of integrating their cur-

## Discussion

This investigation examined age, volume, and sex effects on oropharyngeal swallows of 1 ml and 10 ml liquid in 8 healthy young (age 21–29) and 8 healthy old (age 80–93) women. A few significant differences were observed in terms of age in these women. All durations were prolonged in the older women, though only cricopharyngeal opening significantly so. Laryngeal closure durations were longer for older women, but not significantly. This corresponds with data from Hiss et al. (2001), who found that women had longer swallowing apnea durations (SAD) than men and that women exhibited an increase in SAD with age whereas men exhibited a decrease in SAD with increasing age. Extent of structural movements was generally increased in the older women, particularly the movements related to opening of the upper esophageal sphincter (i.e., anterior hyoid and laryngeal movement and elevation; Jacob, Kahrilas, Logemann, Shah, & Ha, 1989) though only one (laryngeal elevation) significantly so. Increases in hyolaryngeal movement may be a compensation for the lowered position of the larynx with age in women (Robbins et al., 1992). Only tongue base movement diminished significantly with age in women.

Volume effects observed in duration and extent of movement during the 1 ml and 10 ml swallows in this study are similar to those observed in other investigations of swallow changes as bolus volume increases: increased duration and width of cricopharyngeal opening (Cook et al., 1989; Jacob et al., 1989; Kahrilas & Logemann, 1993) and increased duration of airway entrance closure (Logemann et al., 1992), increased extent of posterior pharyngeal wall movement at superior C3, increased laryngeal elevation and anterior movement of the larynx and hyoid. The increases in laryngeal and hyoid movement probably result in the longer and wider cricopharyngeal opening because the movements of these structures "yank" open the upper esophageal sphincter (cricopharyngeal region; Cook et al., 1989; Jacob et al., 1989).

Comparisons of the swallow measures in the young and old men and women resulted in some interesting sex differences in the older groups. As the men aged, the movements of larynx and hyoid generally were reduced, whereas women's movements increased or were relatively stable between the two age groups, as reflected in Figure 2. These data indicate that women in this study maintain muscular reserve better than men. Muscular reserve is the difference between extent of movement needed to accomplish a desired functional result (e.g., UES opening) and the actual extent of movement used (Kenney, 1985). Under normal circumstances, reduced maximal movement would be interpreted as greater efficiency in accomplishing a task, but reserve is most critical when the subject becomes ill and weak (Buchner & Wagner, 1992; Johnson, 1993; Kenney, 1985; Troncale, 1996). With adequate reserve, the mechanism can still swallow safely despite some reduction in maximum movement. With reduced reserve, the necessary movements of swallow are reduced in range, and efficiency and safety of swallow are impaired. Although these results may be confirmed by the statistics provided for vertical laryngeal and hyoid movement in Table 4, the Factor 2 summary measure in Table 7 focuses these results. There was no significant difference in the mean Factor 2 scores between young women and old women ($-.52$ vs $-.27$, $p = 0.57$) but there was between young and old men (.94 vs $-.18$, $p = 0.02$). Cricopharyngeal measures (onset, duration) related to Factor 4 were also reduced in older men, compared with older women. Changes in muscular reserve observed in the hyolaryngeal movement with age in men (Logemann et al., 2000) were not observed in the women in this investigation. Studies of changes in muscular reserve resulting from age have not examined possible sex differences. The results of this present study indicate that older healthy men have greater risk than older women of developing dysphagia when they become weak from illness because of their lost reserve. Data from our studies of aspiration show a preponderance of men with this consequence, even after accounting for sex differences in etiologic incidence (Smith, Logemann, Colangelo, Rademaker, & Pauloski, 1999).

There are some indications from laryngeal function studies involving speech or voicing that women may be better able to compensate for changes resulting from aging. Both Sapienza and Dutka (1996) and Hoit and Hixon (1992) hypothesized that the healthy older women may be capable of making

*(continued)*

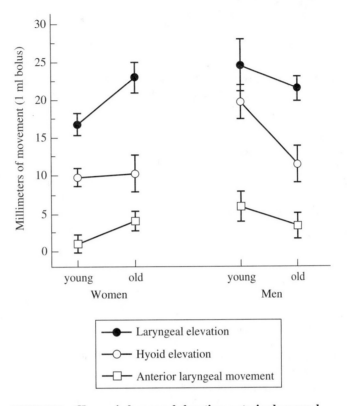

**FIGURE 2   Change in laryngeal elevation, anterior laryngeal movement, and hyoid elevation on 1 ml bolus by age and sex. Error bars present standard errors for each measure.**

behavioral adjustments to counteract the effects of aging on laryngeal structures. In a study of swallowing in normal older and younger men and women, Robbins et al. (1992) found a longer duration of upper esophageal sphincter (UES) opening for women than for men and longer pharyngeal response durations with the manometric tube in place than without it in women. These latter measures may be indicators of greater flexibility in the oropharyngeal mechanism of women so that women can develop more successful behavioral adjustments to compensate for aging than men can. The differences in oropharyngeal swallow in the women and men observed in this study emphasize the need to control for sex and age in the design of studies of normal swallow physiology and to examine the comparative impact of disease and trauma on swallowing in women and men at all ages, but particularly in those over age 60. More research is needed to further define and examine the nature of any differences in the way men and women swallow under various conditions, including volume, viscosity, texture, and taste changes.

From "Oropharyngeal Swallow in Younger and Older Women: Videofluoroscopic Analysis," by J. A. Logemann, B. R. Pauloski, A. W. Rademaker, and P. J. Kahrilas, 2002, *Journal of Speech, Language, and Hearing Research, 45,* pp. 438–441. Copyright 2002 by the American Speech-Language-Hearing Association. Reprinted with permission.

rent results with those from their previous research to generate important new theoretical conclusions along with suggestions for future research that may help to substantiate them.

## Practical Implications of the Research

In addition to the consideration of theoretical implications, the discussion and conclusions often address the question of practical implications of the results. As we mentioned earlier, it is often difficult to draw a true dichotomy between purely basic and applied research. Rather, there is usually a continuum along which research may fall with regard to its basic or applied orientation and with regard to whether practical implications are immediate or further off in the future. What some may consider to be pure research today may, surprisingly, turn out to have a practical implication tomorrow. The transistor, for example, was developed by scientists engaged in basic research in physics rather than by an inventor whose primary goal was to patent an invention for immediate sale.

In some cases an author may have no immediate practical application in mind because the research may have been more basic in its orientation or because applied considerations may have been reserved by the author until the accumulation of sufficient research to make judicious practical decisions. In such a case, the author may eschew the opportunity to discuss practical application if it is believed that such premature speculation would be unjustified or would be misconstrued by readers. On the other hand, authors might speculate about practical implications if they believe that appropriately cautioned speculation can be justified. For instance, authors might hope that this speculation would provoke readers with more practical inclinations to read their research or, perhaps, to begin applied research of their own. Readers should be careful to discern that such speculation is accomplished in a prudent and reasonable fashion. Consumers should also be cognizant of the need for patience in the anticipation of future practical applications when more research is necessary before a particular concept can be applied clinically in an ethical and professional manner.

Some research is undertaken with more immediate practical goals in mind and an author then has a special responsibility to delineate for the audience the implications of the research for assessment and management of communicative disorders. General suggestions for clinical practice may be offered in a few sentences or the author may feel that a more thorough didactic presentation is necessary. Sometimes the author may even write a separate article on the clinical implications of the research, especially at the culmination of a series of related research articles on a particular topic.

Direct practical application of the results of research should be advocated only when the accumulated research has demonstrated the reliability and validity of techniques for assessment and management of communicative disorders. In addition, the limitations of these techniques should be delineated in appropriate caveats to the readers. Unfortunately, some techniques have fallen into disfavor and have been abandoned because practical applications were proffered before sufficient research was completed to ensure clinical success. In such cases, researchers may have suggested clinical application before they had collected sufficient data to warrant immediate use, or clinicians may have attempted to apply techniques that research had not yet confirmed as suitable for clinical use. In some cases *both* researchers and clinicians may have been guilty of overzealous and premature application of inchoate techniques that were destined to fail without extensive research into their proper development. Therefore, it is imperative for both producers and consumers of research to be aware of the limitations inherent in any technique and of the need for cautious clinical application during the development of new techniques.

The next three excerpts, taken from Discussion sections, illustrate the reasonable and cautious discussion of practical implications of research. Excerpt 10.13 contains two paragraphs taken from the Discussion section of an article on the consequences of voice disorders in schoolteachers. Two practical implications are discussed in these paragraphs. The first paragraph considers the implications of teachers' voice disorders for their teaching effectiveness in typical classrooms and the second discusses the need to develop voice disorder prevention programs for teachers. Note how the authors drew on their own results as well as previous research to incorporate practical suggestions for voice treatment and prevention programs.

Excerpt 10.14 contains two practical suggestions for the improvement of speech recognition testing in clinical audiology. The article is a two-part experiment, with the first part concerning the recording and acoustic analysis of speech materials spoken in a noisy background and the second part reporting data on speech recognition for these materials in quiet and in noise. Note how the authors have used the conclusions from both parts of the study to develop their practical implications.

Excerpt 10.15 contains practical suggestions for the enhancement of the speech intelligibility of persons with severe dysarthria who use speech as the primary communication mode. Notice the cautions about generalization that the authors have considered and the suggestions for future research to extend the generalization of these practical implications to clinical situations.

## Implications for Future Research

As we mentioned earlier, no one research article can answer all of the relevant questions on a given topic. In fact, a particular research article may even raise more questions than it answers. Scientific progress depends on the cumulative efforts of a number of investigators and each of their efforts points toward new avenues of research. The Discussion section usually enumerates some of the questions for future research that occur to the author during the course of the investigation.

Future research may be suggested in a number of different areas, including, but not limited to, improvement of internal validity by refinement of the design and execution of the research, extension of external validity, further clarification of the relationship of results to previous research, additional empirical confirmation of theory, and elaboration of practical applications.

Suggestions for future research are often directed toward improvement of the internal validity of the research by refinement of the methods employed. For instance, authors may discuss limitations imposed on their conclusions by aspects of the method of investigation (i.e., threats to internal validity). Authors may also incorporate suggestions for future research to overcome these limitations. These suggestions may be in the form of

EXCERPT  **10.13**

It is also important to recognize that for many teachers, the adverse effects of voice problems were not limited to loss of work. In this study, teachers reported that voice problems interfered with their effectiveness at work and also imposed limitations on job performance. The impact of such dysfunction on teachers and their students may be substantial. Our results indicated that over a third of teachers complained that their voice did not function as it usually does or as they would like it to for more than 5 days of the school year. Despite teachers admitting that voice problems prevented them from doing certain tasks at their job, the majority did not seek help, and most did not take time off work to recover (Roy et al., 2004). One wonders about the possible effects of these voice problems on the quality of instruction the students receive, because the teacher likely limits classroom activities as a result of vocal dysfunction. Furthermore, because the voice is the primary tool of instruction in the classroom, it is essential that students hear and understand the teacher without difficulty. However, poor acoustic environments and high ambient noise levels characterize many elementary and secondary school classrooms, potentially obscuring an already distorted voice signal (Crandell & Smaldino, 1999; Howard & Angus, 2001; Pekkarinen & Viljanen, 1991). In this regard, Morton and Watson (2001) recently evaluated the effect of disordered voice quality on children's ability to process spoken language. A group of 24 school-aged children listened to a series of recorded passages spoken by a female with normal voice and a female with a voice disorder. Children were subsequently tested for their ability to recall words and draw inferences regarding the spoken material. Children performed better on both of these tasks when listening to the normal voice. Thus, the negative effects of a dysphonic voice, combined with voice-related disruptions on students' learning may be substantial.

. . . . . . . . . . .

One purpose of an epidemiologic study is to verify the consistency of prevalence findings. The similarity of our findings with those of other smaller studies suggests that teaching, as an occupation, can produce a high risk of adverse voice problems that seem to cross a variety of geographic boundaries (Jonsdottir, Boyle, Martin, & Sigurdardottir, 2002; Russell et al., 1998; Yiu, 2002). Although epidemiologic studies cannot establish causality, the results reported here and elsewhere suggest that many voice problems are highly occupation-related, making the argument for prevention and early intervention programs compelling. Because of lost workdays, use of sick benefits, replacement costs for substitute teachers, and treatment expenses, Verdolini and Ramig (2001) estimated the societal costs in the United States alone to be $2.5 billion annually for teachers. Although evidence from recent clinical trials research has identified several effective treatment alternatives for teachers with voice disorders, including voice amplification, vocal function exercises, and resonance voice therapy (Roy et al., 2001, 2002, 2003), our results clearly indicate that education, prevention, and treatment programs need to be developed and assessed in order to lessen the occurrence of adverse voice conditions related to this high-risk profession (Russell et al., 1998).

general comments or of specific delineations of procedural steps to be taken in a new study. Indeed, an author may already have such an investigation underway at publication time and readers may anticipate its subsequent publication. The suggestions offered may include replication with larger samples, use of more homogeneous or heterogeneous groups of people depending on the nature of the study, refinements in design or measurement techniques, or improvements in materials or instrumentation. Of course, if too many such suggestions are made, readers may wonder why the study was ever published in the first place. But a few suggestions for improvement are usually warranted because no study can ever be perfectly designed to avoid all of the possible pitfalls of research.

**EXCERPT  10.14**

### Implications

The results of this study have implications for at least two areas of clinical audiology. First, Wiley and Page (1997) argued that, among other things, speech perception tasks should provide results that can be applied to rehabilitation efforts, such as amplification, and the prediction of communication difficulties in everyday listening situations. The results of Part I suggest that the acoustic characteristics of speech spoken in noise are significantly different from those for speech spoken in quiet. These characteristics, therefore, should be considered when using hearing aid prescriptive procedures. For example, many hearing aid prescriptive methods use the long-term spectrum of speech produced in quiet as a reference for all incoming signals (Byrne & Dillon, 1986; Cox & Moore, 1988; Schwartz, Lyregaard, & Lundh, 1988). Hearing aid manufacturers and others recommend a decrease in low-frequency gain and an increase in high-frequency gain for the best perception of speech in noisy environments (Martin, 1996). Although this practice may reduce the effects of upward spread of masking, the results of this study suggest that smaller adjustments may be necessary. Talkers will naturally speak louder in noisy conditions and therefore reduce low-frequency and increase high-frequency energy. If the parameters of a hearing aid are set without this consideration, the acoustic properties of speech may be overcorrected and, in some cases, perception may actually be degraded (e.g., the hearing aid may be forced to operate in saturation). It is important to remember, however, that the talkers in the present study were specifically instructed to speak clearly to a listener. Whether this is fully representative of speech in a typical noise environment is unknown.

The results of Part II suggest that speech-recognition tasks used clinically are of limited value for predicting communication difficulties in everyday situations that involve noise or competing speech because these tasks use speech samples recorded in quiet. The absence of a relation between recognition and the most robust acoustic differences between these speech samples suggests that it may not be possible to predict accurately speech recognition in noise through simple modifications of speech produced in quiet (e.g., increasing the SNR or shaping the frequency response). Rather, these results suggest the need to develop speech samples for recognition tests that incorporate the acoustic characteristics of actual speaking environments, including those with background noise. In this way, the effects of hearing loss on speech recognition can be determined more accurately by closely imitating common communication environments under controlled conditions.

**E X C E R P T   10.15**

### Clinical Implications and Future Directions

Results of the present study have a number of clinical implications for individuals who have severe dysarthria and choose to use speech as their primary mode of communication. First, this study supports previous studies that show provision of top-down linguistic-contextual information to listeners enhances intelligibility. For maximal increases in intelligibility, findings from this study suggest that speakers should employ a combined cueing strategy in which they provide their listeners both with the topic of the message and the first letter of each word as it is spoken. If speakers are unable to employ a combined cueing strategy to supplement their speech, findings from this study suggest that alphabet cues enhance intelligibility to a greater extent than topic cues.

This study was experimental in nature and, as such, findings may not generalize directly to clinical situations. For instance, alphabet cues were experimentally imposed on the habitual speech of the persons with dysarthria for this study. In clinical practice, implementation of alphabet supplementation or a combined cueing strategy would require the speaker to point physically to the first letter of each word as he or she speaks it. The physical act of pointing to an alphabet board may have an effect on speech-production skills for some speakers with motor impairment. In addition, learning demands for employing alphabet and topic cues and the actual effectiveness of these strategies in spontaneous speaking situations are unclear. Further research is necessary to generalize findings from the present study to clinical implementation.

From "Effects of Linguistic Cues and Stimulus Cohesion on Intelligibility of Severely Dysarthric Speech," by K. C. Hustad and D. R. Beukelman, 2001, *Journal of Speech, Language, and Hearing Research, 44,* p. 507. Copyright 2001 by the American Speech-Language-Hearing Association. Reprinted with permission.

Suggestions for future research may also be directed toward external validity. The author may be concerned with extending the generalizability of results to other populations, settings, measures, or treatments. Procedures that are successful with adults may not necessarily work with children; replication with children would be needed to verify the generality of the procedure. By the same token, results obtained with one type of communicative disorder may not necessarily be obtained with another. Results may be limited to a particular setting and a systematic replication may be needed to extend generalization to another setting. Research suggestions aimed at extending external validity are often coupled with caveats discussed in practical implications and readers may be urged to await further research before attempting to generalize results to other populations, settings, measures, or treatments.

Future research may also be suggested as a result of comparison of the results of a particular study to those of previous research. If there are disagreements between the results of a study and previous research, more research may be suggested to resolve the differences. The different results may be due to sampling or procedural differences that can be overcome by procedural comparisons, replications with different samples, or by control studies designed to evaluate the reliability and validity of different procedures with different samples. Agreement of previous research with the results of a particular study may also prompt suggestions for future research as such agreement may indicate that researchers have been pursuing a fruitful approach to the study of the particular phenomenon.

Suggested future research may also be related to the theoretical implications of the results. More research may be needed to firm up the empirical grounding of a theory supported by the results of a particular investigation. On the other hand, further research may be needed to account for discrepancies between the results of a study and existing theory. If a new or modified theory is advanced to explain the results, the new theory or modifications may contain predictions of behavior or phenomena that would need to be confirmed empirically by future research. Changes in population, research materials, instrumentation, or procedures might be necessary to test the predictions of the new theory.

As mentioned previously, the practical implications of a particular research study may not be immediately apparent or feasible and, therefore, further research may be suggested before practical applications can be accomplished. Such suggestions may include standardization of tests on larger samples, gathering of normative data on different populations, development of more efficient or less expensive (i.e., more clinically feasible) methods, or refinements in procedure to improve reliability and validity. Sometimes a procedure may be strongly advocated as useful with a well-defined, closely circumscribed clinical population, but caution is necessary regarding application to other populations until future research confirms the applicability of the measure or technique.

The next four excerpts present examples from Discussion sections that illustrate a variety of thoughtful suggestions for future research. The excerpts concern many of the different kinds of suggestions previously outlined.

Excerpt 10.16 is from a study of problem behavior in children with language delays from low-income families. The authors suggest several avenues for future research, including longitudinal studies, experimental studies of the effects of manipulations of different environmental variables on children's behavior, and more complex correlational studies of factors related to problem behaviors.

E X C E R P T   **10.16**

**Issues for Future Research**

Future research should focus on developing observational methods for assessing problem behaviors of young children from low-income families as an adjunct to informant reports. Longitudinal studies of children with language delays are needed to link more directly language development in preschool to children's academic performance and behavior in kindergarten and first grade. Future studies should be designed to examine the effects of classroom organization, teachers' behaviors, and classroom management styles on children's observed and reported behavior. Finally, research in this area must move beyond simple correlational methods to more sophisticated analyses of the complex relationships among language development, behavior functioning, and social skills in Head Start children.

From "Problem Behaviors of Low-Income Children with Language Delays: An Observation Study," by C. H. Qi and A. P. Kaiser, 2004, *Journal of Speech, Language, and Hearing Research, 47,* p. 606. Copyright 2004 by the American Speech-Language-Hearing Association. Reprinted with permission.

EXCERPT  **10.17**

Additional research needs to be conducted in order to further isolate and define the parameters of the time domain that may affect the intelligibility of esophageal speech. Phone duration, voice onset time, and duration ratios can be manipulated to determine their effect on intelligibility. By incorporating temporal factors into studies that enhance the intelligibility of esophageal speech, more extensive and comprehensive research can be undertaken to improve the overall intelligibility of the esophageal talker.

The perceptual salience of frequency, amplitude, and time reported by Slavin and Ferrand (1995) indicates that there are interactions among these variables, and probably others, that will influence the judgment of esophageal speech. Physically manipulating these variables in a systematic, simultaneous manner, although difficult, will be necessary in order to determine the combinations of variables that are most advantageous for both the talker and the listener. Given the physical limitations of esophageal talkers, research along this line also can provide data concerning the minimum clarity of speech that the esophageal talker needs to provide his/her listener.

Finally, the time domain may be a worthwhile consideration in designing and implementing esophageal speech enhancement devices. For example, a precise acoustical description of injection noise could lead to an algorithm for automatic elimination of these extraneous sounds. In electronic communications this should aid intelligibility substantially, because visual cues are not available (Henry, 1967). Further detailed specification of the esophageal speech signal has the potential to aid these talkers substantially.

From "The Intelligibility of Time-Domain-Edited Esophageal Speech," by R. A. Prosek and L. L. Vreeland, 2001, *Journal of Speech, Language, and Hearing Research, 44*, pp. 532–533. Copyright 2001 by the American Speech-Language-Hearing Association. Reprinted with permission.

Excerpt 10.17, taken from a study of time-domain-edited speech of esophageal speakers, includes several specific suggestions for future research. The authors suggest particular independent variables, such as phone duration and voice onset time, for manipulation to examine their effects on intelligibility and also recommend further examining the effects of interactions among independent variables in determining intelligibility. Clinical implications of future research are also discussed, including suggestions for development of enhancement devices for esophageal speakers.

Excerpt 10.18 from a study of hearing-impaired speakers' intelligibility, includes two specific suggestions for future research. The first suggestion concerns examination of criterion validity of scaling measures in relation to word-identification tests of intelligibility and acoustical characteristics of speech. The second suggestion concerns extension of the external validity of the results to other populations with impaired intelligibility and to other measures (i.e., dimensions of speech that are scaled).

Excerpt 10.19 is from the same article that opened this chapter in Excerpt 10.1 and closes it with an excellent discussion of the theoretical and practical reasons why there is a compelling need for future research in the complex issues of the relationship of personality and voice disorders.

Because the results of this study demonstrate the continuum of our hearing-impaired adults' speech intelligibility to be prothetic, we conclude that direct magnitude estimation has more construct validity than interval scaling for assessing this dimension. Future research should address the criterion validity of direct magnitude estimation by examining its functional relation to word identification tests of speech intelligibility and to acoustical parameters of speech (Monsen, 1978) found to be good predictors of intelligibility.

It is important to test the generalizability of these results to the speech intelligibility of hearing-impaired children, to other populations such as dysarthrics and esophageal speakers with impaired intelligibility, and to other dimensions of speech that are commonly scaled. For example, an interesting parallel is apparent between our results for speech intelligibility and the findings of Berry and Silverman (1972) regarding the inequality of intervals on the *Lewis-Sherman Scale of Stuttering Severity*. They used direct magnitude estimation to judge the widths between adjacent samples of stuttering previously scaled along a

9-point interval scale of stuttering severity and found smaller interval widths at the lower end than at the upper portion of the scale. This finding agrees well with Stevens's (1974) prediction for prothetic continua. Because a number of dimensions like stuttering severity, speech intelligibility, articulatory defectiveness, vocal qualities, etc., are commonly assessed with interval scaling in clinical and research work, it seems imperative that these dimensions be explored to determine whether they constitute metathetic or prothetic continua. A serious reconsideration of the widespread use of interval scaling may be necessary if a number of these continua are found to be prothetic.

As Stevens (1974) has stated:

> The human being, despite his great versatility, has a limited capacity to effect linear partitions on prothetic continua. He does quite well, to be sure, if the continuum happens to be metathetic, but, since most scaling problems involve prothetic continua, it seems that category and other forms of partition scaling generally ought to be avoided for the purposes of scaling. (p. 374)

**Further Suggestions for Future Research**

Although the "Big Three" scales (E, N, CON/P) represent the highest-order traits that reflect the most general level in the hierarchy of dispositions, relying solely on these composite superfactors can be misleading and fail to provide the necessary resolution to adequately describe personality. Because different levels of the trait hierarchy represent different levels of breadth or abstraction in personality description (Briggs, 1989; Costa & McRae, 1995), decomposition of the superfactors into constituent traits affords a clearer analysis of both the type and range of the con-

tent subsumed within each of the broad factors. Analysis at a lower level of the hierarchy, which includes several component traits, can offer important information that is obscured at the highest level. Ideally, then, future personality assessment should be conducted so as to survey different levels of the trait hierarchy (Hull, Lehn, & Tedlie, 1991).

Additional behavioral studies are needed with respect to the operation of both the BAS and BIS and their putative role in behavioral dysregulation in FD and VN. The current study was limited by its exclusive reliance on self-report measures of personality and psychopathology. Future studies should use multi-method assessments of personality and draw on information from multiple sources, such as family members, peers, and clinicians. The relations observed in the current study require replication with multimethod data in order to more effectively separate construct variance from method variance. Further research also is required to determine whether personality differences related to gender exist among these voice-disordered groups. Although males with FD and VN are a minority, it would be interesting to determine whether they share similar personality traits with their female counterparts.

For the past several decades, voice scientists and clinicians have essentially ignored the field of personality psychology. The results of this investigation suggest that the relation between personality and voice disorders merits serious attention for both practical and theo-

retical reasons. For instance, the relation between personality and long-term treatment outcomes in FD and VN needs to be investigated more fully. If personality represents an enduring factor in voice vulnerability, then the lingering question of whether personality influences can be moderated in any significant manner needs to be addressed. Identification of other predisposing anatomical or physiological factors in VN and FD may help define the interaction between personality and voice disorder vulnerability. Most voice treatment techniques focus on the overt disorder of phonation; until more is known of the etiologic factors/triggers, it may be unrealistic to expect great advances in long-term "cure" rates. The results of this investigation seem to suggest, as Moses (1954) did over 40 years ago, that exploring the characteristics of the "person" behind the voice may be as fruitful as studying the structure that produces it.

# EVALUATION CHECKLIST

**Instructions:**   The four-category scale at the end of this checklist may be used to rate the *Discussion* section of an article. The *Evaluation Items* help identify those topics that should be considered in arriving at the rating. Comments on these topics, entered as *Evaluation Notes,* should serve as the basis for the overall rating.

| *Evaluation Items* | *Evaluation Notes* |
| --- | --- |
| 1. Discussion was clearly related to research problem. | |
| 2. Limitations of the method were discussed. | |
| 3. Conclusions were drawn directly and fairly from results. | |
| 4. Reasonable explanations were given for unusual, atypical, or discrepant results. | |
| 5. There was thorough and objective discussion of agreements and disagreements of previous research. | |

*Evaluation Items*                                    *Evaluation Notes*

**6.** The section related results to various theoretical
explanations.

**7.** Implications for clinical practice were stated
fairly and objectively.

**8.** Theoretical or clinical speculations were
identified and justified.

**9.** Suggestions for future research were identified.

**10.** General comments.

*Overall Rating (Discussion):*                  _____    _____    _____    _____
                                                 Poor       Fair       Good     Excellent

# Evaluation of the Complete Research Article: Two Examples

## Overview

In Part II it was necessary to present a somewhat disjointed view of the evaluation process by showing examples of different parts of a research article instead of an integrated evaluation of a complete piece of research. In addition, we provided students with the link between each example in Part II and the principles discussed in Part I. In Part III we provide opportunities to synthesize the evaluation of three complete pieces of research and to find the links between these examples and the principles that were discussed in Part I.

We have reprinted two articles in Part III: one in audiology and one in speech-language pathology. In addition, we have put together the checklists from Chapters 7, 8, 9, and 10 as one reprintable checklist for students to use to guide them in the complete evaluation of each article as an integrating exercise. It then becomes the student's responsibility to draw on the principles in Part I and the examples in Part II and synthesize these resources for the completion of the integrated evaluation.

We chose articles that we believe will illustrate many points discussed in the previous chapters. In general, the articles are examples of good research, but we expect students to make both positive comments and constructive criticisms for the improvement of future research. No single research study is expected to compensate for all possible threats to internal and external validity, given the practical problems of conducting research. Any published paper can profit from suggestions for improvement. The articles we have chosen make important contributions to our knowledge of communicative disorders and are used here to illustrate the process of evaluation: the weighing of positive and negative aspects of the research in order to arrive at a reasonable judgment about the overall adequacy of an article.

# E V A L U A T I O N   C H E C K L I S T — INTRODUCTION

**Instructions:**    The four-category scale at the end of this checklist may be used to rate the *Introduction* section of an article. The *Evaluation Items* help identify those topics that should be considered in arriving at the rating. Comments on these topics, entered as *Evaluation Notes,* should serve as the basis for the overall rating.

*Evaluation Items*                                      *Evaluation Notes*

1. Title identified target population and variables under study.

2. Purpose, procedures, important findings, and implications were summarized in the abstract.

3. A clear statement of the general problem was given.

4. There was a logical and convincing rationale.

5. There was a current, thorough, and accurate review of literature.

6. The purpose, questions, or hypotheses were logical extensions of the rationale.

7. The introduction was clearly written and well organized.

8. General comments.

*Overall Rating (Introduction):*

| Poor | Fair | Good | Excellent |

# E V A L U A T I O N   C H E C K L I S T — M E T H O D

**Instructions:**    The four-category scale at the end of each part of the *Method* section checklist may be used to rate these parts of an article. The *Evaluation Items* help identify those topics that should be considered in arriving at the ratings. Comments on these topics, entered as *Evaluation Notes,* should serve as the basis for the ratings. An additional scale is provided to allow for an overall rating of the *Method* section.

*Evaluation Items (Participants)*                                      *Evaluation Notes*

1. Sample size was adequate.

2. Selection and exclusion criteria were adequate and clearly defined.

3. Participants were randomly selected and randomly assigned.

4. Overall or pair matching was employed.

5. Differential subject-selection posed no threat to internal validity.

6. Regression effect controlled for participants selected on basis of extreme scores.

7. Interaction of subject-selection and treatment posed no threat to external validity.

8. General comments.

*Overall Rating (Participants):*

| | | | |
|---|---|---|---|
| Poor | Fair | Good | Excellent |

### *Evaluation Items (Materials)*

*Evaluation Notes*

1. Instrumentation (hardware and behavioral) was appropriate.

2. Calibration procedures were described and were adequate.

3. Evidence presented on reliability and validity of hardware and behavioral instrumentation.

4. Experimenter and human observer bias was controlled.

5. Test environment was described and was adequate.

6. Instructions were described and were adequate.

7. There were adequate selection and measurement of independent (classification, predictor) variables.

8. There were adequate selection and measurement of dependent (criterion, predicted) variables.

9. General comments.

*Overall Rating (Materials):*

| | | | |
|---|---|---|---|
| Poor | Fair | Good | Excellent |

*Evaluation Items (Procedures)*                                    *Evaluation Notes*

1. Research design was appropriate to purpose
   of study.

2. Procedures reduced threats to internal validity
   arising from:
   (a) history
   (b) maturation
   (c) reactive pretest
   (d) mortality
   (e) interaction of above

3. Procedures reduced threats to external validity
   arising from:
   (a) reactive arrangements
   (b) interactive pretest
   (c) subject-selection
   (d) multiple treatments

4. General comments.

*Overall Rating (Procedures):*

| _____ | _____ | _____ | _____ |
|--------|--------|--------|--------|
| Poor   | Fair   | Good   | Excellent |

*Overall Rating (Method):*

| _____ | _____ | _____ | _____ |
|--------|--------|--------|--------|
| Poor   | Fair   | Good   | Excellent |

# E V A L U A T I O N   C H E C K L I S T — RESULTS

**Instructions:**  The four-category scale at the end of this checklist may be used to rate the *Results* section of
an article. The *Evaluation Items* help identify those topics that should be considered in arriving at the rating.
Comments on these topics, entered as *Evaluation Notes,* should serve as the basis for the overall rating.

*Evaluation Items*                                    *Evaluation Notes*

1. Results were clearly related to research problem.

2. Tables and figures were integrated with text.

3. Summary statistics were used appropriately.

4. Organization of data was clear.

5. Statistical analysis was appropriate to:

   **(a)** level of measurement
   **(b)** number of observations
   **(c)** type of sample
   **(d)** shape of distribution

**6.** There was appropriate use of correlational and inferential analysis.

**7.** There was clear presentation of significant and nonsignificant correlations.

**8.** There was clear presentation of significant and nonsignificant differences and effect sizes.

**9.** General comments.

*Overall Rating (Results):*

            \_\_\_\_\_     \_\_\_\_\_     \_\_\_\_\_     \_\_\_\_\_
            Poor       Fair       Good     Excellent

# EVALUATION CHECKLIST—DISCUSSION

**Instructions:** The four-category scale at the end of this checklist may be used to rate the *Discussion* section of an article. The *Evaluation Items* help identify those topics that should be considered in arriving at the rating. Comments on these topics, entered as *Evaluation Notes,* should serve as the basis for the overall rating.

*Evaluation Items*                                        *Evaluation Notes*

**1.** Discussion was clearly related to research problem.

**2.** Limitations of the method were discussed.

**3.** Conclusions were drawn directly and fairly from results.

**4.** Reasonable explanations were given for unusual, atypical, or discrepant results.

**5.** There was thorough and objective discussion of agreements and disagreements of previous research.

**6.** The section related results to various theoretical explanations.

**7.** Implications for clinical practice were stated fairly and objectively.

**8.** Theoretical or clinical speculations were
identified and justified.

**9.** Suggestions for future research were identified.

**10.** General comments.

*Overall Rating (Discussion):*

| Poor | Fair | Good | Excellent |
|------|------|------|-----------|
| _____ | _____ | _____ | _____ |

# Example Article for Evaluation in Audiology

## Auditory Temporal Order Perception in Younger and Older Adults

**PETER J. FITZGIBBONS**
*Gallaudet University*
*Washington, D.C.*

**SANDRA GORDON-SALANT**
*University of Maryland–College Park*

This investigation examined the abilities of younger and older listeners to discriminate and identify temporal order of sounds presented in tonal sequences. It was hypothesized that older listeners would exhibit greater difficulty than younger listeners on both temporal processing tasks, particularly for complex stimulus patterns. It was also anticipated that tone order discrimination would be easier than tone order identification for all listeners. Listeners were younger and older adults with either normal hearing or mild-to-moderate sensorineural hearing losses. Stimuli were temporally contiguous three-tone sequences within a 1/3 octave frequency range centered at 4000 Hz. For the discrimination task, listeners discerned differences between standard and comparison stimulus sequences that varied in tonal temporal order. For the identification task, listeners identified tone order of a single sequence using labels of relative pitch. Older listeners performed more poorly than younger listeners on the discrimination task for the more complex pitch patterns and on the identification task for faster stimulus presentation rates. The results also showed that order discrimination is easier than order identification for all listeners. The effects of hearing loss on the ordering tasks were minimal.

**KEY WORDS: auditory temporal processing, temporal order discrimination, temporal order identification, age-related processes**

From "Auditory Temporal Order Perception in Younger and Older Adults," by P. J. Fitzgibbons and S. Gordon-Salant, 1998, *Journal of Speech, Language, and Hearing Research, 41,* pp. 1052–1060. Copyright 1998 by the American Speech-Language-Hearing Association. Reprinted with permission.

**411**

This study examines age-related changes in auditory sequential processing in younger and older adults with and without sensorineural hearing loss. Although hearing loss among the elderly population is well documented (Gates, Cooper, Kannel, & Miller 1990; Pearson, Morrell, Gordon-Salant, Brant, & Fozard, 1995), other consequences of aging on perceptual processing of supra-threshold sounds are less well understood. Several recent reports implicate various aspects of temporal processing as being diminished in a number of older listeners. Some of the evidence comes from studies that used temporally altered speech stimuli to compare the recognition performance of young and elderly listeners (Bergman et al., 1976; Gordon-Salant & Fitzgibbons, 1993). Other results come from psychoacoustic experiments with simple stimuli that report age-related differences in temporal gap detection (Moore, Peters, & Glasberg, 1992; Schneider, Pichora-Fuller, Kowalchuk, & Lamb, 1994; Snell, 1997) and duration discrimination (Abel, Krever, & Alberti, 1990; Fitzgibbons & Gordon-Salant, 1994). Some of these results also indicate that age-related deficits in temporal processing may become exaggerated for listening conditions that feature a high degree of stimulus complexity or experimental uncertainty (Fitzgibbons & Gordon-Salant, 1995). Generally, the psychoacoustic temporal measures, show little correlation with audibility factors associated with age-related hearing loss.

The present investigation extends the study of aging and temporal processing to listening tasks that focus on the perception of auditory sequences. The principal experiments use tone sequences and compare the abilities of younger and older listeners to discriminate and identify the temporal order of components within the auditory patterns. The rationale for the experiments is twofold. First, sensitivity to temporal sequencing is a basic aspect of auditory processing that is essential for perceiving a variety of complex time-varying signals, such as speech or music. Second, most of the prevalent theorizing about slowed perceptual processing among the elderly population ascribes the primary difficulties to central and cognitive stages of information processing (Cerella, 1991; Hawkins & Pressen, 1986; Salthouse, 1985). Accurate perception and recall of the temporal order of sounds presented in sequence undoubtedly involves the contribution of various central processing mechanisms that may undergo changes with aging.

There is some evidence that elderly listeners do exhibit significant difficulty with temporal order perception. Trainor and Trehub (1989) compared the performance of younger and older adults on a series of temporal order recognition and discrimination tasks. Listeners were required to distinguish between two contrasting component orders within four-tone sequences of alternating higher and lower frequencies in the region below 1000 Hz. The experiments examined several variables, including stimulus presentation mode (single or recycled patterns), presentation rate, component frequency spacings, and listener practice. The study was designed to examine the disruptive effects of perceptual organization, or auditory stream segregation (Bregman & Campbell, 1971), on temporal ordering performance. It was reasoned that older listeners, with hypothesized slower processing abilities (Salthouse, 1985), might experience perceptual streaming phenomena at lower stimulus rates than would be evident for the younger listeners. Results indicated that the temporal ordering judgments of the older listeners were significantly poorer than those of the younger listeners in each experiment. However, the magnitude of the age-related performance differences appeared to be largely independent of the task (discrimination vs. identification), amount of practice, or the stimulus presentation rate.

Humes and Christopherson (1991) also reported findings indicating that temporal sequencing tasks may be particularly difficult for older listeners. Their study examined various auditory processing abilities in younger and older groups of listeners using the Test of Basic Auditory Capabilities (TBAC), a battery of forced-choice discrimination tasks (Johnson, Watson, & Jensen, 1987). Two of the tests required temporal order judgments, one using four-tone sequences, and the other four-syllable sequences consisting of different consonant-vowel tokens. Each task required listeners to distinguish between standard and comparison sequences that differed by the temporal ordering of the two middle components; presentation rate of sequences was varied within a block of listening trials. Performance of the older listeners on both ordering tasks was significantly poorer than that of the younger listeners, with no apparent influence of audibility factors related to hearing loss.

These few available results indicate the likelihood of an age-related difficulty with sequence perception, although the magnitude and source of the processing deficit are difficult to assess. Thus, for the older listener, it remains unclear whether diminished temporal ordering ability reflects slowed auditory processing or a more general dysfunction in sequential pattern recognition and recall. One purpose of the present investigation is to derive estimates of the minimum stimulus durations that are required by listeners to discriminate tone-order differences within sequences. Observation of significant age-related differences in the measured duration thresholds would give some indication of the extent to which processing speed differs across age groups. Also, it is of interest to know if measured duration thresholds are stable or vary with changes in stimulus attributes. This question was addressed by designing discrimination conditions that featured varying degrees of stimulus complexity and predictability. It was hypothesized that increases in stimulus complexity would have a relatively greater impact on the order discrimination performance of older listeners than on that of younger listeners. This outcome is suggested by previous results showing strong influences of stimulus complexity on duration discrimination performance of older listeners (Fitzgibbons & Gordon-Salant, 1995).

The stimulus sequences used in the order discrimination experiments were also used in a temporal order identification task. One purpose of these measurements was to compare the stimulus durations required for order identification with those required for accurate order discrimination. Additionally, differences in the relative difficulty of the discrimination and identification tasks may have different consequences for ordering judgments of younger and older listeners. Another purpose of the order identification task is to explore possible explanations for age-related performance differences. For example, if the older listeners exhibited a general cognitive difficulty with sequential pattern recognition and recall, then performance deficits for these listeners should be evident across a broad range of stimulus sequence presentation rates. Alternatively, if the age effects are primarily a consequence of slowed auditory processing, then performance differences among the younger and older listeners should be restricted to conditions in which stimulus presentation rates exceed some limiting value. Finally, each experiment is designed to examine the independent and interactive influences of age and sensorineural hearing loss on sequential processing. Toward this goal, performance was compared for four groups of listeners who were matched according to age and degree of hearing loss. Also, the spectral composition of all stimulus sequences was restricted to a narrow region centered at 4000 Hz that coincided with a region of maximal sensitivity loss in the listeners with hearing impairment.

USE THE EVALUATION CHECKLIST TO GUIDE YOUR EVALUATION
OF THE INTRODUCTION

# Method

## Participants

Listeners in the experiments included 40 adults assigned to four groups with 10 participants each, defined according to age and hearing status. These individuals participated in a larger project that included speech experiments, the results of which are reported elsewhere (Gordon-Salant & Fitzgibbons, 1997). The first group included elderly listeners (65–76 years) with normal hearing (pure tone thresholds ≤ 15 dB HL, re: ANSI, 1989, 250–4000 Hz) (Group label = ENH). The second group consisted of young listeners (20–40 years) with normal hearing (pure tone thresholds ≤ 15 dB HL, re: ANSI, 1989, 250–4000 Hz) (Group label = YNH). The third group included elderly listeners (65–76 years) with mild-to-moderate, sloping sensorineural hearing losses (Group label = EHL). These individuals had a negative history for otologic disease, noise exposure, familial hearing loss, and ototoxicity. The presumed etiology of hearing loss for these listeners was presbycusis. Participants in the fourth group were young adults (18–44 years) with sensorineural hearing loss (Group label = YHL). Each listener in this group was matched audiologically on an individual basis to a listener in the EHL group. The etiology of the hearing losses of the younger listeners was either heredity or unknown. Audiometric data for the four subject groups are displayed in Table 1. Immittance measures for all participants showed tympanograms with normal peak pressure (–50 to +50 daPa), normal acoustic admittance at the plane of the tympanic membrane (0.3–1.4 mmho), normal equivalent volume (0.6–1.5 cm$^3$), and normal tympanometric widths (50–110 daPa) (American Speech-Language-Hearing Association, 1990); acoustic reflexes were elicited at levels of 100 dB HL or lower in each ear. These immittance results are consistent with the presence of normal middle-ear function. Additionally, each participant exhibited good general health and passed the Short Portable Mental Status Questionnaire (Pfeiffer, 1975), a screening procedure for cognitive function.

## Stimuli

All stimuli for the experiments were sequences of three pure tones generated using inverse Fast Fourier Transform (FFT) procedures with a digital signal processing board (Tucker-Davis Technologies AP2) and a 16-bit digital-to-analog (D/A) converter (Tucker-Davis Technologies DD1, 20 kHz sampling rate) that was followed by low-pass filtering (Frequency Devices 901F; 6000 Hz cutoff, 90 dB/oct). The tone frequencies for all sequences spanned a 1/3 octave range and were arbitrarily designated as low (L), 3548 Hz; medium (M), 4000 Hz; and high (H), 4467 Hz. The tones within sequences were equal in duration and were presented contiguously in time with each component having a 1-ms cosine-squared rise/fall envelope. Tonal duration

**TABLE 1   Mean pure tone thresholds (and standard deviations) in dB HL (re ANSI, 1989) of the four groups (YNH = young listeners with normal hearing, ENH = elderly listeners with normal hearing, YHL = young listeners with hearing loss, EHL = elderly listeners with hearing loss)**

| | Participant Group | | | |
|---|---|---|---|---|
| *Frequency (Hz)* | *YNH* | *ENH* | *YHL* | *EHL* |
| 250 | 3.9 (3.3) | 11.0 (4.6) | 21.0 (17.6) | 20.0 (12.0) |
| 500 | 2.2 (2.6) | 8.5 (6.3) | 20.5 (17.9) | 21.0 (12.9) |
| 1000 | 2.2 (2.6) | 7.5 (6.3) | 30.0 (21.3) | 23.0 (10.0) |
| 2000 | 0.0 (2.5) | 8.0 (6.7) | 39.5 (20.2) | 33.0 (13.8) |
| 4000 | 2.2 (2.6) | 12.5 (4.9) | 51.0 (14.7) | 51.0 (8.4) |

*Note.* From "Selected Cognitive Factors and Speech Recognition Performance among Young and Elderly Listeners," by S. Gordon-Salant and P. J. Fitzgibbons, 1997, *Journal of Speech, Language, and Hearing Research, 40,* p. 425. Copyright 1997 by American Speech-Language-Hearing Association. Reprinted with permission.

was varied adaptively as an independent variable in the experiments, and changes of duration were implemented equally and simultaneously on all tonal components within sequences.

Three stimulus conditions were used to examine discrimination of tonal temporal order differences. One of these used tone sequences with unidirectional frequency shifts (UNI condition), with the rising sequence LMH and the falling sequence HML serving as the standard and comparison stimuli, respectively, for discrimination trials. A second discrimination condition utilized stimulus sequences containing bidirectional frequency shifts (BI condition), with MHL and HLM used as the respective standard and comparison sequences. For the third discrimination condition, the random (RAN) condition, stimulus sequences changed each trial, with the standard and comparison sequences of a given trial representing different random selections from the pool of six possible tone-order permutations (LMH, LHM, MHL, MLH, HML, HLM). The three discrimination conditions were selected to reflect different degrees of stimulus complexity, with those featuring unidirectional frequency shifts being intended as the least complex, and those with randomly changing frequency patterns the most complex.

Stimulus sequences used for the temporal order identification task were the same randomly ordered tonal patterns as described above for the RAN discrimination condition. However, for identification testing, sequence component durations were fixed within a block of listening trials and were varied across trial blocks.

## Procedures

***Temporal Order Discrimination.***   Temporal order discrimination was measured using adaptive three-interval cued two-alternative forced-choice procedures. For all discrimination conditions, each listening trial included three observation intervals with the standard tone sequence always presented in the first interval; the comparison sequence appeared with equal probability in the second or third interval on each trial, with the remaining interval containing a replication of the standard sequence. Listeners used a keyboard to indicate which interval, 2 or 3, sounded different from interval 1. The intervals of a trial were separated by 500 ms and were marked by a visual display on a computer monitor that also provided feedback on the correctness of response.

Temporal thresholds for the discrimination trials were obtained using an adaptive rule for changing the duration of each tonal component in the standard and comparison sequences on the basis of the listener's response on previous trials. The rule stipulated a decrease in tone durations following two correct-response trials and an increase in durations after each incorrect response. The tracking procedure estimated a threshold duration corresponding to 70.7% correct discrimination (Levitt, 1971). Testing was conducted in 65-trial blocks with initial tone durations of 250 ms and an initial step size for duration changes of 15 ms that was reduced to 2 ms after three reversals in the direction of duration changes. A threshold estimate was calculated by averaging duration values of the reversal points of the final 10 reversals associated with the small step-size changes in the tracking procedure. An average of six separate threshold estimates was used to determine a final estimate for each listener and discrimination condition, with the conditions tested in a different randomly selected order for each listener. Additionally, each listener received 2–3 hrs of practice in each condition before data collection. Although no formal analysis of practice data was undertaken, discrimination performance of listeners in each group showed no systematic improvement after six to eight trial blocks.

***Temporal Order Identification.***     Procedures for the temporal order identification task were implemented subsequent to completion of discrimination testing. The identification trials were single interval, in which one stimulus sequence was presented with a tone order selected randomly from six possible permutations of the three tone frequencies. Using procedures adapted from Divenyi and Hirsh (1974), listeners identified the stimulus sequence for each trial by keyboard response, selecting one of six keys (each labeled with a different sequence frequency order: HML, HLM, MHL, MLH, LMH, LHM); a simple line drawing above each response key was also provided as a visual aid to depict the pitch-shift directions associated with each sequence ordering. The identification trials were listener paced, with a 3-s inter-trial interval following each listener response; and the stimulus presentation interval was marked by visual display on a computer monitor. Percent-correct feedback was provided to listeners following each block of identification trials, but not for individual trials.

There were four order-identification conditions defined by the sequence component tone durations of 750 ms, 500 ms, 250 ms, and 100 ms. The conditions were tested separately in a different randomly selected order across listeners. Each condition was examined using 50-trial blocks, with tone durations fixed within blocks. The results from four trial blocks per condition were averaged to calculate a performance score for each listener. Before data collection, each listener was familiarized and trained with the identification task. Listeners practiced for 6–10 hrs in 2-hr sessions that included 10–12 trial blocks per session using tonal sequences that featured 1-s component durations.

The listeners were tested individually in a sound-attenuating chamber. Stimulus sequences for the discrimination and identification tasks were presented at 85 dB SPL, which corresponded to a minimum sensation level of 25–30 dB at 4000 Hz for the listeners with high-frequency hearing loss. The stimuli were delivered to listeners through an insert ear-phone (Etymotic ER-3A) calibrated in a 2-cm$^3$ coupler (B&K, DB0138). The transducer was selected for listener comfort and to avoid possible collapsing of ear canals, particularly in the older listeners. Testing was monaural in the better ear of listeners with hearing loss and in the preferred ear of listeners with normal hearing. Excluding practice sessions, total time for data collection was about 10 hrs, scheduled in 2-hr sessions. Participants were re-imbursed for their participation in the experiments.

---

USE THE EVALUATION CHECKLIST TO GUIDE YOUR EVALUATION
OF THE METHOD

---

# Results

## Temporal Order Discrimination

Results of the temporal order discrimination experiments are displayed in Figure 1. The figure shows the mean tonal duration thresholds and standard deviations for each group of listeners for the three discrimination conditions: UNI, BI, and RAN. An analysis of variance

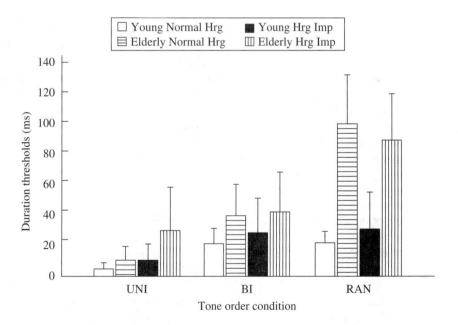

**FIGURE 1** **Mean tonal duration thresholds and standard deviations, obtained from the four listener groups in the three temporal order discrimination conditions (UNI = unidirectional pitch change, BI = bi-directional pitch change, RAN = random pitch change).**

(ANOVA) was performed on the raw data using a repeated-measures design with 2 between-subjects factors (age and hearing status) and 1 within-subjects factor (discrimination condition). The analysis revealed significant main effects of listener age [$F(1, 36) = 43.00$, $p < .01$], discrimination condition [$F(2, 72) = 71.84$, $p < .01$], and a significant interaction between these two factors [$F(2, 72) = 32.29$, $p < .01$]. The main effect of hearing loss on discrimination thresholds was not significant [$F(1, 36) = 1.15$, $p = .29$]. The hearing loss factor was also not involved in any significant interactions.

Subsequent analysis of simple main effects revealed that the thresholds of older listeners were significantly larger than those of the younger listeners for the complex conditions BI and RAN [$F(1, 108) = 5.91$, $p < .01$; $F(1, 108) = 12.41$, $p < .001$, respectively], but not for the UNI condition [$F(1, 108) = 3.48$, $p = .065$]. Simple main-effects analyses also showed that the effect of condition was significant for both younger and older listeners [$F(2, 72) = 4.80$, $p < .01$; $F(2, 72) = 81.49$, $p < .001$, respectively]. Multiple comparison testing (Student-Newman-Keuls) further indicated that the young listeners performed best on the UNI condition and significantly poorer but equivalently on the two more complex conditions BI and RAN ($p < .05$). The older listeners also performed best on the UNI condition and significantly poorer on the BI and RAN conditions ($p < .05$), but there was a further significant performance decrement on the RAN condition compared to the BI condition ($p < .05$).

## Temporal Order Identification

The temporal order identification task proved to be quite difficult for many of the listeners. Despite the slow presentation rate for training sequences (1-s component durations) and the extent of listening practice, 3 listeners from each of the younger groups and 4 listeners from each of the older groups failed to achieve consistent, above-chance identification performance (16.7% correct for the six-choice task). For these listeners, the problem appeared to be specific to difficulties in labeling sequence orders according to relative pitch change; pilot trials using tonal sequences with greater component frequency spacing (e.g., 1 octave) proved equally difficult. Therefore, these listeners were excluded from further testing, and participation in the identification conditions was restricted to those listeners who achieved a performance accuracy of 90% or better on the training trials. Results of the temporal order identification measurements are displayed in Figure 2. The figure shows the mean percent-correct scores and standard deviations from the four stimulus duration conditions for the groups of younger ($n = 7$ each) and older ($n = 6$ each) listeners. An ANOVA was performed on arcsine transforms of the raw percent-correct data (Kirk, 1968), using a repeated-measures design with 2 between-subjects factors (age and hearing status) and 1 within-subjects factor (duration condition). Results of this analysis revealed a significant main effect of condition [$F(3, 66) = 56.94$, $p < .001$] and a significant three-way interaction of the factors age, hearing status, and duration condition [$F(3, 66) = 3.88$, $p < .01$]. The main effects of age and hearing failed to reach significance [$F(1, 22) = 2.63$, $p = .12$; $F(1, 22) = 2.27$, $p = .146$, respectively]. Subsequent analyses of simple main effects revealed a significant condition effects for each listener group [$F(3, 72) > 4.89$, $p < .01$ for all four groups], which multiple-comparison testing confirmed resulted from a progressive decline in performance between almost all successive conditions of decreasing tonal dura-

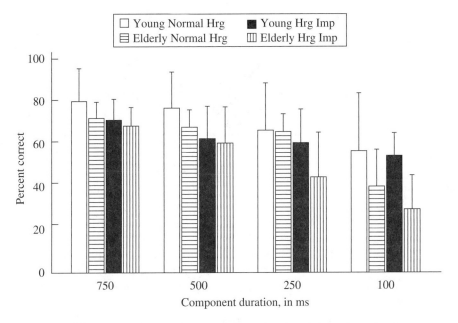

**FIGURE 2   Mean percent correct scores and standard deviations from the four listener groups in four stimulus duration conditions (750 ms, 500 ms, 250 ms, 100 ms).**

tion for each of the four listener groups ($p < .05$). Age effects were restricted to the most difficult condition (100-ms durations), on which older listeners generally performed poorer than younger listeners; this difference, however, reached significance only for the groups of younger and older listeners with hearing loss [$F(3, 72) = 5.84$, $p < .001$]. With one exception, effects of hearing loss were not apparent in the data. The exception was for older listeners in the 250-ms condition, where listeners with hearing loss performed significantly poorer than those with normal hearing ($p < .05$).

## Relationships between Measures

Because identification performance is presumably dependent upon a listener's ability to discriminate relevant stimuli, a correlation analysis was conducted to determine the extent to which discrimination ability is related to recognition performance for tone sequences with equivalent complexity and durations. For the purposes of this comparison, discrimination performance on the RAN condition was compared to identification performance, with the random sequences featuring 100-ms tones. Durations of this magnitude equaled or exceeded those required for accurate performance in the discrimination task for each listener group. The listeners' pure tone thresholds at 4000 Hz were also included in the correlational analysis to examine the extent to which auditory acuity influenced discrimination thresholds and identification performance for stimuli in this frequency region. A significant correlation was observed between duration thresholds for order discrimination and the percent-correct order identification scores ($r = -.54$, $p < .01$). Correlations between the pure tone threshold at 4000 Hz and either the discrimination threshold ($r = .22$) or the identification score ($r = -.20$) were not significant.

---

USE THE EVALUATION CHECKLIST TO GUIDE YOUR EVALUATION
OF THE RESULTS

---

## Discussion

The experiments were designed to examine age-related differences in sequential process-ing by assessing temporal order perception within the context of discrimination and identi-fication tasks. Evidence for age-related differences in temporal order perception emerge in many of the performance measures collected. However, the observed age effects in the data differ somewhat across tasks. The presence of hearing loss did not affect performance for either younger or older listeners. Additionally, the tasks of order discrimination and identi-fication appear to reflect different levels of difficulty for all of the listeners.

The discrimination results reveal the clearest effects of both listener age and stimulus complexity. Stimulus sequence orders featuring rising and falling frequency patterns in the UNI condition proved to be easiest to discriminate for all listeners. For this condition, the young listeners with and without hearing loss produced a mean duration threshold of 7.2 ms, with several individual estimates observed to be as small as 2–3 ms. For these same lis-teners, discrimination performance was poorer and equivalent for the more complex fre-quency patterns of the BI and RAN conditions, with thresholds showing values of 23.7 ms and 25.5 ms, respectively. The older listeners produced a mean duration threshold of 19.8 ms for the UNI condition. However, this value was largely inflated by poor performance of a few older listeners; most others produced threshold estimates comparable to those of the younger listeners. The results were quite different for BI and RAN conditions, in which the older listeners required mean tone durations of 40.1 ms and 94.2 ms, respectively, to dis-criminate order differences. Each of these values reflects significantly diminished perfor-mance relative to that of the younger listeners.

The discrimination results also reveal that some tonal patterns are considerably easier to distinguish than others. This is particularly true for the UNI condition, in which the observed duration thresholds for the majority of younger and older listeners closely ap-proximated reported estimates for auditory temporal acuity (Green, 1971). At these brief durations the rising/falling patterns of the UNI condition are perceived as singular spectral glides, rather than a succession of three tones. However, listeners could still perform the discrimination on the basis of frequency differences between the initial and/or final tones in the standard and comparison sequences of a listening trial. These frequency-difference cues were also available, though less salient, in the BI condition; and they varied in an un-predictable manner in the RAN condition. For these latter two conditions, threshold durations were sufficient to hear tones in succession, and the younger listeners discriminated order differences equally well on both. The much larger duration thresholds of older listeners for BI and RAN conditions are suggestive of both slower processing and a strong influence of stimulus complexity and/or uncertainty.

As stated previously, the temporal order identification task proved to be difficult for all listeners, and several listeners from each of the younger and older groups were not able to perform the task. Of those who met the criterion of 90% accuracy in the training session with 1-s component durations, identification accuracy was observed to decrease progressively from about 75% to 60% across conditions of decreasing tonal durations (from 750 ms to 250 ms). Across this range of tonal durations and/or sequence presentation rates, younger and older listeners performed essentially the same. For the 100-ms condition, age-related performance differences did emerge, with order recognition of the younger listeners showing an accuracy of 55% compared to 34% for the older listeners. However, inspection of the data from all listeners indicates that stimulus durations required for order identification are considerably larger than those required for order discrimination. Most of the listeners required sequence component durations of 250 ms or greater to achieve 60% recognition accuracy. This duration value is about an order of magnitude greater than that required for the young listeners to discriminate order differences with the same RAN sequences. For the elderly listeners, the differences between sequence durations required for identification and discrimination are much smaller, but this is due primarily to their elevated discrimination thresholds for the RAN condition.

It is not unusual in young listeners to observe large differences between component durations required for temporal order identification and discrimination, as revealed in several reviews of the relevant research literature (e.g., Divenyi & Hirsh, 1974; Pinheiro & Musiek, 1985; Warren, 1974). In particular, the duration thresholds associated with temporal order identification tasks can vary widely and depend on a large number of stimulus, procedural, and response factors. If, as in the present study, the identification task requires listeners to name or attach labels to individual components within stimulus sequences, then component durations of 150–500 ms are observed as necessary for moderately trained listeners to achieve accurate ordering performance (Warren, 1974). This range of values is consistent with present results collected from both younger and older listeners in the order identification task.

It is interesting to note that Divenyi and Hirsh (1974) used a procedure similar to the present identification task and observed that young listeners could be trained to identify order within three-tone sequences for component durations of 10 ms or less, depending on the pattern. Their results, however, were collected from a small sample of young adults with musical training who received extensive daily practice on the identification task over the course of many weeks. Divenyi and Hirsh also reported that their listeners were ultimately trained to identify permutations of tone order by discriminating variations in spectral patterns without the need to hear individual tones in succession. Therefore, it is perhaps not surprising that their threshold data for temporal order identification are similar in magnitude to those observed in the present order discrimination task, for the young listeners with normal hearing.

As mentioned above, Trainor and Trehub (1989) observed significant age effects in their temporal ordering tasks, although the magnitude of these effects was similar for order discrimination and identification tasks and were largely independent of changes in stimulus presentation rate. These results suggested that older listeners may exhibit a general difficulty in sequential pattern perception that is not strictly the result of processing speed deficits. It is possible, however, that the lack of strong task and stimulus rate effects in the Trainor and Trehub study may be due in part to the experimental procedures employed. Both the order identification and discrimination tasks that were utilized required listeners to distinguish between two alternatives of a four-tone sequence that differed only by the temporal ordering of two tonal components. Thus, the processing demands associated with each task featured a higher degree of similarity than required for the discrimination and identification tasks of the present study. Additionally, for each ordering task of Trainor and Trehub, stimulus presentation rate was varied randomly among eight values within each block of listening trials. This high level of stimulus uncertainty could have depressed overall listener performance and also have obscured observation of systematic stimulus rate effects. Thus, although the age effects observed by Trainor and Trehub are significant, the source of diminished performance with the older listeners is unclear.

Results of the present experiments indicate that age-related deficits in temporal processing are likely to depend on both stimulus complexity and processing speed. For the order discrimination task, no age effects were apparent for simple rising/falling tone orders, but significant age-related performance decrements existed for the more complex frequency patterns. For temporal order identification there was little or no age effect at the slower sequence presentation rates, although age-related performance differences did emerge at the fastest sequence rate examined. These identification results implicate a processing speed deficit in the older listeners rather than a general cognitive difficulty with serial pattern recognition. Additionally, the longer duration thresholds of the older listeners required for temporal order discrimination also could be interpreted as evidence for slowed processing. However, stimulus attributes play an important role. It seems possible that factors associated with stimulus complexity and stimulus rate interact in unknown ways to promote an information-processing-rate limitation in the older listeners. This limitation in information rate may account for various results from different studies indicating age-related performance deficits on tasks involving sequential processing.

## Acknowledgments

This research was supported by a grant from the National Institute on Aging (R01 AG09191) of the National Institutes of Health. The authors are grateful to Linda Carr-Kraft and Hillary Crowley, for their assistance in data collection for this project, and to John Grose and two anonymous reviewers, for their helpful comments on an earlier version of this paper.

USE THE EVALUATION CHECKLIST TO GUIDE YOUR EVALUATION
OF THE DISCUSSION

# REFERENCES

Abel, S., Krever, E., & Alberti, P. W. (1990). Auditory detection, discrimination and speech processing in ageing, noise-sensitive and hearing-impaired listeners. *Scandinavian Audiology, 19,* 43–54.

American National Standards Institute. (1989). *Specifications for Audiometers* (ANSI S3.6, 1989). New York: Author.

American Speech-Language-Hearing Association. (1990). Guidelines for screening for hearing impairment and middle ear disorders. *ASHA, 32*(Suppl. 2), 17–24.

Bergman, M., Blumenfeld, V. S., Cascardo, D., Dash, B., Levitt, H., & Margulies, M. K. (1976). Age-related decrement in hearing for speech. *Journal of Gerontology, 31,* 533–538.

Bregman, A. S., & Campbell, J. (1971). Primary auditory stream segregation and segregation of order in rapid sequences of tones. *Journal of Experimental Psychology, 89,* 244–249.

Ceralla, J. (1991). Age effects may be global, not local: Comment on Fisk and Rogers (1991). *Journal of Experimental Psychology (General), 120,* 215–223.

Divenyi, P., & Hirsh, I. (1974). Identification of temporal order in three-tone sequences. *Journal of the Acoustical Society of America, 56,* 144–151.

Fitzgibbons, P., & Gordon-Salant, S. (1994). Age effects on measures of auditory temporal sensitivity. *Journal of Speech and Hearing Research, 37,* 662–670.

Fitzgibbons, P., & Gordon-Salant, S. (1995). Duration discrimination with simple and complex stimuli: Effects of age and hearing sensitivity. *Journal of the Acoustical Society of America, 98,* 3140–3145.

Gates, G. A., Cooper, J. C., Kannel, W. B., & Miller, N. J. (1990). Hearing in the elderly: The Framingham cohort, 1983–1985. *Ear and Hearing, 11,* 247–256.

Gordon-Salant, S., & Fitzgibbons, P. (1993). Temporal factors and speech recognition performance in young and elderly listeners. *Journal of Speech and Hearing Research, 36,* 1276–1285.

Gordon-Salant, S., & Fitzgibbons, P. (1997). Selected cognitive factors and speech recognition performance among young and elderly listeners. *Journal of Speech, Language, and Hearing Research, 40,* 423–431.

Green, D. M. (1971). Temporal auditory acuity. *Psychological Review, 78,* 540–551.

Hawkins, H., & Pressen, J. (1986). Auditory information processing. In K. R. Boff, L. Kaufman, & J. P. Thomas (Eds.), *Handbook of perception and human performance: Vol. II. Cognitive processes and performance* (Chapter 6). New York: Wiley-Interscience.

Humes, L. & Christopherson, L. (1991). Speech identification difficulties of hearing-impaired elderly persons: The contributions of auditory processing deficits. *Journal of Speech and Hearing Research, 34,* 686–693.

Johnson, D. M., Watson, C. S., & Jensen, J. K. (1987). Individual differences in auditory capabilities. I. *Journal of the Acoustical Society of America, 81,* 427–438.

Kirk, R. E. (1968). *Experimental design: Procedures for the behavioral sciences.* Belmont, CA: Brooks/Cole.

Levitt, H. (1971). Transformed up-down method in psychoacoustics. *Journal of the Acoustical Society of America, 49,* 467–477.

Moore, B. C. J., Peters, R. W., & Glasberg, B. R. (1992). Detection of temporal gaps in sinusoids by elderly subjects with and without hearing loss. *Journal of the Acoustical Society of America, 92,* 1923–1932.

Pearson, J. D., Morrell, C. H., Gordon-Salant, S., Brant, L., & Fozard, J. L. (1995). Gender differences in a longitudinal study of age-associated hearing loss. *Journal of the Acoustical Society of America, 97,* 1196–1205.

Pfeiffer, E. (1975). A short portable mental status questionnaire for the assessment of organic brain deficit in elderly patients. *Journal of the American Geriatric Society, 23,* 433–441.

Pinheiro, M. L., & Musiek, F. E. (1985). Sequencing and temporal ordering in the auditory system. In M. L. Pinheiro & G. L. Musiek (Eds.), *Assessment of central auditory dysfunction* (pp. 219–238). Baltimore: Williams & Wilkins.

Salthouse, T. A. (1985). *A theory of cognitive aging.* New York: North-Holland.

Schneider, B. A., Pichora-Fuller, M. K., Kowalchuk, D., & Lamb, M. (1994). Gap detection and the precedence effect in young and old adults. *Journal of the Acoustical Society of America, 95,* 980–991.

Snell, K. B. (1997). Age-related changes in temporal gap detection. *Journal of the Acoustical Society of America, 101,* 2214–2220.

Trainor, L. J., & Trehub, S. E. (1989). Aging and auditory temporal sequencing: Ordering the elements of repeating tone patterns. *Perception and Psychophysics, 45,* 417–426.

Warren, R. M. (1974). Auditory temporal discrimination by trained listeners. *Cognitive Psychology, 6,* 237–256.

Received January 16, 1998

Accepted June 15, 1998

Contact author: Sandra Gordon-Salant, PhD, Department of Hearing and Speech Sciences, University of Maryland, College Park, MD 20742. E-mail: sgordon@bssl.umd.edu

# Example Article for Evaluation in Speech-Language Pathology

## Effects of Treatment on Linguistic and Social Skills in Toddlers with Delayed Language Development

**SHARI BRAND ROBERTSON**

*Department of Special Education and Clinical Services*
*Indiana University of Pennsylvania*

**SUSAN ELLIS WEISMER**

*Department of Communicative Disorders and Waisman Center on Mental Retardation and Human Development*
*University of Wisconsin–Madison*

This study investigated the effects of early language intervention on various linguistic and social skills of late-talking toddlers. The 21 children who participated in the investigation were randomly assigned to an experimental group ($n = 11$) or a control (delayed-treatment) group ($n = 10$). The experimental group participated in a 12-week clinician-implemented language intervention program. Groups were compared at pretest and posttest on five linguistic variables: Mean Length of Utterance, Total Number of Words, Number of Different Words, Lexical Repertoire, and Percentage of Intelligible Utterances, as well as on Socialization and Parental Stress. Significant group differences were found for each of the variables, indicating facilitative effects of the treatment. Notably, increases were observed in areas that were not specifically targeted by the intervention. Implications of these results are discussed with respect to considerations regarding clinical management decisions for toddlers with delayed language development.

**KEY WORDS: late talkers, early intervention, treatment efficacy, socialization, parental stress**

Investigation of early language delay has become a focus for research in recent years (Ellis Weismer, Murray-Branch, & Miller, 1994; Paul, 1991, 1996; Paul & Jennings, 1992; Paul, Murray, Clancy, & Andrews, 1997; Paul, Spangle Looney, & Dahm, 1991; Rescorla, 1989; Rescorla & Goossens, 1992; Rescorla, Roberts, & Dahlsgaard, 1997; Thal, 1991; Thal & Tobias, 1992, 1994; Thal, Oroz, & McCaw, 1995; Thal, Tobias, & Morrison, 1991; Whitehurst, Fischel, Arnold, & Lonnigan, 1992). For many children, delays in language development are accompanied by deficits in other areas, such as the sensory system or cognitive abilities. However, researchers have identified a group of toddlers, often described in the literature as "late talkers" (cf. Rescorla, 1989), whose deficits appear to be primarily confined to the linguistic domain. Prevalence rates for this population, as compiled in a study involving middle-class households, have been estimated at 10–15% (Rescorla, 1989).

Late talkers are generally described as having obvious delays in language acquisition, in contrast to seemingly typical development in other areas. Typically, researchers have used two primary methods to identify this group of youngsters. Some have used a cutoff score (usually 10th percentile) on a parental-report assessment protocol, such as the McArthur Communicative Developmental Inventory (Fenson et al., 1993), to identify the linguistic delay (Ellis Weismer et al., 1994; Thal & Tobias, 1992, 1994). Others have defined this population as children who, at 24 months, possess an expressive vocabulary of less than 50 words or demonstrate no multiword utterances in spontaneous conversation (Paul, 1993; Rescorla, 1989; Rescorla & Schwartz; 1990). Despite the linguistic delay, children identified as late talkers demonstrate normal-range performance on sensory, motor, and nonverbal cognitive measures.

Follow-up investigations have indicated that approximately half of the toddlers with late onset of talking at age 2 years catch up to their peers by age 3, with these children being designated "late bloomers" (Paul, 1991; Rescorla & Schwartz, 1990; Rescorla et al., 1997). Even after vocabulary moves into the normal range, a number of late talkers continue to demonstrate production delays in other areas, including phonology, morphology/syntax, and narrative abilities (Paul, 1991; Paul, Hernadez, Taylor, & Johnson, 1996; Paul & Smith, 1993; Rescorla & Schwartz, 1990; Rescorla et al., 1997; Roberts, Rescorla, Giroux, & Stevens, 1998). Several follow-up studies of late talkers have reported that the majority of children meet normative expectations on language assessment measures and measures of early reading skills by the elementary school-age period (Paul, 1996; Paul et al., 1997; Rescorla, 1993; Whitehurst et al., 1991); however, they score significantly below control groups matched on age, SES, and nonverbal cognition in various areas of linguistic functioning (Paul, 1996; Rescorla, 1993). Paul et al. (1997) acknowledge that we may only be beginning to understand the impact that residual linguistic deficits may have on these children as they advance through the higher grades in school. It is important to note that late talkers' participation in language intervention over the course of these follow-up studies has generally not been systematically documented or examined.

# Outcomes and Clinical Management of Late Talkers

Currently, considerable controversy exists regarding appropriate clinical management of children who are classified as late talkers (Ellis Weismer, in press; Olswang & Bain, 1991; Olswang, Rodriguez, & Timler, 1998; Paul, 1996, 1997; van Kleeck, Gillam, & Davis, 1997; Whitehurst et al., 1991; Whitehurst & Fischel, 1994). Uncertainty about clinical decisions regarding intervention for children who are developing normally in all areas except language has arisen because of a lack of clear predictors for spontaneous recovery, uncertainty regarding appropriate diagnosis, and concern for the cumulative effects of early language delay on related areas of development (cf. van Kleeck et al., 1997).

Whitehurst et al. (1991) advocate a "wait and see" approach to the clinical management of late talkers. They investigated the effectiveness of a treatment program in which parents were taught to use milieu teaching techniques to promote language development. Findings indicated that this approach resulted in significant improvements in toddlers' expressive language skills as compared to those of a control group of late talkers who did not receive treatment. However, Whitehurst and colleagues discounted the long-term benefits and importance of early language intervention for these children in light of follow-up findings that indicated no significant group differences at age 5 years on the language assessment measures that were administered (though they acknowledged that the immediate positive effects reassured parents regarding the child's developmental status and probably resulted in improved parent-child interactions). Questions about the conclusions that can be drawn from this investigation have been raised by several investigators given concerns about methodology and interpretation issues (Ellis Weismer et al., 1993; Girolametto, Pearce, & Weitzman, 1996; Olswang & Bain, 1991; Paul, 1991). Potential confounds in this investigation include the lack of random assignment to groups and the lack of control for concurrent therapy provided to participants. Girolametto et al. (1996) have characterized the Whitehurst et al. study as quasi-experimental and contend that the results should be interpreted cautiously (p. 1275).

More recently, for children who exhibit slow expressive language development Paul (1996) has advocated the implementation of a "watch and see" policy given data collected in a longitudinal study that followed children from 20 to 34 months through first grade. She suggests that children who exhibit no additional risk factors beyond slow language development (such as poverty, hearing impairment, exposure to drugs/alcohol, or serious medical problems) could be monitored throughout development as an alternative to direct intervention. If the problem worsens or begins to be manifested in other areas, intervention would then be implemented. Van Kleeck et al. (1997) have expressed concerns about the adoption of a watch-and-see public policy based on the conclusions drawn from Paul's longitudinal investigations because of questions about the heterogeneity of the late-talker sample, lack of clear predictors for spontaneous recovery, and the possible impact of intervention that some children in the cohort received during the study. Paul (1997) has responded to these specific issues and continues to assert that a watch-and-see approach is warranted for toddlers with circumscribed language delays. Although Paul contends that careful monitoring (with guidelines for when to initiate intervention) seems to be the most cost-effective approach, she does not suggest that children who are late to develop language should not receive intervention if necessary resources are available and parents wish to pursue this option. In fact, she argues that treatment may serve a facilitative function as described by Olswang and Bain (1991) or prevent development of future problems in related areas, such as social adjustment and self-esteem. However, she recommends that parents be counseled regarding the probability of the effectiveness of the intervention given the current state of the research in this area (Paul, 1996).

Although there is considerable evidence regarding the effectiveness of a variety of intervention approaches in somewhat older preschoolers, data regarding the efficacy of early intervention for late-talking toddlers is scant (cf. Ellis Weismer, in press). Ellis Weismer, Murray-Branch, and Miller (1993) compared the relative efficacy of two intervention approaches stemming from an interactive approach to language intervention. An alternating treatment, single-case design was used to determine the relative effectiveness of the two treatment methods of interest. Participants in this investigation were 3 toddlers, between the ages of 27 and 28 months, who had been identified as late talkers from a cohort of children involved in a prospective study of language development from the prelinguistic period to multiword productions (Ellis Weismer et al., 1994). The children were taught different sets of words under each of the conditions—modeling and modeling-plus-evoked production—to determine which condition produced a greater degree of vocabulary development. Results revealed that the response to the treatment conditions varied across subjects. One child demonstrated positive gains in the modeling-plus-evoked production condition. The second child produced more target words in the modeling-only format, whereas the third child responded similarly to both intervention techniques. Because of the nature of the experimental design, no direct examination of treatment versus no treatment was undertaken in this study.

Girolametto, Pearce, and Weitzman (1996) studied the effect of a parent-based intervention that used a focused-stimulation approach to promote vocabulary development in late talkers. Children between the ages of 23 and 33 months were randomly assigned to either a treatment or a control (delayed treatment) condition. Following an 11-week intervention adapted from the Hanen Program for Parents, both groups were re-assessed to determine possible differences in both maternal interactional behavior and child linguistic skills. At posttest (3 weeks following the end of the treatment interval) mothers' language input to their toddlers was less complex, presented at a slower pace, and focused more on specific target vocabulary. Children demonstrated significant increases in their vocabulary size, total number of different words used in interactions, number of different target words used in interactions, and number of control words used in interactions. They also demonstrated an increase in multiword utterances. Given these results, Girolametto and his colleagues argue that an interactive model can stimulate positive changes in parental facilitative behaviors as well as in children's linguistic skills.

The notion of a reciprocal relationship between the child and the environment is central to social theories of language learning (Bruner, 1983; Vygotsky, 1978). From this perspective, children operate as participants in various interactive contexts throughout the time that they are learning language. Language, therefore, does not develop in isolation but is heavily dependent on the social context in which it is learned and used. This overlap in the social and linguistic domains during development produces a high correspondence between language impairment and a lack of social competence (Prutting, 1992). In fact, it has been suggested that disorders in the linguistic system are largely defined by the accompanying negative social consequences (Craig, 1996). Paul et al. (1991) found that at age 3 nearly half of a group of children identified as late talkers at age 2 continued to demonstrate significant delays in social skills, regardless of their current level of language functioning. Given these results, Paul and colleagues argue that social skills appear to be vulnerable to disruption even after language deficits have been resolved. Rice (1993) argues that children with language impairment may be victims of a "negative social spiral" (p. 155). Because of their poor communication skills, these children do not interact effectively with their peers and may be rejected socially by them. This leads to a reduction in the number of social interactions these children experience, reducing opportunities to practice and refine their social skills. In this way, language deficits and social deficiencies interact and intensify one another, potentially resulting in long-term negative social consequences.

Similarly, the transactional model of language development (cf. Yoder & Warren, 1993) suggests that the language-learning process involves ongoing reciprocal interactions between child behaviors and parent behaviors. Early disruption in the development of children's language systems can negatively affect the dynamics of this interaction, reducing the potential for learning to occur in this natural social context. Late-talking toddlers may have difficulty responding to their mothers' linguistic input. This may, in turn, make the interactions between parent and child less enjoyable to the mother, who may respond by reducing the number of interactions she initiates with her child. This results in fewer opportunities for children to engage in the very experiences that build language and social competence (Fujiki & Brinton, 1994). Accordingly, remediation of language delay through early intervention efforts provides critical support for the development of skills necessary to support social interactions, maximizing the potential for future learning opportunities.

Disagreements regarding the role of early intervention for late talkers appear to stem from different notions of how "importance" is to be gauged. Whitehurst and colleagues (1991) have stated: "We believe our data, on balance, support the efficacy but not the importance of early intervention" (p. 67). One way to measure importance is to compare long-term outcomes across treated and untreated groups—the approach used in the Whitehurst et al. investigation. Alternatively, importance could be measured by the breadth of short-term changes noted in treated versus untreated groups, which is the view motivating the current investigation. That is, we might assess the value of early intervention not only in terms of its ability to move children into a normal range of linguistic functioning as soon as possible and thereby minimize the potential cumulative effects of the delay, but also with respect to its short-term impact on socialization and parental concerns (cf. Olswang & Bain, 1991, Olswang et al., 1998).

The purpose of this study is to examine the effects of early language intervention on the development of late-talking toddlers across a variety of variables. It is hypothesized that direct, clinician-based language intervention will result in a positive impact on the expressive language abilities of late-talking toddlers as compared to children in a delayed-treatment group. Support for this hypothesis is drawn from previous research suggesting that direct intervention is effective in increasing linguistic functioning in somewhat older preschoolers (cf. Ellis Weismer, in press; Leonard, 1998). In addition, this investigation seeks to examine the role of early language intervention in increasing the socialization skills of late talkers as well as the parents' perceptions of their child's linguistic, social, and behavioral skills. Paul (1991) found that parents of the late talkers in her investigation tended to rate their children as more hyperactive and demonstrating more behavioral problems relative to children in the typically developing group. Although theoretical tenets and some anecdotal evidence support the notion of positive effects of treatment on variables of this nature (e.g., Girolametto et al., 1996), little empirical evidence is available in the current literature. Thus, exploration of the possibility of facilitative effects of language intervention on children's social competence and on parental perceptions of the child is a secondary focus of this investigation.

---

USE THE EVALUATION CHECKLIST TO GUIDE YOUR EVALUATION
OF THE INTRODUCTION

---

# Method

## Participants

Twenty-one late-talking toddlers, 12 boys and 9 girls, participated in this investigation. Children in the experimental group ($n = 11$) ranged in age from 21 to 30 months, with a mean age of 25.6 months at initial recruitment. Children in the control (delayed-treatment) group ($n = 10$) ranged in age from 21 to 28 months, with a mean of 24.6 months. Children in both groups demonstrated significant delays in the acquisition of language, yet normal development in other areas. The cohort included children with expressive delays only as well as those who demonstrated delays in both the expressive and receptive domains, although the majority of children appeared to be experiencing expressive delays only. Ellis Weismer et al. (1994) caution against dividing children whose linguistic systems are at this very early stage of development into a subgroup of those with expressive language delay only and a subgroup of those with delays in both the receptive and expressive domains because of the shifting nature of these abilities and difficulties in language measurement at this stage of development. All children demonstrated normal hearing, oral and speech motor abilities, and no frank neurological impairments. In addition, the toddlers all came from monolingual, English-speaking homes. Children from both groups were from white, middle-class households. Table 1 summarizes the group and individual characteristics of the participants in the investigation.

## Recruitment and Identification of Participants

Because the purpose of this study was to investigate the impact of early intervention on children who had not previously been exposed to therapy, children were actively recruited from the community, rather than enrolling youngsters who were already participating in a program. Potential candidates for the study were located through various means, such as the distribution of flyers to agencies with a high incidence of contact with families of young children (e.g., preschools, pediatricians, day care providers, Head Start centers), articles submitted to local newspapers, and advertising via local radio and public TV stations.

**TABLE 1   Summary of individual and group characteristics of participants**

| Gender | Age (in months) | Receptive language[a] | Expressive language[b] | Cognition[c] | Motor skills[d] | SES[e] |
|--------|-----------------|----------------------|------------------------|--------------|-----------------|--------|
| *Experimental Group* | | | | | | |
| M | 29 | 100 | 74 | 85 | 98 | 16 |
| M | 26 | 96 | 72 | 82 | 101 | 14 |
| M | 28 | 101 | 69 | 81 | 98 | 12 |
| M | 27 | 103 | 68 | 79 | 110 | 16 |
| F | 26 | 93 | 77 | 85 | 90 | 17 |
| F | 22 | 86 | 69 | 88 | 97 | 15 |
| M | 30 | 80 | 63 | 80 | 85 | 12 |
| F | 22 | 116 | 74 | 89 | 121 | 25 |
| F | 27 | 109 | 74 | 85 | 97 | 12 |
| M | 21 | 88 | 70 | 82 | 90 | 16 |
| F | 23 | 77 | 72 | 77 | 87 | 14 |
| *M* | 25.6 | 95.4 | 71.1 | 83.0 | 97.6 | 15.4 |
| *SD* | 3.1 | 12.0 | 3.3 | 3.7 | 10.5 | 3.7 |
| *Control Group* | | | | | | |
| M | 27 | 89 | 72 | 82 | 95 | 12 |
| F | 21 | 98 | 75 | 79 | 101 | 16 |
| M | 27 | 109 | 73 | 86 | 98 | 14 |
| F | 22 | 93 | 69 | 82 | 88 | 20 |
| M | 21 | 104 | 77 | 82 | 112 | 16 |
| M | 26 | 112 | 75 | 86 | 115 | 16 |
| F | 25 | 104 | 70 | 80 | 98 | 20 |
| M | 22 | 85 | 75 | 79 | 90 | 12 |
| F | 28 | 90 | 71 | 81 | 88 | 15 |
| M | 27 | 87 | 69 | 78 | 85 | 20 |
| *M* | 24.6 | 97.1 | 72.6 | 81.5 | 97.0 | 16.1 |
| *SD* | 2.8 | 9.7 | 2.8 | 2.8 | 10.1 | 3.1 |

[a]Standard scores on the receptive portion of the Preschool Language Scale—3 (Zimmerman, Steiner, & Pond, 1992), with a mean of 100 and standard deviation of 15.

[b]Standard scores on the expressive portion of the Preschool Language Scale—3 (Zimmerman, Steiner, & Pond, 1993), with a mean of 100 and standard deviation of 15.

[c]Standard scores on the Mental Scales of the Bayley Scales of Infant Development (BSID-II, Bayley, 1993), with a mean of 100 and standard deviation of 15.

[d]Standard scores on the Motor Scales of the Bayley Scales of Infant Development (BSID-II, Bayley, 1993), with a mean of 100 and standard deviation of 15.

[e]SES indexed by self-report of maternal years in school.

Families of toddlers who responded to these recruitment efforts completed a family background questionnaire and the MacArthur Communicative Developmental inventory—Words and Sentences (CDI; Fenson et al., 1993). Children whose scores on the vocabulary portion of the CDI fell below the 10th percentile (−1.25 *SD*) and whose background information revealed no evidence of developmental delay outside the linguistic realm nor other exclusionary criteria (e.g., evidence of sensory impairment, previous or current intervention, multilingual home environment, evidence of significant physical or cognitive delays, history of frank neurological signs, emotional disturbance, evidence of significant medical involvement) were invited to participate in further assessment to determine eligibility for the study. The 10th percentile was selected as a cutoff given its successful use by researchers in distinguishing late-talking toddlers from children with typically developing language skills (Ellis Weismer et al., 1994; Thal & Tobias, 1992). Instruments used to measure outcome variables were administered immediately before the initiation of intervention (within one week) and again within one week following termination of the treatment.

Children who were eventually identified as participants in the investigation were required to demonstrate normal hearing (per ASHA guidelines, 1997), adequate oral and speech motor skills, scores falling at or below the 10th percentile (−1.25 *SD*) on one or both subscales of the Preschool Language Scale—III (Zimmerman, Steiner, & Pond, 1992), and standard scores within 1 *SD* of the mean on the Motor Scale and within 1.5 *SD* on the Mental Scale of the Bayley Scales of Infant Development—Second Edition (BSID-II; Bayley, 1993). The BSID-II is designed to assess both verbal and nonverbal cognition; consequently, the more liberal eligibility criteria on the mental subscale was implemented in light of the restricted language abilities of late talkers. One of the difficulties researchers who study late talkers experience is accurate identification of the population of interest. By definition, late talkers are assumed to experience delays that are confined primarily to the linguistic domain as opposed to youngsters who demonstrate a more global pattern of developmental delay. Commonly, a measure of cognition is included in the initial assessment protocol to disambiguate between these two groups. Although this is a logical step toward ensuring that the participants are actually drawn from the population of interest, standardized language-free measures of cognition for children of this age are not currently available. Although *t* tests calculated for the Mental Scale of the Bayley suggested no significant differences between the groups' pretreatment, the impact of the verbal component of this subscale was not considered statistically. In order to address this potential confound, the scoreforms of each of the children who participated in this study were compared with an item analysis of verbally loaded items on the MDI compiled by Spitz, Tallal, Flax, and Benasich (1997) as a part of their recent investigation. Children in the control group demonstrated an average of 15.2 (*SD* = 2.82) verbal items correct on the MDI at the beginning of the study. Children in the experimental group achieved an average of 14.63 (*SD* = 3.56) of the verbal items correct. Given these values, group characteristics regarding this area of development were judged to be similar pretreatment.

Although children were not excluded from the study on the basis of their phonological abilities, descriptive information was gathered by means of a checklist of consonants listed by sound class (glides, fricatives, stops, labials) completed by an observer during spontaneous language sampling. Totals were obtained for each child on the number of initial-position consonants produced, the number of final-position consonants produced, and the number of sound classes demonstrated. These data are summarized in Table 2.

**TABLE 2    Number of sounds and sound classes in spontaneous language in terms of means (*M*) and standard deviation (*SD*)**

|  | Sound classes demonstrated | Consonants used in initial position | Consonants used in final position |
|---|---|---|---|
| Experimental |  |  |  |
| *M* | 3.45 | 10.00 | 7.54 |
| *SD* | .82 | 4.15 | 2.95 |
| Control |  |  |  |
| *M* | 3.50 | 11.50 | 7.60 |
| *SD* | .71 | 3.79 | 3.27 |

## Experimental Design

This investigation consisted of a pretest-posttest control group design utilizing an experimental and a control (delayed-treatment) group. Following pretesting, children in the experimental group were provided with 12 weeks of direct clinician-implemented intervention. At the end of the treatment period, the 21 children were reassessed with respect to the experimental variables.

A delayed-treatment group, rather than a treatment/no-treatment design, was employed in this investigation. Although there is currently no empirical evidence that withholding intervention will negatively affect the ultimate language functioning of late talkers, the theoretical framework upon which this investigation is based would suggest that this could put children at risk for negative consequences in linguistic development as well as in related developmental areas. Consequently, children who were originally assigned to the control group were given the opportunity to participate in the same treatment program that was provided to the experimental group following the conclusion of the study. The 12-week treatment interval was deliberately chosen to maximize the potential of finding significant treatment effects for children in the experimental group (as was demonstrated in Girolametto et al., 1996) as well as to minimize the possibility of lasting negative consequences as a result of an overly long delay between identification and treatment for children in the control group.

## Dependent Variables

Although the primary focus of language intervention was to facilitate gains in a child's linguistic behaviors, possible facilitative effects of treatment on related domains were also of interest. Data gathered from direct assessment as well as from parent report were used to measure the linguistic and social/behavioral functioning of the toddlers participating in this study.

*Linguistic Variables.*    Five variables measuring linguistic growth and speech intelligibility were investigated in this study. To obtain data for four of the variables, audiotaped transcripts of 15-min spontaneous language samples gathered at pre- and posttest intervals were transcribed and analyzed using Systematic Analysis of Language Transcripts (SALT; Miller & Chapman, 1996). These four variables were mean length of utterance (MLU), total number of words (TNW), number of different words (NDW), and percentage of intelligible utterances. MLU, which provided an overall estimate of linguistic complexity, is well established as a valid and developmentally sensitive index of language growth for children at this stage. TNW within a set time interval (15 min) provided a general measure of verbal output or talkativeness. NDW was chosen as a measure of vocabulary growth. Watkins, Kelly, Harbers, and Hollis (1995) reported that NDW is a sensitive and informative estimate of lexical diversity in children with language impairments. Percentage of intelligible utterances was used as an index of the intelligibility of children's communicative attempts. Data regarding reported vocabulary size was obtained from pre- and posttest scores obtained on the CDI.

***Social/Behavioral Variables.*** Two variables related to social/behavioral characteristics were explored to determine the possibility of facilitative effects of early language intervention with late talkers. The first variable, socialization, was measured through pre- and posttesting on the Socialization Domain of the Vineland Adaptive Behavior Scales (VABS, Interview Edition, Expanded Form; Sparrow, Balla, & Ciccetti, 1984). This instrument was selected for the protocol because it includes items that were likely to reflect socialization gains associated with increases in communication skills, provided standard scores in 2-month increments, and has been used effectively to assess socialization skills in prior investigations involving late-talking toddlers (Paul et al., 1991). The second variable, parental stress, was assessed through scores obtained at pre- and posttest on the child domain of the Parenting Stress Index–Child Domain (PSI; Abidin, 1995). The PSI has been used in early intervention research studies (Tannock, Girolametto, & Siegel, 1992) to assess the effect of treatment on parental stress levels. The PSI includes a Defensive Responding score derived from specific items that are phrased in different ways across the test to identify respondents who may be responding in a biased manner.

## Treatment

Treatment consisted of an interactive, child-centered intervention that provided general stimulation emphasizing vocabulary development and use of early 2- or 3-word combinations within a social context. Treatment was provided by three ASHA-certified speech-language pathologists in a center-based birth-to-3 program. Each of these professionals had at least 2 years of experience in assessment and intervention with infants and toddlers who demonstrate language delay. Children in the experimental group attended therapy sessions twice a week throughout the 12-week treatment interval. Each therapy session lasted 75 min, with no more than 4 children enrolled in any particular group. Clinicians were paired with the same children throughout the course of the treatment.

To provide organization and structure, intervention was incorporated around a familiar routine or "script" (Constable, 1986). Once the script was established, specific components were manipulated, such as a deliberate violation of the routine, to increase opportunities for linguistic input or to encourage children to use language (cf. Bunce &

Watkins, 1995). In conjunction with this daily routine, a unit or "theme" was designated on a weekly or biweekly basis. The themes were designed to help children organize information by providing a unifying concept to which all newly presented vocabulary could be linked. Linguistic input was naturally paired with hands-on activities and visual cues that encouraged mapping of the new information through cross-modal referencing. Clinicians systematically employed reduction of the rate of input, manipulation of stress to emphasize particular linguistic targets, and positioning of targeted vocabulary at the beginning or end of an utterance (cf. Paul, 1995) to increase the saliency of the linguistic input.

A key component of the treatment was to encourage communicative attempts and to facilitate increases in the children's linguistic skills through specific techniques summarized in Table 3. Often referred to as scaffolding (Bruner, 1983) or mediation (Vygotsky, 1978), these techniques elicit the targeted behavior by focusing the child's attention on specific aspects of the communicative context. When a portion of the child's communicative attempt is incorporated into the adult response, only the modified portion of the adult model is novel information enabling more of the cognitive resource to be directed toward the new learning. Specific techniques were selected for individual children based on their current level of functioning (e.g., clinicians initially used parallel talk for children who were not yet using words; expansion and/or expatiation were implemented when a child began to verbalize).

Bricker (1986) argues that children's participation in real conversations and real interactions allows them to gain experience with language that cannot be duplicated in a structured lesson targeting a particular discrete language skill. Consequently, another key component of the therapeutic intervention was the organization of the intervention environment to provide multiple opportunities for the child to share information, participate in naturally occurring interactions (e.g., greetings exchanged when children enter room), regulate the behavior of others (e.g., "juice please"), and receive appropriate feedback and reinforcement (e.g., child provided with cookie following production of word *cookie*) (Norris & Hoffman, 1990). Rice and Wilcox (1995) provide a detailed description of a social-cognitive intervention similar to the treatment protocol used in this investigation.

**TABLE 3    Treatment techniques used to promote linguistic growth**

| Technique | Description | Example |
|---|---|---|
| Parallel Talk (no verbalization by child) | Clinician provides verbal description of child's actions | "Hug the bear" "Sweep the floor" |
| Expansion/Expatiation (following verbalization by child) | Repetition of child's utterance with the addition of relevant semantic or grammatical information to extend child's meaning | Child: "Doggie" Clinician: "Hug Doggie" or "Big Doggie" |
| Recast (following verbalization by child) | Repetition of child's utterance with modification of modality or voice | Child: "Want juice" Clinician: "You want some juice?" |

Parents were not directly involved in treatment but were obviously aware of the group to which their children were assigned. Parents were also not prohibited from observing their children during the intervention sessions. An informal log indicated that most parents limited their visits to the first one or two sessions in which the child participated. Given this, it is conceivable that observation of some of the treatment sessions may have influenced the parents of children in the treatment group to change their communicative behaviors during interactions with their child. However, given the minimal number of observations compared to the number of therapy sessions and the absence of formal training for parents, this impact is likely to be fairly small.

## Scoring Agreement

To ensure agreement for spontaneous language sample transcripts, 15% of the total number of transcripts (6) were randomly selected from the experimental and control groups, and the child utterances were retranscribed from the original audiotapes by an independent ASHA-certified speech-language pathologist. A word-by-word comparison percentage of 96.6% (116/120) was calculated by computing the number of agreements divided by the total number of judgments, then multiplying by 100.

Computation of MLU and NDW was obtained through SALT; consequently, accuracy of the input encoded into the computer system, such as coding for bound morphemes, was essential in order to obtain accurate data-analysis output. Fifteen percent (6) of the total number of transcripts (42) were re-entered into the SALT Editor program (SED) by an independent transcriber (selected independently from those used to determine scoring agreement). A morpheme-by-morpheme agreement percentage of 99% (120/121) was obtained by dividing the total number of agreements by the total number of judgments and multiplying by 100.

To assess scoring agreement on the test protocols (CDI, VABS, PSI), 5% of the total number of scoreforms (2 of each protocol) were independently re-scored in the same manner as described above. A comparison percentage was obtained by dividing the total number of points calculated by the first scorer by the total number of points calculated by the second scorer and multiplying by 100. The agreement percentages obtained were 98.9%, (190/192), 100% (99/99), and 99.5% (206/207) for the CDI, VABS, and PSI respectively.

## Treatment Fidelity

Before the implementation of treatment, clinicians providing intervention participated in two 50-minute training sessions to familiarize themselves with the assessment protocol and treatment. A combination of videotaping and observation of 13 (5%) of the treatment sessions was undertaken to assess the treatment fidelity. Adherence to the predetermined performance standards for the therapeutic techniques described previously was assessed via a specially designed checklist (see Appendix). Point scores of 9 to 12 on the checklist were predetermined to be within the high range. A mean fidelity score of 10.53 ($SD = .96$) was obtained across with scores ranging from 9 to 12. Thus, clinicians were closely adhering to the prescribed intervention procedures.

USE THE EVALUATION CHECKLIST TO GUIDE YOUR EVALUATION
OF THE METHOD

# Results

## Pretest Comparisons

Comparisons of the two groups on a range of variables were conducted before the initiation of treatment to assess possible differences using two-tailed $t$ tests with an alpha of .05. No significant differences were found between the experimental and control groups on the following independent variables: chronological age, receptive language level, expressive language level, mental scale of the BSID-II, motor scale of the BSID-II, and SES ($t$s = $-1.03$ to $1.05$, $p$s > .30). This suggests that the characteristics of both groups were similar in terms of the variables that were measured before intervention.

## Pretest-Posttest Comparisons

An analysis of covariance (ANCOVA) was calculated for each of the variables of interest in this investigation, with group (experimental, control) as the between-subjects variable. The dependent variable was the posttreatment score and the covariant was the pretreatment score. Because multiple ANCOVAs were calculated on the data, a conservative alpha level of .01 was selected. A summary of the data obtained for each of the dependent variables is presented in Table 4.

***Mean Length of Utterance.*** The ANCOVA calculated for MLU revealed a significant difference between groups, $F(1, 18) = 10.33$, $p = .003$, $\eta^2 = .37$. Children who participated in the experimental (treatment) group demonstrated significantly greater increases in MLU than the children in the control (delayed-treatment) group. Most children were not yet combining words pretreatment (9/11 in the experimental group, 8/10 in the control group). Two children from the experimental group did not produce any spontaneous language at all during the language sampling attempts. Posttreatment, all children in the experimental group had begun to demonstrate multiword utterances, a net increase of 9. Two additional children from the control group began combining words during the 12-week interval.

***Total Number of Words.*** The results of the ANCOVA for TNW indicated that there was a significant difference between the groups, $F(1, 18) = 46.83$, $p = .000$, $\eta^2 = .72$. Children in the experimental group produced significantly more words in the 15-min posttreatment language samples than the control group, controlling for pretreatment TNW. Children in the experimental group averaged an increase of 21 words, with individual children using 0–40 words pretreatment and 18–76 words posttreatment. Children who did not participate in treatment demonstrated a mean increase of 5 words, using 2–26 words pretreatment and 4–38 words posttreatment.

**TABLE 4   Summary data for dependent variables in terms of means (*M*) and standard deviations (*SD*)**

|  | Pretreatment | | Posttreatment | |
| --- | --- | --- | --- | --- |
|  | *M* | *SD* | *M* | *SD* |
| Mean Length of Utterance (MLU) | | | | |
| Experimental | 1.04 | .09 | 1.32 | .32 |
| Control | 1.03 | .07 | 1.09 | .11 |
| Total Number of Words (TNW) | | | | |
| Experimental | 11.8 | 12.4 | 33.3 | 16.6 |
| Control | 11.3 | 8.7 | 16.6 | 12.5 |
| Number of Different Words (NDW) | | | | |
| Experimental | 5.9 | 4.8 | 15.1 | 5.2 |
| Control | 6.4 | 3.3 | 8.5 | 5.3 |
| Lexical Repertoire (CDI) | | | | |
| Experimental | 39.4 | 40.5 | 76.2 | 37.5 |
| Control | 41.1 | 30.0 | 51.4 | 40.8 |
| Percent Intelligible Utterances | | | | |
| Experimental | 69.8 | 11.3 | 88.1 | 7.5 |
| Control | 69.2 | 21.6 | 71.5 | 11.9 |
| Socialization (VABS) | | | | |
| Experimental | 45.3 | 5.9 | 50.5 | 6.1 |
| Control | 44.3 | 5.5 | 46.2 | 5.3 |
| Parental Stress (PSI) | | | | |
| Experimental | 117.6 | 16.8 | 103.6 | 15.1 |
| Control | 112.4 | 17.9 | 110.2 | 17.3 |

***Number of Different Words.***   The results of the ANCOVA for NDW used in a 15-min language sample again revealed significant differences between the two groups, $F(1, 18) = 41.05$, $p = .000$, $\eta^2 = .69$. This suggests that children who participated in treatment demonstrated significantly greater increases in their lexical diversity than children who had not yet begun treatment. The experimental group increased the number of different words used to communicate by an average of 10. In contrast, children from the control group averaged 2 additional different words in their spontaneous language sample at posttest. Given that the groups also differed significantly in TNW, an additional analysis was conducted to determine whether the results for NDW simply reflected their difference in verbal output. An ANCOVA was conducted in which the pretreatment/posttreatment difference scores were used as the dependent variable and posttreatment TNW served as the covariate. These findings again revealed that the experimental group used a significantly greater number of different words than the control group, controlling for TNW, $F(1, 18) = 24.03$, $p = .000$, $\eta^2 = .57$.

***Lexical Repertoire.***   Children in the experimental group demonstrated significantly greater gains in their reported vocabulary size than children in the control group. Results of the ANCOVA indicated that significant differences exist between the two groups posttreatment, $F(1, 18) = 46.86$, $p = .000$, $\eta^2 = .72$. Children who participated in treatment increased their expressive vocabularies by an average of 37.73 words over the 12-week interval, with a range of 27 to 56 new words being reported. Parents of children in the control group reported an average gain in expressive vocabulary of 10.3 words, ranging from a low of 3 new words to a high of 26 new words. Note that the highest reported gain by children in the control group is lower than the lowest reported gain by children in the experimental group, suggesting robust treatment effects on this variable.

***Percentage of Intelligible Utterances.***    The ANCOVA for percentage of intelligible utterances revealed a significant group difference, $F(1, 18), = 24.44, p = .000, \eta^2 = .60$. Children in the experimental group produced significantly more intelligible spontaneous utterances in the 15-min samples than those in the control group, controlling for pretreatment intelligibility. It should be noted that the two children in the experimental group who produced no spontaneous speech during the pretreatment assessment were excluded from this analysis. The mean percentage of intelligibility was relatively high for both the experimental and control groups before intervention (69.8% and 69.2% respectively); however, there was a great deal of variability among individual children. It ranged from 60% to 91% intelligibility pretreatment in the experimental group (excluding children who did not produce any words) and from 38% to 100% intelligibility in the control group. Following the treatment interval, children in the experimental group averaged 88.1% intelligible utterances, with a range of 75–100%. Children who did not participate in treatment demonstrated 71.5% intelligibility posttreatment, with intelligibility ranging from 54% to 90%.

***Socialization.***    The ANCOVA computed for socialization, as measured by the Socialization Scale of the VABS, revealed a significant difference between the experimental and the control group following treatment, $F(1, 18) = 12.15, p = .003, \eta^2 = .40$. Although not specifically targeted during the treatment phase, an increase in the socialization skills of children in the experimental group appears to be an indirect effect of early language intervention programming. Because of the close relationship between language and social skills, some of the items used to measure social functioning on the VABS included linguistic components. Thus, increases identified on the Socialization subdomain of the VABS may actually reflect the linguistic growth stimulated by the treatment rather than documenting indirect treatment effects. Although increased linguistic proficiency is obviously a desired result of language intervention, conclusions regarding indirect treatment effects on social skills are clearly weakened if the documented gains occurred only on items that are related to communication.

To address this potential confound, an analysis of the assessment items included on the VABS was conducted to identify the tasks that tapped the linguistic domain. The socialization portion of this test is divided into three subdomains: Interpersonal Relationships, Play and Leisure Time, and Coping Skills. The highest item completed by children from both groups was identified for each subdomain. Two independent raters then judged all items up to and including these ceiling items as either language or nonlanguage tasks. Items judged by either or both raters as language-loaded were designated as language items for the purpose of this analysis. The points assigned to nonlanguage items versus the total score were calculated for each child, for each subdomain, pre- and posttreatment. A difference ratio was calculated by dividing the total gain score for nonlanguage items by the total gain score for each group. The experimental group demonstrated a difference ratio of .830, with 44 of the 53 net points gained by the group on the VABS attributed to nonlanguage items. The difference ratio for the control group was .578, with 11 points of the net gain of 19 points attributed to change in nonlanguage areas. These results suggest that the changes noted in the socialization skills of the experimental group were not merely reflective of the language increases already noted.

***Parental Stress.*** The ANCOVA calculated for the Child Domain of the Parental Stress Index (PSI) revealed significant differences between the two groups, $F(1, 18) = 53.32$, $p = .000$, $\eta^2 = .75$. On this test instrument, improvements in parental perceptions of their child are indicated by reduced scores. For the experimental group, a mean reduction in stress indicators of 13.9 points for the experimental group was noted, with individual parents reporting changes from 7 to 21 points. Parents of children in the control group reported less dramatic changes (in which a mean difference of 2.0 was obtained), with scores ranging from –2 to 6. These findings appear to be the result of a facilitative effect of the language intervention program on family dynamics despite the absence of therapeutic goals or techniques specifically targeting this area.

***Correlation Between Intake Characteristics and Progress.*** Partial correlation analyses were conducted to determine the association between intake characteristics of the children and posttreatment assessments, partialling out the effects of pretreatment performance. An alpha level of .05 was adopted for this analysis. For the total sample ($N = 21$), the only significant correlation was between SES and VABS scores ($r^2 = -.485$, $p = .030$). Separate correlational analyses of the experimental and control groups revealed that a significant negative correlation between SES and VABS scores for the experimental group ($r^2 = -.711$, $p = .02$) accounted for the significant finding for the total sample; there were no significant correlations for the control group for any variables ($r^2$s < .61, $ps > .08$). SES was also negatively correlated with NDW for the experimental group ($r^2 = -.658$, $p = .039$), and CA at entry was positively correlated with NDW posttreatment ($r^2 = .641$, $p = .046$). Finally, entry CA was negatively correlated with PSI for the experimental group ($r^2 = .640$, $p = .046$).

---

USE THE EVALUATION CHECKLIST TO GUIDE YOUR EVALUATION
OF THE RESULTS

---

# Discussion

The purpose of this study was to provide preliminary data regarding efficacy of intervention models that use clinician-implemented intervention for late talkers. A secondary intent was to determine if intervention aimed at increasing language skills provided indirect treatment effects on related areas of development.

## Linguistic Variables

Variables used in this study to measure language growth included four direct measures—mean length of utterance, number of different words, total number of words, and intelligibility in spontaneous speech—and one indirect measure: total number of words in vocabulary as reported by parents on the CDI. Children in the experimental group demonstrated increased complexity and increased verbal output within a set time interval compared to the controls. Lexical diversity of the children in the experimental group was also significantly higher posttreatment for children in the experimental group even when differences in total number of words was taken into account. Although not specifically targeted in treatment, intelligibility of spontaneous speech improved significantly for the experimental children compared to the controls, although both groups exhibited relatively high levels of intelligibility and there was considerable variability among the children. These findings parallel those of the investigation by Girolametto et al. (1996) that documented gains in vocabulary, the use of multiword phrases, grammatical complexity, and general talkativeness following a parent-delivered intervention program. Phonological improvements, in terms of expanded speech sound inventories and gains in the variety of complex syllable shapes, following this lexical training program were also reported (Girolametto, Pearce, & Weitzman, 1997). Whitehurst and his colleagues (1991) reported gains following treatment in overall vocabulary growth as well as an increase in the spontaneous use of targeted words. Combined with the findings of the current investigation, strong support for the efficacy of language intervention is evidenced, at least in terms of short-term increases.

## Socialization

Results of this investigation suggest that late talkers can benefit from early intervention in areas that are not directly targeted during treatment. These results argue for the importance of intervention in providing a facilitative or preventive function relative to the child's eventual performance levels. Children in the experimental group demonstrated significantly greater changes in their socialization skills, with a greater proportion of the change being attributed to nonlanguage items than the change noted for children in the control group. This suggests that the increase in socialization cannot be attributed solely to the change in linguistic skills exhibited by these toddlers. Visual examination of the data regarding the VABS suggests that treatment effects for two of the subdomains, Interpersonal Relationships and Play and Leisure Time, were robust for children in the experimental group whereas no apparent treatment effects were noted for these children in the area of Coping Skills. This observation is not unexpected given gains noted on the linguistic variables and the nature of the intervention provided to children in the experimental group. An increase in the interpersonal relationships domain for children in the experimental group might be expected because these children demonstrated both increased language skills and better parental perceptions of their behavior as measured by the PSI. Gains noted in the Play and Leisure Skills subdomain may have been facilitated by the treatment program itself. Children who took part in the treatment were given time, materials, modeling, and reinforcement for playing with other children. For many children who took part in this investigation, the early intervention center served as a first play-group experience. Some of the therapy techniques used in treatment paralleled items from this subdomain of the VABS (e.g.,

Plays with others with minimal supervision; Participates in at least one game or activity with others). Not unexpectedly, children in the control group, who were not exposed to these play experiences, did not demonstrate substantial increases in this area. These observations are compatible with the social interactionist theory of language development, which posits a strong interrelationship between the linguistic and social domains.

## Parental Stress

Results of the current investigation suggest that benefits of intervention may transcend within-child characteristics and facilitate positive changes of parental perceptions of their children's skills and behaviors. The Child Domain of the PSI is divided into 6 subtests that assess parents' perception of various aspects of their children's behavior: Distractibility, Adaptability, Reinforces Parent, Demandingness, Mood, and Acceptability. Although statistical analysis indicates a significant difference between experimental and control groups in terms of total scores, visual inspection of the data revealed relatively greater gains on two subtests: Acceptability and Reinforces Parent. This observation may provide additional support for the notion of an interdependent relationship among language, social skills, and environment. It may be argued that as children's communicative proficiency increases, parents begin to perceive their child as being more like their typically developing peers. This influences parents' perceptions regarding their children's acceptability both within the family and in the community and may facilitate more opportunities for interactions within these systems. In addition, because of the child's increased ability to participate in verbal exchanges, parents receive more reinforcement from the interactions they have with their child. This positive reinforcement encourages parents to engage in more frequent and longer interaction sequences with their children—the very behaviors that are widely believed to stimulate development in all areas (Bruner, 1983; Vygotsky, 1978).

## Relation Between Intake Characteristics and Progress

Selected intake characteristics were found to be related to certain gains observed for children who received treatment. Correlational analyses revealed a negative correlation between SES and VABS scores. This suggests that children in the experimental group with relatively lower SES had higher VABS scores at posttreatment. Language stimulation provided by treatment may have been more influential for the lower SES children (although it is important to note that the range of SES was relatively restricted). This assumption is also supported by the negative correlation between SES and NDW. Lower SES levels were associated with higher gains in vocabulary diversity. Chronological age at entry was associated with outcome on two variables. Older age at entry was associated with greater vocabulary diversity posttreatment, and parents of children who were older at entry reported a greater decrease in their concerns on the PSI.

## Clinical Implications

The results of this study have important implications regarding the clinical management of late talkers. Some researchers have suggested that although early language intervention has been shown to produce increases in vocabulary and linguistic complexity, these are merely short-term results that have little lasting impact on the overall development of the child (Whitehurst et al., 1991). However, evidence that children who are slow to develop language are at risk for related problems in social skills and disruption in the parent-child relationship (cf. Rice, 1993; Yoder & Warren, 1993, 1998) argues for the importance of early intervention that moves children toward normal linguistic functioning as quickly as possible. The current investigation did not attempt to address the issue of long-range outcomes following language intervention; rather, it assessed the breadth of short-term effects of early language intervention across a number of variables. Results of this investigation indicated that children in the experimental group demonstrated benefits not only in vocabulary and multiword combinations, but also in areas that were not specifically targeted for intervention, such as social skills, speech intelligibility, and parental stress. These preliminary data suggest that clinician-implemented language intervention can produce significant short-term results within a relatively short treatment interval, stimulating positive changes across a number of variables. Children who were provided with early intervention demonstrated gains in vocabulary and grammatical and phonological skills, improved their socialization skills, and elicited more positive perceptions of their skills and behaviors by their parents—in turn reflecting decreased parental stress.

Olswang et al. (1998) have recently offered guidelines concerning when to recommend treatment for late-talking toddlers and when to adopt a watch-and-see approach. The current investigation provides evidence for the effectiveness of early intervention in facilitating short-term linguistic gains as well as affecting more broadly such other areas as socialization and parental concerns, which may weigh into the decision regarding appropriate clinical management. Given the number of toddlers who demonstrate delayed acquisition of language and the potential for continued problems for at least some of the children, further investigation regarding the efficacy and importance of early intervention and the role of early intervention in both short-term change and long-term outcomes would be warranted.

> USE THE EVALUATION CHECKLIST TO GUIDE YOUR EVALUATION
> OF THE DISCUSSION

## Acknowledgments

This investigation was funded in part by a grant from the Doctoral Committee of the Department of Communication Disorders, University of Wisconsin–Madison. The authors wish to express their thanks to the parents and children who so willingly participated in this investigation. In addition, the authors are extremely grateful to the staff at Early Intervention Services for their enthusiastic cooperation. Portions of this work were presented at the Treatment Research in Communication Disorders–Special Interest Group (TRCD-SIG) Conference, Nashville, TN, in April 1998 and at the ASHA Convention in San Antonio, TX, in November 1998.

# REFERENCES

Abidin, R. (1995). *The Parenting Stress Index.* Charlottesville, VA: Pediatric Psychological Press.

American Speech-Language-Hearing Association. (1997). *Guidelines on audiological screening.* Rockville, MD: Author.

Bayley, N. (1993). *Scales of Infant Development.* New York: Psychological Corporation,

Bricker, D. (1986). *Early education of at-risk and handicapped infants, toddlers, and preschool children.* Glenview, IL: Scott Foresman.

Bruner, J. (1983). Child talk. Learning how to use temperament, and the risk of childhood behavioral problems: I. Relationship between parental characteristics and changes in children's temperament over time. *American Journal of Orthopsychiatry, 47,* 568–576.

Bunce, G., & Watkins, R. (1995). Language intervention in a preschool classroom: Implementing a language-focused curriculum. In M. Rice & K. Wilcox (Eds.), *Building a language-focused curriculum for the preschool classroom* (pp. 39–72). Baltimore: Paul H. Brookes Publishers.

Constable, C. (1986). The application of scripts in the organization of language intervention contexts. In K. Nelson (Ed.), *Event knowledge: Structure and function in development* (pp. 205–230). Hillsdale, NJ: Lawrence Erlbaum Associates.

Craig, H. (1996). Specific language impairment: A changing role for normal developmental language theories during the 1990's. In M. Smith & J. Damico (Eds.), *Childhood language disorders.* New York: Thieme Medical Publishers, Inc.

Ellis Weismer, S. (in press). Language intervention for young children with language impairments. In L. Watson, T. Layton, & E. Crasi (Eds.), *Handbook of early language impairments in children: Volume II. Assessment and treatment.* Albany, NY: Delmar Publishers.

Ellis Weismer, S., Murray-Branch, J., & Miller, J. (1993). Comparison of two methods for promoting vocabulary in late talkers. *Journal of Speech and Hearing Research, 36,* 1037–1050.

Ellis Weismer, S., Murray-Branch, J., & Miller, J. (1994). A prospective longitudinal study of language development in late talkers. *Journal of Speech and Hearing Research, 36,* 1037–1062.

Fenson, L., Reznick, S., Thal, D., Bates, E., Hartung, J., Pethick, S., & Reilly, J. (1993). *The MacArthur Communicative Developmental Inventory.* San Diego, CA: Singular Publishing Group, Inc.

Fujiki, M., & Brinton, B. (1994). Social competence in language impaired children. In R. Watkins & M. Rice (Eds.), *Specific language impairments in children* (pp. 123–143). Baltimore: Paul H. Brookes.

Girolametto, L., Pearce, P., & Weitzman, E. (1996). Interactive focused stimulation for toddlers with expressive language delays. *Journal of Speech and Hearing Research, 39,* 1274–1283.

Girolametto, L., Pearce, P., & Weitzman, E. (1997). Effects of lexical intervention on the phonology of late talkers. *Journal of Speech, Language, and Hearing Research, 40,* 338–348.

Leonard, L. (1998). *Children with specific language impairment.* Cambridge: MIT Press,

Miller, J., & Chapman, R. (1996). *SALT: Systematic Analysis of Language Transcripts* [Computer program]. Language Analysis Laboratory, Waisman Center, University of Wisconsin–Madison.

Norris, J., & Hoffman, P. (1990). Comparison of adult-initiated versus child-initiated interaction styles with a handicapped prelanguage child. *Language, Speech, and Hearing Services in the Schools, 21,* 28–36.

Olswang, L., & Bain, B. (1991). Intervention issues for toddlers with specific language impairments. *Topics in Language Disorders, 11*(4), 69–86.

Olswang, L., Rodriguez, R., & Timler, G. (1998). Recommending intervention for toddlers with specific language learning difficulties: We may not have all the answers, but we know a lot. *American Journal of Speech-Language Pathology, 7*(1), 23–32.

Paul, R. (1991). Profiles of toddlers with slow expressive language development. *Topics in Language Disorders, 11*(4), 1–14.

Paul, R. (1993). Patterns of development in late talkers: Preschool years. *Journal of Childhood Communication Disorders, 15,* 7–14.

Paul, R. (1995). *Language disorders from infancy through adolescence: Assessment and intervention.* Boston: Mosby.

Paul, R. (1996). Clinical implications of the natural history of slow expressive language development. *American Journal of Speech-Language Pathology, 5*(2), 5–21.

Paul, R. (1997). Understanding language delay: A response to van Kleeck, Gillam, and Davis. *American Journal of Speech-Language Pathology, 6*(2), 40–49.

Paul, R., Hernadez, R., Taylor, L., & Johnson, K. (1996). Narrative development in late talkers: Early school age. *Journal of Speech and Hearing Research, 39,* 99–107.

Paul, R., & Jennings, P. (1992). Phonological behavior in toddlers with slow expressive language development. *Journal of Speech and Hearing Research, 35,* 99–107.

Paul, R., Murray, C., Clancy, K., & Andrews, D. (1997). Reading and metaphonological outcomes in late talkers. *Journal of Speech, Language, and Hearing Research, 40,* 1037–1047.

Paul, R., & Smith, R. (1993). Narrative skills in 4-year-olds with normal, impaired, and late-developing language. *Journal of Speech and Hearing Research, 36,* 592–598.

Paul, R., Spangle Looney, S., & Dahm, P. (1991). Communication and socialization skills at age 2 and 3 in "late talking" young children. *Journal of Speech and Hearing Research, 34,* 858–865.

Prutting, C. (1992). Pragmatics as social competence. *Journal of Speech and Hearing Disorders, 47,* 123–134.

Rescorla, L. (1989). The language development survey: A screening tool for delayed language in toddlers. *Journal of Speech and Hearing Disorders, 54,* 587–599.

Rescorla, L. (1993). *Outcome of toddlers with specific expressive delay (SELD) at ages 3, 4, 5, 7, & 8.* Poster presented at the Biennial Meeting of Society for Research in Child Development, New Orleans.

Rescorla, L., & Goossens, M. (1992). Symbolic play development in toddlers with expressive specific language, impairment (SLI-E). *Journal of Speech and Hearing Research, 35,* 1290–1302.

Rescorla, L., Roberts, J., & Dahlsgaard, K. (1997). Late talkers at age 2: Outcome at age 3. *Journal of Speech, Language, and Hearing Research, 40,* 556–566.

Rescorla, L., & Schwartz, E. (1990). Outcome of toddlers with specific expressive language delay. *Applied Psycholinguistics, 11,* 393–407.

Rice, M. (1993). "Don't talk to him, he's weird." A social consequences account of language and social interactions. In A. P. Kaiser & D. B. Gray (Eds.), *Communication and language intervention issues: Volume 2. Enhancing children's communication: Research foundations for intervention* (pp. 139–158). Baltimore: Paul H. Brookes Publishers.

Rice, M., & Wilcox, K. (1995). *Building a language-focused curriculum for the preschool classroom.* Baltimore: Paul H. Brookes Publishers.

Roberts, J., Rescorla, L., Giroux, J., & Stevens, L. (1998). Phonological skills of children with specific expressive language impairment (SLI-E): Outcome at age 3. *Journal of Speech, Language, and Hearing Research, 41,* 374–384.

Sparrow, S. S., Balla, D. A., & Ciccetti, D. V. (1984). *Vineland Adaptive Behavior Scales.* Circle Pines, MN: American Guidance Service.

Spitz, R., Tallal, P., Flax, J., & Benasich, A. (1997). Look who's talking: A prospective study of familial transmission of language impairments. *Journal of Speech, Language, and Hearing Research, 40,* 990–1001.

Tannock, R., Girolametto, L., & Siegel, L. (1992). Language intervention with children who have developmental delays: Effect of an interactive approach. *American Journal on Mental Retardation, 97,* 145–160.

Thal, D. (1991). Language and cognition in normal and late talking toddlers. *Topics in Language Disorders, 11*(4), 33–43.

Thal, D., Oroz, M., & McCaw, V. (1995). Phonological and lexical development in normal and late-talking toddlers. *Applied Psycholinguistics, 16,* 407–424.

Thal, D., & Tobias, S. (1992). Communicative gestures in children with delayed onset of oral expressive language use. *Journal of Speech and Hearing Research, 35,* 1281–1289.

Thal, D., & Tobias, S. (1994). Communication gesture in normally developing and late-talking toddlers. *Journal of Speech and Hearing Research, 37,* 157–170.

Thal, D., Tobias, S., & Morrison, D. (1991). Language and gesture in late-talkers: A 1-year follow-up. *Journal of Speech and Hearing Research, 34,* 604–612.

van Kleeck, A., Gillam, R., & Davis, B. (1997). When is "watch and see" warranted? A response to Paul's 1996 article, "Clinical implications of the natural history of slow expressive language development." *American Journal of Speech-Language Pathology, 6*(2), 34–39.

Vygotsky, L. (1978). *Mind in society.* Cambridge: MIT Press.

Watkins, R., Kelly, D., Harbers, H., & Hollis, W. (1995). Measuring children's lexical diversity: Differentiating typical and impaired language learners. *Journal of Speech and Hearing Research, 38,* 1349–1355.

Whitehurst, G., & Fischel, J. (1994). Early developmental language delay: What, if anything, should the clinician do about it? *Journal of Child Psychology and Psychiatry, 35,* 613–648.

Whitehurst, G., Fischel, J., Arnold, D., & Lonigan, C. (1992). Evaluating outcomes with children with expressive language delay. In S. Warren & J. Reichle (Eds.), *Causes and effects in communication and language intervention* (pp. 277–313). Baltimore: Paul H. Brookes Publishing.

Whitehurst, G., Fischel, J., Lonigan, C., Valdez-Menchaca, M. C., Arnold, D., & Smith, M. (1991). Treatment of early expressive language delay: If, when, and how. *Topics in Language Disorders, 11,* 55–68.

Yoder, P., & Warren, S. (1993). Can prelinguistic intervention enhance the language development of children with developmental delays? In A. Kaiser & D. B. Gray (Eds.), *Enhancing children's communication: Research foundations for early language intervention* (pp. 35–63). Baltimore: Paul H. Brookes.

Yoder, P., & Warren, S. (1998). *Investigation of secondary and tertiary effects of treatment in a complex world.* Paper presented at the Treatment Efficacy Conference, Nashville, TN.

Zimmerman, I., Steiner, V., & Pond, R. (1992). *Preschool Language Scale—3.* Chicago: The Psychological Corporation.

Received August 10, 1998

Accepted March 31, 1999

Contact author: Shari Brand Robertson, PhD, Department of Special Education and Clinical Services, Indiana University of Pennsylvania, 203 Davis Hall, Indiana, PA 15705-1087. E-mail: srobert@grove.iup.edu

---

**A P P E N D I X .  Treatment Fidelity Index**

---

Date of Treatment Session _____

I. Structure                                                          Points Assigned

   A. Evidence of an established daily **routine.**

| Yes | Partial | No | |
|-----|---------|-----|---|
| (2) | (1) | (0) | _____ |

   B. Evidence of **theme-based** activities.

| Yes | Partial | No | |
|-----|---------|-----|---|
| (2) | (1) | (0) | _____ |

II. Linguistic Input

   A. **Increased Saliency**—observed instances of manipulation of stress, position, rate.

_____                    _____

Tally (10 or above = 2, 5–9 = 1, 4 or below = 0).

   B. **Language Models**—observed instances of expansion, focused repetition, scaffolding.

_____                    _____

Tally (15 or above = 2, 7–14 = 1, 6 or below = 0).

III. Interaction and Feedback

   A. **Interaction Opportunities**—observed attempts by clinician to manipulate environment to engage children in verbal interactions (e.g., sharing, regulation, greeting).

_____                    _____

Tally (15 or above = 2, 7–14 = 1, 6 or below = 0).

   B. **Feedback**—observed instances of feedback tied to communicative task.

_____                    _____

Tally (15 or above = 2, 7–14 = 1, 6 or below = 0).

                               **TOTAL FIDELITY SCORE**   _____

# Proclamation of the Association of American Medical Colleges and the National Health Council

**Clinical Research:** A Reaffirmation of Trust Between Medical Science and the Public—Proclamation and Pledge of Academic, Scientific, and Patient Health Organizations

WHEREAS the future of medicine and health depends on an enduring collaboration and trust between scientific researchers and patients, and

WHEREAS recent, widely reported problems in clinical research have shaken public trust, and

WHEREAS research integrity is paramount to achieving good science and valid results, and

WHEREAS the ethical and responsible conduct of research involving human beings is essential in order to develop tomorrow's therapies and cures, and

WHEREAS by volunteering to participate in clinical research, patients make an essential and irreplaceable contribution to science and society, agreeing to take part in procedures that often have no known direct benefit to them as individuals while at times putting themselves at some measure of risk, and

WHEREAS in return for this contribution and for the trust that they place in researchers, research volunteers have a right to expect that they be treated with beneficence, justice and respect, and

WHEREAS the health and welfare of patients must always be placed above all other concerns,

BE IT THEREFORE RESOLVED that the undersigned medical schools, teaching hospitals, patient groups, health care associations, scientific societies, and other organizations reaffirm their commitment to the safe and ethical pursuit of the new knowledge necessary for the development of treatments and cures. We are committed to the protection and preservation of the rights and welfare of all the individuals who volunteer to participate in human subjects research.

We pledge ourselves, our institutions, and our researchers to uphold and ensure:

- The principles of beneficence, justice, and respect for individuals;
- The rights of patients and the responsibilities of researchers;
- The inviolable trust of informed consent, freely given by anyone who volunteers to participate in research. Informed consent means:
  - That patients are informed of any reasonably foreseeable risks and benefits of participating in the research activity; and
  - That patients understand that research procedures are not necessarily treatment and, in given instances, may not benefit themselves in any way and may possibly harm them.
  - That no coercion whatsoever, financial or otherwise, is used to induce patients to enter into or to remain in a research project; and that patients have complete freedom of choice as to whether to withdraw from a research activity;
- The central importance of, and adherence to, the procedures mandated by federal human subjects regulations, which prescribe a process by which research protocols are reviewed with attention to safety, ethics, and the protection of human participants;
- That the potential benefits to the individual and society exceed any known risks before studies involving human subjects research begin;
- The provision of adequate resources, training, and oversight for, and the creation of, a climate of support and respect for Institutional Review Boards (IRBs), which play a critical role in ensuring the integrity of human subjects research and in the federally mandated process for monitoring research protections; and
- Respect for and adherence to other rules, laws, and recognized codes that guide the ethical conduct of research generally. Such rules include those pertaining to conflicts of interest, misconduct, privacy and confidentiality, genetics research, and others.

The undersigned institutions and organizations stand committed to these principles and take public responsibility for keeping the ethical conduct of research involving human beings high on the national agenda.

# AUTHOR INDEX

# SUBJECT INDEX